Textbook of **PATHOLOGY** *for Allied Health Sciences*

Textbook of PATHOLOGY *for Allied Health Sciences*

Ramadas Nayak MBBS MD
Professor and Head
Department of Pathology
Yenepoya Medical College
Yenepoya University (Accredited by NAAC with "A" grade)
Mangaluru, Karnataka, India
Formerly, Head
Department of Pathology
Kasturba Medical College
Manipal University
Mangaluru, Karnataka, India

Foreword
Poornima Baliga B

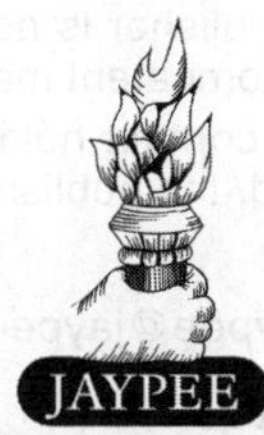

JAYPEE BROTHERS MEDICAL PUBLISHERS
The Health Sciences Publisher
New Delhi | London

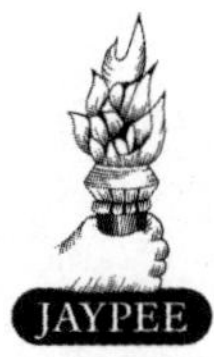

Jaypee Brothers Medical Publishers (P) Ltd

Headquarters
EMCA House
23/23-B, Ansari Road, Daryaganj
New Delhi - 110 002, India
Landline: +91-11-23272143, +91-11-23272703
+91-11-23282021, +91-11-23245672
E-mail: jaypee@jaypeebrothers.com

Corporate Office
4838/24, Ansari Road, Daryaganj
New Delhi - 110 002, India
Phone: +91-11-43574357
Fax: +91-11-43574314
E-mail: jaypee@jaypeebrothers.com

Overseas Office
J.P. Medical Ltd
83 Victoria Street, London
SW1H 0HW (UK)
Phone: +44 20 3170 8910
E-mail: info@jpmedpub.com

EU GPSR Authorised Representative
Logos Europe, 9 rue Nicolas Poussin
17000, La Rochelle, France
Phone: +33 (0) 6 67 93 73 78
E-mail: contact@logoseurope.eu

Website: www.jaypeebrothers.com
Website: www.jaypeedigital.com

Inquiries for bulk sales may be solicited at: jaypee@jaypeebrothers.com

Textbook of Pathology for Allied Health Sciences

First Edition: 2017

Reprint: 2025, **2026**

ISBN: 978-93-5270-107-0

Printed at: Samrat Offset Pvt. Ltd.

Dedicated to

Students who inspired me,
Patients who provided the knowledge,
and
My parents, family members, friends and colleagues
who encouraged and supported me.

Foreword

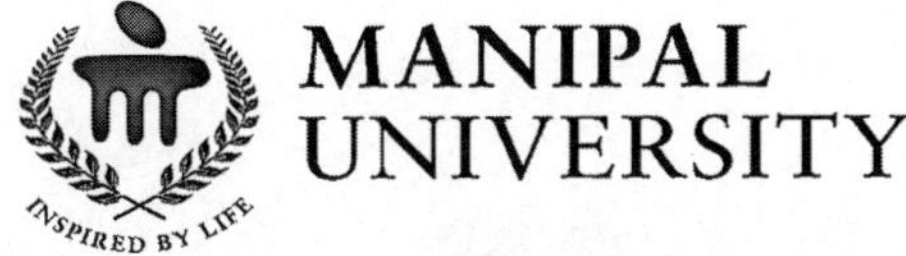

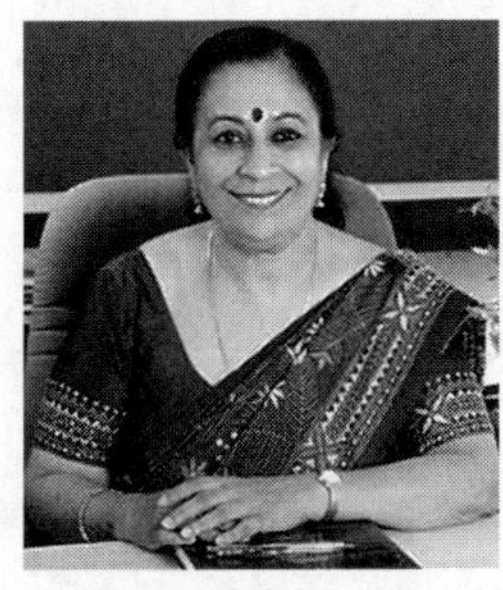

I am pleased to offer my comments on this book *Textbook of Pathology for Allied Health Sciences*. The science graduates undertaking the paramedical course need to be familiar with the concepts and terminology in addition to the knowledge of this vast, ever-expanding and developing branch of basic sciences. This book imparts the necessary knowledge in easy language, elaborating the basic theoretical background. The content is well organized with simple illustrations making it easy to understand for the reader.

If a reader has a question in his/her mind as to whether this book is good, my answer is Yes. This is a textbook written by an expert who knows his pathology, an experienced teacher, a well-informed academician who knows how to present pathology for the allied health sciences students.

In the words of the great Clinician William Oster, one of the founders of modern medicine, our clinical practice will be as good as our understanding of pathology.

Poornima Baliga B MD
Pro Vice-Chancellor
(Faculty of Health Sciences)
Manipal University
Manipal, Karnataka, India

Preface

Pathology is a rapidly-expanding and ever-changing field and lays the foundation for understanding diseases. This textbook is an endeavor to present the vast knowledge of pathology in a lucid manner for allied health science students. My aim is to provide a sound knowledge of pathology and hence, give insight into etiology, pathogenesis, pathology and the disease course. Every attempt has been made to present information in a simplified text augmented with the use of illustrations.

Organization

This book consists of 39 chapters and is organized into three sections namely *General Pathology, Systemic Pathology* and *Clinical Pathology*.

Section 1 (Chapters 1–10): It consists of general pathology and provides an overview of the basic pathologic mechanisms underlying diseases including cellular adaptations, inflammation, tissue repair, chronic inflammation, hemodynamic disorders, immunological disorders, neoplasia, genetics and radiation.

Section 2 (Chapters 11–29): It deals with systemic pathology with chapters devoted to diseases of various organ systems including vascular, cardiac, hematology, lymph nodes, respiratory, head and neck, gastrointestinal, liver and biliary tract, pancreas, urinary, male genital tract, female genital tract, breast, bones, joints and soft tissue tumors, endocrines, diabetes mellitus, skin, peripheral nervous system and skeletal muscles, central nervous system, and eye.

Section 3 (Chapters 30–39): It deals with clinical pathology with chapter on anticoagulants and hemoglobin estimation, blood cell counts, hematocrit, ESR estimation and peripheral blood smear examination, reticulocyte count, bone marrow examination, cerebrospinal fluid examination, body fluids, gastric analysis, and sputum examination, semen analysis, urine analysis and stool examination.

After many years (more than 36 years) of teaching students of allied health sciences, I found there is no textbook meant solely only for these students. These students struggle to read textbooks meant for medical and dental students and end up in getting poor results in examination. I also observed that students of allied health sciences find it difficult to understand, remember and answer the questions during examinations, in a satisfying way. This encouraged me to write a book to fill the niche, to provide basic information to students of allied health sciences in a nutshell. The text provides all the basic information, the student will ever need to know. Key points are shown in bold letters so that student can rapidly go through the book on the previous day or just before the examination. Most students are fundamentally "visually oriented." As the saying "one picture is worth a thousand words", it encouraged me to provide many illustrations.

Courses for Which this Book is Intended

It is difficult and economically not feasible to have separate textbooks of pathology for each course. So, this book is prepared in such a way that it can be used by all the 13 BSc courses mentioned below. The contents of Bachelor of Science of this book includes the course contents for the following courses:

- Bachelor of Science in Anesthesia Technology (BSc Anesthesia Technology)
- Bachelor of Audiology, Speech and Language Pathology (BASLP)
- Bachelor of Science in Cardiac Care Technology (BSc Cardiac Care Technology)

- Bachelor of Cardiovascular Technology (BCVT)
- Bachelor of Science in Medical Laboratory Technology (BMLT)
- Bachelor of Science in Medical Radiological Technology (BSc MRT)
- Bachelor of Science in Operation Theater Technology (BSc OT Technology)
- Bachelor of Science in Optometry (BSc OPT)
- Bachelor of Science in Perfusion Technology (BSc Perfusion Technology)
- Bachelor of Physiotherapy (BPT)
- Bachelor of Science in Radiotherapy Technology (BSc RTT)
- Bachelor of Science in Renal Dialysis Technology (BSc Renal Dialysis Technology)
- Bachelor of Science in Respiratory Care Technology (BSc Respiratory Care Technology)

In addition, this textbook includes the course contents needed for the following courses:

- Bachelor of Ayurveda Medicine and Surgery (BAMS) (Ayurvedacharya)
- Bachelor of Homoeopathic Medicine and Surgery (BHMS)
- Bachelor of Siddha Medicine and Surgery (BSMS)

This textbook can also be used as a last minute reading (LMR) even by medical and dental students.

How to Use this Book

I recommend this textbook to all students of allied health sciences for understanding the basic knowledge and refresh their knowledge during examinations. Firstly, the students are required to go through the course contents of their respective course (which may vary with their university to which it is affiliated). Secondly, they should mark the course contents in each chapters which they are intended to study. Thirdly, they are requested to give more emphasis on words in bold letters that represent the key points to be remembered. Finally, and not the least they are requested to study all the usually asked questions given under self-assessment exercises.

Numerous illustrations, gross photographs, photomicrographs, tables, flowcharts and X-rays have been incorporated for easy understanding of the subject.

Ramadas Nayak

Acknowledgments

My sincere thanks to all my family members, especially my wife Smt Rekha Nayak, my daughter Ms Rashmitha Nayak and my son-in-law Mr Ramnath Kini, who have patiently accepted my long preoccupation with this work. A special thanks to my grandson master Rishab Kini.

- I am grateful to Dr Poornima Baliga B, Pro Vice-Chancellor (Faculty of Health Sciences), Manipal University, Manipal, Karnataka, for writing the foreword and encouragement and support.
- I wish to express our gratitude to Mr Yenepoya Abdulla Kunhi, Honorable Chancellor, and Mr Farhaad Yenepoya, Director of Finance, Yenepoya University (Accredited by NAAC with "A" grade), Mangaluru, Karnataka, India, for their inspiration and encouragement.
- I would like to express my gratitude to all my friends and colleagues, who helped, inspired and supported me in the different stages of preparing this textbook.

I am grateful to all those who provided support, talked things over, read, offered comments and assisted in the editing, proofreading and designing. My special thanks to the following:

- Dr Rakshatha Nayak, Tutor, Department of Pathology, Yenepoya Medical College, a constituent of Yenepoya University, Mangaluru.
- Dr Krishnaraj Upadhyaya, Professor, Department of Pathology, Yenepoya Medical College, a constituent of Yenepoya University, Mangaluru.
- Shri Jitendar P Vij (Group Chairman), Mr Ankit Vij (Group President), Ms Ritu Sharma (Director–Publishing), and Ms Chetna Malhotra Vohra (Associate Director–Content Strategy) of M/s Jaypee Brothers Medical Publishers (P) Ltd, New Delhi, India, for publishing the book in the same format as wanted, well in time.
- Ms Sunita Katla (Publishing Manager), Ms Samina Khan (Executive Assistant to Director–Publishing), Mr Rajesh Sharma (Production Coordinator), Ms Seema Dogra (Cover Designer), Ms Geeta Rani Barik (Proofreader), Mr Rajesh Ghurkundi (Graphic Designer) and Mr Raj Kumar (DTP Operator) of M/s Jaypee Brothers Medical Publishers (P) Ltd, New Delhi, India.
- Mr Venugopal V (Bengaluru) and Mr Vasudev H (Mangaluru) of M/s Jaypee Brothers Medical Publishers (P) Ltd, Bengaluru Branch, Karnataka, for taking this book to every corner of Karnataka.
- Last but definitely not least, a thank you to my undergraduate and postgraduate students. Without you, I would not write. You make all my books possible.
- There are many more people I could thank, but space, and modesty compel me to stop here.

Contents

SECTION 1: GENERAL PATHOLOGY

SECTION 2: SYSTEMIC PATHOLOGY

Course Contents

Bachelor of Science in Anesthesia Technology (BSc Anesthesia Technology), Bachelor of Science in Cardiac Care Technology (BSc Cardiac Care Technology), Bachelor of Science in Operation Theater Technology (BSc OT Technology), Bachelor of Science in Perfusion Technology (BSc Perfusion Technology) and Bachelor of Science in Respiratory Care Technology (BSc Respiratory Care Technology).

Applied Pathology

I. Cardiovascular System

- Atherosclerosis: Definition, risk factors, briefly pathogenesis, morphology, clinical significance and prevention.
- Hypertension: Definition, types and briefly pathogenesis and effects of hypertension.
- Aneurysms: Definition, classification, pathology and complications.
- Ischemic heart diseases (IHD): Definition, types. Briefly pathophysiology, pathology and complications of various types of IHD.
- Pathophysiology of heart failure.
- Cardiac hypertrophy: Causes, pathophysiology and progression to heart failure.
- Valvular heart diseases: Causes, pathology and complication. Complications of artificial valves.
- Cardiomyopathy: Definition, types, causes and significance.
- Congenital heart diseases: Basic defect and effects of important types of congenital heart diseases.
- Pericardial effusion: Causes, effects and diagnosis.

II. Hematology

- Anemia: Definition, morphological types and diagnosis of anemia. Brief concept about hemolytic anemia and polycythemia.
- Leukocyte disorders: Briefly leukemia, leukocytosis, agranulocytosis, etc.
- Bleeding disorders: Definition, classification, causes and effects of important types of bleeding disorders. Briefly various laboratory tests used to diagnose bleeding disorders.

III. Respiratory System

- Chronic obstructive airway diseases (COPD): Definition and types. Briefly causes, pathology and complications of each type of COPD.
- Briefly concept about obstructive versus restrictive pulmonary disease.
- Pneumoconiosis: Definition, types, pathology and effects in brief.
- Pulmonary congestion and edema.
- Pleural effusion: Causes, effects and diagnosis.

IV. Renal System

- Clinical manifestations of renal diseases. Briefly causes, mechanism, effects and laboratory diagnosis of acute renal failure (ARF) and cardiorenal syndrome (CRS).
- Briefly glomerulonephritis and pyelonephritis.
- End stage renal disease: Definition, causes, effects and role of dialysis and renal transplantation in its management.
- Brief concept about obstructive uropathy.

Course Contents for Bachelor of Audiology, Speech and Language Pathology (BASLP)

Pathology of Speech and Hearing Systems

Unit 1

- Normal cell: Introduction to pathology.
- Cell injury: Etiology of cell injury and pathogenesis of cell injury.
- Cellular adaptations: Atrophy, hypertrophy.
- Pigments and cellular aging.

Unit 2

- Inflammation and healing, chemical mediators of inflammation, morphology of inflammation, regeneration, factors influencing healing.
- Immune pathology: Components of immune system, diseases of immunity; inflammation.

Unit 3

- Infectious diseases with reference to speech and hearing systems.
- Environmental and nutritional diseases.

Unit 4

- Pathologies of the laryngeal, articulatory and phonatory systems, inflammatory conditions, tumors, developmental anomalies, carcinoma.

Unit 5

- Pathologies of the auditory systems: Inflammatory lesions of the ear, tumors.

Course Contents for Bachelor of Ayurveda Medicine and Surgery (BAMS) (Ayurvedacharya)

Basic Pathology

- Introduction to pathology and its subdivisions.
- Introduction to cell injury and cellular adaptations.
- Definition and brief description of inflammation, healing/repair.
- Definition and brief description of edema, shock, hemorrhage, thrombosis, embolism, ischemia and infarction.
- Types of immunity, different types of immune responses in the body, basic knowledge of autoimmune diseases, acquired immune deficiency disease and hypersensitivity.
- Nomenclature and classification of tumors, difference between benign and malignant tumors.
- Introduction to nutritional disorders, disorders of macro- and micronutrients.
- Introduction to infections.
- Introduction and classification of microorganisms such as virus, bacteria and fungus.

Course Contents for Bachelor of Cardiovascular Technology (BCVT)

Cardiovascular System

- Coronary artery disease and myocardial infraction.
- Rheumatic fever.
- Valvular heart disease: Mitral stenosis, mitral regulation, aortic stenosis, aortic regulation, tricuspid value disease, combined valvular diseases.
- Pericardial, myocardial disease including end myocardial disease.
- Hypertension.
- Pulmonary hypertension.
- Congenital heart disease: Acyanotic, cyanotic, shunts, left-to-right shunts.

Course Contents for Bachelor of Homoeopathic Medicine and Surgery (BHMS)

General Pathology

- Cell injury, cellular adaptation (hyperplasia, hypertrophy, atrophy and metaplasia), degeneration, necrosis and gangrene, disorders of pigmentation, calcification.
- Inflammation, regeneration and repair (healing).
- Leprosy.
- Immunity, amyloidosis.
- Hyperemia, hemorrhage, edema, thrombosis, embolism, ischemia, infarction and shock.
- Disorders of metabolism.
- Neoplasia: Definition, variation in cell growth, nomenclature and taxonomy, characteristics of neoplastic cells, anaplasia, etiology and pathogenesis, grading and staging, diagnostic approaches, interrelationship of tumor and host, course and management.
- Infection, pyrexia, hospital infection, hyperlipidemia and lipidosis.
- Malnutrition and deficiency diseases.
- Effects of radiation.

Course Content for Bachelor of Homoeopathic Medicine and Surgery (BHMS)

Systemic Pathology

- Diseases of blood vessels and lymphatics.
- Diseases of cardiovascular system.
- Diseases of the respiratory system.
- Diseases of the oral cavity and salivary glands.
- Diseases of the gastrointestinal (GI) system.
- Diseases of liver, gallbladder and biliary ducts.
- Diseases of the pancreas (including diabetes mellitus).
- Diseases of kidney and lower urinary tract.
- Diseases of male reproductive system and prostate.
- Diseases of the female genitalia and breast.
- Diseases of hemopoietic system, bone marrow and blood.
- Diseases of eye, ear, nose and throat (ENT) and neck.
- Diseases of endocrine glands: Pituitary, thyroid, parathyroid and adrenals.
- Diseases of the skin and soft tissue.
- Diseases of the musculoskeletal system.
- Diseases of the nervous system.

Course Contents for Bachelor of Science in Medical Laboratory Technology (BMLT)

Hematology and Clinical Pathology

- Origin, development, maturation, function and fate of blood cells.
- Various anticoagulants, their functions, uses, advantages and disadvantages. Capillary and venous blood, methods of blood collection.
- Different types of hemocytometers and their rulings. Total count of red blood cells (RBCs), white blood cells (WBCs) (with correction of nRBC), eosinophils and platelets. Micropipette methods and bulk dilution technique, their advantages and disadvantages. Composition, function, preparation and storage of various diluting fluid. Errors in sampling, mixing, diluting and counting. Automatic blood cell counters. Quality control methods in cell counts.
- Principles of staining, Romanowsky stains, preparations and staining properties of various Romanowsky stains with emphasis to Leishman's stain. Preparation and use of buffer solutions in staining.

- Preparation of blood smears. Thin smear, thick smear, wet preparations and buffy coat preparation. Leishman's staining. Different leukocyte count in blood smears with recognition of abnormal blood cells.
- Collection of bone marrow and preparation of bone marrow smears, morphologic study of marrow films and its differential count. Indications of bone marrow aspiration.
- Hemoglobin and estimation of hemoglobin. Principles, techniques, advantages and disadvantages of different methods. Normal and abnormal values. Errors and quality control in various methods.
- Abnormal hemoglobin method of identification of abnormal hemoglobin. Sickling phenomenon. Hb-F and its demonstration.
- Principles and different methods of determining erythrocyte sedimentation rate (ESR) and packed cell volume (PCV). Advantages and disadvantages of each method. Clinical significance of ESR and PCV, normal values.
- Methods of determination of red cell indices [mean corpuscular volume (MCV), mean corpuscular volume (MCH), mean corpuscular hemoglobin concentration (MCHC) and indices] and its significance.
- Supravital staining technique. Principles and uses, demonstration and counting of reticulocytes. Composition and preparation.

Course Contents for Bachelor of Science in Medical Radiological Technology (BSc MRT)

General Pathology

- Regenerative changes: Fatty change, necrosis, gangrene and pathogenic calcification.
- Mechanism and changes in inflammation.
- Disorders of circulation: Edema, thrombosis, embolism, shock, infarction.
- Neoplasia: Detailed study of tumors, characteristics, classification, etiology and pathogenesis. All the common benign and malignant tumors.
- Common infection: Common acute bacterial infection. Detailed study of tuberculosis, leprosy and syphilis. Commonest fungal infection with a short account of opportunistic fungal infection. Brief account of all viral infections including acquired immune deficiency syndrome (AIDS), common protozoa and helminths.
- Detailed study of biological effects of radiation.
- Genetic diseases: Down's syndrome and hemophilia.
- Immunology: Autoimmune diseases, rheumatoid arthritis, systemic lupus erythematosus (SLE) and AIDS.
- Brief study of nutritional diseases.

Systemic Pathology

- ***Cardiovascular system (CVS):*** Ischemic heart diseases (IHD), rheumatic heart disease (RHD), infective endocarditis, hypertension, valvular diseases.
- ***Respiratory system:*** Pneumonias, tuberculosis (TB), bronchial asthma and tumors.
- ***Gastrointestinal tract (GIT):*** Oral cavity, esophageal carcinoma, peptic ulcer, carcinoma of stomach, malabsorption, inflammatory bowel diseases, dysentery, appendicitis and peritonitis.
- ***Gallbladder:*** Gallstones and cholecystitis.
- ***Pancreas:*** Pancreatitis, stones and diabetes mellitus.
- ***Male reproductive system:*** Hydrocele, orchitis, epididymitis and benign prostatic hypertrophy.
- ***Female reproductive system:*** Cervicitis, carcinoma of cervix, carcinoma of endometrium, disorders of menstruation, leiomyoma, brief account of ovarian tumors, disease of pregnancy and ectopic pregnancy.
- ***Breast:*** Fibroadenoma and carcinoma of breast.
- ***Hematology:*** Anemias, leukemia and bleeding disorders.
- ***Lymphoreticular systems:*** Lymphadenitis and lymphomas.
- ***Bones:*** Congenital disorders, osteomyelitis, rickets, osteomalacia, bone tumors and arthritis.
- ***Endocrine:*** Pituitary, thyroid, parathyroid and adrenal.
- ***Eye and ear:*** Brief account of eye and ear infection.
- ***Skin:*** Psoriasis, eczema, skin tumors (basal, squamous, malignant melanoma)
- ***Renal system:*** Glomerulonephritis, nephrotic syndrome pyelonephritis, renal failure, stones and tumors.

Course Content for BSc Optometry (BSc OPT)

- Introduction and etiology.
- Degeneration, apoptosis, disturbances of metabolism.
- Inflammation and repair.
- Circulatory disturbances: Edema, thrombosis, embolism, shock, infarction.
- Acute bacterial infection: Specific infection, tuberculosis, leprosy, fungal infection, viral, and chlamydial infection.
- Neoplasia: Definition, classification, behavior of benign and malignant neoplasm, spread of tumors, etiopathogenesis and diagnostic methods.
- Hematology: Introduction and RBC disorders, WBC disorders, plasma cell dyscrasia, bleeding and coagulation disease, clinical pathology, introduction, functioning of laboratory, collection of blood sample, hematology technique, examination of urine.
- Ocular pathology: Infection, degenerative conditions, ocular manifestation in systemic disease, cataract and tumors.

Course Contents for Bachelor of Physiotherapy (BPT)

General Pathology

1. Introduction to Pathology

2. Cell Injuries
- Reversible and irreversible cell injuries, types, sequential changes, cellular swellings; types of necrosis, gangrene, and autolysis; pathological calcification—dystrophic and metastatic, intracellular accumulations.

3. Inflammation and Repair
- Acute inflammation: Features, causes, vascular and cellular events. Inflammatory cells and mediators.
- Chronic inflammation: Causes, types, classification nonspecific and granulomatous with examples.
- Repair wound healing by primary and secondary unions, factors promoting and delaying the process. Healing in specific site including bone healing.

4. Immunopathology
- Immune system: General concepts.
- Hypersensitivity: Type and examples, antibody and cell-mediated tissue injury with examples.
- Secondary immune deficiency including HIV infection.
- Autoimmune disorder: Basic concepts and classification, SLE, AIDS—etiology, modes of transmission, diagnostic procedures.

5. Infectious Disease
- Mycobacterial diseases: Tuberculosis, leprosy and syphilis.
- Bacterial disease: Pyogenic, diphtheria, gram-negative infection, bacillary dysentery.
- Viral diseases: Poliomyelitis, herpes, rabies, measles, HIV infection.
- Fungal disease and parasitic diseases: Malaria, filaria, amebiasis.

6. Circulatory Disturbances
- Hyperemia/ischemia and hemorrhage.
- Chronic venous congestion: Lung, liver, spleen.
- Edema: Pathogenesis and types.
- Thrombosis and embolism: Formation, fate and defects.
- Infarction: Types, common sites.
- Shock: Pathogenesis, types.

7. Growth Disturbances and Neoplasia
- Neoplasia: Definition, classification, biological behavioral benign and malignant, carcinoma and sarcoma.
- Malignant neoplasia: Grades and stages, local and distant spread.

- Carcinogenesis: Environmental carcinogens, chemical, viral, occupational, heredity and cellular oncogenes and prevention of cancer.
- Benign and malignant tumors.

8. Urinary System
- Glomerular nephritis, nephrotic syndrome.
- Urinary tract infection.
- Renal calculi.
- Renal carcinomas.

9. Nutritional Disorders
- Vitamin deficiency disorders.
- Protein-energy malnutrition: Marasmus, kwashiorkor.
- Obesity and bulimia.

10. Genetic Disorders
- Basic concepts of genetic disorders and some common examples and congenital malformation and hemophilia.

11. Hematology
- Constituents of blood and bone marrow.
- Regulation of hematopoiesis.
- Anemia: Classification, clinical features and laboratory diagnosis. Thalassemia, spherocytosis and enzyme deficiencies.
- Leukocyte disorders: Leukocytosis, leukopenia, leukemoid reaction, leukemia.
- Blood transfusion: Grouping and cross matching, untoward reactions, transmissible infections including HIV and hepatitis.

12. Respiratory System
- Pneumonia.
- Bronchitis.
- Bronchiectasis.
- Asthma.
- Tuberculosis.
- Occupational lung diseases and their effect on physical activity.
- Carcinoma of lungs.

13. Cardiovascular Pathology
- Atherosclerosis.
- Aneurysm.
- Arteritis.
- Tumors of blood vessels.
- Ischemic heart disease: Myocardial infarction.
- Endocarditis, rheumatic heart disease, vascular diseases.
- Hypertension and hypertensive heart disease.
- Congenital heart disease: Atrial septal defect, ventricular septal defect, Fallot's tetralogy, patent ductus arteriosus.

14. Alimentary Tract
- Oral pathology: Ulcers, carcinoma.
- Esophagus: Inflammatory and carcinoma.
- Stomach and intestine: Gastritis, ulcer and tumors.

15. Hepatobiliary Pathology
- Jaundice: Types, etiopathogenesis and diagnosis.
- Hepatitis: Acute, chronic, and neonatal.
- Alcoholic liver disease common clinical conditions.

16. Lymphatic System
- Lymphadenitis, causes of lymph node enlargements, common clinical conditions.

17. Musculoskeletal System
- Osteomyelitis.
- Metabolic diseases: Rickets, osteomalacia, osteoporosis.
- Hyperparathyroidism, Paget's disease.
- Tumors classification: Benign, malignant, metastatic and synovial sarcoma.
- Arthritis: Suppurative, rheumatoid, osteoarthritis, gout, tuberculous, hemarthropathies.
- Diseases of muscles.

18. Endocrine Pathology
- Diabetes mellitus: Types, pathogenesis and pathology.
- Thyroid: Non-neoplastic and neoplastic lesions.

19. Neuropathology
- Inflammations and infections: Tuberculous meningitis, pyogenic meningitis, viral meningitis.
- Brain abscess.
- Vascular lesions of central nervous system.
- CNS tumors.
- Poliomyelitis.
- Peripheral neuropathies including diabetic neuropathies.
- Parkinsonism dementia, Alzheimer's disease.
- Disorders of spinal cord: Subacute combined degeneration (SCD), trauma, syringomyelia, tabes dorsalis.

20. Dermatopathology
- Common clinical conditions.

Course Contents for Bachelor of Science in Radiotherapy Technology (BSc RTT)

Pathology of Common Malignant Disease of Individual Sites (in brief)
- Skin cancer.
- Head and neck tumors.
- Brain tumors.
- Gastrointestinal tract tumors (esophagus, rectum, and anus).
- Lung cancer.
- Lymphomas.
- Breast cancer.
- Gynecological cancers.
- Prostate cancer.
- Bladder cancer.
- Seminoma.
- Pediatric tumors and others.

Course Contents for Bachelor of Science in Renal Dialysis Technology (BSc Renal Dialysis Technology)

Applied Pathology
- Congenital abnormalities of urinary system.
- Classification of renal diseases.
- Glomerular diseases: Causes, types and pathology.
- Tubulointerstitial diseases.
- Renal vascular disorders.

- End stage renal diseases: Causes and pathology.
- Pathology of kidney in hypertension, diabetes mellitus, pregnancy.
- Pathology of peritoneum: Peritonitis—bacterial, tubular and sclerosing peritonitis, dialysis-induced changes.
- Pathology of urinary tract infections.
- Pyelonephritis and tuberculous pyelonephritis.

Course Contents for Bachelor of Siddha Medicine and Surgery (BSMS)

Principles of Modern Pathology including Clinical Pathology

- Cell response to injury, common causes, degeneration, fatty changes, etc.
- Disorders of cell growth, hypertrophy, hyperplasia, aplasia.
- Inflammation and wound healing.
- Disease due to trauma, burns and their classifications, effect of radiation.
- Circulatory disturbances: Hemorrhage (cause, pathology, types, clinical features), venous congestion, pathology of fluid compartment, normal distribution of water, exudates, transudate fluid, edema (definition, etiology), thrombosis, embolism, infarction.
- Gene and chromosomal pathology, diseases due to abnormalities of gene.
- Metabolic disease: Pigmentation, hemosiderin, porphyrin, jaundice, diabetes mellitus.
- Deficiency disease.
- Hemopoietic system: Blood formation, anemia, leukemia, leukopenia, disease caused by platelets abnormalities, purpura, blood group, abnormal blood transfusion.

Clinical Pathology

- Hematology: Red blood cells, erythrocyte sedimentation rate, hemoglobin, blood group, coagulation of blood, white blood cells.
- Blood smear examination: Malarial parasites, *Wuchereria bancrofti*.
- Examination of sputum for acid-fast bacilli (AFB).
- Examination of urine: Normal characteristics, normal constituents and abnormal constituents.
- Examination of feces: Morphology, life cycle, pathogenicity and laboratory investigations of the following worms: *Ascaris lumbricoides, Ancylostoma duodenale, Enterobius vermicularis, Trichuris trichiura, Strongyloides stercoralis, Trichinella spiralis, Taenia saginata, Taenia solium*, protozoan, *Entamoeba histolytica*.
- Vaginal smear for *Trichomonas vaginalis*.
- Blood: Widal test, venereal diseases research laboratory (VDRL), enzyme-linked immunosorbent assay (ELISA) test, HbsAg.
- Skin: Demonstration of lepra bacilli.
- Rheumatoid arthritis (RA) factor, antistreptolysin O (ASO) titer.

SECTION

1

General Pathology

CHAPTER

1

Introduction

CHAPTER OUTLINE

- ➤ Normal Cell Structure and Functions
- ➤ Introduction to Pathology

NORMAL CELL STRUCTURE AND FUNCTIONS

- A cell is a fundamental unit of life.
- All cells are tridimensional, although when viewed under the light microscope on a glass slide, they appear to be flat.

Components of the Cell (Fig. 1.1)

All cells share the fundamental structural components. Each cell has three essential components: (A) Cell membrane, (B) Cytoplasm and (C) Nucleus.

A. Cell Membrane/Unit Membrane

It is the outer boundary of the cell.

Light microscopy: The membrane appears at the periphery as a thin condensation.

Function of cell membrane: Cell membrane plays a critical role in virtually every aspect of cell function.

B. Cytoplasm

Cytoplasm or cytosol is the component of the cell, located between the nucleus and the cell membrane.

Light microscopy: Various products of cell metabolism may be seen in the cytoplasm, and appear as granules or vacuoles.

Cytoplasmic organelles

Ultrastructurally, the cytoplasm is composed of: (1) organized cell components, or organelles; (2) the cytoskeleton, and (3) cytoplasmic matrix.

1. Organized components of the cytoplasm: They mainly consists of: (i) membranous systems, (ii) ribosomes, (iii) mitochondria, (iv) lysosomes, and (v) centrioles.

i. **Membranous system:** It is composed of: (a) the endoplasmic reticulum, and (b) the Golgi complex.

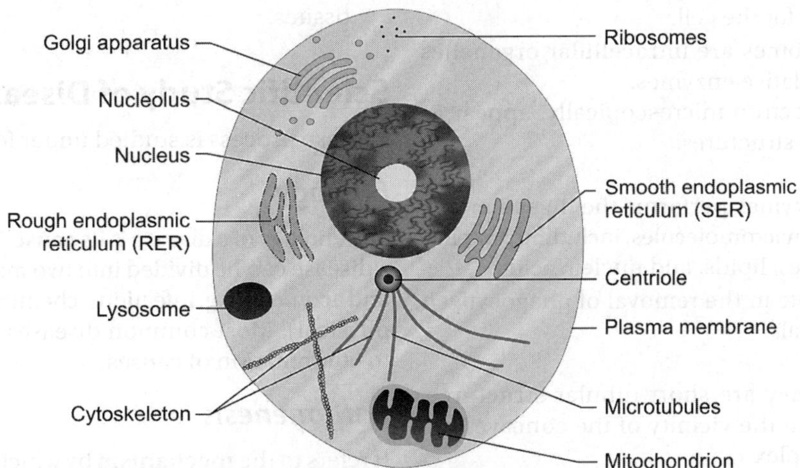

Fig. 1.1: Various constituents of cell

a. **Endoplasmic reticulum:**
   - **Appearance:** It is a closed system of unit membranes forming tubular canals and flattened sacs or cisternae. It subdivides the cytoplasm into a series of compartments.
   - **Types:** The membranes of the endoplasmic reticulum may be "rough," i.e. rough endoplasmic reticulum (RER) (i.e. covered with numerous attached granules), or "smooth" i.e. smooth endoplasmic reticulum (SER) (i.e. free of any particles).
   - **Function:** Rough endoplasmic reticulum is abundant in metabolically active cells.

b. **Golgi complex:**
   - **Appearance:** It consists of a series of parallel, doughnut-shaped flat spaces or cisternae and spherical or egg-shaped vesicles demarcated by smooth membranes.
   - **Function:** They synthesize and package cell products for the cells' own use and for export.

ii. **Ribosomes**
   - They are found in all cells.
   - Two types of ribosomes namely free and attached.
   - **Functions:**
     - Free ribosomes produce proteins for the cell's own use.
     - Attached ribosomes produce proteins for export.

iii. **Mitochondria:** They are present in all eukaryotic cells.
   - **Appearance:** Each mitochondrion is composed of two membranes. The outer membrane is a continuous, closed-unit membrane. Running parallel to the outer membrane is the inner membrane that forms numerous crests or invaginations.
   - **Function:** Most important function is the formation of energy-producing adenosine triphosphate (ATP) from phosphorus and adenosine diphosphate (ADP). ATP is exported into the cytoplasm and is an essential source of energy for the cell.

iv. **Lysosomes:** Lysosomes are intracellular organelles that contain degradative enzymes.
   - **Appearance:** Electron microscopically, appear as spherical or oval structures.
   - **Function:**
     - Lysosomal enzymes performs the digestion of a wide-range of macromolecules, including proteins, polysaccharides, lipids, and nucleic acids.
     - They participate in the removal of phagocytized foreign material.

v. **Centrioles**
   - **Appearance:** They are short tubular structures, usually located in the vicinity of the concave face of the Golgi complex.
   - **Function:** Play a key role during cell division.

2. The cytoskeleton: The cytoskeleton of the cells is mainly composed of three types of fibrillar proteins namely (1) the actin filaments (microfilaments, tonofilaments), (2) intermediate filaments, and (3) microtubules. Cytoskeleton maintains the physical shape of cells, involved in motion of the cells, and provide structural support to all cell functions.

3. Cytoplasmic matrix: The space within the cytoplasm, not occupied by the membranous system, the cell skeleton, or by the organelles, is called as the cytoplasmic matrix. It is composed of proteins and free ribosomes.

C. Nucleus

It is present within the cytoplasm.
- **Content:** It contains mainly deoxyribonucleic acid (DNA) that governs the genetic and functional aspects of cell activity.
- **Nucleolus:** In normal resting nuclei, the nucleoli are seen as round or oval structures occupying a small area within the nucleus.

INTRODUCTION TO PATHOLOGY

Definition: Pathology is the **scientific study (logos) of disease (pathos)**. It mainly focuses on the study of the structural and functional changes in cells, tissues, and organs in disease.

Learning Pathology

Study of pathology can be divided into general pathology and systemic pathology.
- **General pathology:** It deals with the study of mechanism, basic reactions of cells and tissues to abnormal stimuli and to inherited defects.
- **Systemic pathology:** This deals with the changes in specific diseases/responses of specialized organs and tissues.

Scientific Study of Disease

Disease process is studied under following aspects:

Etiology

The etiology of a disease is its **cause**. The causative factors of a disease can be divided into two major categories: genetic and acquired (e.g. infectious, chemical, hypoxia, nutritional, physical). Most common diseases are multifactorial due to combination of causes.

Pathogenesis

It refers to the **mechanism** by which the causative factor/s produces structural and functional abnormalities.

Pathogenesis deals with sequence of events that occur in the cells or tissues from the beginning of any disease process.

Morphologic Changes

All diseases start with structural changes in cells. **Rudolf Virchow** (known as the **Father of modern pathology**) proposed that injury to the cell is the basis of all diseases. Morphologic changes refer to the **gross and microscopic structural changes** in cells or tissues affected by disease.

Gross

Many diseases have characteristic gross pathology and a fairly confident diagnosis can be given before light microscopy. For example, cirrhosis of liver is characterized by total replacement of liver by regenerating nodules.

Microscopy

Light microscopy: Abnormalities in tissue architecture and morphological changes in cells can be studied by light microscopy.

- **Histopathology:** Sections are routinely cut from tissues and processed by pararffin-embedding. The sections are cut from the tissue by a special instrument called microtome and examined under light microscope. In certain situations (e.g. histochemistry, rapid diagnosis), sections are cut from tissue that has been hardened rapidly by freezing (frozen section). The sections are stained routinely by hematoxylin and eosin.
  - **Pathognomonic abnormalities:** If the **structural changes are characteristic of a single disease or diagnostic of an etiologic process,** it is called as **pathognomonic.** Pathognomonic features are those features which are restricted to a single disease, or disease category. The diagnosis should not be made without them. For example, **Aschoff bodies** are pathognomonic of **rheumatic heart disease** and **Reed Sternberg cells** are pathognomonic of **Hodgkin lymphoma**.
- **Cytology:** The cells from cysts, body cavities, or scraped from body surfaces or aspirated by fine needle from solid lesions can also be studied under light microscope. This study of cells is known as cytology and is used widely, especially in diagnosis and screening of cancer.
- **Histochemistry (special stains):** Histochemistry (refer Table 2.4) is the study of the chemistry of tissues, where tissue/cells are treated with specific reagent so that the features of individual cells/structure can be visualized, e.g. **Prussian blue reaction for hemosiderin.**
- **Immunohistochemistry and immunofluorescence:** They utilize antibodies (immunoglobulins with antigen specificity) to visualize substances in tissue sections or cell preparations. Former uses **monoclonal antibodies** linked chemically to enzymes and later **fluorescent dyes**.

Electron microscopy: Electron microscopy (EM) is useful to the study changes at ultrastructural level, and to the demonstration of viruses in tissue samples in certain diseases.

Functional Derangements and Clinical Manifestations

- **Functional derangements:** The effects of genetic, biochemical, and structural changes in cells and tissues are **functional abnormalities**. For example, insufficient secretion of a cell product (e.g. insulin lack in diabetes mellitus).
- **Clinical manifestations:** The functional derangements produce two clinical manifestations of disease, namely symptoms and signs. Diseases characterized by **multiple abnormalities** (symptom complex) are called syndromes.
- **Prognosis:** The prognosis forecasts (predicts) the known or likely **course (outcome) of the disease**, and therefore, the fate of the patient.
- **Complications:** It is a **negative pathologic process** or event occurring **during the disease** which is not an essential part of the disease. It usually aggravates the illness. For example, perforation and hemorrhage are complications which may develop in typhoid ulcer of intestine.

SELF-ASSESSMENT EXERCISE

I. Short Note

1. Components of cell.

CHAPTER 2

Cell Injury and Adaptation

CHAPTER OUTLINE

- Types of Cellular Responses to Injury
- Cellular Adaptations
- Definitions
- Cell Injury
- Intracellular Accumulations
- Necrosis
- Apoptosis
- Pathologic Calcification
- Other Tissue Changes
- Pigments

TYPES OF CELLULAR RESPONSES TO INJURY

Depending on the nature of stimulus/injury, cellular responses can be mainly divided into four types.

- Cellular adaptations.
- Cell injury.
  - Reversible cell injury: Cellular swelling, fatty change
  - Irreversible cell injury: Necrosis, apoptosis
- Intracellular accumulations.
- Pathologic calcification.

CELLULAR ADAPTATIONS

When the cell is exposed to pathological stimuli, it undergoes a series of metabolic changes known as cell stress. The cells can undergo adaptation to damaging stimuli, and achieve **a new, steady altered state that allows the cells to survive** and continue to function in an abnormal environment. Cells can adapt to certain pathologic stimuli by changes in size, number or differentiation of cells in affected tissue. These are reversible changes and constitute **cellular adaptations**.

Types of Adaptations (Fig. 2.1)

The types adaptations include: Hypertrophy, hyperplasia, atrophy and metaplasia.

Hypertrophy

Definition: Hypertrophy is defined as an **increase in the size of the tissue or organ due to increase in the size of cells**.

It develops in organs composed of nondividing cells such as muscles, e.g. cardiac and skeletal muscles.

Causes

Hypertrophy can be physiological or pathological.

Physiological: It occurs when there is increased functional demand/workload.

- **Hypertrophy of skeletal muscle:** For examples, the bulging muscles of bodybuilders, manual laborer and athletes and those engaged in "pumping iron".
- **Hypertrophy of smooth muscle:** For example, growth of the **uterus during pregnancy** from estrogenic **(hormone)** stimulation.

Pathological: It is caused by increased functional demand/workload.

- **Hypertrophy of cardiac muscle:** For examples, **left ventricular hypertrophy** (Fig. 2.2) due to hypertension or damaged heart valves (aortic stenosis, mitral incompetence).
- **Hypertrophy of smooth muscle:** For examples, **hypertrophy of urinary bladder muscle** (Fig. 2.3) in response to urethral obstruction (e.g. prostate hyperplasia).

Morphology

- **Gross:** The involved **organ is enlarged**.
- **Microscopy:** There is **increase in size of the cells** as well as the nuclei.

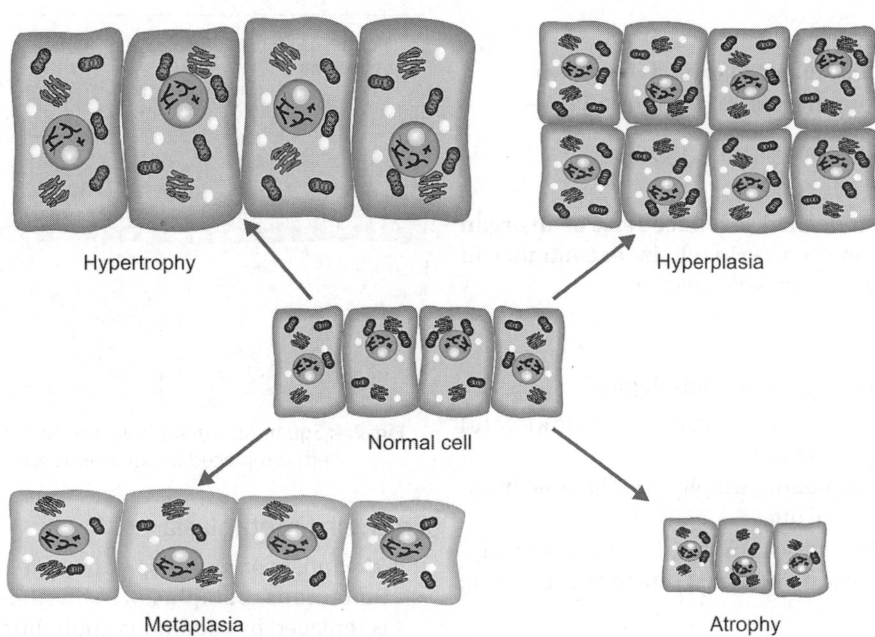

Fig. 2.1: Different types of cellular adaptations

Hyperplasia

Definition: Hyperplasia is defined as an **increase in the number of cells in an organ or tissue**, usually resulting in **increased size/mass of the organ or tissue**.

Causes

Hyperplasia can be physiological or pathological.

Physiological: It can be caused by hormonal stimulation, or as compensatory process.

- **Hyperplasia due to hormones:** For examples, hyperplasia of glandular epithelium of the **female breast at puberty, pregnancy and lactation**, hyperplasia of the uterus during pregnancy.
- **Compensatory hyperplasia:** For example, in liver following partial hepatectomy (removal of part of liver) the remaining normal liver cells proliferate and may grow back to its original size.

Pathological: It may be due to **excessive** endocrine stimulation or chronic injury/irritation.

- **Excessive hormonal stimulation:** For example, **endometrial hyperplasia** (due to estrogen) and benign prostatic hyperplasia [due to androgens (Fig. 2.3B)].
- **Chronic injury/irritation:** Long-standing inflammation or chronic injury may lead to hyperplasia especially in skin or oral mucosa.

Pathological hyperplasia can progress to cancer. For example, **endometrial hyperplasia can develop into endometrial cancer**.

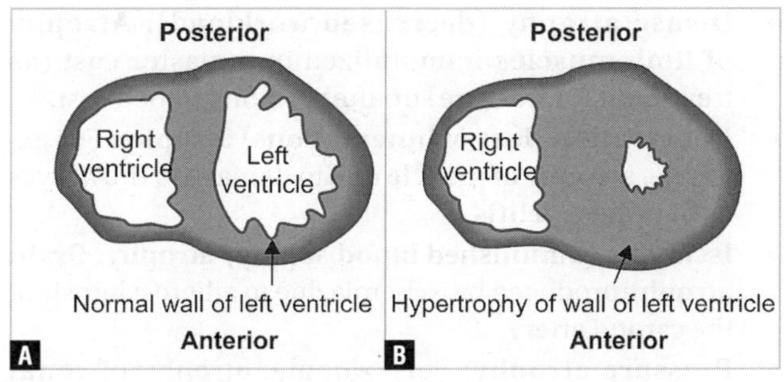

Figs 2.2A and B: (A) Transverse section of normal heart, (B) Transverse section of heart with hypertrophy of left ventricle characterized by the thickening of the left ventricle wall

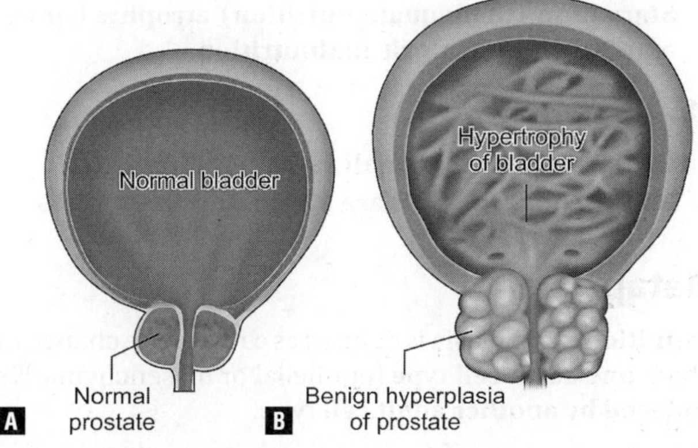

Figs 2.3A and B: Cut section of prostate along with urinary bladder. (A) Normal prostate; (B) Benign hyperplasia of prostate leading to enlargement of the prostate

Morphology

- **Gross:** The **size** of the affected organ is **increased**.
- **Microscopy:** Shows **increased number of cells**.

Atrophy

Definition: Atrophy is defined as **reduced size of an organ or tissue** resulting from decrease in cell size and number. In atrophy, function of an organ is also reduced.

Causes

Atrophy may be physiological or pathological.

Physiological: It is common during normal fetal development, and in adult life.

- **During fetal development:** Atrophy of embryonic structures, e.g. thyroglossal duct.
- **During adult life:** For examples, involution of thymus, **atrophy of brain and heart due to aging** (senile atrophy).

Pathological: It can be local or generalized.

Local

- **Disuse atrophy (decreased workload): Atrophy of limb muscles** immobilized in a plaster cast (as treatment for fracture) or after prolonged bed rest.
- **Denervation (loss of innervations) atrophy:** For example, **atrophy of muscle** due to damage to the nerves as in **poliomyelitis**.
- **Ischemic (diminished blood supply) atrophy: Brain atrophy** produced by ischemia due to atherosclerosis of the carotid artery.
- **Pressure atrophy:** For example, atrophy of **renal parenchyma in hydronephrosis** (distention of the pelvis and calices of the kidney with urine, as a result of obstruction of the ureter).

Generalized

- **Starvation (inadequate nutrition) atrophy:** For example, **protein-calorie malnutrition**.

Morphology

- **Gross:** The **organ is small** and often shrunken.
- **Microscopy:** The **cells are smaller** in size.

Metaplasia

Definition: Metaplasia is defined as a reversible change in which **one adult cell type** (epithelial or mesenchymal) is **replaced by another adult cell type**.

Types of Metaplasia

There are two types namely epithelial and mesenchymal.

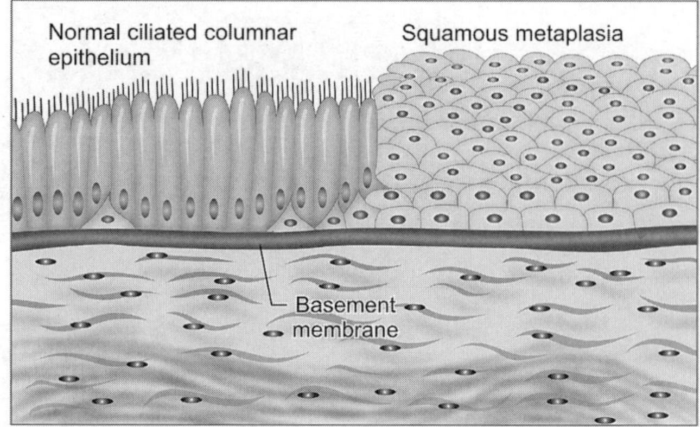

Fig. 2.4: Squamous metaplasia in which columnar epithelium (left) is replaced by squamous epithelium (right)

Epithelial metaplasia

It is the most common type of metaplasia.

- **Squamous metaplasia:** In this the original epithelium is replaced by squamous epithelium.
  - **Respiratory tract: Chronic irritation due to tobacco smoke**, the normal ciliated columnar epithelial cells of the trachea and bronchi are replaced by squamous epithelium (Fig. 2.4).
  - **Cervix:** Squamous metaplasia in cervix is associated with chronic infection.
- **Columnar metaplasia:** The subtypes are:
  - **Squamous to columnar:** In **Barrett esophagus,** the squamous epithelium of the esophagus replaced by columnar cells.
  - **Intestinal metaplasia:** The gastric glands are replaced by cells resembling those of the small intestine.

Connective tissue metaplasia

- **Osseous metaplasia:** Formation of new bone at sites of tissue injury is known as osseous metaplasia. Bone formation in muscle, known as **myositis ossificans**, occasionally occurs after intramuscular hemorrhage.

DEFINITIONS

- **Congenital anomaly (birth defect/congenital defect/congenital disorder):** The term congenital means "born with". All types of the **structural abnormality** or defect that is present at birth are termed as **congenital anomaly**.
- **Malformation:** It is a primary (or intrinsic) **structural defect** occurring during the development of an organ or tissue.
- **Agenesis:** It refers to the **complete absence of an organ** and its associated primordium.

- **Aplasia:** It refers to the **absence of an organ** that occurs due to failure of growth of the existing primordium.
- **Hypoplasia:** It refers to **incomplete development or decreased size of an organ** with decreased numbers of cells.
- **Dysplasia:** This term **in the context of malformations** (versus neoplasia) describes an **abnormal organization of cells.**

CELL INJURY

Causes of Cell Injury

Reduced Oxygen Supply

Hypoxia refers to inadequate oxygenation of tissues. Hypoxia is an important and common cause of cell injury and cell death. Hypoxia may be due to decreased blood flow (called ischemia) or inadequate oxygenation of the blood.

Physical Agents

These include: Mechanical trauma, radiation, electric shock, sudden atmospheric pressure changes and thermal injury.

Chemical Agents

This includes a wide variety of agents such as:

- Heavy metals and poisons (e.g. arsenic, mercuric salts or cyanide)
- Chemicals, strong acids and alkalies
- Environmental and air pollutants (e.g. insecticides and herbicides)
- Industrial and occupational hazards (carbon monoxide and asbestos)
- Other chemicals like alcohol and cigarette smoking
- Iatrogenic, i.e. the consequence of taking a drug prescribed by the physician can produce undesirable effects.

Infectious Agents

These include: Viruses, bacteria, fungi, rickettsiae and parasites.

Abnormal Immunologic Reactions

The immune system is required for defense against infectious pathogens. However, abnormal immune reactions itself may cause cell injury.

- **Autoimmunity:** Immune reactions to self-antigens can result in autoimmune diseases.
- **Hypersensitivity reactions:** Exaggerated immune reactions may cause cell injury.

Nutritional Imbalances

It may result from either **nutritional deficiencies** (deficiencies of specific vitamins) or **nutritional excesses** (excess of cholesterol predisposes to atherosclerosis). Obesity is associated with several diseases, such as diabetes.

Genetic Factors

Diseases may result from abnormal mutated genes or chromosomal abnormalities (e.g. Down syndrome). Genetic defects may cause cell injury.

Idiopathic

Idiopathic diseases are those in which the cause is not known.

Types of Cell Injury

The cell injury may be mainly divided into reversible and irreversible. Reversible injury may progress to an reversible stage and result in cell death.

Reversible Cell Injury

If the stimulus is acute and brief or mild, the cell injury produces changes in the cells which are reversible up to a certain point.

Light microscopic features of reversible cell injury

There are two patterns of reversible cell injury namely cellular swelling and fatty change.

- **Cellular (hydropic) swelling:** It is due to changes in ion concentrations and fluid homeostasis. There is increased flow of water into the cells and results in increased water content of injured cells.
- **Fatty change:** (Discussed under fatty change on page no 10).

Irreversible Cell Injury

If the cell is exposed to continuous injurious stimulus or if the injury is severe, the cells undergo cell death. There are two main types cell death namely **necrosis and apoptosis.**

- **Necrosis:** Necrosis is always a pathologic process.
- **Apoptosis:** Apoptosis may be physiological or pathological.

INTRACELLULAR ACCUMULATIONS

Metabolic derangements may result in retention or excess accumulation of various substances inside the cells. Intracellular accumulation of substance may occur by two mechanisms.

Accumulation of excess amount of normal cellular constituent: This occurs when normal substance is produced at a normal or increased rate, but the rate of metabolism is inadequate to remove it. For examples, water, lipids, proteins, carbohydrates (glycogen), etc.

Accumulation of an abnormal substance: The abnormal substance may be:

- **Exogenous:** Abnormal substances accumulate because the cell can neither degrade the substance nor has the ability to transport it to other sites. For examples, **accumulations of carbon particles, inhaled silica, injected tattoo pigments**.
- **Endogenous:** Substances that cannot be metabolized because of deficiency or defect of the enzyme and thus accumulate in cells. These are usually due to the genetic defect, e.g. hereditary storage diseases.

Cloudy Swelling (Hydropic Change, Vacuolar Degeneration)

- It was originally applied to the gross appearance of organ involved, but is now applied to the microscopic appearance.
- It is closely related to hydropic change, vacuolar degeneration. They represent disturbances in protein and water metabolism. Being a manifestation of a disturbance in protein metabolism, it is also called albuminous degeneration.

Causes: It may be caused by many forms of mild injury but usually due to bacterial toxins, chemical poisons and malnutrition. It is due to changes in ion concentrations and fluid homeostasis. There is an increased flow of water into the cells which results in increased water content of injured cells.

Organs involved: Kidney, liver, heart and muscle.

Gross: Organ affected is slightly enlarged due to swelling of its cells. Organ appears pale because of compression of blood vessels by the swollen cells. Cut surface has a cloudy appearance and opaque.

Microscopy: Best example is cloudy swelling of highly specialized cells of the convoluted tubule of the kidney. The cell is swollen and projects unevenly into the lumen of the tubule. As the process advances the cytoplasm breaks down and its granular material gets discharged into the lumen of the tubule. These granules are proteinaceous in nature.

Steatosis (Fatty Change)

Definition: Steatosis or fatty change is defined as abnormal accumulations of triglycerides within parenchymal cells.

Organs Involved

Fatty change is seen in organs involved in fat metabolism. **Liver** being the major organ is commonly involved. It may also occur in heart, muscle and kidney.

Fatty Liver

Definition: Steatosis (fatty change) of liver is defined **as abnormal accumulations of triglycerides within parenchymal cells of liver**.

Mild fatty change may not have any effect on cellular function. But more severe fatty change may impair cell function and lead to cell death.

Causes: The causes of steatosis include:

Disorders with hepatocyte damage: Alcohol abuse, protein malnutrition, starvation, hypoxia/anoxia (anemia, cardiac failure), **toxins** (carbon tetrachloride, chloroform, etc.). **Alcohol is the most common cause** of fatty change in the liver.

Disorders with hyperlipidemia: Obesity, diabetes mellitus or congenital hyperlipidemia.

Morphology of fatty liver

Gross: Liver is **enlarged** and becomes **yellow, soft and greasy to touch**.

Microscopy: Accumulation of fat is first seen as **small vacuoles in the cytoplasm** around the nucleus. As the process progresses the vacuoles coalesce, creating cleared spaces that **displace the nucleus to the periphery of the cell** (Fig. 2.5). Occasionally contiguous cells rupture and the enclosed fat globules coalesce, producing so-called fatty cysts.

Demonstration of fat

In fatty change, the fat appears as clear vacuoles within parenchymal cells of the involved organ when stained with Hematoxylin and Eosin. The clear vacuole can be demonstrated as fat by **frozen sections stained with Sudan IV or Oil Red-O**, both stains **give an orange-red color to the contained fat**. Osmic acid can also used which gives a black color.

Heart

Lipid in the cardiac muscle can have two patterns.

Alternate involvement: Prolonged moderate hypoxia (e.g. severe anemia), causes intracellular deposits of fat, which create grossly apparent bands of involved yellow myocardium alternating with bands of darker, red-brown, uninvolved myocardium (**tigered effect, tabby cat appearance**).

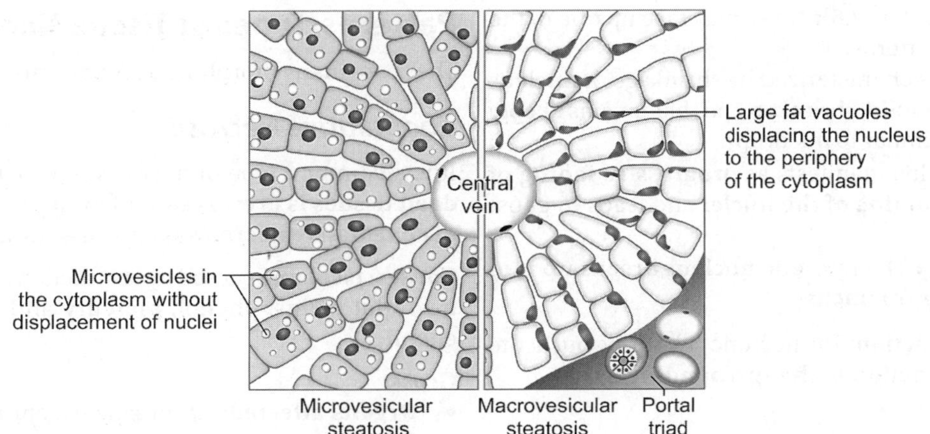

Fig. 2.5: Fatty liver (hepatic steatosis). Diagrammatic appearance of microvesicular (left half) and macrovesicular fatty change/steatosis (right half)

Uniform involvement: More severe hypoxia or some types of myocarditis (e.g. diphtheria infection) shows more uniform involvement of myocardial fibers.

Proteins Accumulations

Proteins usually appear as rounded, eosinophilic droplets, vacuoles, or aggregates in the cytoplasm.

Conditions

- **Reabsorption of protein droplets in proximal renal tubules:** Increased reabsorption of the protein by the proximal renal tubules is observed in kidney diseases associated with heavy protein loss in the urine (proteinuria).
- **Russell bodies:** These are plasma cells distended with excessive amounts proteins due to active synthesis of immunoglobulins.
- **Defective intracellular transport and secretion of critical proteins:** For example α1-antitrypsin deficiency.
- **Accumulation of cytoskeletal proteins:** Alcoholic hyaline is an eosinophilic cytoplasmic inclusion in liver cells that is characteristic of alcoholic liver disease.
- **Aggregation of abnormal proteins:** For example certain forms of **amyloidosis**.

Glycogen Accumulations

- Glycogen is a readily available energy source stored in the cytoplasm of normal cells.
- Excessive intracellular accumulation of glycogen is found with an abnormal glucose or glycogen metabolism.
- **Demonstration of glycogen:** Glycogen dissolves in aqueous fixatives and appears as clear vacuoles within the cytoplasm. It is identified when tissues are **fixed in absolute alcohol** and stained with **PAS reaction** which imparts a rose-to-violet color to the glycogen.

Conditions

- **Diabetes mellitus:** It is a disorder of glucose metabolism in which glycogen is found in renal tubular epithelial cells, liver cells, β cells of the islets of Langerhans, and heart muscle cells.
- **Glycogen storage diseases (glycogenoses):** These genetic disorders are associated with enzymatic defects in the synthesis or breakdown of glycogen. Thus, they are associated with massive accumulation of glycogen within the cells causing cell injury and cell death.

NECROSIS

Definition: Necrosis is the **morphological changes indicative of cell death in a living tissue** following extremely harmful injury.

Causes of Necrosis

All the causes of cell injury if severe, persistent can cause necrosis (refer page no. 9).

Morphology

The general changes occurring in necrotic cell, irrespective of type of necrosis are as follows:

Cytoplasmic changes: Increased eosinophilia.

Nuclear changes (Fig. 2.6)**:** These may take up one of the three following patterns.

- **Pyknosis:** It is characterized by shrinkage of nucleus which appears **solid, shrunken** and (blue) stains **deeply basophilic** (similar to ink drop).
- **Karyolysis:** This manifests as **progressive fading of basophilic staining of the nuclei** and leads to ghost nuclei.
- **Karyorrhexis:** The pyknotic **nucleus breaks up into many smaller fragments**.

Inflammatory reaction: The necrotic cells bring out acute **inflammatory reaction in the surrounding tissue**.

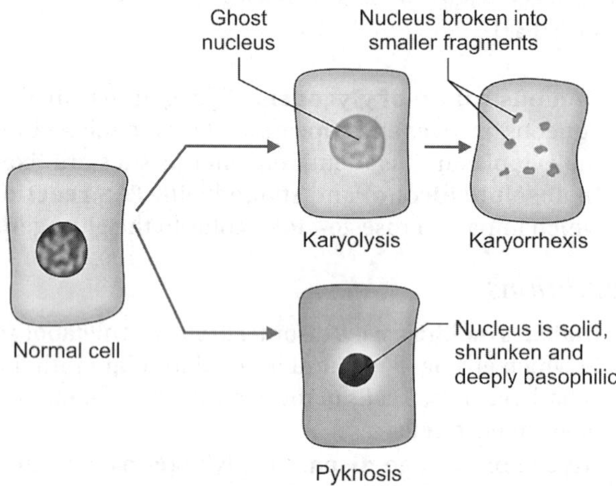

Fig. 2.6: Nuclear changes in necrosis

Patterns/Types of Tissue Necrosis

There are many morphological patterns of necrosis.

Coagulative Necrosis

It is a common type of necrosis in which the **outline of dead tissues is preserved** for few days. A **localized area of coagulative necrosis** is known as **infarct**.

Causes: Ischemia caused by obstruction in a vessel, potent bacterial toxins, phenol, mercury and other corrosive chemicals.

Gross:

- **Organs affected:** All organs except the brain. More frequently involved are **heart, kidney and spleen.**
- **Appearance:** The involved tissue has an opaque appearance similar to that of boiled meat. The **necrotic tissues appear dry, pale, yellow and soft** in consistency (Fig. 2.7A).

Microscopy: The **outline of dead tissue is preserved** for some days (Figs 2.7B and C). Nuclear and cytoplasmic changes take place as described under necrosis above.

Liquefactive Necrosis (Colliquative Necrosis)

The term is applied in which the **dead tissue rapidly undergoes softening** and transformed into a liquid viscous mass.

Causes:

- **Ischemic injury to central nervous system** (CNS)
- **Suppurative infections:** Focal infections by bacteria which stimulate the accumulation of leukocytes.

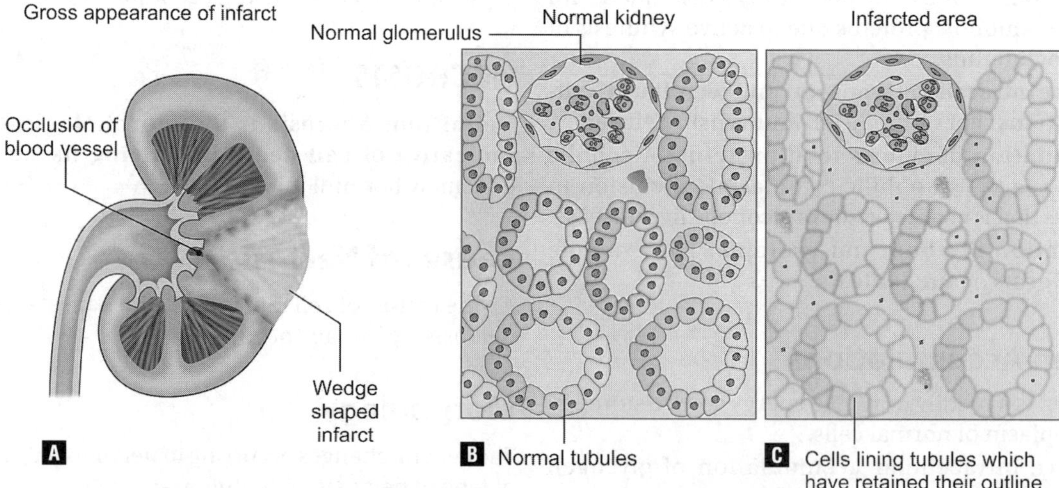

Figs 2.7A to C: (A) Renal infarct; (B) Normal glomeruli and tubules; (C) Acute tubular necrosis. The tubules are lined by epithelial cells showing eosinophilic cytoplasm and nuclear changes of coagulative necrosis. The outline of the necrotic epithelial cells can be made out

Organs affected: Brain, abscess (any organ or tissue). The necrotic area in the brain is soft and center is liquefied.

Microscopy: Abscess is localized collection of pus. It consists of a cavity containing pus formed by liquefactive necrosis and inflammatory cells in a solid tissue. **Pus** consists of liquefied necrotic cell debris, dead leukocytes and macrophages (scavenger cells). Abscess shows a cavity containing pus and surrounding wall with granulation tissue and inflammatory cells.

Caseous Necrosis

It is a distinctive type of necrosis. This shows **combined features of both coagulative and liquefactive necrosis.**

Cause: It is characteristic of **tuberculosis** and is due to hypersensitivity reaction.

Gross:
- **Organs affected:** Tuberculosis may involve any organ. Most common are **lung and lymph nodes**.
- **Appearance:** The necrotic area appears **yellowish-white, soft, granular, friable** and sharply circumscribed.

The **necrotic tissue resembles** dry, clumpy **cheese**, hence the name caseous (cheese-like) necrosis.

Microscopy:
- It is characterized by a focal lesion known as a **granuloma** (refer Fig. 4.2). The granuloma in tuberculosis is tuberculous granuloma or tubercle. The granulomas may be caseating (soft granuloma) or noncaseating (hard granuloma).
- The caseating granulomas show a **central area of caseous necrosis**. Caseous necrosis appears as a shapeless, eosinophilic, coarsely granular material. The necrotic area is **surrounded by epithelioid cells; Langhans type giant cells** (nuclei arranged in a horse-shoe pattern), **lymphocytes and fibroblasts.**
- The caseous necrotic material may undergo dystrophic calcification.

Fat Necrosis

It refers to a **focal areas of fat destruction**, which affect adipose tissue.

Types: The two types are **enzymatic** and **traumatic**. The most common is enzymatic necrosis resulting from pancreatitis.

Enzymatic fat necrosis

It is peculiar to adipose tissue around acutely inflamed pancreas (**in acute pancreatitis**).

Mechanism: In pancreatitis, the enzymes leak from the injured pancreatic acinar cells and cause tissue damage. The activated lipase enzyme destroys fat cells and liberates free fatty acids. These fatty acids combine with calcium and are precipitated as calcium soaps (fat saponification).

Gross: Fat necrosis appears as **chalky-white areas.**

Microscopy: The necrotic foci appear as **fat cells with pale, shadowy outlines**, surrounded by an inflammatory reaction.

Traumatic fat necrosis

It occurs in tissues with high fat content (like in breast and thigh) following severe trauma.

Fibrinoid Necrosis

It is a special form of necrosis characterized by deposition of pink-staining (fibrin-like) proteinaceous material. It usually involves arteries and walls of arterioles and glomeruli of the kidney. It is usually seen in immune mediated vascular injury.

Gangrene (Gangrenous Necrosis)

Definition: Gangrene is defined as **massive necrosis with superadded putrefaction.**

Putrefaction is decomposition by microorganisms, resulting in production of foul smelling substances and gas.

Types: It is mainly of two types namely dry and wet gangrene. A variant of wet gangrene known as gas gangrene is caused by clostridia (Gram positive anaerobic bacteria).

Dry gangrene

Causes: Arterial occlusion (e.g. atherosclerosis).

Sites: It usually involves a limb, generally the distal part of lower limb (leg, foot and toe).

Gross: The affected part is **dry, shrunken, shriveled, (mummified) and dark brown or black** in color resembling the foot of a mummy. The black color is due to the iron sulfide. A **line of demarcation** is usually seen between gangrenous and adjacent normal area (Fig. 2.8).

Microscopy: The necrosis shows smudging of soft tissue and overlying skin. The line of demarcation consists of granulation tissue with inflammatory cells.

Wet gangrene

Sites: Usually occurs in moist tissues or organs (e.g. **bowel, lung, mouth,** etc.).

Causes: Usually **due to the venous blockage** (e.g. strangulated hernia, intussusception or volvulus). In **diabetics**, the gangrene foot is of wet type because of the high sugar content in the necrotic tissue which favors growth of bacteria.

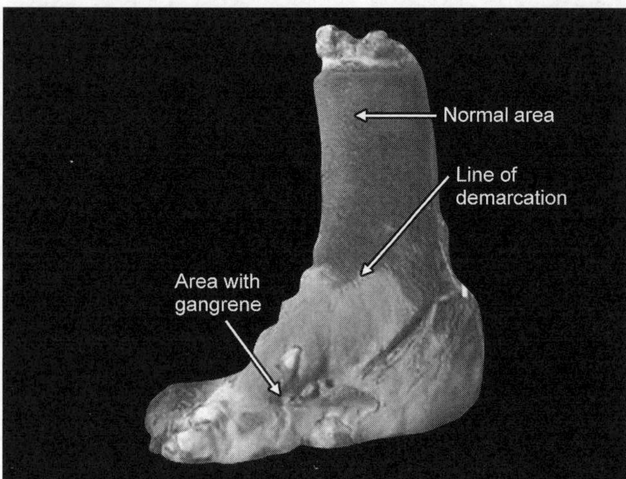

Fig. 2.8: Dry gangrene of left leg shows dry shrunken discolored gangrenous foot separated from adjacent normal area by a line of demarcation

Table 2.1: Differences between dry and wet gangrene

Features	Dry	Wet
General features		
Common site	Limbs	Bowels
Examples	Gangrene due to atherosclerotic occlusion	Volvulus, intussusception
Etiological factors		
Cause of ischemia	Arterial obstruction	Commonly venous obstruction
Rate of obstruction	Slow	Abrupt
Pathogens	Absent	May be present and may be the causative agent
Gross features		
Appearance of involved part	Shriveled, dry (mummification) and black	Swollen, soft and moist
Line of demarcation	Clear cut	Not clear cut
Putrefaction	Minimal	Marked, may be foul swelling
Spread	Slow	Rapid
Prognosis	Fair	Poor due to severe septicemia

Gross: The affected part is **soft, swollen, putrid, rotten and dark**. There is **no clear line of demarcation** between the gangrenous part and viable part.

Microscopy: It is usually **liquefactive** type of necrosis.

Differences between dry and wet (moist) gangrene are shown in Table 2.1.

Gas gangrene

It is a special type of wet gangrene caused by infection with gas forming anaerobic clostridia.

Gummatous Necrosis

The necrotic tissue is firm and rubbery and the original architecture can be seen on histological examination. It is usually found in syphilis.

APOPTOSIS

Definition: Apoptosis is a **type cell death** in which **cells activate enzymes that degrade the cell's own nuclear DNA and nuclear and cytoplasmic proteins.**

Causes of Apoptosis

Apoptosis may be physiological or pathological.

Physiological Situations

Apoptosis is a physical process during embryogenesis, development and throughout adulthood. Important physiologic situations associated with apoptosis are:

- **Removal of excess cells during embryogenesis and developmental processes:** For example, disappearance of web tissues between fingers and toes.
- **Elimination of cells after withdrawal of hormonal stimuli:** For example, endometrial cell breakdown during the menstrual cycle.
- **Elimination of cells after withdrawal of tropic stimuli:** For example, neutrophils in an acute inflammatory response, lymphocytes after immune response.
- **Elimination of potentially harmful cells:** In immunology, the clones of self-reactive lymphocytes that recognize normal self-antigens are deleted by apoptosis.

Pathological Conditions

Apoptosis is responsible for cell loss in many pathologic states. For example, elimination of cells with damaged DNA, killing of viral infected cells, elimination of neoplastic cells and elimination of parenchymal cells in pathologic atrophy.

Morphology

Electron Microscope

The ultrastructural features of apoptosis (Fig. 2.9) are:

Cell shrinkage: Cells shrink and cytoplasm becomes dense.

Nuclear condensation and fragmentation: Chromatin aggregates peripherally, under the nuclear membrane.

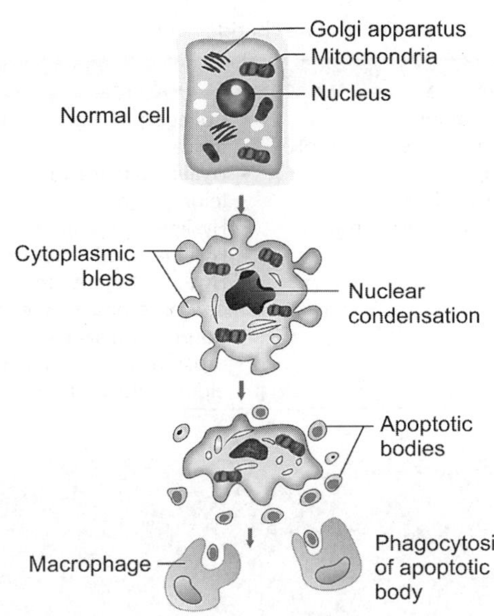

Fig. 2.9: Electron microscopic changes in apoptosis

The nucleus may break-up to produce two or more nuclear fragments.

Formation of cytoplasmic blebs and apoptotic bodies: The cell first shows extensive surface blebbing followed by fragmentation into membrane-bound apoptotic bodies. The apoptotic bodies are composed of cytoplasm and tightly packed organelles, with or without nuclear fragments.

Phagocytosis of apoptotic cells/bodies: The apoptotic bodies are rapidly ingested by phagocytes **(usually by macrophages)** and degraded by the lysosomal enzymes of phagocytes.

Light Microscopy

The **apoptotic cells** appear as a **round or oval** mass having intensely **eosinophilic** cytoplasm. The **nucleus appear as fragments of dense nuclear chromatin** and pyknotic. Apoptosis does not elicit an inflammatory reaction in the host.

Differences between necrosis and apoptosis (Table 2.2).

Autolysis: Autolysis (auto = self, lysis = digestion) is disintegration of the cell by its own hydrolytic enzymes released from lysosomes in the cytoplasm. This term is usually used for postmortem change in which there is no surrounding inflammatory reaction.

PATHOLOGIC CALCIFICATION

Definition: Pathologic calcification is the **abnormal deposition of calcium salts** (together with minute quantities of other mineral salts) in tissues other than osteoid or enamel.

Table 2.2: Differences between apoptosis and necrosis

Features	Apoptosis	Necrosis
Cause	Physiological or pathological	Invariably pathological
Morphology		
Extent	Single or small cluster of cells	Involves group of cells
Nucleus	Undergoes fragmentation	Pyknosis, karyorrhexis, karyolysis
Cellular contents	Intact; may be released in apoptotic bodies	Enzymatic digestion; may leak out of cell
Inflammatory response	Absent	Usual in the adjacent tissue
Fate of dead cells	Ingested (phagocytosed) by neighboring cells	Ingested by neutrophils and macrophages

Types

There are two categories of pathologic calcification namely **dystrophic calcification** and **metastatic calcification.**

Dystrophic Calcification

Definition: Deposition of calcium salts in dying or dead tissues is known as dystrophic calcification.

Causes

Necrotic tissue: Dystrophic calcification is encountered in areas of necrosis, e.g. **caseous, enzymatic fat necrosis**. Calcification can occur in **dead eggs** of *Schistosoma*, cysticercosis, hydatid cysts.

Degenerating tissue: Examples include:

- **Heart valves:** Dystrophic calcification may occur in **aging or damaged heart valves.**
- **Atherosclerosis:** Calcification is common in the atheromas of advanced atherosclerosis.
- **Monckeberg's medial calcific sclerosis:** Calcification in the media of the muscular arteries in old people.
- **Psammoma bodies: Single necrotic** cells on which **several layers of mineral** progressively get deposited to create lamellated shape, are called psammoma bodies.

Metastatic Calcification

Definition: Deposition of calcium salts in apparently normal tissues is known as metastatic calcification. Metastatic calcification is almost always **associated with an increased serum calcium** concentration (hypercalcemia) secondary to deranged calcium metabolism.

Causes

Calcification is seen in various disorders, including chronic renal failure, vitamin D intoxication, and hyperparathyroidism. There are four principal causes of hypercalcemia:

1. **Increased secretion of parathyroid hormone** (PTH) with subsequent bone resorption.
2. **Destruction of bone tissue:** Secondary to primary tumors of bone marrow (e.g. multiple myeloma, leukemia).
3. **Vitamin D–related disorders:** Vitamin D intoxication.
4. **Renal failure:** It causes retention of phosphate, leading to secondary hyperparathyroidism.

Sites

Any disorder with hypercalcemia can lead to metastatic calcification in any normal tissue throughout the body, but principally affects the following locations:

- **Lungs**
- **Kidney**
- **Blood vessels**
- **Stomach.**

Morphology of Calcification

Gross: Calcium salts appear as fine, white granules or clumps. On palpation they feel gritty and sandlike deposits.

Microscopy: Calcium salts have a **basophilic, amorphous granular**, sometimes clumped appearance.

OTHER TISSUE CHANGES

Hyaline Change

Hyaline refers to **an alteration within cells or in the extracellular space**, which gives a **homogeneous, glassy, pink appearance** in routine histological sections.

Examples of Hyaline Change (Table 2.3)

Intracellular hyaline

- **Mallory body** in the liver is alcoholic hyaline **composed of cytoskeletal filaments**.
- **Russell bodies** are **excessive accumulation of immunoglobulins in the plasma cells**.

Extracellular hyaline

- Collagenous fibrous tissue in **old scars**.
- Hyaline change in **uterine leiomyoma** (Fig. 2.10).
- In **chronic glomerulonephritis,** the **glomeruli** show hyalinization.

Table 2.3: Examples of hyaline change

Intracellular hyaline	Extracellular hyaline
• Mallory bodies • Russell bodies (e.g. multiple myeloma) • Crooke's hyaline • Zenker's hyaline change	• Collagenous fibrous tissue in scar • Hyaline change in uterine leiomyoma • Hyaline membrane in newborn • Hyaline arteriosclerosis • Hyalinization of glomeruli in chronic glomerulonephritis • Corpora amylacea in prostate, brain, spinal cord in elderly, old infarct of lung

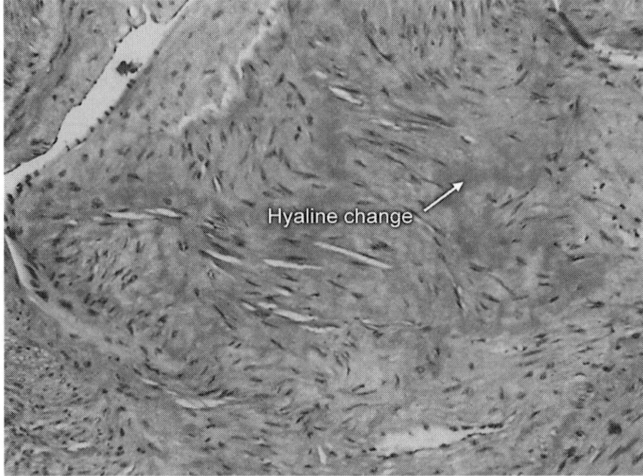

Fig. 2.10: Hyaline change in leiomyoma of uterus

Mucoid Degeneration

- Mucus is the viscid watery secretion produced by mucous glands. It consists of loose combination of proteins and mucopolysaccharides. Its main constituent is a glycoprotein called mucin.
- Mucus is produced by mitochondria and then they move to Golgi apparatus, where they are converted into mucin. When this process is exaggerated with excessive secretion of mucus it is termed mucoid degeneration.
- Mucin is normally produced by both epithelial cells of mucus membranes and mucous glands and also by certain connective tissue cells, especially in the fetus (e.g. umbilical cord). Mucoid degeneration may involve both epithelial and connective tissue mucin. Usually, connective tissue mucin is termed as myxoid, i.e. mucus like.
- Both epithelial and connective tissue mucin are stained by alcian blue. Epithelial mucin stains positively with

Table 2.4: Different types of pigments

Endogenous pigments	Exogenous pigments
• Bilirubin • Melanin • Hemosiderin • Hemoglobin derived pigments • Lipofuscin	• Carbon (anthracotic) • Tattooing • Arsenic • β-carotene

periodic acid-Schiff (PAS) and connective tissue mucin is PAS negative and stains positively with colloidal iron.

Epithelial mucin: Examples of excessive epithelial mucin secretion are:
- Catarrhal inflammation of the mucus membrane, e.g. inflammation of mucosa of respiratory tract and gastrointestinal (GI) tract.
- Obstruction, e.g. mucocele of gallbladder, appendix, and oral cavity.
- Cystic fibrosis of pancreas.
- Mucus secreting tumors, e.g. GI tract and ovary.

Connective tissue mucin: Examples:
- Mucoid or myxoid degeneration: Examples of tumors include myxoma, neurofibroma, fibroadenoma and sarcomas.
- Dissecting aneurysm of aorta.
- Myxedema: Myxomatous changes in dermis.
- Myxoid change in ganglion.

PIGMENTS

Pigments are **colored substances**, which are either normal constituents of cells (e.g. melanin), or are abnormal and accumulate in cells. Different types of pigments are listed in Table 2.4.

Melanin

The term melanin is derived from the Greek (*melas*, black).
- It is the only endogenous, brown-black pigment.
- It formed in melanocytes by the oxidation of tyrosine to dihydroxyphenylalanine by the enzyme tyrosinase.

Hemosiderin

It is a hemoglobin-derived, golden yellow-to-brown, granular or crystalline pigment and is one of the major storage forms of iron.

Causes of Excess Hemosiderin

Local or systemic excess of iron cause hemosiderin to accumulate within cells.

- **Local excesses:**
  - **Bruise**
  - **Brown induration of lung** in chronic venous congestion of lung.
- **Systemic excesses: Systemic overload of iron** is known as **hemosiderosis**. The main causes are:
  - **Increased absorption of dietary iron.**
  - **Excessive destruction of red cells,** e.g. hemolytic anemias.
  - **Repeated blood transfusions.**

Morphology

Site of accumulation

- **Localized:** Found in the macrophages of the involved area.
- **Systemic:** Initially found in **liver, bone marrow, spleen, and lymph nodes**. Later deposited in macrophages of other organs (e.g. skin, pancreas and kidney).

Microscopy

Appears as a **coarse, golden, granular pigment within the cytoplasm**.

Special stain

Prussian blue histochemical reaction in which hemosiderin converts colorless potassium ferrocyanide to **blue-black** ferric ferrocyanide.

Other Pigments

- **Hemochromatosis:** Severe accumulation of iron is associated with damage to liver, heart, and pancreas. The triad of cirrhosis of liver, diabetes mellitus (due to pancreatic damage) and brown pigmentation of skin constitute **bronze diabetes**.
- **Hemozoin:** It is a brown-black pigment containing heme in ferric form. This pigment is seen in chronic malaria and in mismatched blood transfusions.
- **Bilirubin** is the normal major pigment found in bile. It is non-iron containing pigment derived from hemoglobin.
- **Lipofuscin:**
  - Lipofuscin is an **insoluble endogenous pigment, also called as lipochrome or wear-and-tear pigment.**
  - **Composition:** It is composed of lipids, phospholipids and protein. The term lipofuscin is derived from the Latin (*fuscus*, brown), and refers to brown lipid.
  - **Significance:** It **indicates a product of free radical injury and lipid peroxidation**. Lipofuscin does not injure cell or its functions. It is observed in cells undergoing slow, regressive changes and is particularly prominent in the liver and heart (often

called brown atrophy of heart) of aging patients or patients with severe malnutrition and cancer cachexia.

- **Appearance:** Microscopically, it appears as a yellow-brown, finely granular cytoplasmic pigment, often present in the perinuclear region.

SELF-ASSESSMENT EXERCISES

I. Essay

1. Define necrosis. Describe the various types of necrosis with suitable examples. Add a note on autolysis.

II. Short Notes

1. Hypertrophy.
2. Hyperplasia.
3. Atrophy.
4. Metaplasia.
5. Causes of cell injury.
6. Fatty liver/steatosis of liver.
7. Pathogenesis of steatosis/fatty liver.
8. Special stains for fat.
9. Gross and microscopic features of fatty liver/steatosis of liver.
10. Types of necrosis.
11. Coagulative necrosis.
12. Liquefactive necrosis.
13. Caseous necrosis.
14. Fat necrosis.
15. Define and classify gangrene.
16. Gangrene.
17. Differences between dry and wet gangrene.
18. Apoptosis.
19. Mention the types of calcification.
20. Pathologic calcification.
21. Dystrophic calcification with examples.
22. Metastatic calcification with examples.
23. Hyaline change.

CHAPTER 3

Inflammation and Repair

CHAPTER OUTLINE

- Introduction
- Acute Inflammation
- Sequence of Events in Acute Inflammation
- Chemical Mediators of Inflammation
- Outcomes of Acute Inflammation
- Morphological Types/Patterns of Acute Inflammation
- Systemic Effects of Inflammation
- Chronic Inflammation
- Granulomatous Inflammation
- Repair and Healing
- Cutaneous Wound Healing
- Factors that Influence Wound Healing
- Complications of Wound Healing
- Healing of a Fracture

INTRODUCTION

Definition: Inflammation is a **complex local response of the living vascularized tissues to injury**. It mainly consists of responses of blood vessels and leukocytes.

Type of Inflammation

Inflammation may be divided into **acute** or **chronic**. The differences between acute and chronic inflammation are shown in Table 3.1.

Inflammation is **usually** a **protective** beneficial response. It localizes the cause of cell injury such as microorganism, foreign particles, or any other injurious agents. **Sometimes** inflammation may be **harmful**. For example, destruction of joint in septic arthritis, hypersensitivity reactions and autoimmune diseases.

Cardinal Sign of Inflammation

Cornelius Celsus first described the **four** cardinal signs of inflammation**: Rubor (redness), tumor (swelling), calor (heat), and dolor (pain).** A **fifth** clinical sign, **loss of function** (functio laesa) was later added by Rudolf Virchow.

ACUTE INFLAMMATION

Causes of (Stimuli for) Acute Inflammation

- **Infections** (bacterial, viral, fungal, parasitic) **and microbial toxins**

Table 3.1: Differences between acute and chronic inflammation

	Acute inflammation	Chronic inflammation
Onset	Rapid in onset (usually in minutes)	May follow acute inflammation or be insidious in onset
Duration	Short duration. Last for hours or a few days	Longer duration; may be months
Predominant cells	Neutrophils (also called polymorphonuclear leukocytes)	Lymphocytes, macrophages and sometimes plasma cells
Characteristics	Exudation of fluid and plasma proteins (edema) and the emigration of leukocytes	Inflammatory cells associated with the proliferation of blood vessels, tissue destruction and fibroblast proliferation
Fate	When causative agent is removed, the reaction subsides. If not it can progress to a chronic phase	Fibrosis and scar formation
Example	Acute appendicitis	Chronic pyelonephritis

- **Tissue necrosis:** This may develop due to ischemia
- **Physical agents include:** Mechanical trauma, radiation, electric shock and sudden changes in atmospheric pressure.
- **Chemical injury include:** Strong acids and alkalis, insecticides, etc.
- **Foreign bodies.**
- **Immune reactions.**

SEQUENCE OF EVENTS IN ACUTE INFLAMMATION

Two major components of acute inflammation are:
- Reactions of blood vessels (vascular changes)
- Reactions of leukocytes (cellular events).

Reactions of Blood Vessels (Vascular Events)

Purpose

Reactive changes in the blood vessels deliver the circulating cells, fluid and plasma proteins from the blood circulation to sites of tissue injury (e.g. infection).

Changes in Blood Vessel

It consists of (1) **changes in the vascular flow and caliber (hemodynamic changes)** and (2) **increased vascular permeability.**

1. **Changes in vascular flow and caliber** (Fig. 3.1): The changes are as follows:
   - **Vasodilatation and increased blood flow:** The earliest change of acute inflammation is dilatation of the arterioles in the injured site. Vasodilatation results in increased blood flow and is responsible for the local heat (**calor**) and redness (**rubor**).
   - **Increased vascular permeability:** Vasodilatation is followed by increased permeability of the microvasculature (which consists of arteriole, capillaries and venules). Increased vascular permeability leads to escape of protein-rich fluid from the blood circulation into the extravascular tissues (causing **edema**).
   - **Slowing of blood flow:** The loss of fluid along with vasodilatation results in slowing of blood flow, and concentration of RBCs in small vessels.
   - **Stasis:** In the dilated small vessels with slowed blood flow, the slow moving **RBCs get packed**, a condition named stasis. It is responsible for localized redness (**rubor**).

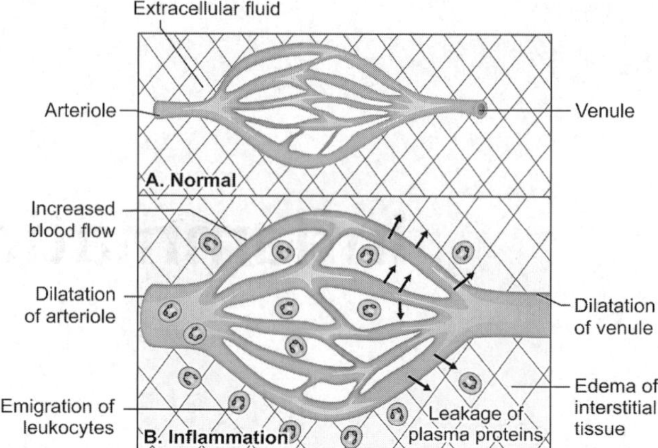

Figs 3.1A and B: (A) Blood flow in the normal microvasculature. (B) During acute inflammation. (1) Vascular dilatation and increased blood flow causes redness and warmth; (2) Leakage of plasma fluid and proteins causes edema; (3) Leukocyte emigrate out of microvasculature and accumulate at the site of injury

   - **Reaction of leukocytes (leukocyte events):** Refer below.
2. **Increased vascular permeability (vascular leakage):** It results in escape of protein-rich fluid from the blood circulation into the extravascular tissues (Fig. 3.2).

   Definitions:
   - **Exudation:** It is the process of escape of fluid, proteins and circulating blood cells from the blood vessels into the interstitial tissue or body cavities. Increased vascular permeability causes escape of a protein-rich fluid (exudate) resulting in edema (**tumor**).
   - **Edema:** It is defined as accumulation of excess of fluid in the interstitial tissue or serous cavities. It can be either an exudate or a transudate. Differences between exudate and transudate are shown in Table 3.2.

Leukocytic/Cellular Events

This process **delivers leukocytes** capable of phagocytosis (neutrophils and macrophages) **to the site of injury**. The leukocyte events can be divided into: Leukocyte recruitment and leukocyte activation.

Leukocyte Recruitment/Extravasation

Normally, leukocytes move rapidly in the blood. During inflammation, they slow down and escape to the site of injury/causative agent in the extravascular space. Leukocyte extravasation is the **process of migration of leukocytes from the lumen of the vessel to the site of injury in the extravascular tissues**.

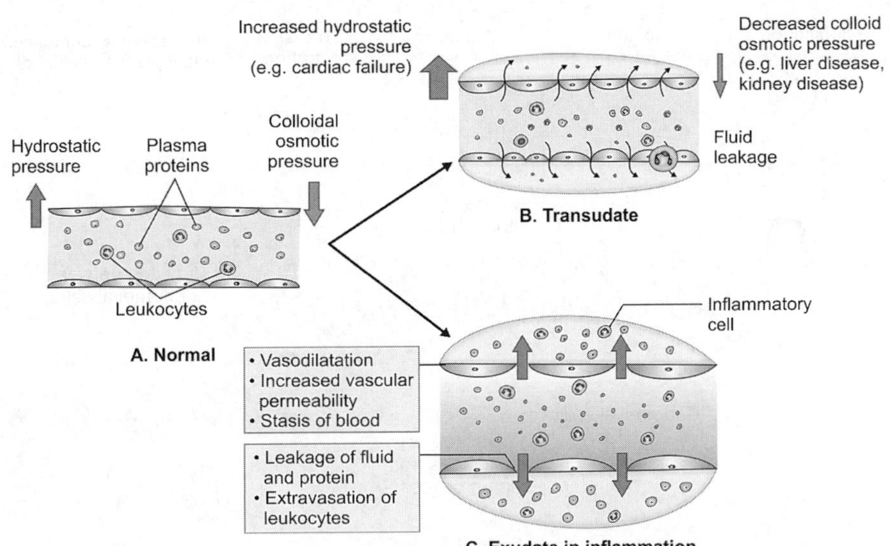

Figs 3.2A to C: Formation of transudates and exudates. (A) Normal. The force that drives the fluid out of vessel is hydrostatic pressure and the force that draws the fluid in is colloid osmotic pressure; (B) A transudate is formed when fluid leaks out either due to increased hydrostatic pressure or decreased osmotic pressure; (C) An exudate is formed in inflammation, because of increased vascular permeability vasodilatation and stasis of blood

Table 3.2: Differences between transudate and exudate

Characteristics	Transudate	Exudate
Mechanism	Due to non-inflammatory process (increased hydrostatic pressure) with normal vascular permeability	Increased vascular permeability due to inflammatory process
Appearance	Clear, serous	Cloudy/purulent/hemorrhagic
Color	Straw yellow	Yellow to red
Specific gravity	<1.018	>1.018
Protein	Low, <2 g/dL, mainly albumin	High, >2 g/dL
Clot	Absent	Clots spontaneously because of high fibrinogen
Cell count	Low	High
Type of cells	Few lymphocytes and mesothelial cells	Neutrophils in acute and lymphocytes in chronic inflammation
Bacteria	Absent	Usually present
Lactate dehydrogenase	Low	High

Steps in leukocyte recruitment/extravasation (Fig. 3.3)

In the vascular lumen:

1. **Margination:** When the blood flow slows down (stasis), leukocytes (mainly neutrophils) move towards the peripheral column and **accumulate along on the endothelial surface** of vessels.
2. **Rolling:** Marginated leukocytes attach weakly to the endothelium, detach and bind again with a mild jumping movement. It causes rolling of leukocyte along the endothelial surface.
3. **Adhesion of leukocyte to endothelium:** Endothelium gets activated and leukocytes bind more firmly.

Across the vessel wall and the endothelium:

1. **Transmigration or diapedesis:** Leukocytes migrate through the vessel wall by squeezing through the intercellular junctions between the endothelial cells.
2. **Migration across the basement membrane:** Leukocytes penetrate the basement membrane of the vessel.

Outside the vessel wall:

1. **Chemotaxisis** defined as process of **migration of leukocytes toward the inflammatory stimulus** in

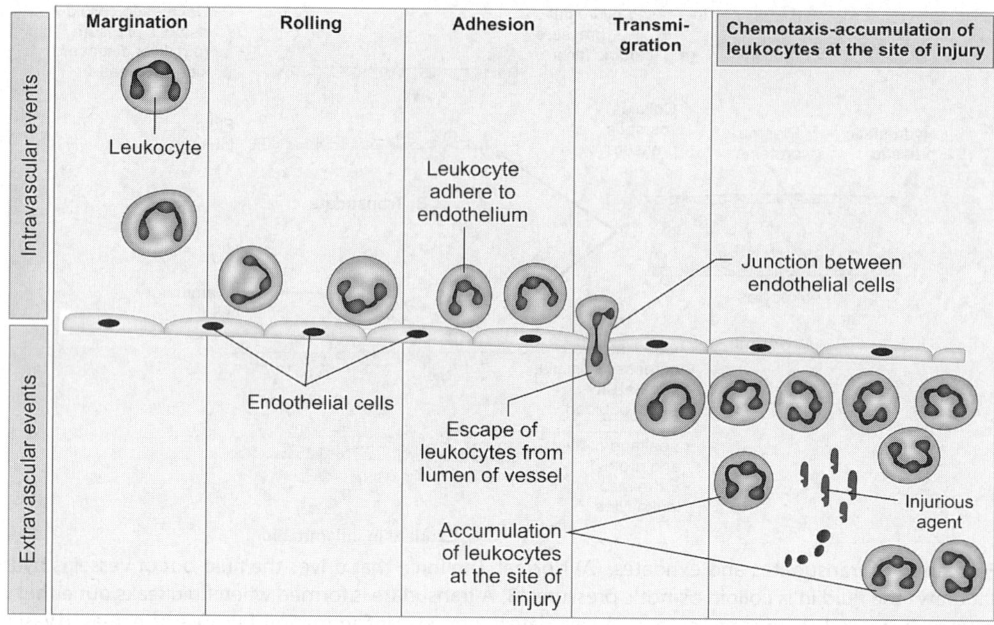

Fig. 3.3: Reaction of leukocyte in inflammation. The leukocytes first marginate, roll, then become activated and adhere to endothelium, then transmigrate across the endothelium, pierce the basement membrane, and migrate toward chemoattractants from the source of injury

the **direction of the gradient** of locally produced chemoattractants. **Chemoattractants** are chemical which attract leukocytes to site of injury and may be exogenous (e.g. bacterial products) or endogenous.

2. **Accumulation of leukocytes at the sites of infection and injury.**

Leukocyte Activation

Activation of leukocytes: Recognition of microbes or dead cells by the leukocyte initiates several responses in leukocytes together known as leukocyte activation. The most important feature of **leukocyte activation** is **phagocytosis and intracellular killing.**

Phagocytosis and clearance of the offending agent

Many leukocytes **recognize, internalize, and digest** foreign material, microorganisms, or cellular debris. This process is termed phagocytosis. It consists of three steps (Figs 3.4A to C):

1. **Recognition and attachment:** The phagocytic cells recognize components of microbes and necrotic cells.
2. **Engulfment:** Next step in phagocytosis is engulfment and formation of a phagocytic vacuole.
   - **Phagosome:** Extensions of the **cytoplasm of leukocyte form pseudopods surrounding the particle to be ingested** and forms a vesicle or vacuole called a phagosome.
   - **Phagolysosome:** The membrane of **phagosome fuses** with membrane of **lysosome to form a phagolysosome**. Lysosomal **granules present in the lysosomes of leukocytes are discharged** into this phagolysosome.
3. **Killing and degradation of the ingested material:** Occurs within neutrophils and macrophages. Most important microbicidal agents are:
   - **Reactive oxygen species:** Microbial killing is mainly performed by free radicals generated by reactive oxygen species (ROS). The ROS generated by **H_2O_2-MPO-halide system** is the most efficient bactericidal system of neutrophils. The enzyme myeloperoxidase (MPO) present in the neutrophils can convert weak ROS into a powerful ROS. Types of ROS are:
     - Superoxide anion ($O_2^{\bar{\cdot}}$, one electron)—**weak**
     - Hydrogen peroxide (H_2O_2 two electrons)—**weak**
     - Hydrogen peroxide ($^{\bullet}OH$), three electrons—**highly reactive.**

Reactive nitrogen species derived from nitric oxide (NO), and **Lysosomal enzymes.**

CHEMICAL MEDIATORS OF INFLAMMATION

Definition: Substances that initiate and regulate inflammatory reactions are called as **mediators of inflammation.**

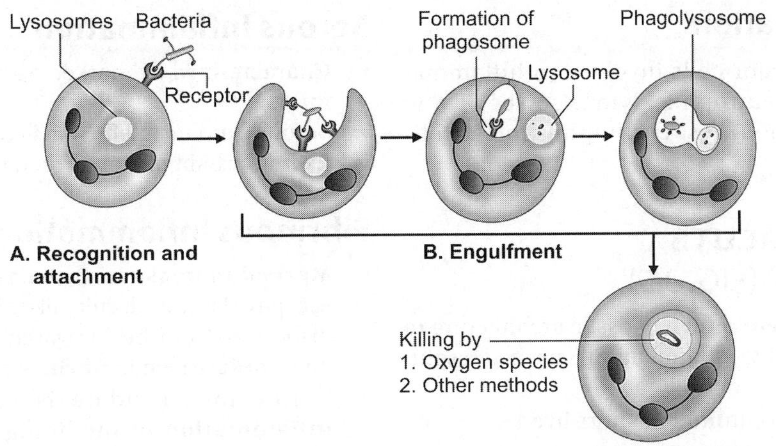

Figs 3.4A to C: Phagocytosis and intracellular killing/degradation of microbes/injurious agents. (A) **Phagocytosis** involves recognition and binding of the injurious agent to receptors on the leukocyte membrane; (B) Next step is **engulfment**, formation of a phagosome. The phagosome fuses with lysosomes to form phagolysosome; (C) **Killing/degradation**. During this the ingested particles within the phagolysosomes is destroyed by lysosomal enzymes and by reactive oxygen species

Numerous chemical mediators are responsible for inflammatory reactions.

General Features of Mediators

- **Source of mediators:** Mediators are derived either from cells or from plasma proteins.
- **Chemical mediators have hightly regulated actions.**
- **Short-lived:** Most of these mediators have a short-lifespan.

Main mediators involved in the inflammatory reaction are listed in Table 3.3.

Most important mediators involved in acute inflammation are summarized in Table 3.4.

Table 3.3: Main chemical mediators of acute inflammation

Cell-derived	Plasma protein-derived
• **Vasoactive amines** – Histamine – Serotonin	• **Complement components** – C3a – C5a – C3b – C5b-9 (MAC)
• **Arachidonic acid (AA) metabolites** – Prostaglandins – Leukotrienes	• **Kinins** – Bradykinin – Kallikrein
• **Platelet-activating factor (PAF)**	• **Coagulation/fibrinolytic system**
• **Reactive oxygen species (ROS)**	
• **Nitric oxide (NO)**	
• **Cytokines (TNF, IL-1) and chemokines**	

Abbreviations: IL-1, interleukin-1; TNF, tumor necrosis factor; MAC, membrane attack complex.

Table 3.4: Important mediators involved in acute inflammation

Action of the mediator	Name of the mediator	Source of the mediator
Vasodilation	Prostaglandins	Mast cells, all leukocytes
	Histamine	Mast cells, basophils, platelets
Increased vascular permeability	Histamine	Mast cells, basophils, platelets
	Serotonin	Platelets
	C3a and C5a (liberate vasoactive amines from mast cells, other cells)	Plasma (produced in liver)
	Bradykinin	
	Leukotrienes C_4, D_4, E_4	Mast cells, all leukocytes
Chemotaxis and leukocyte activation	Cytokines (TNF, IL-1, IL-6)	Macrophages, lymphocytes, endothelial cells, mast cells
	Chemokines	Leukocytes, activated macrophages
	C3a, C5a	Plasma (produced in the liver)
	Leukotriene B_4	Mast cells, leukocytes
	Bacterial products (e.g. *N*-formyl methyl peptides)	Bacteria
Fever	IL-1 TNF	Macrophages, endothelial cells, mast cells
	Prostaglandins	Mast cells, leukocytes
Pain	Prostaglandins	
	Bradykinin	Plasma protein

Abbreviations: IL-1, interleukin-1; IL-6, interleukin-6; TNF, tumor necrosis factor.

Cells of Inflammation

Leukocytes are the major cells involved in inflammation. These include neutrophils, lymphocytes (T and B), monocytes, macrophages, eosinophils, mast cells and basophils.

OUTCOMES OF ACUTE INFLAMMATION (FIG. 3.5)

- **Resolution: Complete return** of tissue architecture **to normal** following acute inflammation is termed resolution. It occurs:
  - When the injury is limited or short-lived.
  - With no or minimal tissue damage.
  - When injured tissue is capable of regeneration.
- **Organization/healing by fibrosis:** Process of **replacement of dead tissue by living tissue,** which matures to form scar tissue is known as **organization.**
- **Progression to chronic inflammation:** Chronic inflammation may follow acute inflammation, or it may be chronic from the beginning itself. Acute progress to chronic when the acute inflammatory response cannot be resolved. This may be due to:
  - Persistence of the injurious agent.
  - Abnormality in the process of healing.

  Examples:
  - **Bacterial infection of the lung** may begin as acute inflammation (pneumonia). But when it fails to resolve, it can cause extensive tissue destruction and form a cavity with chronic inflammation known as lung abscess.
  - Acute osteomyelitis if not treated properly **may progress to chronic osteomyelitis**.

MORPHOLOGICAL TYPES/PATTERNS OF ACUTE INFLAMMATION

Gross and microscopic appearances can often provide clues about the cause.

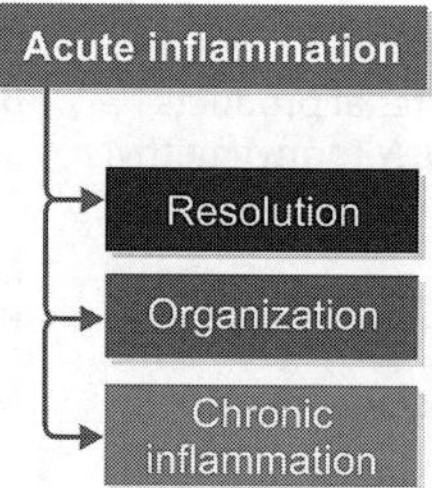

Fig. 3.5: Outcomes of acute inflammation: 1. Resolution, 2. Organization (healing by fibrosis and scarring), or 3. Chronic inflammation

Serous Inflammation

- Characterized by marked outpouring of a thin serous fluid.
- Serous exudate or effusion is yellow, straw-like in color.
- Example: Skin blister formed in burn or viral infection.

Fibrinous Inflammation

- **Marked increase in vascular permeability** leads to escape of large molecules like fibrinogen from the lumen of the vessel into the extravascular space and forms fibrin. The **exudate rich in fibrin** is called fibrinous exudate.
- A fibrinous exudate is mostly observed with **inflammation in** the lining of body cavities, such as the **meninges, pericardium and pleura**. When a fibrinous exudate develops on a serosal surface, such as the pleura or pericardium, it is known as fibrinous pleuritis or fibrinous pericarditis, respectively.
- For example fibrinous pericarditis (Fig. 12.10) is seen in rheumatic fever and classically known as "**bread and butter**" pericarditis.

Suppurative or Purulent Inflammation: Abscess

- It is characterized by the production of large amounts of pus or purulent exudate.
- For example acute appendicitis.
- **Abscess:** It is the **localized collections of purulent inflammatory exudates in a tissue**, an organ, or a confined space. Abscesses have a central necrotic focus (consisting of necrotic leukocytes and necrotic parenchymal cells) surrounded by a zone of preserved neutrophils. If pus accumulates in hollow organs or pleural cavity, it is known as empyema, e.g. Boil caused by *Staphylococcus aureus.*

Membranous Inflammation

In this type, epithelium is covered by membrane consisting of fibrin, desquamated epithelial cells and inflammatory cells, e.g. pharyngitis or laryngitis due to *Corynebacterium diphtheria.*

Fistula

It is an abnormal or surgically made tract/passage open at both ends, through which abnormal communication between two surfaces is established. The passage may be:

- Between a hollow or tubular organ and the body surface (e.g. fistula in ano) or
- Between two hollow or tubular organs (from one cavity to another).

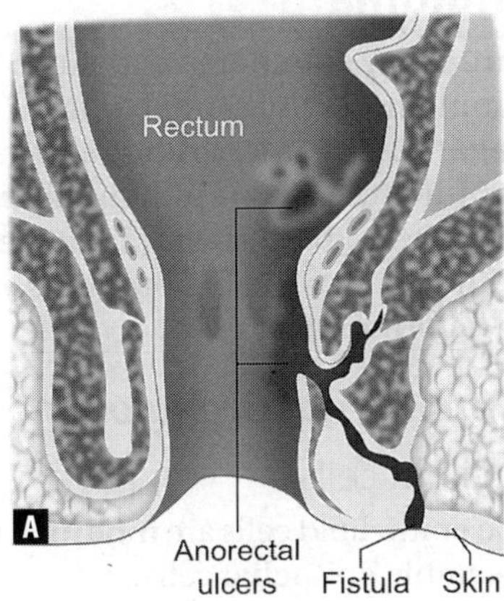

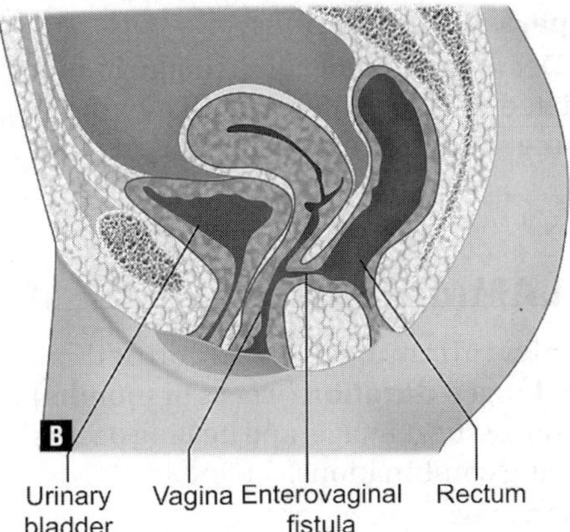

Figs 3.6A and B: (A) Fistula in ano; (B) Enterovaginal fistula

Types

1. **Congenital:** It may be due to developmental abnormality (e.g. tracheoesopahgeal fistula between trachea and esophagus).
2. **Acquired due to:** (1) Trauma/surgery (e.g. biliary fistula), (2) inflammation (e.g. fistula between intestines in Crohn disease) and (3) necrosis (e.g. fistula in ano charcterized by a fistula between rectum and anal skin (Fig. 3.6A), fistula between rectum and vagina (Fig. 3.6B), vesicovaginal fistula following radiotherapy induced necrosis for the treatment of carcinoma of cervix).

Sinus

- It is a tract/passage leading from a chronically inflamed cavity to surface. It most of the cases, it is due to the presence of foreign body or necrotic material.
- **Example:** Sinuses associated with chronic osteomyelitis (inflammation of bone) in which necrosis of bone is followed by sinuses. These sinuses connect the skin to the necrotic area of bone (Fig. 3.7).

Cellulitis

It develops when the inflammation spreads in the connective tissue planes.

Ulcer

An ulcer is defined as a local defect, or excavation of the surface of an organ or tissue. Common sites:

1. Mucosa of the mouth, stomach (e.g. peptic ulcer of the stomach or duodenum) intestines, or genitourinary tract.
2. Skin and subcutaneous tissue of the lower extremities (e.g. varicose ulcers).

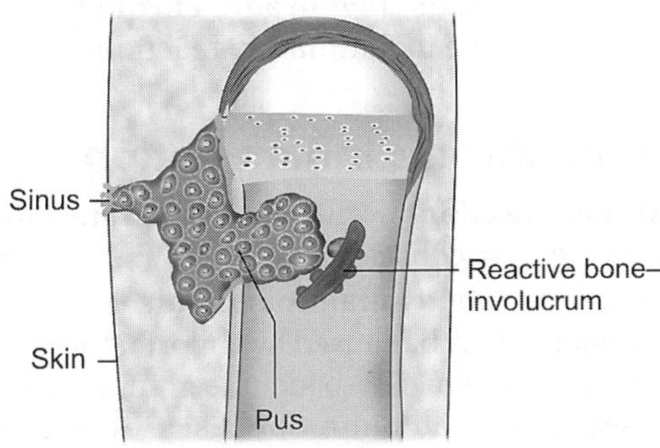

Fig. 3.7: Chronic osteomyelitis with sinus

SYSTEMIC EFFECTS OF INFLAMMATION

Systemic changes in acute inflammation are collectively known as **acute-phase response, or the systemic inflammatory response syndrome (SIRS)**.

The clinical and pathologic changes of acute-phase response are:

1. **Fever.**
2. **Raised plasma levels of acute-phase proteins:** These are plasma proteins synthesized in the liver and may be markedly raised in response to inflammatory stimuli. These include: **(1) C-reactive protein (CRP), (2) fibrinogen, (3) serum amyloid A (SAA) protein.**
3. **Changes in the leukocytes:**
   - **Leukocytosis:** Total leukocyte count more than 11,000 cells/μL are termed as leukocytosis. Common in inflammatory reactions, especially those caused by bacterial infections.
   - **Lymphocytosis:** It is seen in **viral infections** (e.g. infectious mononucleosis, mumps, and German measles).

- **Eosinophilia:** It is seen in **bronchial asthma, allergy, and parasitic infestations**.
- **Leukopenia:** Decreased number of circulating white cells is associated with few infections like **typhoid fever and some viruses, rickettsia, and certain protozoa**.

CHRONIC INFLAMMATION

Definition: Chronic inflammation is defined as **inflammation of prolonged duration** (weeks or months) in which inflammation, tissue damage, and healing occurs at same time, in varying combinations.

Chronic inflammation may:

- **Follow an acute inflammation,** which does not resolve (e.g. chronic osteomyelitis) or
- **Begin as insidious, low-grade, chronic**, response without any acute inflammatory reaction.

Causes of Chronic Inflammation

- **Persistent infections** by microbes which are difficult to eradicate, e.g. mycobacteria.
- **Immune-mediated inflammatory diseases:** Chronic inflammation may be caused by abnormal activation of the immune system. These include immune-mediated diseases such as autoimmune diseases and allergic reactions.
- **Prolonged exposure to potentially toxic agents:** When a toxic agent (either exogenous or endogenous) cannot be degraded, it may result in chronic inflammation. For example, silicosis caused by inhalation of silica particles which cannot be degraded.

Morphologic Features

Chronic inflammation is characterized by:

- **Mononuclear cells infiltrate:** Macrophages, lymphocytes, and plasma cells.
- **Tissue destruction:** Due to the persistence of causative agent or by the inflammatory cells.
- **Healing by fibrosis.**

GRANULOMATOUS INFLAMMATION

Granulomatous inflammation is a **distinctive pattern of chronic inflammation**. It is produced by limited number of infectious as well as noninfectious conditions and involves immune reactions. The **microscopic feature is the presence of granuloma**.

Granuloma

Definition: A granuloma is defined as a distinctive type of chronic inflammation characterized by **microscopic aggregation of macrophages** that are transformed into epithelium-like (epithelioid) cells, surrounded by lymphocytes and occasional plasma cells. Older granulomas in addition shows rim of fibroblasts and connective tissue as the outermost layer.

Components of Granuloma

Epithelioid cells

- The epithelioid cells are **modified macrophages** which resemble epithelial cells.
- They have a pale pink granular cytoplasm with indistinct cell borders, often appearing to merge into one another.
- The nucleus is oval or elongate, and may show folding of the nuclear membrane. The nucleus is less dense than that of a lymphocyte.

Giant cells

Epithelioid cells frequently fuse to form giant cells and are found in the periphery or sometimes in the center of granulomas. Nuclei may be as many as 20 or more (in number) which may be arranged either peripherally (**Langhans-type giant cell**) or haphazardly (**foreign body-type giant cell**).

Types of Granuloma

Granulomas are divided into two types according to pathogenesis.

Foreign body granulomas

It is caused by inert foreign bodies. For examples, foreign body granulomas form around material such as sutures and talc.

Immune granulomas

They are caused by poorly degradable or particulate agents which can induce cell-mediated immune response. For example, the most common immune granuloma is seen in infection with *Mycobacterium tuberculosis*.

REPAIR AND HEALING

Injury to cells and tissues **results in loss of cells and tissues.** It sets in inflammation (restrict the tissue damage) and initiate replacement of lost tissue by living tissue.

Definition: Healing is a process of replacement of dead tissue by living tissue.

It can be broadly divided into regeneration and repair.

- **Regeneration:** It is defined as a process in which lost/damaged tissue is completely replaced by tissue of similar type. Regeneration occurs in tissues consisting of cells with regenerative activity. These include hematopoietic cells, epithelium of the skin and gastrointestinal (GI) tract.
- **Repair:** It is defined as a process in which lost/damaged tissue is replaced by fibrous tissue or scar, e.g. healed myocardial infarction (coagulative necrosis of heart muscle). The term healing and repair is commonly used synonymously (equivalent in meaning).

Factors Deciding the Pattern of Healing

Mostly healing occurs by a combination of both regeneration and repair. The proportion of regeneration and repair in healing process depends on the **regenerative capacity of the lost/damaged tissue.** According to regenerative capacity of the cells, the tissues of the body can be divided into three groups.

- **Continuously dividing (labile) tissues:** They proliferate (divide) throughout life. For examples, **stratified squamous epithelium** of the skin, oral cavity, vagina and cervix; **columnar epithelium** of the GI tract and uterus.
- **Quiescent (stable) tissues:** They normally do not proliferate. However, they can rapidly **proliferate in response to stimuli** or demand. For example, **parenchymal cells** (of liver).
- **Nondividing (permanent) tissues:** These consist of cells which **cannot divide after birth**, e.g. **neurons, skeletal muscle** cells and **cardiac muscle** cells.

Granulation Tissue (Fig. 3.8)

- During the first 24–72 hours of the healing process, the proliferation of fibroblasts and vascular endothelial cells begins. It forms a specialized type of tissue known as **granulation tissue**, which is characteristic of tissue repair.
- The term granulation tissue is derived from its **pink, soft, granular** gross appearance on the surface of healing wounds. **Microscopically**, it consists of **new small blood vessels** (angiogenesis) and **proliferation of fibroblasts**. The new blood vessels are **leaky**, and are responsible for edema seen in granulation tissue.
- Granulation tissue progressively grows into the **incision space/wound.** The **amount of granulation tissue** is more prominent in healing by secondary union. The amount of granulation tissue **depends on the size of the tissue deficit** created by the wound and **intensity (severity) of inflammation.**
- The granulation tissue **fills the wound area** by about 5–7 days.

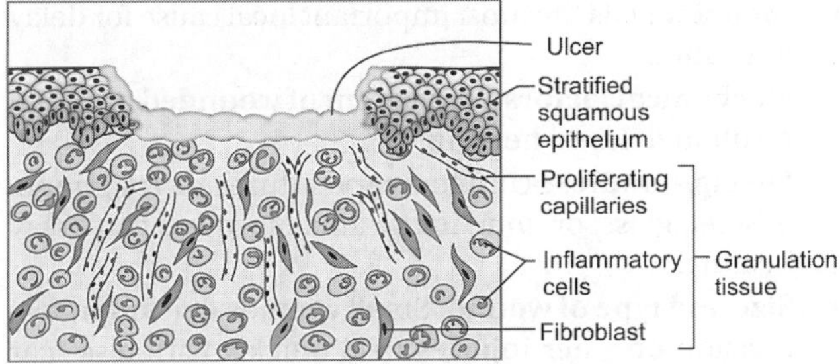

Fig. 3.8: Microscopic appearance of granulation tissue which consists of proliferating capillaries, fibroblasts and inflammatory cells

CUTANEOUS WOUND HEALING

Healing by Primary Union or by First Intention (Fig. 3.9)

Healing of a clean, uninfected surgical incision in the skin approximated by surgical sutures is known as healing by primary union or by first intention. Surgical incision causes **death of a minimum number** of epithelial and connective tissue **cells.** The **disruption (separation or division) of epithelial basement membrane** continuity is also **minimal**. Re-epithelialization occurs with a **relatively thin scar**. This is simplest type of cutaneous wound healing. Various **stages in the healing by first intention are:**

- **First 24 hours:** Blood clots in the space between sutured margins. **Neutrophils** appears at the margins of incision. Epithelial cells at the edges undergo proliferation and migration across the wound.
- **Day 2: Macrophages** begin to appear. Surface epithelial continuity is re-established in the form of a thin surface layer.
- **Day 3–7: Granulation tissue** begins to invade tissue spaces. Surface epithelial achieves (attains) normal thickness. Collagen is progressively laid down. Acute inflammatory response begins to subside.
- **Day 10–14:** Wound normally gains about 10% strength of normal skin. Further fibroblast proliferation occurs with **collagen deposition.**
- **Weeks to months:** Collagen deposition along the line of stress and wound gradually achieves **maximal 80% of tensile strength** of normal skin.

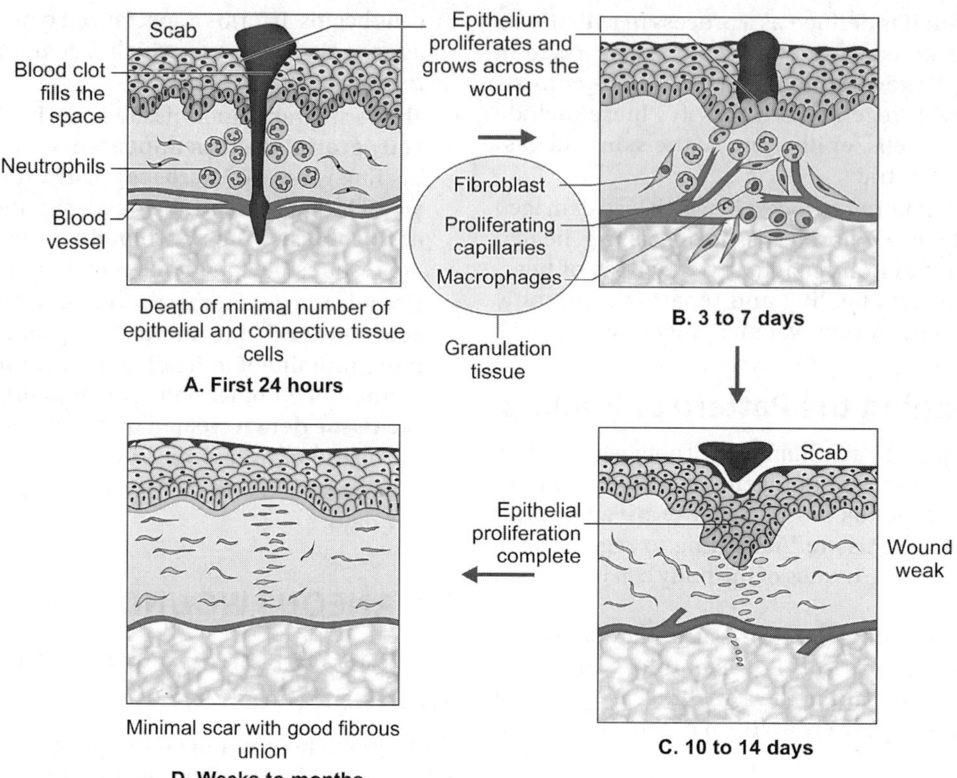

Figs 3.9A to D: Healing by primary intention. (A) A wound with closely apposed edges and minimal tissue loss. The blood clot fills the gap between the edges of the wound; (B) Epithelium at the edges proliferates. Minimal amount of granulation tissue is formed; (C) The epithelial proliferation is complete and the wound is weak; (D) Fibrosis results in a small scar

Healing by Secondary Union or by Second Intention (Fig. 3.10)

When injury produces **large defects** on the skin surface with **extensive loss of cells** and tissue, the healing process is known as healing by secondary union or by second intention. Healing in such cutaneous wound is more complicated. Basic mechanisms of healing by primary (first intention) and secondary (second intention) union are same. The features of **healing by secondary intention** are:

- The **inflammatory reaction is severe**.
- There is formation of **abundant granulation tissue**.
- It also shows **extensive deposition of collagen**, with substantial scar formation, which may contract.
- Presence of **wound contraction**.

Wound Contraction

Wound contraction generally occurs in large surface wounds and is an important feature in healing by secondary union.

Advantages of the wound contraction

It decreases the gap between dermal edges of the wound and **reduces the wound surface area. Myofibroblasts** of granulation tissue have ultrastructural features of smooth muscle cells. They contract in the wound tissue and are responsible for wound contraction.

FACTORS THAT INFLUENCE WOUND HEALING

Local Factors

- **Infection:** It is the most important local cause for delay in healing.
- **Mechanical factors: Movement of wounded area** can result in delayed healing.
- **Foreign bodies:** Unnecessary sutures or fragments of steel, glass, or bone in the area of wound can delay healing.
- **Size and type of wound:** Small wounds due to surgical incision or other injuries heal quickly with less scar formation than large wounds.
- **Location:** Wound healing is delayed at sites in which **skin covers bone with little intervening tissue** where skin cannot contract (e.g. skin over the anterior tibia).

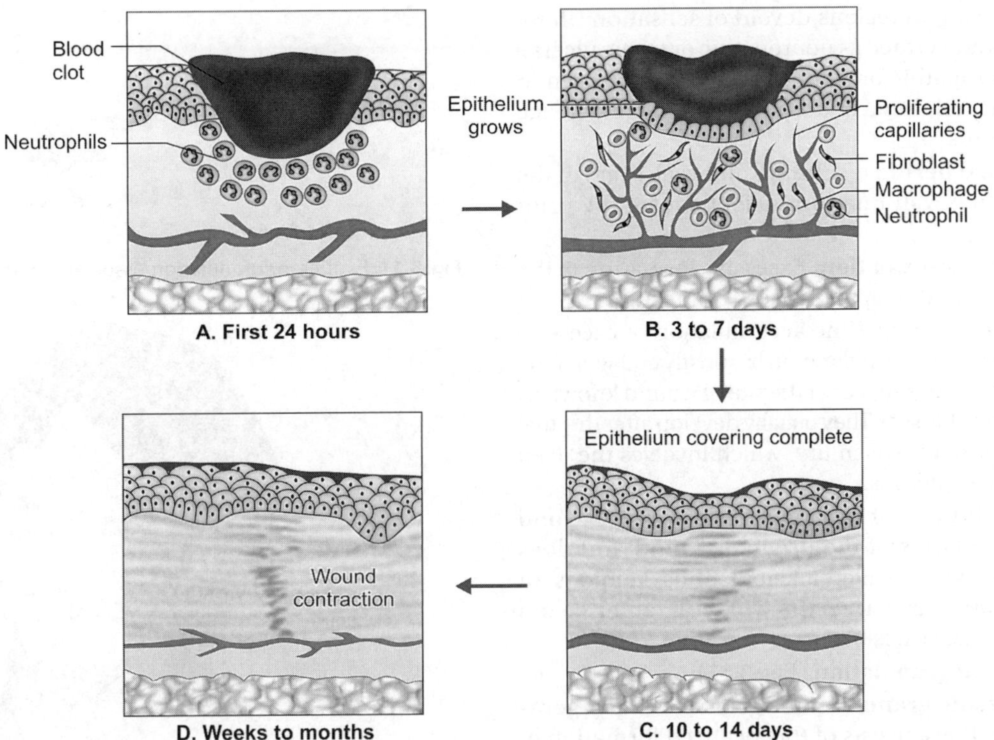

Figs 3.10A to D: Healing by secondary intention. (A) There is significant loss of tissue and the edges are far apart. Acute inflammation develops both at the edges and base; (B) The cell proliferation starts from the edges and large amount of granulation tissue is formed; (C) The wound is covered on the entire surface by the epithelium. The collagen fibers are deposited; (D) Granulation tissue is replaced by a large scar. There is significant wound contraction

- **Blood supply:** Wounds in areas with **good blood supply**, such as the face, **heal faster** than those with **poor blood supply**, such as the foot. For example, **varicose veins** of the legs decrease the venous drainage and can cause nonhealing of ulcers.
- **Ionizing radiation:** Exposure of wound to ionizing radiation **decreases healing** process.
- **Complications of wound healing** (refer pages 29-30): They may delay wound healing.

Systemic Factors

- **Nutrition: Protein deficiency, vitamin C deficiency**, inhibits collagen synthesis and diminishes healing process.
- **Age:** Wound healing is rapid in young compared to in aged individuals.
- **Metabolic status: Diabetes mellitus** is associated with delayed healing.
- **Circulatory status: Inadequate blood supply** (e.g. arteriosclerosis) or **venous abnormalities** (e.g. varicose veins) that retard venous drainage delay healing.
- **Hormones:** Steroids inhibit collagen synthesis, thereby impair wound healing.
- **Hematological abnormalities:** Defects in neutrophils and bleeding disorders may slow the healing process.

COMPLICATIONS OF WOUND HEALING

- **Inadequate granulation tissue formation:** Inadequate formation of granulation tissue or a deficient scar formation can cause wound dehiscence, ulceration and incisional hernia.
  - **Dehiscence** (the wound splitting open) or rupture of a wound is most common life-threatening complication after abdominal surgery. It is due to increased abdominal pressure/mechanical stress on the abdominal wound from vomiting, coughing, or ileus.
  - **Ulceration:** Wounds can ulcerate due to inadequate new blood vessel formation (angiogenesis) during healing. For example, wounds in the leg of patients with atherosclerotic peripheral vascular disease or varicose veins usually ulcerate. Nonhealing wounds

also develop in regions devoid of sensation (these wounds are termed as neuropathic or tropic ulcers). The neuropathic or trophic ulcers may be seen in diabetic peripheral neuropathy and nerve damage from leprosy.
  - **Incisional hernia** resulting from weak scars of the abdominal wall due to a defect caused by prior surgery.
- **Excessive scar formation:** Excessive formation of the components of the repair process can result in:
  - **Hypertrophic scar:** The accumulation of excessive amounts of extracellular matrix, mostly collagen may give rise to a raised scar at the site of wound known as a hypertrophic scar. They usually develop after thermal (burn) or traumatic injury, which involves the deep layers of the dermis.
  - **Keloid:** If the scar tissue grows/progress beyond the boundaries of the original wound and does not regress, it is called a keloid. Thus, keloid is an exuberant scar that recurs with still larger keloid after surgical excision.
  - **Exuberant granulation** (Fig. 3.11):
    - **Pyogenic granuloma or granuloma pyogenicum:** This consists of the localized formation of excessive amounts of granulation tissue. Such exuberant granulation tissue projects above the level of the surrounding skin and prevents re-epithelialization. This mass formed is often named as **proud flesh**.
    - **Desmoids or aggressive fibromatoses:** Incisional scars or traumatic injuries may be followed by excessive proliferation of fibroblasts and other connective tissue elements. They are known as desmoids, or aggressive fibromatoses, which may recur after excision.
- **Excessive contraction:** A decrease in the size of a wound is known as contraction. **An exaggeration of** this **contraction is termed contracture** and results in deformities of the wound and the surrounding tissues. This will compromise/reduce movements (e.g. contractures that follow severe burns can compromise the movement of the involved region (Fig. 3.12) and joint movements) or obstruction (e.g. in GI tract contracture/stricture can cause intestinal obstruction).
- **Others:**
  - Infection of wound by microbes.
  - Epidermal cysts can develop due to persistence of epithelial cells at the site of wound healing.
  - Pigmentation may develop due to either colored particle left in the wound or due to hemosiderin pigment.

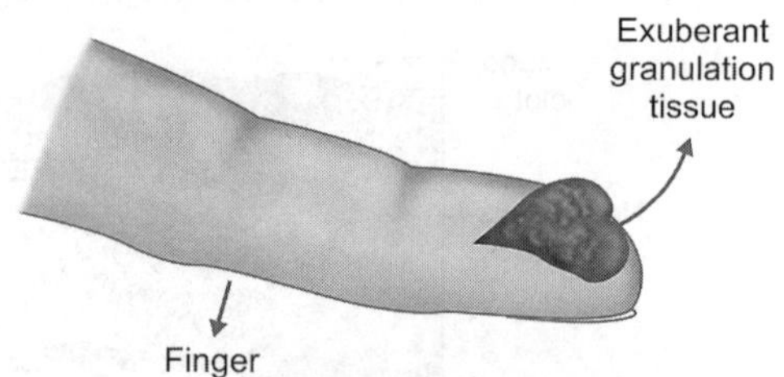

Fig. 3.11: Exuberant granulation tissue at the tip of the finger

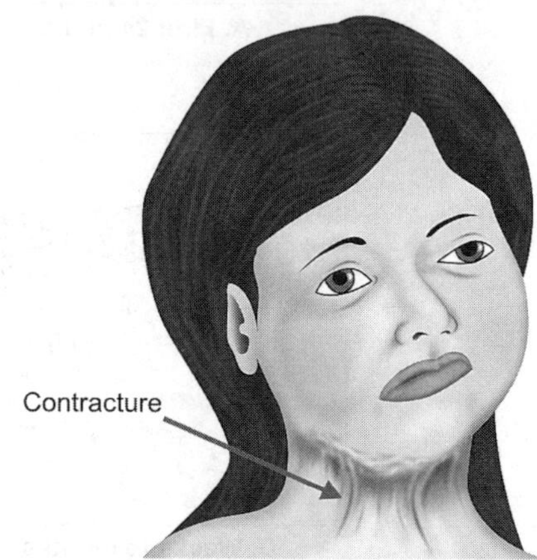

Fig. 3.12: Wound contracture—severe contracture of a wound on the right side of neck, following burns

  - Neoplasia: For example, squamous cell carcinoma may develop in Marjolin's ulcer, which is the scar that follows burns in skin.

HEALING OF A FRACTURE

Phases of Fracture Healing (Figs 3.13A to E)

Bone can repair by reactivating processes that normally takes place during embryogenesis. There are three major phases of fracture healing.

Inflammatory Phase

- **Fracture and hemorrhage:** Soon **after fracture, blood vessels** (in the periosteum, cortex and medullary cavity) **rupture** leads to extensive hemorrhage (hematoma), at the fracture site and surrounding tissue.
- **Inflammatory cells:**
  - **Fibrin mesh work** in the clotted blood **helps**.
    - To seal the fracture site.
    - Influx of inflammatory cells (neutrophils and macrophages) to the area.

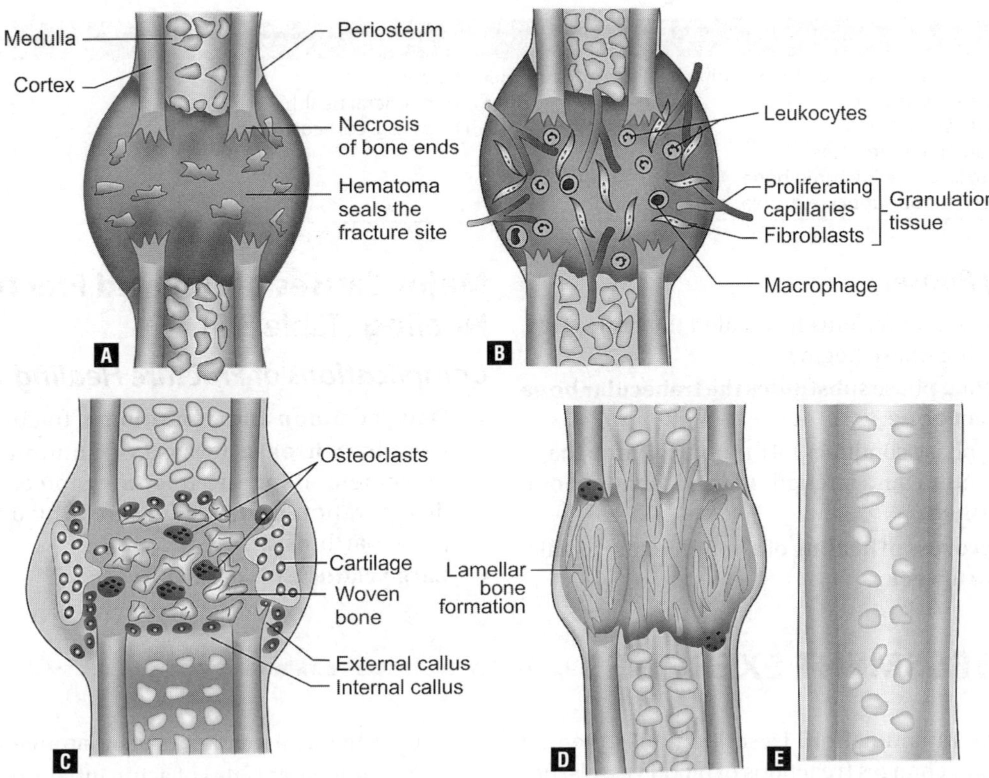

Figs 3.13A to E: Healing of a fracture. (A) Immediately after a fracture, blood clot/hematoma forms at the site of fracture; (B) During the inflammatory phase of fracture healing, the inflammatory cells (neutrophils and macrophages) migrate to the area of fracture and neovascularization develops; (C) The reparative phase of fracture healing is characterized by the formation of a callus near the fracture site; (D) In the remodeling phase, the reactive bone (lamellar or woven) develops; (E) Healing is complete and bone attains its original contour

- ◆ Ingrowth of fibroblasts and new capillary vessels (neovascularization) to the site, producing granulation tissue between the fracture fragments.
- **Formation of granulation tissue:** It consists of proliferating capillaries and fibroblasts and are formed at the site of fractures.
- **Soft-tissue callus or procallus formation:**
  - **Osteoblasts migrate into the granulation tissue** and **differentiate into osteoid synthesizing units.** They **deposit** large quantities of **osteoid collagen in a haphazard pattern** producing **woven bone** (unmineralized bone is called osteoid).
  - **Granulation tissue containing** (mineralized or unmineralized) **bone or cartilage** is termed a **callus.**
  - At this stage, **callus** is predominantly **uncalcified** and is called **soft-tissue callus or procallus,** which **provides a type of temporary connection between the ends of the fractured bones.** However, procallus does not have any structural rigidity for any weight-bearing. The callus depending on its site and appearance can be divided into external and internal callus.
  - The **repair tissue** attains **maximal thickness at the end of the second or third week** and consists of hyaline cartilage and woven bone.

Reparative Phase

- **Lamellar bone formation:** As the healing advances, the hyaline cartilage and woven bone of the original fracture **callus are replaced by lamellar bone.** This is stronger and consists of **parallel collagen fibers**.
- **Endochondral ossification:** It is the replacement process in which the hyaline cartilage is replaced by woven bone.
- **Bony callus:** At this stage, the **callus is mineralized** (calcified) and is known as **bony (osseous) callus.** As the mineralization proceeds, the stiffness and strength of the callus increases. By the second or third week, controlled weight-bearing can be tolerated.

Table 3.5: Major causes of delayed fracture healing

Local factors	General factors
• Excessive movement of fractured bone during healing process • Infection of the fractured site • Severe local soft tissue injury • Wide separation of fracture ends • Extensive necrosis of the fractured bone • Poor or impaired blood supply (e.g. tibia, head of femur)	• Old age • Poor general health • Drugs, e.g. corticosteroids

Remodeling Phase

- Several weeks after a callus has sealed the bone ends, the remodeling phase begins.
- The remodeling phase **substitutes the trabecular bone with compact bone**.
- Remodeling phase continues till the original bone shape (contour), outline and strength of the fractured bone is re-established.

The **whole process of healing** of a bone fracture usually takes **about 6 to 8 weeks**.

Major Causes of Delayed Fracture Healing (Table 3.5)

Complications of Fracture Healing

- **Delayed union and nonunion** of fracture.
- **Pseudoarthrosis:** In case of nonunion, too much movement along the fracture gap can cause cystic degeneration in the callus, creating a false joint or pseudoarthrosis.
- **Large callus with deformity**.

SELF-ASSESSMENT EXERCISES

I. Essay

1. Define inflammation. Describe the sequential vascular changes (reactions of blood vessels/hemodynamic changes) of acute inflammation.
2. Describe the leukocyte/cellular events in acute inflammation.
3. Describe the healing of a clean surgical wound/healing by first intention.
4. Describe the process of wound healing. List the factors that affect wound healing.
5. Describe the mode of healing of wound by second intention.
6. Describe the healing of fractures in long bones.

II. Short Notes

1. Cardinal signs of inflammation.
2. Causes of acute inflammation.
3. Differences between transudate and exudate.
4. Chemotaxis.
5. Phagocytosis.
6. Chemical mediators of inflammation.
7. Outcomes (fate) of acute inflammation.
8. Morphological types/patterns of acute inflammatory reaction.
9. Systemic effects of inflammation.
10. Differences between acute and chronic inflammation.
11. Causes of chronic inflammation.
12. Cells of chronic inflammation.
13. Chronic granulomatous inflammation.
14. Define and classify granuloma.
15. Granulation tissue.
16. Factors that influence wound healing.
17. Complications of wound healing.
18. Fracture healing.
19. Sinus.
20. Fistula.

CHAPTER

4

Infectious Diseases

CHAPTER OUTLINE

- Mycobacterial Diseases
- Tuberculosis
- Leprosy
- Syphilis
- Bacterial Diseases
- Viral Diseases
- Rickettsial Infections
- Chlamydial Infections
- Fungal Infections and Opportunistic Infections
- Parasitic Diseases

MYCOBACTERIAL DISEASES

Mycobacterium is bacteria, which appear as slender aerobic rods that grow in straight or branching chains. Mycobacteria have a waxy cell wall composed of mycolic acid, which is responsible for their **acid-fast nature**. Mycobacteria are weakly Gram-positive.

TUBERCULOSIS

Tuberculosis, also called as Koch's disease, is a chronic granulomatous disease caused by *Mycobacterium tuberculosis*.

Etiology

Characteristics of Mycobacteria

The most common and important mycobacteria causing human disease is *M. tuberculosis*. It is a thin **rod-shaped aerobic bacterium** which is **not stained by Gram's** staining. However, they are seen as pink bacteria when stained by Ziehl–Neelsen stain. Once stained, the bacilli cannot be decolorized by acid alcohol and retain stains (carbol fuschin of Ziehl–Neelsen stain). Due to this characteristic mycobacteria are classified as **acid-fast** (and **alcohol-fast**) bacilli (AFB). Acid fastness is mainly due to the high content of mycolic acids in the waxy (lipid) cell wall of the mycobacteria.

Predisposing Factors

Tuberculosis is common in India.

- Incidence of tuberculosis is high wherever there is poverty, overcrowding, and chronic debilitating illness.
- Some of the diseases are associated with increased risk. These include diabetes mellitus, Hodgkin lymphoma, malnutrition, immunosuppression, alcoholism, chronic lung disease (e.g. silicosis), and chronic renal failure.
  - HIV is the most important risk factor.

Mode of Infection

The various modes of transmission of tuberculosis are:

- **Inhalation:** Airborne spread is the most common mode of transmission. The most common source of infection is patients suffering from active open pulmonary tuberculosis. Patients whose sputum contains AFB visible by microscopy are known as **open case of tuberculosis**. The bacilli are released during coughing, sneezing, or speaking by these patients.
- **Ingestion:** Tuberculosis may be transmitted by drinking nonpasteurized milk from cows infected with *M. bovis*.
- **Inoculation:** This is extremely rare mode of transmission and may develop during handling of postmortem material with tuberculosis.

Primary Tuberculosis

- **Initial** (first) **infection with tubercle bacilli** (*Mycobacterium tuberculosis*) in an unsensitized (previously unexposed) individual is known as primary tuberculosis.
- Source of the organism is always exogenous.

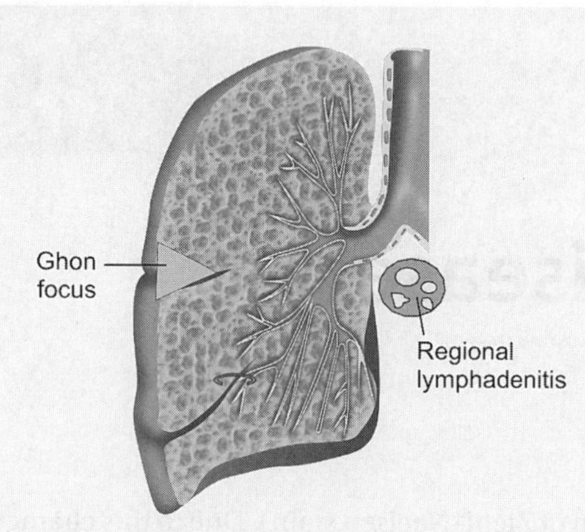

Fig. 4.1: Primary tuberculosis of lung with Ghon focus in the subpleural region of upper lobe. Ghon complex consists of combination of Ghon focus and regional lymphadenitis

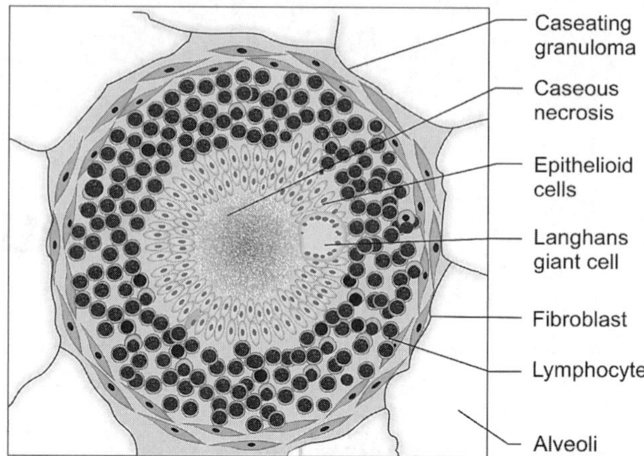

Fig. 4.2: Microscopic appearance of tuberculous lung diagrammatic. Central area of caseation surrounded by epithelioid and multinucleated giant cells

Morphology

Sites of primary tuberculosis: Lung, intestine, tonsils, skin (very rare).

Lung

It is the **commonest site** of primary tuberculosis. Usually involved are the **lower part of the upper lobe or the upper part of the lower lobe**. This is because most of the inspired air is distributed to the middle and lower lung zones. The primary lesion is usually seen at the periphery of the lung near the pleural surface. About 2–4 weeks after the infection, a circumscribed **gray-white** area of about 1–1.5 cm develops in the **subpleural parenchymal region of the lung.** This lung lesion is known as the **Ghon focus.** The center of Ghon focus may undergoes caseous necrosis. Tubercle bacilli are carried along the lymphatics to the regional draining nodes.

- **Ghon complex:** The combination of subpleural parenchymal primary lesion in the lung (**Ghon focus**) and **regional lymph nodal involvement** is known as the **Ghon complex** (Fig. 4.1). The primary focus along with regional lymphadenitis in other organs is called primary complex.
- **Fate of Ghon complex:** In **most (90%)** of the individuals, primary tuberculosis **heals by fibrosis and calcification.** In others (less than 10% of infected adults) it may develop into progressive primary tuberculosis or may progress and spread by lymphatics and blood to other organs or parts of the body.

Other sites of primary complex

- **Intestine:** Primary focus in the small intestine (usually ileal region) along with mesenteric lymphadenitis.
- **Tonsils:** Primary focus in the pharynx and tonsil with cervical lymphnode enlargement.
- **Skin:** Primary focus in the skin along with regional lymphnode involvement.

Microscopy

Granuloma in tuberculosis is called as tubercle (Fig. 4.2). Granuloma with caseous necrosis is called soft tubercle and granuloma without caseation is called hard tubercle. The typical caseating granuloma consists of:

- Central area of **caseous necrosis**. The necrotic material resembles soft cheese and hence is known as caseous necrosis.
- It is surrounded by **epithelioid cells** (modified macrophages), some of which may fuse to form multinucleate giant cells. The **giant cells** may be **Langhans type** (nuclei arranged in horse-shoe pattern) or foreign body type (nuclei in the center).
- The epithelioid cells are surrounded by a **rim of lymphocytes.**
- These granulomas are usually enclosed by fibroblasts.

Secondary Tuberculosis (Synonym: Post primary Tuberculosis, Reactivation Tuberculosis)

Clinical illness developing in a **previously sensitized individual** due to reactivation of initial infection or fresh infection is called as **secondary (or post primary) tuberculosis.**

Source of infection: Most common source is reactivation of a latent infection. Rarely, it may be exogenous reinfection.

Any organ may be involved in secondary tuberculosis, but the lungs are by far the most common site.

Morphology

Gross (Fig. 4.3)**:** In the lungs, secondary tuberculosis usually involves the **apex of the upper lobes** of one or both lungs. These areas have higher mean oxygen tension (compared to that in the lower zones) which favors mycobacterial growth.

The lesions are seen **within 1–2 cm of the apical pleura. The lesions may undergo cavitations** (Fig. 4.3). The erosion of the cavities into an airway is an important source of infection because the infected person expels bacilli during coughing. The **regional lymph nodes are less prominently involved** in secondary tuberculosis than in primary tuberculosis.

Microscopy

The active lesions show characteristic tubercles with central caseous necrosis known as caseating granulomas (Fig. 4.2). Acid-fast stains may show tubercle bacilli.

Fate of Secondary Tuberculosis

Healing: It may heal with fibrosis and calcification, rarely ossification.

Progress: The disease may progress along several different pathways (Refer spread of tuberculosis below).

Spread of Tuberculosis (Fig. 4.4)

If the treatment is inadequate or if host defenses are impaired, the infection may spread via airways, lymphatics and blood vessels.

- **Pleural spread:** It results in serous pleural effusion or tuberculous empyema.
- **Spread along mucosal lining:** Spread from expectorated infectious material may lead to **endobronchial**, **endotracheal** and **laryngeal tuberculosis**.
- **Miliary tuberculosis:** It is the disseminated form of tuberculosis and the **lesions resemble millet seeds**, hence named "miliary". It may occur when the organisms gain entry into systemic circulation. The most commonly involved organs are liver, bone marrow, spleen, adrenals, meninges, kidneys, fallopian tubes and epididymis.
- **Isolated tuberculosis:** Commonly involved organs are: Meninges (tuberculous meningitis), kidneys (renal tuberculosis), adrenals, fallopian tubes (salpingitis) and bones (osteomyelitis): When tuberculosis involves the vertebrae, the disease is referred to as **Pott disease**.
- **Lymphadenitis:** It is the most frequent presentation of extrapulmonary tuberculosis, and usually occurs in the cervical region ("scrofula").
- **Intestinal tuberculosis.**

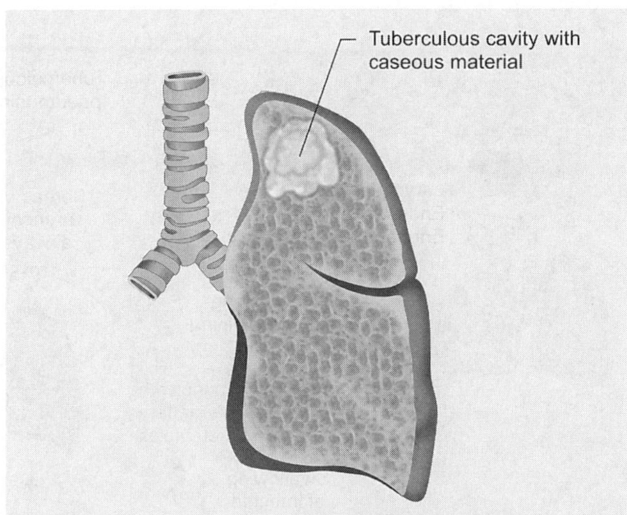

Fig. 4.3: Secondary tuberculosis of lung with cavitation in the upper lobe. Diagrammatic representation

Clinical Features

- Localized secondary tuberculosis may remain asymptomatic; later manifestations may appear insidiously.
- **Systemic symptoms:**
  - **Nonspecific symptoms include:** Malaise, anorexia, weight loss and fever.
  - Low-grade fever which is remittent (appearing late each afternoon and then subsiding-commonly known as **evening rise of temperature**) and night sweats.
  - **Cough with sputum** which is first mucoid and later purulent.
  - Hemoptysis is present in 50% of cases of pulmonary tuberculosis.

Diagnosis of Pulmonary Tuberculosis

- Based on the history, physical and radiographic findings of consolidation or cavitation in the apices of the lungs.
- **Sputum for AFB:** Identification of acid-fast tubercle bacilli in the sputum.
- **Tuberculin (Mantoux) skin test:** Intradermal injection of purified protein derivative (PPD) of *M. tuberculosis* produces a visible and palpable induration of 10 mm diameter or more at the site of injection of PPD. The induration peaks in 48–72 hours. A positive tuberculin test signifies T cell-mediated immunity to mycobacterial antigens. Thus, positive Mantoux test indicates that the patient is exposed to mycobacterial antigen.
- **Cultures of the sputum:** Conventional cultures require up to 10 weeks.
- **PCR amplification of** *M. tuberculosis.*

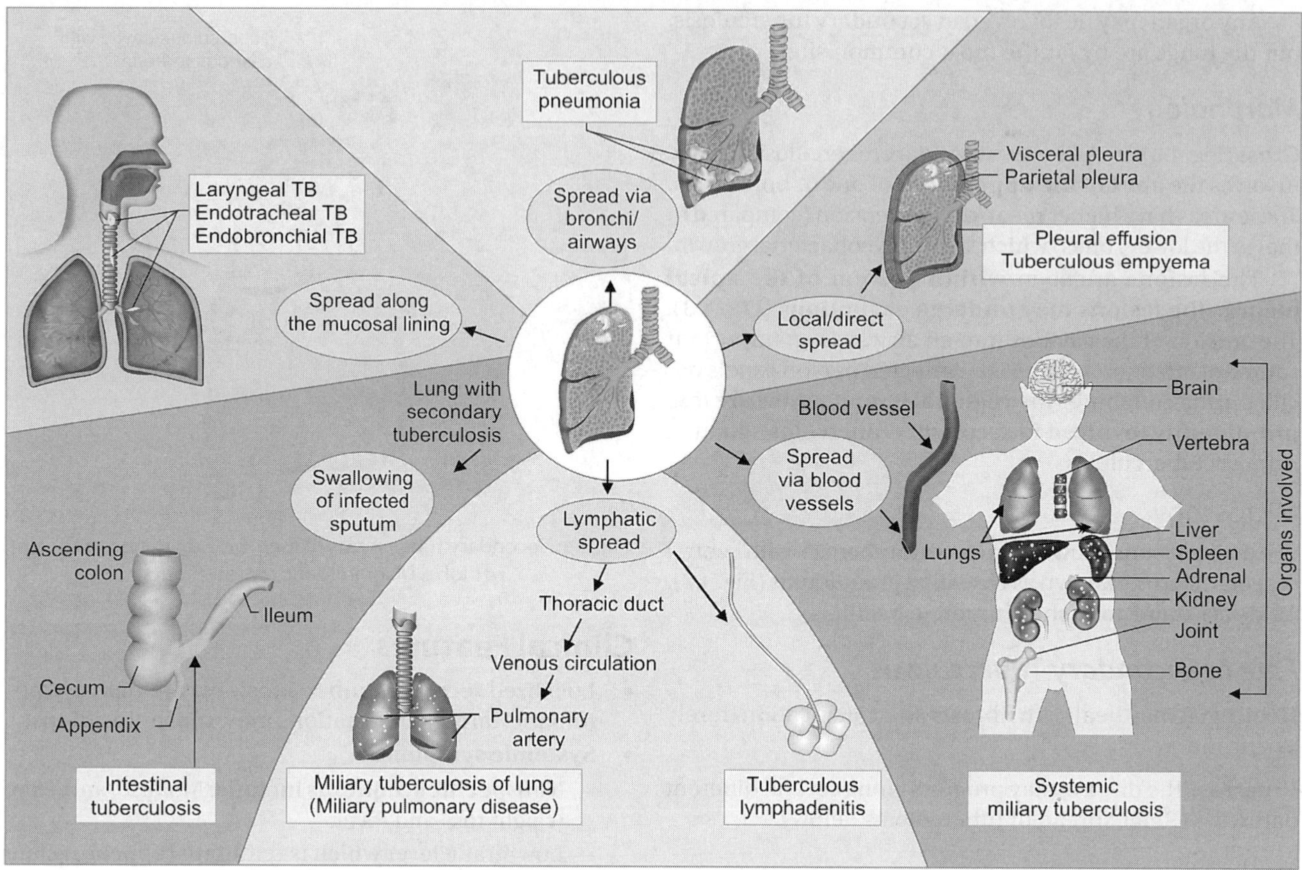

Fig. 4.4: Progress and complications of secondary tuberculosis of lung

Prognosis

Generally good if infections are localized to the lungs. All stages of HIV infection are associated with an increased risk of tuberculosis.

LEPROSY

Leprosy (Hansen disease), is a **chronic**, **granulomatous**, slowly progressive, destructive infection caused by ***Mycobacterium leprae***.

Sites of involvement: Mainly involves the **peripheral nerves**, **skin and mucous membranes** (nasal) and results in disabling deformities.

Leprosy is one of the oldest human diseases and lepers were isolated from the community in the olden days.

***Mycobacterium leprae*:** It is a slender, weakly acid-fast intracellular bacillus. It proliferates at low temperature of the human skin.

Mode of transmission: *Mycobacterium leprae* has comparatively low communicability.

1. **Inoculation/inhalation:** Likely to be transmitted from person-to-person through aerosols from asymptomatic lesions in the upper respiratory tract of leprosy patients. Inhaled *M. leprae*, is taken up by alveolar macrophages and disseminates through the blood, but replicates (multiply) only in relatively cool tissues of the skin and extremities.
2. **Intimate contact:** For many years of intimate contact with leprosy patients.

Source of infection: *M. leprae* is present in nasal secretions or ulcerated lesions of patients suffering from leprosy.

Incubation period: Generally 5 to 7 years.

Classification

- **Ridley-Jopling (1966) classification:** It depends on the clinicopathological spectrum of the disease, which

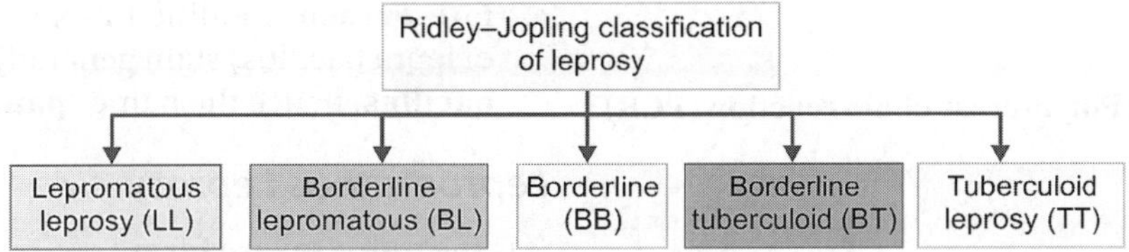

Fig. 4.5: Ridley–Jopling classification of leprosy

Table 4.1: Differences between lepromatous and tuberculoid leprosy

Opportunistic infections	Lepromatous leprosy	Tuberculoid leprosy
Clinical features		
Skin lesions	Symmetrical, multiple, ill-defined, macular, nodular	Asymmetrical, hypopigmented, well-defined macular
Disfigurement	Leonine facies, loss of eyebrows, pendulous ear lobes, claw-hands, saddle nose	Minimal disfigurement
Nerve involvement	Seen, but with less severe sensory loss than tuberculoid	Common with sensory disturbances
Microscopy of skin lesions		
Type of lesion	Nodular or diffuse collections of lepra cells within dermis	Noncaseating granulomas composed of epithelioid cells and giant cells
Grenz/clear zone between inflammatory cells and epidermis	Present	Absent
Lepra bacilli	Plenty within the lepra cells as globular masses (globi)	Rare if any
Bacillary index	4 or 5	0
Other features		
Immunity	Suppressed—low resistance	Good immunity—high resistance
Lepromin test	Negative	Positive

is **determined by the immune resistance of the host** (Fig. 4.5). They are classified into five groups with two extremes or polar forms, namely tuberculoid and lepromatous types.
- **Tuberculoid leprosy (TT):** It is the polar form that has maximal immune response.
- **Borderline tuberculoid (BT):** In this type, the immune response falls between BB and TT.
- **Borderline leprosy (BB):** It exactly falls between two polar forms of leprosy.
- **Borderline lepromatous (BL):** It has the immune response that falls between BB and LL.
- **Lepromatous leprosy (LL):** It is the other polar form with least immune response.

- **WHO classification:**
  - **Paucibacillary:** All cases of tuberculoid leprosy and some cases of borderline type.
  - **Multibacillary:** All cases of lepromatous leprosy and some cases of borderline type.

Lepromin Test

It is **not a diagnostic test** for leprosy. It is **used for classifying** the leprosy based on the immune response.

- **Procedure:** An antigen extract of *M. leprae* called lepromin is intradermally injected.
- **Reaction:**
  - An **early positive reaction** appears as an indurated area in 24 to 48 hours is called **Fernandez reaction**.
  - A **delayed granulomatous reaction** appearing after 3 to 4 weeks is known as **Mitsuda reaction**.
- **Interpretation:**
  - **Lepromatous leprosy**—shows **negative lepromin test**.
  - **Tuberculoid leprosy—**show **positive lepromin test**.

Differences between lepromatous and tuberculoid leprosy are presented in Table 4.1.

Diagnosis of Leprosy

- **Clinical examination:**
  - **Sensory testing**.
  - Examination of peripheral nerve.
- **Demonstration of acid-fast bacilli**.
  - Skin smears prepared by **slit and scrape method**.
  - **Nasal swabs stained by Ziehl-Neelsen method**.

- **Skin biopsy.**
- **Nerve biopsy.**
- **Molecular method: Polymerase chain reaction (PCR).**

Morphology

Two extremes or polar forms of the diseases are the tuberculoid and lepromatous types.

Tuberculoid Leprosy

- **Lesion in skin:**
  - **Site:** Usually on the **face, extremities, or trunk**.
  - **Type: Localized, well-demarcated, red or hypopigmented, dry, elevated**, skin **patches** having raised outer edges and depressed pale centers (central healing).
- **Nerve involvement:**
  - **Dominating feature** in tuberculoid leprosy.
  - Nerve involvement causes **loss of sensation** in the skin and results in atrophy of skin and muscle. These affected parts are liable to trauma, and lead to the development of chronic skin ulcers.
  - **Consequences:** It may lead to **contractures, paralyses, and autoamputation** of fingers or toes. Involvement of facial nerve can lead to paralysis of the eyelids, with keratitis and corneal ulcerations.

Microscopy (Fig. 4.6)

- **Granuloma:** These are well-formed, circumscribed and **non-caseating** (no caseation). Termed tuberculoid leprosy because the granulomas resemble those found in tuberculosis. Granulomas are composed of epithelioid cells (modified macrophages), Langhans giant cells, and lymphocytes.
- **Absence of Grenz zone:** Granulomas in the dermis extend to the basal layer of the epidermis (without a clear/Grenz zone).

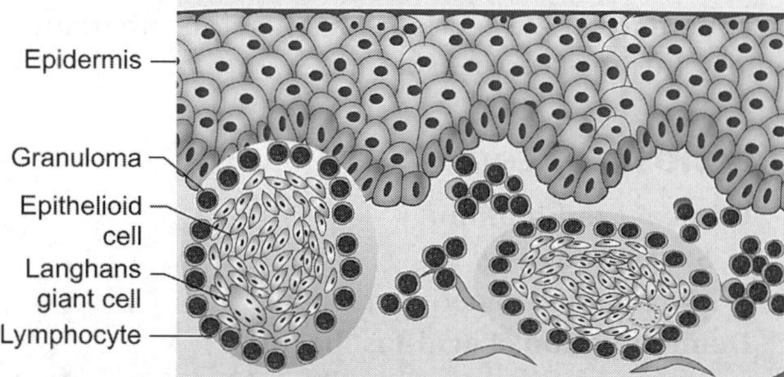

Fig. 4.6: Microscopy of tuberculoid leprosy with circumscribed noncaseating granulomas (diagrammatic)

- **Fite-Faraco** (modified Z-N stain for demonstration of lepra bacillus) stain generally **does not show lepra bacillus**, hence the name "**paucibacillary**" leprosy.

Lepromatous Leprosy

It is the **more severe form**.

- **Lesion in skin:**
  - **Thickening of skin** and **multiple, symmetric, macular, papular, or nodular lesions**. The nodular skin lesions may ulcerate. Most skin lesions are **hypoesthetic or anesthetic**.
  - More severe involvement of the **cooler areas of skin** (e.g. earlobes, wrists, elbows, and knees, and feet).
  - With progression, the nodular lesions produce a lion-like appearance known as **leonine facies** (Fig. 4.7).
- **Peripheral nerves:**
  - Particularly the **ulnar and peroneal nerves** are symmetrically invaded with mycobacteria.
  - **Loss of sensation and trophic changes** in the hands and feet may follow the damage to the nerves.

Microscopy of skin lesion (Fig. 4.8)

- **Flattened epidermis**.
  - **Grenz** (clear) **zone:** It is a characteristic **narrow, uninvolved dermis** (normal collagen) which separates the epidermis from nodular accumulations of macrophages.
  - **Lepra cells:** The nodular lesions contain large aggregates of lipid-laden foamy macrophages (lepra

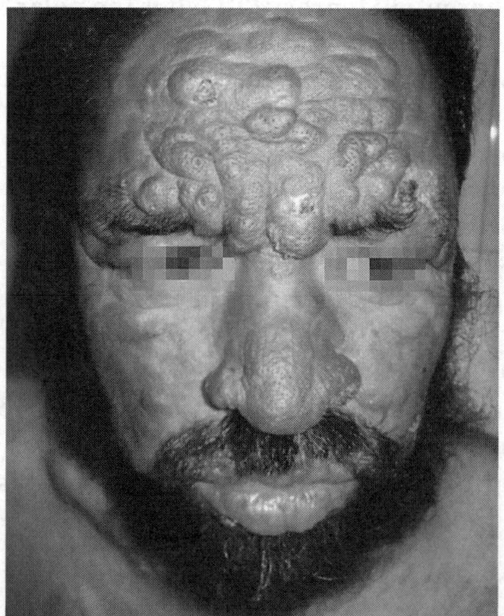

Fig. 4.7: Leonine facies of lepromatous leprosy

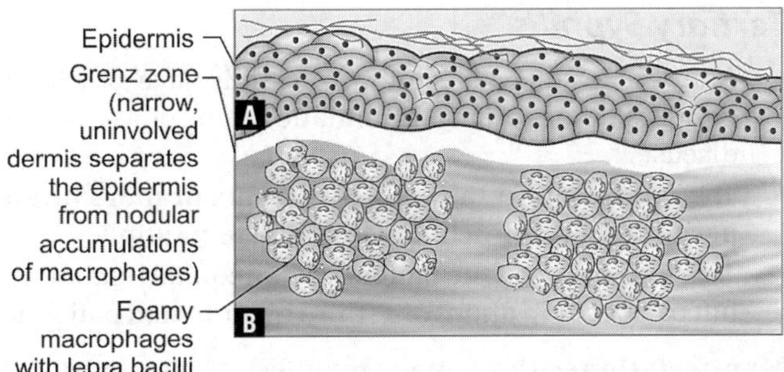

Figs 4.8A and B: (A) Microscopic appearance of lepromatous leprosy. (B) Diagrammatic. The epidermis is thinned and the dermis shows dense collections of lepra cells. The epidermis is separated from the collections of lepra cells by an uninvolved Grenz zone

cells, Virchow cells), filled with aggregates ("globi") of acid-fast lepra bacilli (*M. leprae*).
- **Fite-Faraco (acid-fast) stain:** It shows **numerous lepra bacilli** ("red snappers") within the foamy macrophages. They may be arranged in a parallel fashion like **cigarettes in a pack**.
- Due to the presence of numerous bacteria, lepromatous leprosy is also referred to as **"multibacillary"**.

SYPHILIS

Syphilis (lues) is a **chronic, sexually transmitted** disease **caused by spirochete *Treponema pallidum*.**

Etiology

- ***Treponema pallidum*** *(Fig. 4.9)***:**
  - It is a **thin, delicate, corkscrew-shaped spirochete**, with tapering ends.
  - Actively motile.
  - **Staining:** It can be visualized by **silver stains, dark-field examination and immunofluorescence techniques**.
- **Source of infection:** An open lesion of **primary or secondary syphilis**. These lesions include those in the mucous membranes or skin of the genital organs, rectum, mouth, fingers, or nipples.
- **Mode of transmission:**
  - **Sexual contact:** It is the usual mode of spread.
  - **Transplacental transmission:** From mother with active disease to the fetus (during pregnancy) results in congenital syphilis.
  - **Blood transfusion**.
  - **Direct contact:** With the open lesion of syphilitic patients is rare mode of transmission.

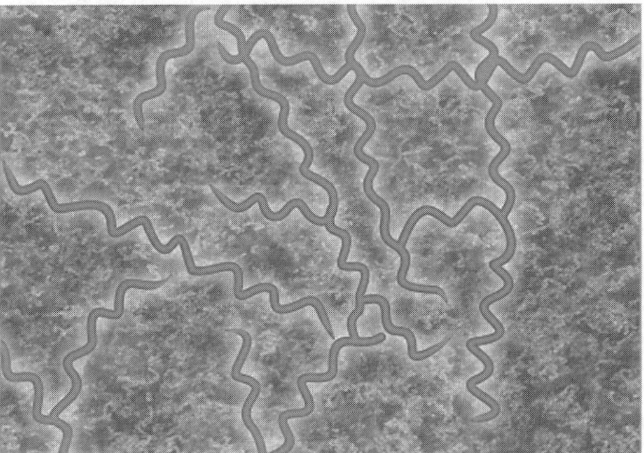

Fig. 4.9: Appearance of *Treponema pallidum* under dark-field examination

Stages of Syphilis (Fig. 4.10)

Treponema pallidum passes from the site of inoculation to regional lymph nodes. From here it enters to the systemic circulation, and disseminate throughout the body. Syphilis can be **(1) congenital or (2) acquired**. The course of acquired syphilis is divided into three stages:

1. Primary syphilis.
2. Secondary syphilis.
3. Tertiary syphilis.

Primary Syphilis

Develops about **3 weeks after contact** with an infected individual and the lesion is primary chancre.

Primary chancre

It is the classical lesion of primary syphilis.

- **Sites: Penis or scrotum** in men and **cervix, vulva** and **vaginal** wall in women. It may also be seen in the anus or mouth.
- **Gross features:** It is single, firm, **nontender (painless)**, slightly raised, **red papule** small circumscribed, superficial, solid elevation of the skin (chancre). It erodes to create a clean-based shallow ulcer. Because of the induration surrounding the ulcer, it is designated as **hard chancre.**
- **Demonstration of treponema:** Plenty of treponemes can be demonstrated in the chancre.

Regional lymphadenitis

It is due to nonspecific acute or chronic inflammation.

Symptoms: Usually painless and often unnoticed.

Fate: It heals in 3 to 6 weeks with or without therapy.

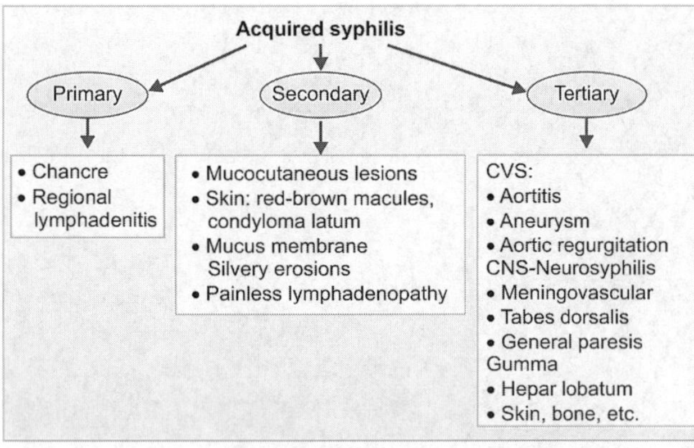

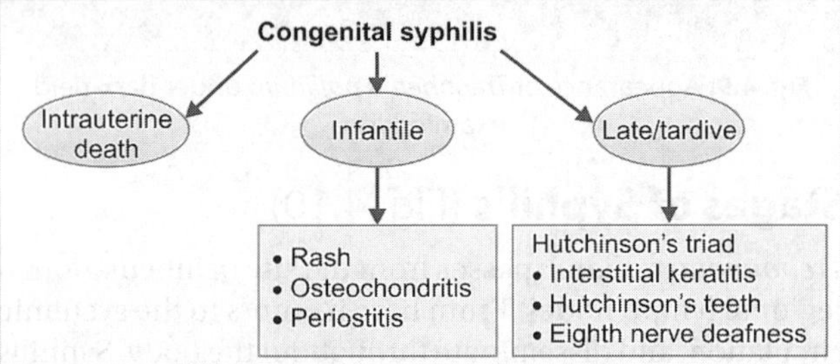

Fig. 4.10: Various manifestations of syphilis

Secondary Syphilis

It develops 2–10 weeks after the primary chancre in approximately 75% of untreated patients.

Lesions of secondary syphilis

Mucocutaneous lesions: These are painless, and contain spirochetes and are infectious.

- **Skin lesions:**
  - **Skin rashes:** Consist of **discrete red-brown macules** (discolored skin lesion that is not elevated above the surface). They are more frequent on the **palms** of the hands, or **soles** of the feet.
  - **Condylomata lata:** These are **broad-based, elevated plaques** (superficial, solid, skin lesion) with numerous spirochetes. They are seen in moist areas of the skin, such as the **anogenital region (perineum, vulva, and scrotum),** inner thighs, and axillae.
- **Mucosal lesions:** Usually occurs in the mucous membranes of **oral cavity or vagina as silvery-gray superficial erosions. Rarely, they may coalesce to produce characteristic "snail track" ulcers in the mouth.** These are **highly infectious.**

Painless lymphadenopathy: Especially involves **epitrochlear nodes** and shows plenty of spirochetes.

Tertiary Syphilis

- After the lesions of secondary syphilis have subsided patients enters an asymptomatic latent phase of the disease.
- The latent period may last for 5 years or more (even decades), but spirochetes continue to multiply.
- This stage is rare if the patient gets adequate treatment, but can occur in about one-third of untreated patients.

Manifestations: Three main manifestations of tertiary syphilis are: **cardiovascular syphilis, neurosyphilis, and so-called benign tertiary syphilis.** These may occur alone or in combination.

Cardiovascular syphilis

Most **frequently involves the aorta** and known as syphilitic aortitis.

- **Syphilitic aortitis:** Affects the **proximal aorta**.
- **Saccular aneurysm and aortic valve insufficiency:** On gross examination, the aortic intima appears rough and pitted (**tree-bark appearance**).
- **Myocardial ischemia:** Due to narrowing of the coronary artery ostia (at the origin from aorta).

Neurosyphilis

It may be asymptomatic or symptomatic.

Asymptomatic neurosyphilis: It is detected by CSF examination, which shows pleocytosis (increased numbers of inflammatory cells), elevated protein levels, or decreased glucose. Antibodies can also be detected in the CSF, which is the most specific test for neurosyphilis.

Symptomatic disease: Takes one of several forms.

- **Chronic meningovascular disease:** Chronic meningitis involves base of the brain, cerebral convexities and spinal leptomeninges.
- **Tabes dorsalis:** It is characterized by **demyelination of posterior column, dorsal root and dorsal root ganglia**.
- **General paresis of insane:** Shows generalized brain parenchymal disease with **dementia**; hence called as general paresis of insane.

Benign tertiary syphilis

It is characterized by the formation of nodular lesions called **gummas** in any organ or tissue.

Syphilitic gummas

- May be single or multiple.
- **White-gray and rubbery**.
- Vary in size from microscopic lesions to large tumor-like masses.

- **Site:** They occur in most organs but mainly involve the following:
  - **Skin, subcutaneous tissue** and the mucous membranes of the upper airway and mouth.
  - **Bone and joints:** It causes local pain, tenderness, swelling, and sometimes pathologic fractures.
  - In the **liver,** scarring due to gummas may cause a distinctive hepatic lesion known as **hepar lobatum**.
- **Microscopy:** Center of the gammas show **coagulative necrosis** surrounded by plump, **palisading macrophages**, fibroblasts and plenty of **plasma cells**. Treponemes are scant in gummas.

Congenital Syphilis

Transplacental Transmission

- *T. pallidum* can cross placenta and spread from infected **mother to the fetus** (during pregnancy).
- Transmission occurs, when **mother is suffering from primary or secondary syphilis** (when the spirochetes are abundant). Because of routine serologic testing for syphilis is done in all pregnancies congenital syphilis is rare.

Manifestations of congenital syphilis can be divided into:

- **Intrauterine death and perinatal death.**
- **Early (infantile) syphilis:** It occurs in the **first 2 years of life** and often manifested by **nasal discharge** and congestion (**snuffles**).
  - A **desquamating or bullous eruption/rash**, mainly in the hands, feet, around the mouth and anus.
  - **Skeletal abnormalities:**
    - **Syphilitic osteochondritis:** Inflammation of bone and cartilage is more distinctive in the nose produces characteristic **saddle nose deformity**.
    - **Syphilitic periostitis:** Leads to anterior bowing, or **saber shin**.
  - **Liver: Diffuse fibrosis** in the liver.
  - **Lungs:** Diffuse interstitial fibrosis causes lungs to appear pale and airless (**pneumonia alba**).
- **Late (tardive) syphilis:** Manifests **2 years after birth** and about 50% of untreated children with neonatal syphilis will develop late manifestations.
  - **Manifestations:** Distinctive manifestation is **Hutchinson's triad** and consists of:
    - **Interstitial keratitis.**
    - **Hutchinson's teeth:** They are like small screw-drivers or peg-shaped incisors, with notches in the enamel.
    - **Eighth-nerve deafness.**

Laboratory Diagnosis

- **Immunofluorescence of exudate.**
- Microscopy and PCR are also useful.
- **Serological tests:**
  - **Nontreponemal antibody tests:** These tests measure antibody to cardiolipin, a phospholipid present in both host tissues and *T. pallidum*. These antibodies are detected by the rapid plasma reagin and **Venereal Disease Research Laboratory (VDRL) tests.**
  - **Antitreponemal antibody tests:** These measure antibodies, which react with *T. pallidum*.

BACTERIAL DISEASES

Pyogenic Bacteria

- **They produce suppurative/purulent inflammation.** Pyogenic inflammation is a type of inflammation characterized by increased vascular permeability and leukocytic infiltration, mainly of neutrophils. The neutrophils accumulate at the site of infection due to release of chemoattractants from the "pyogenic" (pus-forming) bacteria. These bacteria are mostly extracellular Gram-positive cocci and Gram-negative rods.
- **Gross:** Size of the lesion depends on the location of the lesion and the organism involved. The size of purulent lesions may range from tiny microabscesses to diffuse involvement of the involved organ or tissue.
- **Microscopy:** It consists of pus, which is formed by masses of dying and dead neutrophils and liquefactive necrosis of the involved tissue.
- **Consequences:** Depends on the site and causative organism. Examples include:
  - Pneumococcal infection of lung usually spares alveolar walls and cause lobar pneumonia that resolves completely.
  - Staphylococci and *Klebsiella* infection of lung destroy alveolar walls and form abscesses that heal with scar formation.
  - Bacterial pharyngitis resolves without sequelae.
  - Untreated acute bacterial infection of a joint destroys the joint.
- **Bacteremia:** Is an invasion of the bloodstream by bacteria and occurs when bacteria enter the blood. It occurs commonly as an integral part of some infections.
- **Pyemia:** Septicemia is the presence of infective agents in the bloodstream. Pyemia is **septicemia due to pyogenic organisms**. Pyemia occurs when pathogenic organisms enter into the bloodstream and form small aggregates (microemboli). They result in either pyemic abscesses or septic infarct in various organs.

Diphtheria

- Diphtheria is caused by *Corynebacterium diphtheria*.
- *Corynebacterium diphtheria* is a slender Gram-positive rod with clubbed ends.
- **Mode of spread:** From person-to-person in respiratory droplets (respiratory diptheria) or skin exudate (cutaneous diptheria).
- **Incubation period:** Commonly 3–4 days.
- **Types:** Common types include:
  - **Respiratory diphtheria:** It causes pharyngeal infection. Inhaled *C. diphtheria* is carried in respiratory droplets proliferate at the site of attachment on the mucosa. It produces exotoxin which causes necrosis of the epithelium and formation of a dense fibrinosuppurative exudate. The coagulation of this exudate on the ulcerated necrotic surface creates a tough, dirty gray to black, superficial membrane known as **pseudo-membrane** (because it is not formed by viable tissue). When the membrane sloughs off, there is bleeding and may lead to asphyxia. With control of the infection, the pseudomembrane is either coughed-up or dissolved by enzymatic digestion. The toxin also damages the heart, nerves, and other organs.
  - **Cutaneous diphtheria:** It causes chronic ulcers with a dirty gray membrane without any systemic damage.
- **Immunization with diphtheria toxoid (formalin-fixed toxin):** It stimulates production of toxin-neutralizing antibodies which protect persons from the lethal effects of the toxin.

Gram-Negative Bacterial Infections

Whooping Cough or Pertussis

Pertussis or whooping cough is a highly communicable acute bacterial disease of childhood, caused by the Gram-negative coccobacillus ***Bordetella pertussis***. The wide use of DPT vaccine has reduced the prevalence of whooping cough.

Incubation period: About 1–2 weeks.

Pathogenesis

- *Bordetella pertussis* has strong affinity for the bronchial epithelium and also invades macrophages. *B. pertussis* proliferates and stimulates the bronchial epithelium to produce abundant tenacious mucus causing **laryngotracheobronchitis**.
- In severe cases, it causes bronchial mucosal erosion, hyperemia, and copious mucopurulent exudate.
- The toxin produced by the organism inhibits neutrophils and macrophages and paralyze cilia. Within 7–10 days after exposure, catarrhal stage of whooping cough begins and is the most infectious stage.
- Peripheral blood shows **marked lymphocytosis** (up to 90%) and enlargement of lymphoid follicles in the bronchial mucosa and peribronchial region.

Clinical features: It is characterized by **paroxysms of violent coughing** followed by a characteristic **loud inspiratory "whoop."** Other features include low-grade fever, rhinorrhea, conjunctivitis and excess tear production. The condition is self-limiting but may cause death due to asphyxia in infants.

Bacillary dysentery (refer pages 209).

VIRAL DISEASES

Poliovirus Infection

- Poliovirus causes an acute systemic viral infection. It can produce a wide range of clinical manifestations ranging from mild, self-limited infections to paralysis of limb muscles and respiratory muscles.
- Poliovirus is a spherical, unencapsulated **RNA virus** belonging to the enterovirus genus.
- **Mode of infection:** Poliovirus infects only humans and is transmitted by the **fecal-oral route**.
- The vaccines [Salk formalin fixed (killed) vaccine and the Sabin oral, attenuated (live) vaccine] have eradicated polio in India.

Pathogenesis

- **Incubation period:** About 10 days.
- The polio virus is ingested and replicates in the mucosa of the pharynx, tonsils and gut (Peyer patches in the ileum).
- From the mucosa, it spreads through lymphatics to lymph nodes and eventually the blood. Most poliovirus infections are asymptomatic.
- In nonimmunized patients poliovirus infection causes a subclinical or mild gastroenteritis. In about 1% of infected patients, poliovirus secondarily invades the CNS and replicates in motor neurons of the spinal cord (spinal poliomyelitis) or brain stem (bulbar poliomyelitis).

Morphology

- Acute cases show mononuclear cell perivascular cuffs in the **anterior horn motor neurons of the spinal cord**.

Clinical Features

- **Spinal cord involvement:** When polio affects the motor neurons of the spinal cord, it destroys motor neurons and leads to paralysis.
- **CNS infection:** It causes meningeal irritation and shows features of aseptic meningitis.

Herpes Virus Infections

- Herpes viruses are large encapsulated viruses with double-stranded DNA genome.
- Herpes viruses cause acute infection followed by latent infection. During latent infection, the viruses persist in a noninfectious form with periodic reactivation and shedding of infectious virus. Reactivation of the virus causes dissemination of the infection and tissue injury.
- There are eight types of human herpes viruses, belonging to three subgroups: α-group (e.g. HSV-1, HSV-2); β-group (e.g. CMV, human herpesvirus-6) and the γ-group (EBV and KSHV/HHV-8).

Herpes Simplex Viruses

There are two types of Herpes simplex viruses (HSV) namely **HSV-1 and HSV-2.** They **differ serologically but are closely related genetically and cause a similar set of primary and recurrent infections.**

1. **Mucocutaneous lesions**
   - HSV-1 and HSV-2 cause self-limited cold sores and gingivostomatitis.
   - **Blisters or cold sores:** Both viruses replicate at the site of entry of the virus (namely the skin and the mucous membranes usually oropharynx or genitals). They cause vesicular lesions of the epidermis. Fever **blisters or cold sores** are observed in the facial skin around mucosal orifices (lips and nose).
   - **Gingivostomatitis:** It is usually observed in children and is caused by HSV-1.
   - The viruses spread to sensory neurons and are transported along axons to the neuronal cell bodies, where they establish latent infection.
   - **Genital herpes** is more often caused by HSV-2 than by HSV-1.
   - In immunocompetent individuals, primary HSV infection resolves, although the virus remains latent in nerve cells. During latency period, the viral DNA remains within the nucleus of the neuron. Reactivation of HSV-1 and HSV-2 may occur with or without symptoms, and this reactivation causes the spread of virus from the neurons to the skin or to mucous membranes.
2. **Ophthalmic lesions:** Two forms of **corneal lesions may be produced: (1) herpes epithelial keratitis and (2) herpes stromal keratitis** (can lead to corneal blindness).
3. **Nervous system:** HSV-1 can also produce encephalitis.

Morphology

- HSV-infected cells contain large, pink to purple **intranuclear inclusions** (Cowdry type A).
- HSV also produces inclusion-bearing multinucleated syncytia.

Rabies

Rabies is a viral disease causing **severe encephalitis** and transmitted to humans by the **bite of a rabid animal (usually a dog).**

Rabies virus is sensitive to and killed by ethanol, iodine preparations, and soap detergents.

Morphology of Brain

Gross

External examination of the brain shows edema and vascular congestion.

Microscopy

- It shows widespread neuronal degeneration and an inflammatory reaction which is most severe in the brainstem.
- **Negri bodies:** These are the **pathognomonic** microscopic features. They are cytoplasmic, round to oval, eosinophilic inclusions that can be found in pyramidal neurons of the hippocampus and Purkinje cells of the cerebellum. Rabies virus can be identified within the Negri bodies by ultrastructural and immunohistochemical methods.

Clinical Features

- Rabies virus enters the CNS by ascending along the peripheral nerves from the wound site.
- **Incubation period** usually ranges from **1 to 3 months** and it depends on the distance between the wound and the brain.
- **Symptoms**
  - **Nonspecific symptoms:** Rabies presents with nonspecific symptoms such as malaise, headache, and fever. **Local paresthesia around the wound** along with above symptoms is diagnostic.
  - **CNS excitability:** As the infection progresses, patient develops severe CNS excitability. The slightest touch is painful and causes violent motor responses or even

convulsions. Signs of meningeal irritation and flaccid paralysis may develop as the disease progresses.
- **Hydrophobia:** Contracture of the pharyngeal muscles on swallowing produces foaming at the mouth. This causes aversion/fear to swallow even water (hydrophobia).
- Produces coma and death from respiratory failure.

Measles (Rubeola)

- Measles is an **acute viral infection** caused by measles (rubeola) virus.
- It **affects multiple organs** and causes a wide range of disease ranging from mild, self-limited infections to severe systemic manifestations. It can produce severe disease in patients with defects in cellular immunity (e.g. with HIV or hematologic malignancy).
- Measles can be prevented by vaccine. Epidemics of measles occur among unvaccinated individuals.
- Diagnosis is by clinical features, by serology, or by detection of viral antigen in nasal exudates or urinary sediments.

Pathogenesis

- Measles virus is a single-stranded RNA virus of the paramyxo virus family.
- **Mode of transmission:** Measles virus is transmitted by respiratory droplets.
- **Incubation period:** 9–11 days.
- Measles can replicate in many cell types such as epithelial cells and leukocytes. Initially virus multiplies within the respiratory tract and then spreads to local lymphoid tissues. Replication of the virus in lymphoid tissue is followed by viremia and systemic dissemination to many tissues. The tissues involved are conjunctiva, skin, respiratory tract, urinary tract, small blood vessels, lymphatic system, and CNS.
- Most children develop T-cell–mediated immunity to the virus which control the viral infection and produces the measles rash. Hence, the measles rash is less common in patients with deficiencies in cell-mediated immunity. In malnourished, it may cause croup, pneumonia, diarrhea and protein-losing enteropathy, keratitis (producing scarring and blindness), encephalitis, and hemorrhagic rashes ("black measles").
- Measles can cause transient immunosuppression, resulting in secondary bacterial and viral infections.
- Antibody-mediated immunity to measles virus protects against reinfection.

Morphology

- **Measles rash:** It is blotchy, reddish-brown and observed on the face, trunk, and proximal extremities. It is produced by dilated skin vessels, edema, and a mononuclear perivascular infiltrate.
- **Koplik spots:** These are pathognomonic of measles and consist of ulcerated mucosal lesions in the oral cavity near the opening of the Stensen (parotid) ducts. They appear as small, irregular, bluish-white dots measuring 1 mm in diameter surrounded by erythema.
- **Lymphoid organs—Warthin–Finkeldey cells:** Lymphoid organs show marked follicular hyperplasia, enlarged germinal centers, and randomly distributed multinucleate giant cells, called **Warthin–Finkeldey cells** (pathognomonic of measles). These giant cells have eosinophilic nuclear and cytoplasmic inclusion bodies. These are also found in the lung and sputum.

RICKETTSIAL INFECTIONS

Rickettsiales are vector-borne obligate intracellular bacteria. These organisms have the structure of Gram-negative, rod-shaped bacteria. However, they stain poorly with Gram stain.

Diseases Produced

They cause epidemic and scrub typhus, spotted fevers (*Rickettsia rickettsia*), ehrlichiosis, and anaplasmosis.

1. **Epidemic typhus**
   - Caused by *Rickettsia prowazekii.*
   - **Mode of transmission:** Transmitted from person-to-person by body lice.
   - **Clinical features:** Include macular rash that progresses to a petechial, maculopapular rash on the entire body except the face, palms, and soles.
2. **Scrub typhus**
   - Caused by *Orientia tsutsugamushi.*
   - **Mode of transmission:** By chiggers.
   - **Clinical features:** Include fever, headache, myalgia and cough and associated lymphadenopathy from the chigger bite.
3. **Rocky Mountain spotted fever**
   - Caused by *Rickettsia rickettsia.*
   - **Mode of transmission:** By dog ticks.
   - **Clinical features:** Begins as a nonspecific severe illness with fever, myalgias, and gastrointestinal distress. As the disease progresses widespread macular then petechial rash involving the palms and soles develop.

Pathogenesis

- The manifestations of rickettsial infections are mainly due to infection of endothelial cells (especially those in the lungs and brain) which results in endothelial dysfunction and injury.
- Widespread endothelial dysfunction/injury can cause shock, peripheral and pulmonary edema, and disseminated intravascular coagulation, renal failure and CNS manifestations (e.g. coma).

Morphology

Characterized by small vessel lesions and focal areas of hemorrhage and inflammation in many organs and tissues.

Diagnosis

- Rickettsial diseases are usually diagnosed clinically.
- Diagnosis is confirmed by serology or immunostaining of the organisms.

CHLAMYDIAL INFECTIONS

Chlamydia trachomatis

- It is a small Gram-negative bacterium and exists in two forms during its unique life cycle.
  - **Elementary body:** It is infectious, metabolically inactive form and has a spore like structure. Host cells take up the elementary body by endocytosis and form endosome. The bacteria prevent fusion of the endosome and lysosome.
  - **Reticulate body:** Inside the endosome of the host cell, the elementary body differentiates into a metabolically active form, called the reticulate body. The reticulate body replicate and forms new infectious elementary bodies.
- **Diseases produced:** *C. trachomatis* infection cause (1) urogenital infections, (2) inclusion conjunctivitis (3) lymphogranuloma venereum, (4) ocular infection of children, trachoma.
- Genital infection by *C. trachomatis* is the most common sexually transmitted bacterial infection in women.

Morphology

- *C. trachomatis* **urethritis** appears identical to gonorrhoea. It produces mucopurulent discharge containing mainly neutrophils.
- **Lymphogranuloma venereum** contains a mixed granulomatous and neutrophilic inflammatory response. Chlamydial inclusions are seen in the cytoplasm of epithelial cells or inflammatory cells. Regional lymphadenopathy is common and shows granulomatous inflammatory reaction associated with irregularly shaped foci of necrosis containing neutrophils (**stellate abscesses**). With time, extensive fibrosis may cause local lymphatic obstruction, lymphedema, and strictures.

FUNGAL INFECTIONS AND OPPORTUNISTIC INFECTIONS

Fungi grow as multicellular filaments (mold) or individual cells alone or in chains (yeast). They have cell wall which gives them a shape.

- **Yeasts** are round to oval and reproduce by budding. Some yeasts (e.g. *Candida albicans*) produce buds that fail to detach and become elongated, producing a chain of elongated yeast cells called **pseudohyphae**.
- **Molds** are thread-like filaments (hyphae) that grow and divide at their tips. They can produce round cells known as **conidia**, which can easily become airborne, disseminating the fungus.
- Many fungi are dimorphic, i.e. they exist as yeast or molds, depending on environmental conditions (yeast form at human body temperature and a mold form at room temperature).

Types of Fungal Infections

Fungal infections are also known as *mycoses*. Human fungal infections are divided into four major types:

1. **Superficial and cutaneous mycoses:** Common and limited to the skin, hair, and nails.
2. **Subcutaneous mycoses:** Involve the skin, subcutaneous tissues, and lymphatics.
3. **Endemic mycoses:** Caused by dimorphic fungi and can produce serious systemic illness in healthy individuals.
4. **Opportunistic mycoses:** They can cause life-threatening systemic diseases in individuals who are immunosuppressed.

Diagnosis

1. Histological examination.
2. **Culture:** Definitive identification of some requires culture.

PARASITIC DISEASES

Protozoa

- Protozoa are unicellular eukaryotic organisms. The protozoa are transmitted by insects or by the fecal-oral route.

Malaria

- Malaria, caused by the intracellular parasite *Plasmodium.*
- *Plasmodium falciparum* (causes severe cerebral malaria) and the four other malaria parasites that infect humans (*P. vivax, P. ovale, P. knowlesi,* and *P. malariae*) are all transmitted by female anopheles mosquitoes.

Life Cycle and Pathogenesis

The life cycles of the *Plasmodium* species are similar.

- *P. vivax, P. ovale, P. knowlesi,* and *P. malariae:* They produce low levels of parasitemia, mild anemia.
- ***P. falciparum* infection:** It **produces high levels of parasitemia** and may lead to severe anemia, cerebral symptoms, renal failure, pulmonary edema, and death.

The life cycle of *Plasmodium* species is simple because it involves only humans and mosquitoes. However, the development of the parasite is complex, because it passes through several morphologically distinct forms. Malarial parasites pass their life cycle in two different hosts namely: (1) human (intermediate host) and (2) female anopheles mosquito (definitive host).

1. **Human cycle:** It starts with the introduction of infectious stage of *Plasmodium*, the *sporozoite* by the bite of infected female anopheles mosquito. The *sporozoite* is found in the salivary glands of mosquitoes. During mosquito bite, the mosquito takes a blood meal and sporozoites are released into the human's blood. The different stages of human cycle are:
   - **Exoerythrocytic stage:** Within minutes of entry of sporozites into the human blood, they attach to and invade liver cells. Within liver cells, malaria parasites multiply, releasing about 30,000 *merozoites* (asexual, haploid forms) when each infected liver cells ruptures.
     - During *P. falciparum* infection, rupture of liver cells usually occurs within 8 to 12 weeks.
     - In contrast, *P. vivax* and *P. ovale* releases weeks to months after initial infection.

     The infection of the liver and development of merozoites is referred to as the exoerythrocytic stage. This stage is asymptomatic.
   - **Erythrocytic stage** (Fig. 4.11)**:** Once released from the liver, *Plasmodium* merozoites bind to the surface of red cells and invade RBC by penetration of the membrane. Within the red cells (erythrocytic stage) the parasites grow and hydrolyze hemoglobin through its enzymes.
     - **Asexual forms:** In the red cells, parasite passes through the stages of asexual forms namely trophozoite, schizont and merozoite. These asexual forms of parasite can be demonstrated in the thick blood smears.
       - ◊ *Trophozoite* is the first stage of the parasite in the red cell and is characterized by the presence of a single chromatin mass.
       - ◊ *Schizont:* It is the next stage and shows multiple chromatin masses, each of which develops into a merozoite.
       - ◊ *Merozoites*: Lysis of the red cell containing merozoites occurs and the new merozoites infect additional red cells. The characteristic clinical features of malaria such as paroxysmal fever, chills, and rigors develop during the release of these merozoites into the blood. The periodicity of such paroxysms (every 48–72 hours) varies with the species of the malarial parasite.
     - **Sexual forms:** Most malaria parasites within the red cells develop into merozoites. However, some parasites under specific conditions develop into sexual forms called gametocytes. These gametocytes infect the mosquito when mosquito bites the infected human and takes its blood meal.
     - **Malaria** is more severe when caused by *Plasmodium falciparum* than the other Plasmodium species.
2. **Mosquito cycle:** A female anopheles mosquito during its blood meal from an infected patient ingests both sexual and asexual forms of parasite, but it is only the mature sexual forms (gametocytes) capable of development. In the mosquito, the gametocytes mature into sporozoite in their gut. They are then transported to the salivary glands of mosquitoes.

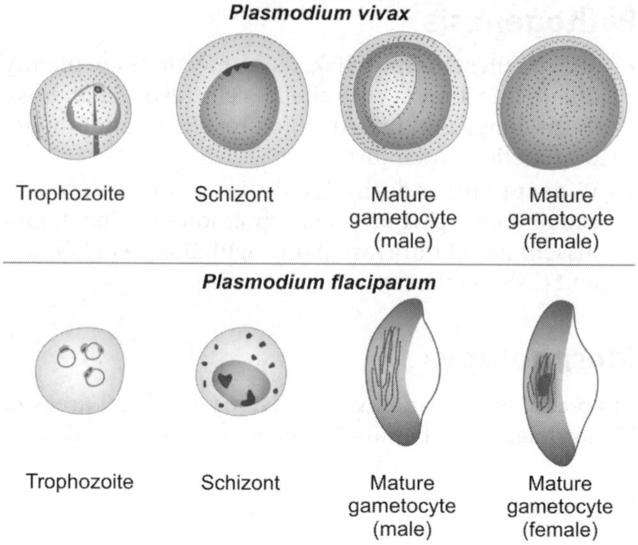

Fig. 4.11: Diagrammatic appearance of malarial parasite (*Plasmodium vivax and falciparum*) in human

Morphology

- **Peripheral blood smear:** Diagnosis of malaria infection can be made by examination of a Giemsa-stained peripheral blood smear (Fig. 4.11). It **shows the asexual stages of the parasite within infected red cells.**
- **Spleen:** *Plasmodium falciparum* infection produces **splenomegaly**. In chronic infections, the spleen becomes fibrotic and brittle, with a thick capsule. The parenchyma appears gray or black because of the granular, brown-black, faintly birefringent hemozoin pigment.
- **Liver:** It is enlarged and pigmented. Kupffer cells contain malarial pigment, parasites, and cellular debris.
- **Brain:** In **cerebral malaria** caused by *P. falciparum*, blood vessels of the brain show plugging of parasitized red cells. Around the vessels there are ring hemorrhages and small focal inflammatory reactions called as **malarial** or **Dürck granulomata**.

Amebiasis (refer pages 209-10).

Tapeworms (Cestode Parasites)

Cysticercosis

- Cysticercosis is infection caused by larvae that develop after ingestion of eggs of tapeworm namely ***Taenia solium*** (pork tapeworm/armed tape worm). **Cysticercus is the resting stage of larva in the intermediate host**.
- *Taenia solium* has a complex life cycle and requires two mammalian hosts: (1) a definitive host (in which the worm reaches sexual maturity—humans) and (2) an intermediate host (in which the worm does not reach sexual maturity—humans and pigs).

Mode of infection

T. solium can be transmitted to humans in two ways with distinct outcomes.

1. Ingestion of larval cysts called cysticerci (present in uncooked pork) or
2. Ingestion of eggs present in contaminated food/water.

Pathogenesis (Fig. 4.12)

- **Ingestion of cysticerci** (larval cysts)**:** When larval cysts are ingested in undercooked pork by human beings, they attach to the intestinal wall and develop into mature adult tapeworms. They can grow to many meters in length. The life cycle of parasite is completed with this mode of infection and cysticercosis does not develop. Adult tapeworms shed eggs in the feces of human beings.
- **Ingestion of eggs:** When intermediate hosts (pigs or humans) ingest eggs in food or water contaminated with human feces, the eggs develop into larvae, penetrate the gut wall and enter the blood circulation. They spread to various sites like muscle, brain and form **cystic larvae termed cysticercus cellulosae.**

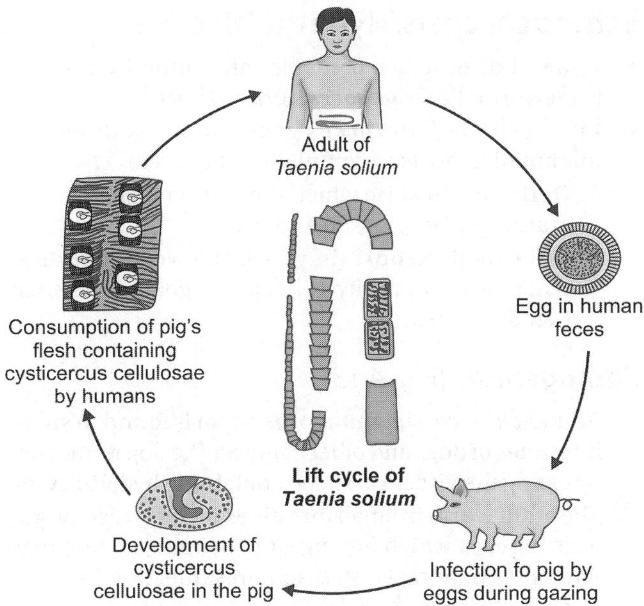

Fig. 4.12: Life cycle of *Taenia solium*

Morphology of cysticercus

- **Organs affected:** Cysticerci may be found in any organ, but the more common locations include the **brain, skeletal muscles, skin, and heart**.
- **Number:** The cysticercus can be single or multiple.
- **Appearance:** Cysticercus consists of round to oval white to opalescent cyst, 0.5–1 cm (often grape-sized) in diameter containing little, clear cyst fluid. It contains an invaginated scolex (which has four suckers) and circle of birefringent hooks on its wall. They remain viable for long time. Once the embryo dies, it induces granulomatous reaction with eosinophils and may later show scarring and calcification, which may be visible by radiography.

Clinical features

- **Adult tape worm** in the intestine can produce abdominal pain, diarrhea and loss of appetite.
- **Cysticercus cellulosae**
  - **Neurocysticercosis:** The most serious manifestations of cysticercosis are due to involvement of the brain (neurocysticercosis). Cerebral symptoms depend on the location of the cysts. It can produce epilepsy (convulsions), hydrocephalus, increased intracranial pressure, blurred vision and other neurologic disturbances.

Echinococcosis/Hydatid Disease

- Hydatid disease is a parasitic infestation by cestode (tapeworms) ***Echinococcus granulosus***.
- **Life cycle: *Echinococcus granulosus*** requires two mammalian hosts to complete its life cycle.
  - **Definitive host** (in which the worm reaches sexual maturity)**:** Dog, jackal, and fox.
  - **Intermediate host** (in which the worm does not reach sexual maturity)**:** Sheep, pig, goat, cattle, man (dead end host).

Pathogenesis (Fig. 4.13)

- Adult *Echinococcus granulosus* worm is found in small intestines of dogs and other canines. The dog is infected by eating the viscera of sheep containing hydatid cysts.
- The adult worm in small intestines of dogs, discharges eggs in feces which are ingested by man, sheep, pigs and other mammals. Man acquires infection by:
  - Handling dogs.
  - Eating food/vegetables contaminated with eggs shed by dogs or foxes.
- The eggs hatch in the human duodenum and are carried to the liver by portal venous system and other sites through systemic circulation. Those which are trapped in the hepatic sinusoids develop into hydatid cyst.

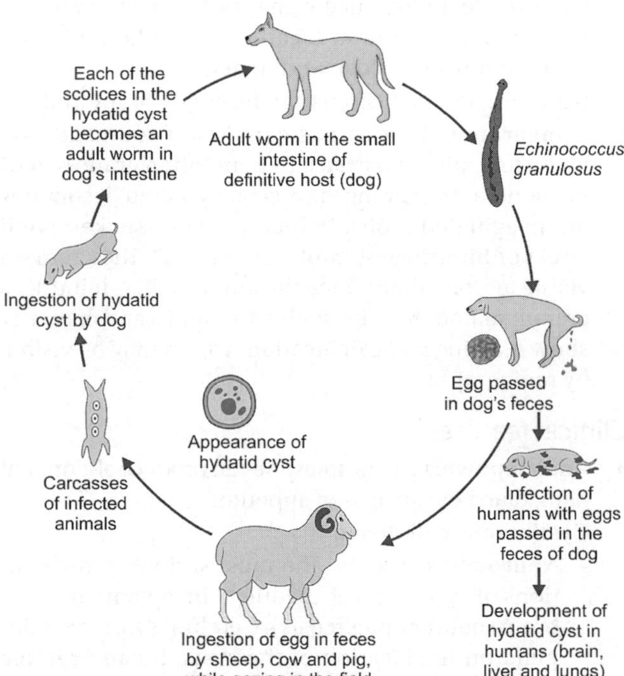

Fig. 4.13: Life cycle of *Echinococcus granulosus*

Morphology

- **Sites:** About 65% human *E. granulosus* cysts are found in the liver and 5 to 15% in the lung, and the remaining 10 to 20% in bones and brain or other organs.
- **Hydatid cysts** begin at microscopic levels and grow slowly. They may eventually attain a size over 10 cm in diameter in about 5 years. *E. granulosus* usually produces unilocular hydatid cyst while *E. multiloularis* produces multilocular hydatid disease in the liver.
- **Microscopy:** The cyst wall consists of 3 distinguishable zones enclosing an opalescent fluid:
  1. **Pericyst (outer, capsular layer):** It shows inflammatory reaction and consists of fibroblasts, giant cells, and mononuclear and eosinophils.
  2. **Ectocyst(intermediate opaque, non-nucleated layer):** It is distinctive and has innumerable delicate laminations.
  3. **Endocyst** (inner, nucleated, germinative layer with daughter cysts and scolices projecting into the lumen)**:** Daughter cysts can develop within the large mother cyst. They appear first as minute projections of the germinative layer that develop central vesicles and thus form tiny brood capsules. Degenerating scolices of the worm produce a fine, grain-like (sand-like) sediment within the hydatid fluid (hydatid sand).

Clinical Features

- Liver: Produces pressure effects due to cyst.
- Cerebral: Epilepsy.
- Renal: Hematuria.
- Rupture of cyst: The liberation of antigenic proteins in the hydatid fluid into the circulation produces eosinophilia and may even cause anaphylactic reactions.

Laboratory diagnosis

Casoni test.

Filariasis

Filariasis is transmitted by mosquitoes and is caused by closely related nematodes, *Wuchereria bancrofti* and *Brugia* species (*B. malayi*).

Diseases

Filariasis causes a spectrum of diseases.

1. Asymptomatic.
2. Recurrent lymphadenitis.
3. Chronic lymphadenitis with elephantiasis.
4. Tropical pulmonary eosinophilia.

Pathogenesis

- Definitive host is man and intermediate host is mosquito.
- During the mosquito bite to humans, the infective larvae are released by mosquitoes into the tissues. They develop within lymphatic channels into adult males and females which mate and release microfilariae into the bloodstream.
- During the mosquito bite of the infected persons, the mosquitoes can take up the microfilariae. These microfilariae undergo further development in the mosquito and they become infective and transmit the disease to humans.

Morphology

- In chronic filariasis, the adult parasites lodge in the lymphatics and stimulate fibrosis and the formation of granulomas around the adult parasites. Thus, chronic filariasis is leads to **persistent lymphedema** of the extremities, scrotum, penis, or vulva.
- In severe and long-standing swollen leg may develop tough subcutaneous fibrosis and epithelial hyperkeratosis, termed **elephantiasis** (Fig. 4.14A). Adult filarial worms (live, dead, or calcified) are observed in the draining lymphatics or nodes. Microfilaria (Fig. 4.14B) is the embryo of *Wuchereria bancrofti* and can be seen in blood and body fluids.
- Filariasis can also cause hydrocele.

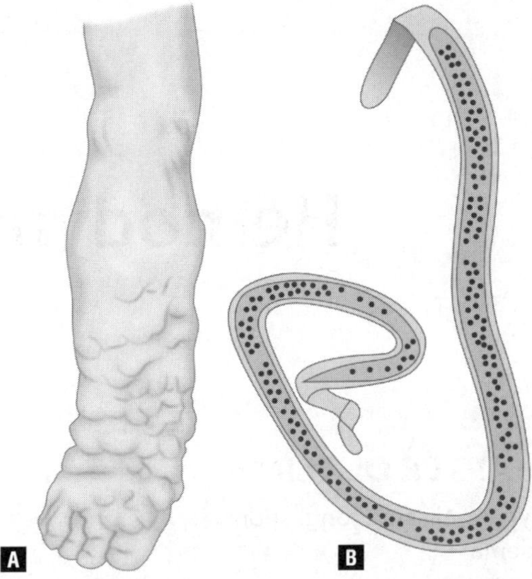

Figs 4.14A and B: (A) Elephantiasis of leg; (B) Diagrammatic apperance of Microfilaria (embryo of *Wuchereria bancrofti*)

SELF-ASSESSMENT EXERCISE

I. Short Notes

1. Primary tuberculosis and its fate.
2. Ghon focus/Ghon complex.
3. Epithelioid cells.
4. Granuloma.
5. Miliary tuberculosis.
6. Pulmonary tuberculosis.
7. Classify leprosy.
8. Tuberculoid leprosy.
9. Lepromatous leprosy.
10. Congenital syphilis.
11. Gumma.
12. Poliomyelitis.
13. Malaria.
14. Hydatid cyst.

CHAPTER

5

Hemodynamic Disorders

CHAPTER OUTLINE

- Hyperemia and Congestion
- Edema
- Thrombosis
- Embolism
- Infarction
- Shock

HYPEREMIA AND CONGESTION

Hyperemia and congestion are characterized by **locally increased blood volume.**

Hyperemia

Definition: Hyperemia is an **active process** in which **arteriolar dilation** leads to increased **blood flow to a tissue/organ**.

- Seen in **inflammation** and is responsible for the two cardinal signs of inflammation namely **heat** (calor) and **redness** (rubor/**erythema**).

Congestion

Definition: Congestion is a **passive process** resulting from **reduced venous outflow of blood** from a tissue/organ.

Types and Causes

1. **Systemic:** For example, in congestive heart failure, congestion involves liver, spleen, and kidneys.
2. **Local:** For example, congestion of leg veins due to deep venous thrombosis → edema of the lower extremity.

Chronic Venous Congestion (CVC) of Lung

Causes

- **Mitral stenosis:** For example, rheumatic mitral stenosis.
- **Left-sided heart failure:** It develops secondary to coronary artery disease or hypertension.

Consequences

Four major consequences of CVC lung are:

- **Microhemorrhages:** The wall of alveolar capillaries may rupture causing minute hemorrhages into the alveolar space with release of RBCs into the alveoli. The hemoglobin of these RBCs breakdown and **liberate iron-containing hemosiderin pigment** (brown color). The alveolar macrophages phagocytose hemosiderin. **Hemosiderin-laden macrophages** are known as **heart failure cells**. When stained by Perl's stain, the hemosiderin in these cells appear blue-black in color.
- **Pulmonary edema**.
- **Fibrosis** in the interstitium of lung.
- **Pulmonary hypertension**.

Morphology

Gross

- Lung is **heavy**.
- Cut section (c/s) **rusty brown color** (due to hemosiderin pigment), **firm in consistency** (due to fibrosis) and is known as **brown induration of lung**.

Microscopy (Fig. 5.1)

- **Distension** and **congestion of capillaries** in the alveolar septa of lung.

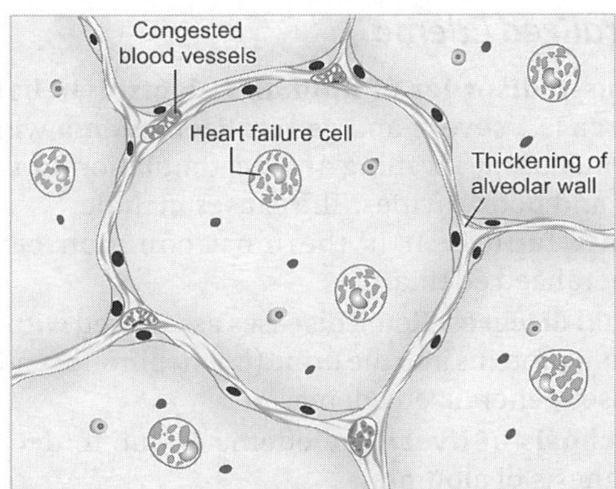

Fig. 5.1: Chronic venous congestion lung (diagrammatic) with thickened alveolar walls and hemosiderin laden macrophages (heart failure cells) in the alveolar lumen

- **Thickened alveolar septa** due to increase in the fibrous connective tissue and is responsible for the firm consistency of the lung.
- **Heart failure cells** are seen in the alveoli.

Chronic Passive (venous) Congestion (CVC) of Liver

Cause

For example, **right-sided heart failure** is the most common cause.

Morphology

Gross

- **Liver increases in size** and weight and the **capsule appears tense.**
- **Cut section** shows **alternate** (combination of) **dark and light areas** (Fig. 5.2) and resembles cross-section of a nutmeg (**nutmeg liver**).

Microscopy (Fig. 5.3)

- **Centrilobular region:**
  - **Congestion and hemorrhage** in the central veins (terminal hepatic venule) and adjacent sinusoids.
  - The **severe central hypoxia may produce centrilobular hepatocyte necrosis**.
  - **Thickening of central veins and fibrosis** in prolonged venous congestion.
  - **Cardiac sclerosis/cardiac cirrhosis** may occur with sustained chronic venous congestion (e.g. due to constrictive pericarditis or tricuspid stenosis).
- **Periportal region:** It shows **fatty change** in hepatocytes.

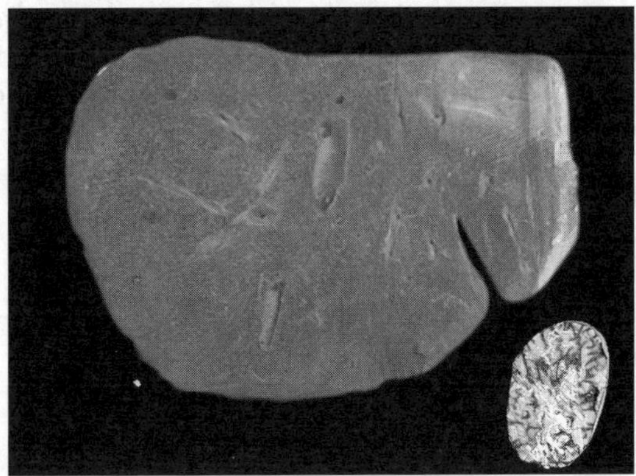

Fig. 5.2: Gross appearance of chronic venous congestion of liver, which shows alternate dark and light area and resembles the cut surface of a nutmeg (inset)

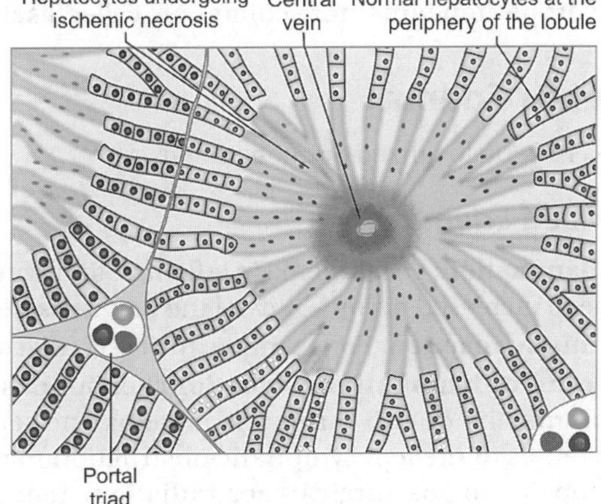

Fig. 5.3: Chronic venous congestion of liver shows centrilobular necrosis with degenerating hepatocytes surrounded by apparently normal hepatic parenchyma in the periportal region

Congestive Splenomegaly (CVC Spleen)

Congestion and enlargement of spleen is called as congestive splenomegaly.

Cause

Cirrhosis of the liver is the main cause (e.g. alcoholic cirrhosis, pigment cirrhosis).

Morphology

Gross

- Spleen is **enlarged, firm and tense. Capsule is thickened.**
- Cut section may show **Gamna-Gandy bodies,** which consist of **iron-containing, fibrotic, and calcified foci of old hemorrhage**.

- Enlarged spleen **may show excessive functional activity** termed as **hypersplenism** and leads to hematologic abnormalities (e.g. thrombocytopenia, pancytopenia).

Microscopy

- Red pulp
  - **Dilatation and congestion** in the early stages.
  - Hemorrhage and fibrosis in later stages.
- **Thickened fibrous capsule and trabeculae**.

EDEMA

Definition: Edema is defined as an abnormal **increase in interstitial fluid** within tissues. The abnormal fluid collections in the different body cavities are called as hydrothorax (pleural cavity), hydropericardium (pericardial cavity), and hydroperitoneum (more commonly called **ascites**).

Types of Edema

Edema may be localized or generalized.

Localized Edema

- **Inflammation:** Local edema in inflammation is mainly due to increased permeability of the blood vessels.
- **Immune reaction:** For example, urticaria (hives).
- **Venous or lymphatic obstruction:** Venous obstruction may be due to thrombus in veins and usually develops in the leg. Lymphatic obstruction may develop due to postsurgical, postradiation, neoplastic or filariasis.

Generalized Edema

It is due to **disorder of fluid and electrolyte balance**. **Anasarca** is a **severe** and **generalized edema** with subcutaneous tissue swelling and accumulation in visceral organs and body cavities. The causes include:

- **Heart failure:** It is the most common cause of generalized edema.
- **Renal diseases:** Renal diseases associated with loss of serum proteins into the urine (e.g. nephrotic syndrome) causes generalized edema.
- **Cirrhosis of liver:** The edema is due to decreased synthesis of albumin.

Transudate Versus Exudate

Edema caused by increased hydrostatic pressure or reduced plasma proteins is typically a protein-poor fluid and is called as transudate. Transudate is seen in patients suffering from heart failure, renal failure and hepatic failure. In contrast, edema fluid found in inflammation is protein-rich and is called as exudate. The differences between transudate and exudate are shown in Table 3.2.

Causes of Edema

The various pathophysiologic categories of edema are shown in Box 5.1.

Pathogenesis of Edema (Fig. 5.4)

Edema develops when there are disturbances in the normal fluid balance. It is mainly due to either **increased**

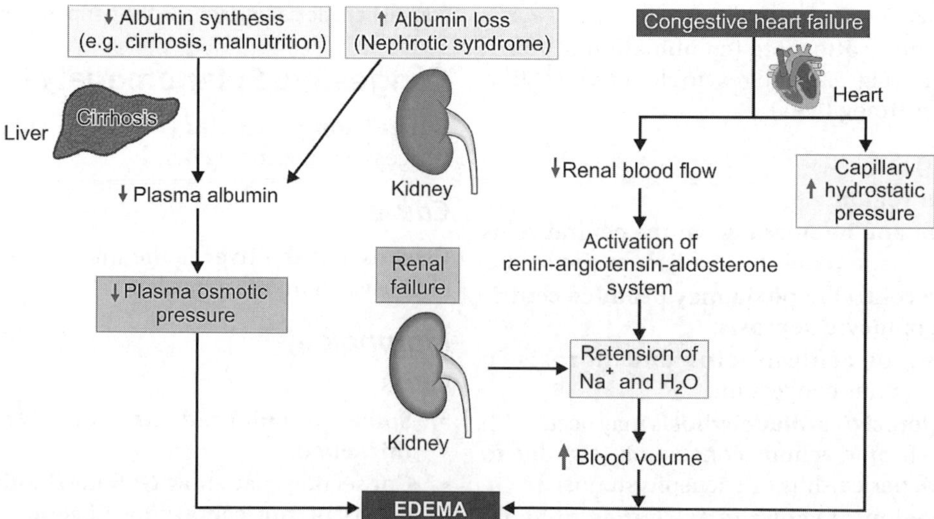

Fig. 5.4: Pathogenesis of systemic edema from congestive heart failure, renal failure, or reduced plasma osmotic pressure

Box 5.1: Pathophysiologic categories of edema

Increased hydrostatic pressure • Impaired venous return: Congestive heart failure, ascites (cirrhosis), venous obstruction or compression (thrombosis, external pressure)
Reduced plasma osmotic pressure (Hypoproteinemia) • Nephrotic syndrome • Cirrhosis of liver (ascites) • Malnutrition
Lymphatic obstruction • Inflammatory: For example, filariasis • Postsurgical/post irradiation • Neoplastic
Sodium retention • Excessive salt intake with renal insufficiency
Inflammation • Acute inflammation and chronic inflammation

hydrostatic pressure or **diminished plasma** colloid **osmotic pressure**.

Increased Hydrostatic Pressure

The increased hydrostatic pressure may cause edema which may be localized or generalized.

- **Localized increase in hydrostatic pressure:** It may develop when there is local obstruction to the venous blood flow (e.g. **deep venous thrombosis** of lower limbs).
- **Generalized increase in venous hydrostatic pressure:** It occurs most commonly in **congestive heart failure**. Congestive heart failure may be due to failure of the left ventricle, right ventricle or both.

Reduced Plasma Osmotic Pressure

Plasma albumin is mainly responsible for the plasma osmotic pressure. The plasma osmotic pressure is reduced when there is decreased synthesis or loss of albumin from the circulation.

- **Reduced albumin synthesis:** Causes include **severe liver diseases** (e.g. cirrhosis) or **protein malnutrition** (with decreased protein intake).
- **Loss of albumin:** Urinary loss of albumin occurs in **nephrotic syndrome**.

Consequences of reduced plasma osmotic pressure

- Reduced plasma osmotic pressure causes an **increased movement of fluid from the circulation into interstitial tissue spaces.** This reduces the plasma volume.
- The **reduced intravascular volume in turn** leads to **decreased perfusion of the kidneys.**
- Decreased kidney perfusion stimulates **increased** production of **renin, angiotensin, and aldosterone by the kidney**. This, in turn leads to **retention of salt (sodium) and water**.

Sodium and Water Retention

Salt (sodium) and water retention may also be a primary cause of edema. Increased salt retention is usually associated with retention of water and leads to:

- Increased hydrostatic pressure (due to increased plasma volume).
- Decreased plasma colloid osmotic pressure (due to dilution effect on albumin).
- Increased sodium retention may be primary (e.g. renal failure, glomerulonephritis) or secondary (e.g. congestive heart failure).

Lymphatic Obstruction

Obstruction to the lymphatic drainage causes localized edema known as lymphedema.

Causes

- **Inflammatory:** In parasitic infestation, **filariasis** (caused by *Wuchereria bancrofti*) the parasite causes lymphatic obstruction. It can result in edema of the external genitalia and lower limbs. If massive, lower limb may resemble the elephant leg and is known as **elephantiasis.**
- **Postsurgical/post irradiation:** In patients with breast cancer, severe edema of the upper arm may complicate **surgical removal and/or irradiation of the breast** and associated axillary lymph nodes.
- **Invasive malignant tumors:** For example, blocking of subcutaneous lymphatics by malignant tumors may be seen in breast concer [peau d'orange (orange skin) appearance].

Morphology

Edema can be **easily detected on gross examination**. It may involve any organ or tissue, but is **most common in subcutaneous tissues, the lungs,** and the **brain**.

Generalized Edema

It is seen mainly in the subcutaneous tissues.

- **Subcutaneous edema:** In most cases, the distribution of **edema is dependent on gravity** and is termed **dependent edema**. Thus, it is prominent in the legs when standing, and in the sacrum when recumbent. **If pressure is applied** by a finger over substantially edematous subcutaneous tissue, it **displaces the**

interstitial fluid and leaves a depression. This sign is called as **pitting edema**.

- **Edema of renal origin:** It can **affect all parts of the body**. Initially, it is observed **in tissues with loose connective tissue matrix**, such as the **eyelids (periorbital edema) and scrotal region**.

Pulmonary Edema

- **Gross:** The **weight of lungs is increased** 2 to 3 times of normal weight. **Cut section** shows frothy, **blood-tinged fluid** (due to mixture of air, edema, and extravasated red cells) **oozing from the lung**.

THROMBOSIS

Definition: Thrombosis is defined as the **process of formation of a solid mass in the circulating blood from the constituents of flowing blood**. The mass formed is called thrombus.

Etiology

Three primary abnormalities (Fig. 5.5) that can form thrombus (called **Virchow's triad**) are:

- Endothelial injury (changes in blood vessel)
- Alterations in normal blood flow (changes in blood flow)
- Hypercoagulability of the blood (changes in blood itself).

Endothelial Injury (Changes in Blood Vessel)

- **Physical endothelial injury**
  - The endothelial cell injury in the **heart** may be due to **myocardial infarction**, catheter trauma, **vegetations** (wart-like thrombi) on cardiac valves.
  - In the **arteries**, it may be due to ulceration of **atherosclerotic plaques**, traumatic or inflammatory vascular injury (vasculitis).
- **Endothelial dysfunction:** This may be caused by hypertension, turbulent blood flow, toxins (bacterial endotoxins, toxins from cigarette smoke), radiation injury and metabolic abnormalities (e.g. homocystinemia or hypercholesterolemia).

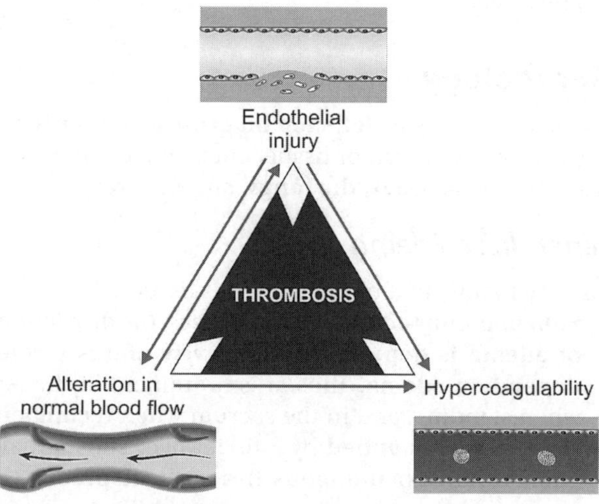

Fig. 5.5: Virchow's triad in thrombosis

Alterations in Normal Blood Flow (Changes in Blood Flow)

Normally, blood flows in a laminar pattern or in a streamline in which fluid plasma flows in parallel layers, with no disruption between the layers. In this laminar flow, platelets (and other blood cellular elements) flow centrally in the vessel lumen and separated from endothelium by a slower moving layer of plasma. Turbulence (disturbed movement of blood) and stasis (slowing of blood flow) contributes to thrombosis.

- **Turbulence** causes **endothelial injury or dysfunction**. The causes of turbulence are:
  - **Heart: Acute myocardial infarction,** arrhythmias (a disturbance in or loss of regular rhythm of heart)/ atrial fibrillation (arrhythmia characterized by fibrillary contractions) and **rheumatic mitral stenosis.**
  - **Blood vessels: Atherosclerosis, aneurysms (abnormal dilatation of blood vessel) or varicose veins.**
- **Stasis** is a major contributor for **venous thrombi.** The various causes of venous stasis are: heart failure, chronic venous insufficiency, postoperative immobilization, and prolonged bed rest.

Hypercoagulability (Changes in Blood Itself)

Hypercoagulability state (also known as thrombophilia) is defined as a systemic disorder associated with increased tendency to develop thromboembolism. The various causes are shown in Table 5.1.

Morphology

Composition of thrombi: Both gross and microscopy of thrombi show alternating light (pale or white) and dark areas. These alternating laminations of light and dark areas are called **lines of Zahn** (Fig. 5.6).

Site and types: Thrombi can develop anywhere in the cardiovascular system.

- **Heart:** Common sites in the heart are atrial appendages and heart valves (called as **vegetations**).
- **Blood vessels:**
  - **Arteries:** Aorta or larger vessels usually develop **mural thrombi (attached to the wall and projects into the lumen, without complete occlusion of the**

Table 5.1: Various causes of hypercoagulable states

Type of disorder	Common causes
Primary (genetic)	• **Deficiency of antithrombotic (anticoagulant factors):** For example, antithrombin III deficiency, protein C and S deficiency • **Increased prothrombotic factors:** Factor V mutation (factor V Leiden) prothrombin mutation, homocystinuria
Secondary (acquired)	• **High-risk for thrombosis:** Prolonged bed rest or immobilization, myocardial infarction, tissue injury (e.g. surgery, fracture, burn), disseminated intravascular coagulation, cancer, prosthetic cardiac valves • **Lower risk for thrombosis:** Nephrotic syndrome, hyperestrogenic states (pregnancy and postpartum), oral contraceptive use, smoking, sickle cell anemia

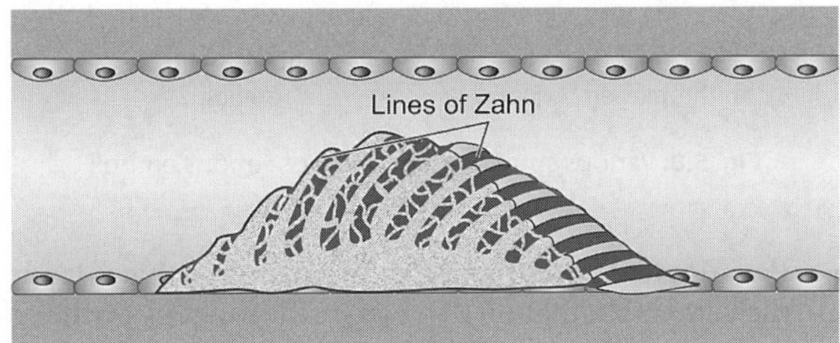

Fig. 5.6: Diagrammatic appearance of thrombus showing alternating dark and light areas (lines of Zahn)

lumen), whereas thrombi in the medium or smaller vessels are usually **occlusive (occludes the lumen of the blood vessel).**

- **Venous thrombosis (phlebothrombosis):** It is invariably **occlusive** and develops at sites of stasis. Deep veins of the lower extremity is the commonest site (90% of cases).

Fate of the Thrombus (Fig. 5.7)

- **Dissolution/lysis:** The thrombi may undergo lysis.
- **Propagation (process of spreading):** Thrombi may grow and increase in size in the direction of blood flow and this process is known as propagation.
- **Embolization:** Thrombus may get detached or separated from its site of origin and travel as emboli to other sites in the vasculature.
- **Organization (replacement of thrombus by fibrous tissue):** Older thrombi become organized by the ingrowth of endothelial cells, smooth muscle cells and fibroblasts.
- **Recanalization:** New capillary channels (pathways) may form in an organized thrombus. These channels can re-establish the continuity of the original lumen and is known as recanalization.

Clinical Consequences

Thrombi may cause **obstruction of arteries and veins,** and are **sources of emboli**. Venous thrombi can cause

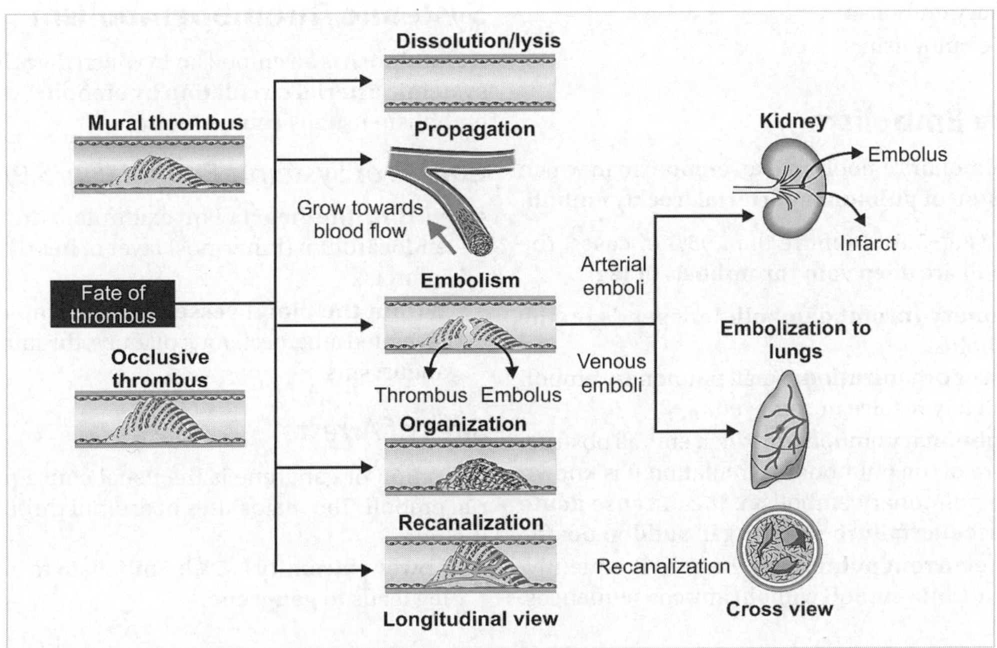

Fig. 5.7: Fate of thrombus

edema in vascular beds distal to site of obstruction by thrombi. Thrombi can detach and **embolize** to the lungs and cause death. The arterial thrombi can embolize and cause **infarctions** in the organs in which it lodges.

Venous Thrombosis (Phlebothrombosis)

Most venous thrombi develop in the superficial or deep veins of the leg. **Deep venous thrombosis (DVT)** occurs in popliteal, femoral, and iliac veins. They more frequently embolize to the lungs which causes pulmonary infarction. Small thrombi may be asymptomatic. Some patients have calf tenderness, with forced dorsiflexion of the foot (**Homan sign**).

EMBOLISM

Definition: An **embolus is a detached intravascular solid, liquid, or gaseous mass** that is **carried in the circulation to a site distant from its point of origin**.

Classification

- **Depending on physical nature of the emboli:**
  - **Solid:** Thromboemboli, atheromatous material, tumor emboli
  - **Liquid:** Fat, bone marrow and amniotic fluid emboli
  - **Gaseous:** Air or other gases.
- **Depending on source:** It may be **cardiac emboli, arterial emboli, venous emboli or lymphatic emboli**.
- **Depending on the site of arrest of emboli:**
  - Pulmonary embolism
  - Systemic embolism.

Pulmonary Embolism

Definition: Pulmonary embolism is an **embolism** in which there is **occlusion of pulmonary arterial tree by emboli**.

Site of origin (Fig. 5.8)**:** In more than 95% of cases, the source of emboli are **deep vein thrombosis of leg**.

Fate of pulmonary thromboemboli: It depends on the size of the embolus.

- **Resolution or organization:** Small pulmonary emboli may completely resolve or removed.
- **Massive pulmonary embolism:** When emboli obstruct 60% or more of the pulmonary circulation it is known as massive pulmonary embolism. It can cause **acute right ventricular failure resulting in sudden death**.
- **Multiple, recurrent pulmonary emboli:** Frequently, there are **multiple emboli** without any consequences.

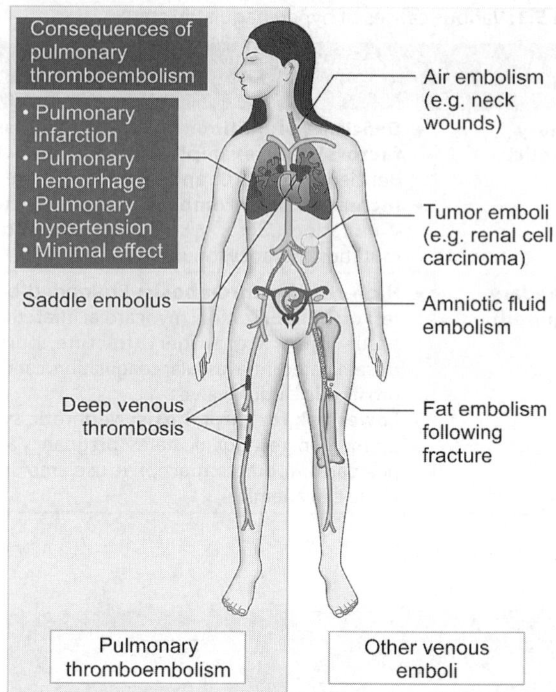

Fig. 5.8: Various sources and effects of venous emboli

- **Paradoxical embolism:** It refers to emboli that arise in the venous circulation and bypass the lungs by traveling through an interatrial (incompletely closed foramen ovale) or interventricular defect.

Systemic Thromboembolism

Definition: It is an embolism in which there is **occlusion of systemic arterial circulation by emboli**. Systemic arterial embolism usually causes infarcts.

Causes of Systemic Emboli (Fig. 5.9)

- **Within the heart:** For example, thrombi over the endocardium (innermost layer of heart) of myocardial infarcts.
- **Within the blood vessels:** For example, thrombi on ulcerated atherosclerotic plaques, thrombi within aortic aneurysms.

Sites of Arrest

Infarction or gangrene is the usual consequence of arterial emboli. The major sites of arterial thromboembolism include:

- **Lower extremity** (75%)**:** Embolism to an artery of the leg leads to **gangrene**.

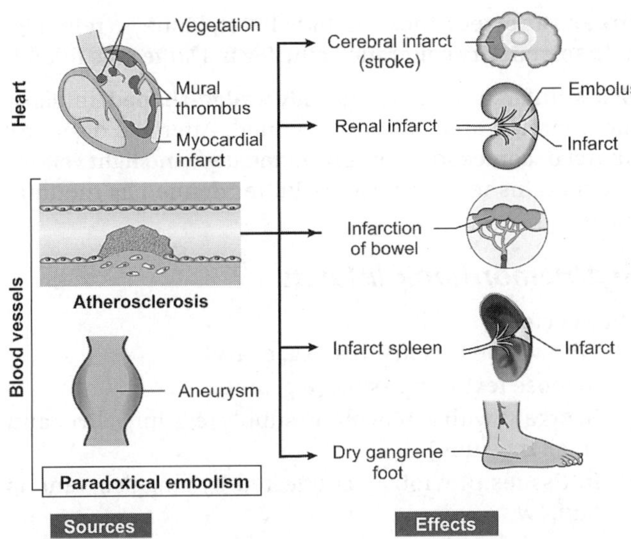

Fig. 5.9: Various sources and effects of systemic arterial emboli

- **Brain:** Arterial emboli to the brain cause **ischemic necrosis** (stroke).
- **Intestine:** In the mesenteric circulation, emboli cause bowel **infarction**.
- **Kidney:** Renal artery embolism may cause renal **infarct**.
- **Blood vessels:** Cause inflammation of arteries leading to **mycotic aneurysm**.
- Others including spleen and upper extremities are involved to a lesser extent.

Fat and Marrow Embolism

Fat embolism is release of **emboli of fat globules** (from adipose tissue injury), and fatty marrow into ruptured blood vessels. **Fat embolism syndrome** is the term applied to patients who become symptomatic due to severe fat embolism. It occurs in only minority of patients.

Causes

- **Severe trauma to fat-containing tissue**, particularly accompanying **bone fractures**
- Rarely, soft tissue trauma and burns.

Pathogenesis

Probably involves both mechanical obstruction and biochemical injury.

- **Mechanical obstruction:** Fat microemboli favors aggregation of red cell and platelet with fat emboli. These aggregates can occlude the pulmonary and cerebral microvasculature.
- **Biochemical injury:** Free fatty acids released from fat globules/fat emboli may cause local toxic injury to endothelium, and platelet activation.

Sites of arrest of fat emboli: Lungs, brain, kidneys and other organs.

Clinical presentation: Fat embolism may be asymptomatic or in its most severe form manifest as fatal fat embolism syndrome.

Air Embolism

Air embolism develops when **air is introduced** into venous or arterial **circulation.**

Causes: Air may enter the venous circulation through **neck wounds, chest wall injury, thoracocentesis** (surgical puncture of thoracic cavity with a needle for aspiration of pleural fluid), or punctures of the great veins during **surgery/invasive procedures** or hemodialysis (type of dialysis for the removal of certain elements from the blood). It may also develop during criminal abortion.

Decompression Sickness

It is a form of gas embolism. It may be acute or chronic.

Cause

It occurs when an individual is exposed to sudden decrease in atmospheric pressure. Such sudden change of pressure can develop in **scuba** and **deep sea divers** and **underwater construction workers** (e.g. tunnels, drilling platform construction). Decompression sickness may also develop in individuals in unpressurized aircraft.

Mechanism

- At high pressure (e.g. during a deep sea dive), when air is inhaled large amounts of inert gas (nitrogen) are dissolved in the blood, body fluids and tissues.
- When the deep sea diver ascends (depressurizes), the gas (particularly nitrogen) is released from solution in the tissues. However, if they ascend too rapidly, gas bubbles form in the circulation and within tissues, obstructing blood flow and directly injure the cells.

Effects

- **Musculoskeletal system:** The gas bubbles in the vasculature of muscle and joints causes muscular and joint pains. This painful condition is called the **bends.**
- **Respiratory system:** In the lungs, gas bubbles in the vasculature, lead to respiratory distress called the **chokes.**
- **Nervous system:** Severe involvement of cerebral blood vessels obstruction by gas may cause delerium, coma or death.

Caisson Disease

Chronic form of decompression sickness is called caisson disease. The gas emboli in vessel lead to vascular obstruction and cause multiple foci of **ischemic (avascular) necrosis of bone**, the more common sites are the head of the femur, tibia and humerus.

Amniotic Fluid Embolism

It is characterized by the **entry of amniotic fluid** containing fetal cells and debris **into the maternal circulation** through open uterine and cervical veins (veins of uterine cervix). Amniotic fluid embolism is a rare maternal dangerous complication which occurs at the end of labor and the immediate postpartum period.

Mechanism: Amniotic emboli are composed of the solid epithelial constituents (squames) which enter the pulmonary circulation of the mother. The amniotic fluid has a high thromboplastin (**thrombogenic** substances) activity which **initiates** a potentially fatal **disseminated intravascular coagulation.**

Clinical features: It is characterized by sudden onset of severe dyspnea, cyanosis, neurologic impairment ranging from headache to seizures, shock, followed by coma and death.

INFARCTION

Definition: An infarct is defined as a **localized area of ischemic necrosis** caused by **occlusion of either the arterial supply or the venous drainage**. The process is known as infarction.

Common and important infarcts: Myocardial infarction (heart), cerebral infarction (brain) and pulmonary infarction (lung).

Causes: Arterial occlusion is the most important cause of infarction. The common cause is occlusion of vessel by **thrombus or emboli**.

Morphology

Classification: Infarcts are classified according to the color as white/pale (anemic) or red (hemorrhagic).

White/Pale Infarcts

They occur:

- With arterial occlusions
- In solid organs
- With end-arterial circulation (e.g. heart, spleen and kidney), without a dual blood supply.

Organs affected: These include heart, kidneys (refer Fig. 2.7), spleen. Dry gangrene of the leg is a large pale infarct.

Gross: Infarcts tend to be usually **wedge-shaped.** Initially, the infarcted area is poorly defined. After 1–2 days, the infarct becomes soft, sharply delineated, and light yellow. The margins tend to become better defined as the time passes.

Red/Hemorrhagic Infarcts

They occur:

- With venous occlusions (e.g. ovary)
- In loose textured tissues (e.g. lung)
- In organs with a dual blood supply (e.g. lung, liver and small intestine)
- In tissues previously congested by sluggish venous outflow.

Gross: Red infarcts are sharply circumscribed, firm and dark red to purple.

Microscopy of Infarct

Both pale and red infarct show **ischemic coagulative necrosis.** However, **infarct in brain shows liquefactive necrosis.**

Factors that Influence Development of an Infarct

The major factors that determine the outcome are:

- Nature of the vascular supply
- Rate of occlusion development
- Vulnerability to hypoxia
- Oxygen content of blood.

SHOCK

Definition: Shock is a pathological process characterized by **intense failure of the circulatory system to maintain an appropriate blood supply to the microcirculation.** This results in life-threatening inadequate perfusion (**hypoperfusion**) of vital organs.

Types of shock: The causes of shock fall into three general categories (Table 5.2).

Pathogenesis of Cardiogenic Shock

Cardiogenic shock is due to **failure of myocardial pump.** The various causes (Table 5.2) lead to decrease in the cardiac output and perfusion of tissue. The left-sided failure also obstructs the entry of blood from pulmonary vein into the left atrium. This causes movement of fluid from

Table 5.2: Three major types of shock

Type	Causes
Cardiogenic	• Myocardial infarction • Ventricular rupture • Arrhythmia • Cardiac tamponade (pathologic compression of heart) • Pulmonary embolism
Hypovolemic	Fluid loss (e.g. hemorrhage, vomiting, diarrhea, burns)
Septic	Severe microbial infections (bacterial and fungal)
Less common types Neurogenic shock Anaphylactic shock	During anesthetic accident or a spinal cord injury IgE–mediated (type I) hypersensitivity reaction

pulmonary vessels into the pulmonary interstitial space and later into the alveoli (pulmonary edema).

Pathogenesis of Hypovolemic Shock

Inadequate blood or plasma volume due to various causes leads to **hypovolemia** (abnormal decrease in the volume of circulating blood) and hypotension. The result is inadequate perfusion of tissues.

Pathogenesis of Septic Shock

Causative Organisms

Septic shock is most commonly due to infections by Gram-positive bacteria, followed by Gram-negative bacteria and fungi.

Major Pathogenic Pathways in Septic Shock (Fig. 5.10)

The major factors contributing to pathophysiology of septic shock are: Inflammatory mediators, endothelial cell activation and injury, metabolic abnormalities, immune suppression and organ dysfunction.

Inflammatory mediators: Microbial components can activate the following:

- **Activation of neutrophils and macrophages**
- **Activation of the complement cascade.**

Endothelial cell activation and injury: Microbial constituents, inflammatory mediators produced by leukocytes, hypoperfusion and activation of complement cascade cause endothelial activation or injury. This leads to thrombi in small vessels, increased vascular permeability and vasodilatation. The net result is **decreased oxygen and nutrient supply to the tissues** due to hypoperfusion and dysfunction of many organs.

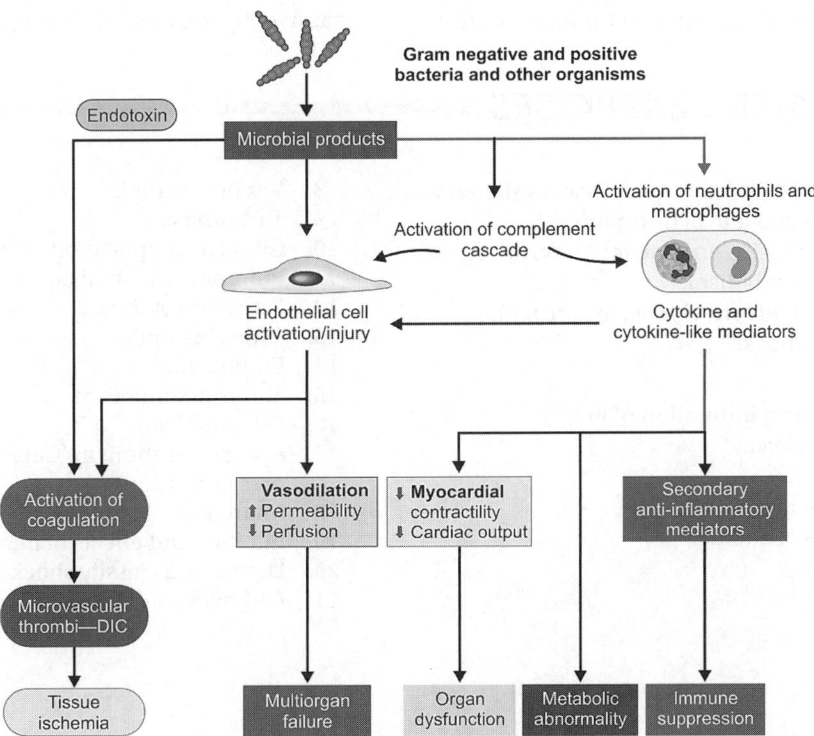

Fig. 5.10: Major pathogenic mechanisms in septic shock. Microbial products activate endothelial cells and cascade of events that lead to end-stage multiorgan failure

Metabolic abnormalities: Septic patients show hyperglycemia due to the action of cytokines. The hyperglycemia decreases neutrophil function and suppresses bactericidal activity.

Immune suppression: The hyperinflammatory state initiated by sepsis can suppress the immune system.

Organ dysfunction: High levels of cytokines and secondary mediators may **diminish myocardial contractility and cardiac output**. Ultimately, there may be **failure of multiple organs**, such as the kidneys, liver, lungs and heart, terminating in death.

Stages of Shock

Shock is a progressive disorder. If not corrected, it can lead to death. The exact mechanism(s) of death from sepsis is not clear. Shock evolves through three general phases:

Nonprogressive (Compensated/Reversible) Phase

During the initial phase, various compensatory mechanisms develop and **redistribute the blood** in such a way that the **perfusion of vital organs is maintained**.

Progressive Phase

If the underlying causes are not corrected, shock passes to the progressive phase. During this phase, there is widespread tissue hypoperfusion, tissue **hypoxia** and **blood** begins to **pool in the microcirculation.** This **worsens the cardiac output** and there will be widespread hypoxic damage to the vital organs and they begin to fail.

Irreversible Phase

Without intervention, the shock enters an irreversible stage. Widespread cell injury further aggravates the shock state. **Acute renal failure** may develop and cause death.

Morphology

- **Kidney: Acute tubular necrosis** (acute renal failure).
- **Lungs:** Lungs may show **diffuse alveolar damage** which can result in acute respiratory distress syndrome **(ARDS)** also called shock lung. On microscopic examination, **hyaline membrane** is seen lining the alveolar surface.
- **Disseminated intravascular coagulation (DIC)** with **widespread** deposition of fibrin-rich **microthrombi**, particularly in the brain, heart, lungs, kidney, adrenal glands and gastrointestinal tract.

Prognosis

- Patients with hypovolemic shock survive with appropriate management.
- Septic shock, or cardiogenic shock associated with massive myocardial infarction, prognosis is worse.

SELF-ASSESSMENT EXERCISES

I. Essay

1. Define thrombus/thrombosis. Discuss the etiopathogenesis and fate of thrombus.
2. Define and classify embolism. Describe types and sequel of embolism.
3. Define and classify shock. Discuss the pathogenesis of septic shock.

II. Short Notes

1. CVC lung/brown induration of lung.
2. Nutmeg/CVC liver.
3. Define edema.
4. Localized edema.
5. Pathogenesis of edema.
6. Renal edema.
7. Transudate.
8. Virchow's triad.
9. Thrombosis.
10. Clinical complications of thrombosis.
11. Pulmonary embolism.
12. Fate of thrombus.
13. Types of emboli.
14. Embolism.
15. Thromboembolism.
16. Fat embolism.
17. Air/gas embolism/Caissons disease/decompression sickness.
18. Infarction.
19. Etiology and effects of infarct.
20. Define and classify shock.
21. Pathogenesis of shock.

CHAPTER 6

Immunopathology

CHAPTER OUTLINE

- Immunity
- Hypersensitivity: Immunologically Mediated Tissue Injury
- Immediate (Type I) Hypersensitivity
- Antibody-Mediated (Type II) Hypersensitivity
- Immune Complex–Mediated (Type III) Hypersensitivity
- T Cell-Mediated (Type IV) Hypersensitivity
- Autoimmune Diseases
- Systemic Lupus Erythematosus
- Acquired Immunodeficiency Syndrome
- Amyloidosis

The normal immune system is essential for protection against infection. Immune system is like a double-edged sword. Though it is protective in most of the situations, sometimes an hyperactive immune system may cause fatal diseases.

IMMUNITY

Definition: Immunity is **resistance** (defense mechanism) exhibited **by host against invasion by any foreign antigen**, including microorganisms.

Types: There are two types namely innate and adaptive immunity.

Innate (Natural/Native) Immunity

General Features

- **First line of defense present by birth.**
- **Does not depend on the prior contact** with foreign antigen or microbes.
- **Lacks specificity**, but **highly effective**. No memory, and no self/non-self recognition.
- **No memory** is seen.
- It functions in stages: (1) recognition of microbes and damaged cells, (2) activation of various mechanisms, and (3) elimination of the unwanted substances.

Functions of Innate Immune Response

- **Inflammation** and destruction of invading microbe.
- **Antiviral defense.**

Adaptive Immunity

If the innate immune system fails to provide effective protection against invading microbes, the adaptive immune system is activated.

General Features

- **Second line of defense** acquired during life.
- **Takes more time to develop** and is **more powerful than innate immunity**.
- **Long-lasting protection.**
- Prior exposure to antigen is present.
- Three **characteristic features** are: (1) **specificity**, (2) **diversity,** and (3) **memory.**

Functions of Adaptive Immune Response

- **Antibodies:** Protection against extracellular microbes in the blood, mucosal secretions and tissues.
- **T-lymphocytes:** Defense against viruses, fungi and intracellular bacteria either by direct killing of infected cells.

HYPERSENSITIVITY: IMMUNOLOGICALLY MEDIATED TISSUE INJURY

Immune response is usually a protective process but sometimes it may be injurious. Hypersensitivity means that

Table 6.1: Classification of hypersensitivity reaction according to the effector immune mechanism

Types	Effectors
1. Immediate hypersensitivity reaction (type I hypersensitivity) 2. Antibody-mediated disorders (type II hypersensitivity) 3. Immune complex-mediated disorders (type III hypersensitivity)	Antibody molecules
4. Cell-mediated immune disorders (type IV hypersensitivity)	Antigen-specific effector T-cells

the body responds to a particular antigens in an exaggerated fashion, which does not happen in normal circumstances. **Injurious immune reactions are called *hypersensitivity*.**

Definition: Hypersensitivity reaction is a **pathological, excessive, and injurious immune response to antigen leading to tissue injury**, **disease** or sometimes death **in a sensitized individual**. The resulting diseases are named as hypersensitivity diseases.

Classification of Hypersensitivity Reactions (Table 6.1)

Hypersensitivity diseases are classified on the basis of the immunologic mechanism that mediates the disease. This classification helps in distinguishing the manner in which the immune response causes tissue injury and disease, and also the pathological and clinical manifestations. However, multiple mechanisms may be operative in any one hypersensitivity disease.

IMMEDIATE(TYPE I)HYPERSENSITIVITY

Usually known as **allergic or atopic disorders** and the environmental antigens that elicit these reactions are known as **allergens**.

Definition: Type I hypersensitivity reaction is a type of immunological tissue reaction, which **occurs rapidly (within 5–10 minute) after the interaction of antigen** (allergen) **with a IgE antibody on the surface of the mast cells in a previously sensitized person** (refer pages 316–319).

Characteristics

- **Immediate** reaction occurring within 5–10 minutes.
- **Antibodies:** Mediated by IgE antibody.
- **Develops after the interaction of an antigen with IgE bodies** bound to **mast cells.**
- **Genetic susceptibility:** Occurs in genetically susceptible individuals **previously sensitized** to the antigen.
- **Antigens (allergens):** Many allergens (e.g. house dust mites, pollens, animal danders or moulds) in the environment are **harmless for majority of individuals.** Allergens elicit significant IgE reactions only in **genetically predisposed individuals**, who are said to be **atopic**.

Sequence of Events (Flowchart 6.1)

During Initial Exposure to Antigen (Sensitization)

In a genetically susceptible individual, the following events occur:

- **Exposure to sensitizing antigen:** Individuals are exposed to environmental allergens and may be introduced by: **(1) inhalation, (2) ingestion, or (3) injection.**
- **Production of IgE antibody:** By B cells.
- **Sensitization of mast cells by IgE antibody:** IgE antibodies produced by B cells, attach to the mast cells.

During Subsequent Exposure to Antigen

In sensitized individual (the mast cell has attached IgE antibodies), during subsequent re-exposure to the specific allergen, following events occur:

Flowchart 6.1: Sequence of events in type I hypersensitivity. A. It is initiated by the exposure to an allergen, which stimulates IgE production. IgE binds to mast cells; B. On re-exposure to the allergen, antigen binds to IgE on the mast cells and activates it to secrete the mediators. These mediators produce the manifestations of type I hypersensitivity

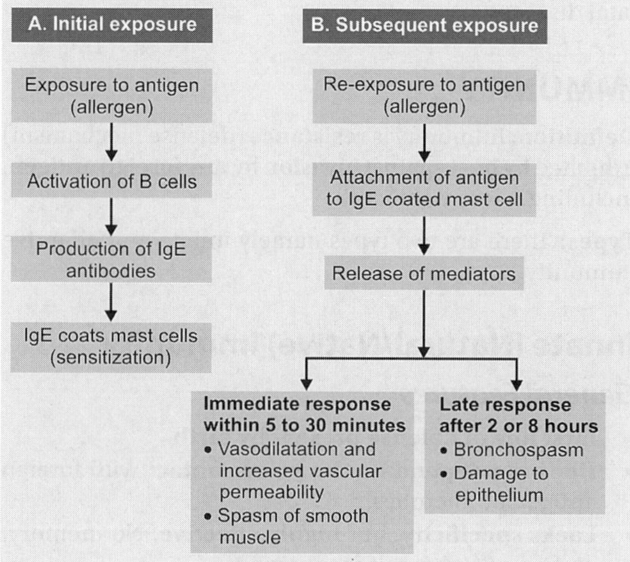

- **Mast cell activation:** The **antigen (allergen) binds** to the more than one **IgE antibody molecules on mast cells** and generate signals that **causes mast cell degranulation.** It results in **secretion of mediators**.
- **Two phases:** IgE triggered reactions can be divided into two phases:
  1. **Immediate response:** Develops **within 5–30 minutes** after exposure to an allergen and **subside in 60 minutes**. Characterized by **vasodilation, vascular leakage**, and **smooth muscle spasm or glandular secretions**.
  2. **Late-phase reaction:** Develops in **2–8 hours after** the exposure to antigen which may **last for several days**.

Clinical Manifestations

Systemic Anaphylaxis

- **Acute, potentially fatal form** and known as anaphylaxis (ana = without, phylaxis = protection).
- Usually **follows injection of an antigen into a sensitized individual**.
- **Causes:** It develops:
  - After **administration of foreign proteins** (e.g. antisera), **drugs** (e.g. penicillin), hormones, and enzymes.
  - Following exposure to **food allergens** (e.g. peanuts, shellfish) or **insect toxins** (e.g. bee venom).
- **Clinical features:**
  - Itching, hives, and skin erythema appear within minutes after exposure.
  - Followed by difficulty in breathing and respiratory distress due to contraction of respiratory bronchioles.
  - Laryngeal edema results in hoarseness and laryngeal obstruction, which further aggravates respiratory difficulty.
  - Vomiting, abdominal cramps, diarrhea may follow.
  - May lead to shock and death within the hour.

Local Reactions

- Recurrent and nonfatal. Site of local reaction depends on the portal of entry of the allergen.
- **Causes:** Develop against common environmental allergens, such as pollen, animal dander, house dust, and foods.

Atopy

Susceptibility to type I hypersensitivity reactions is genetically determined. Atopy refers to a familial predisposition to produce an **exaggerated localized immediate hypersensitivity** (IgE-mediated) **reactions to inhaled and ingested environmental** substances (allergens) that are otherwise harmless.

Examples of type I hypersensitivity reactions are listed in Table 6.2.

Table 6.2: Examples of type I hypersensitivity reactions

Localized type I hypersensitivity	Systemic type I hypersensitivity
• Bronchial asthma (extrinsic) • Hay fever/allergic rhinitis • Allergic conjunctivitis • Urticaria • Atopic dermatitis/eczema	Anaphylaxis due to: • Antibiotics: Most commonly penicillin • Bee stings • Insect bite • Foreign proteins (e.g. antisera)

ANTIBODY-MEDIATED (TYPE II) HYPERSENSITIVITY

Definition: Type II hypersensitivity disorders are **caused by antibodies (IgG/IgM)**, which react with **target antigens on the surface of cells or fixed in the extracellular matrix.**

Characteristics

Antibodies: IgG (usually) and IgM (rarely) type of antibodies mediate type II reactions.

Antigen: It may be endogenous or exogenous.

- **Endogenous antigens:** It may be normal molecules intrinsic to the cell membrane or extracellular matrix (e.g. autoimmune diseases).
- **Exogenous antigens:** These antigens may get adsorbed on a cell surface or extracellular matrix and may cause altered surface antigen (e.g. drug metabolite).

Mechanisms of Injury

Mechanism of tissue injury can be broadly divided into: **(1) complement dependent** (autoimmune hemolytic anemia, immune thrombocytopenic purpura, transfusion of incompatible blood) **and (2) antibody-dependent** (myasthenia gravis, Graves, disease).

IMMUNE COMPLEX–MEDIATED (TYPE III) HYPERSENSITIVITY

Definition: Type III hypersensitivity reactions are **characterized by formation of immune** (antigen and antibody) **complexes in the circulation** and may **get deposited in blood vessels, leading to complement activation and acute inflammation**. The inflammatory cells recruited (neutrophils and monocytes) **release**

lysosomal enzymes which generate toxic free radicals and cause tissue damage.

Characteristics

Antibodies: Complement-fixing antibodies namely IgG, IgM, and occasionally IgA.

Antigen:

- **Exogenous:** Various **foreign proteins**, e.g. foreign serum protein injected (e.g. diphtheria antitoxin, horse antithymocyte globulin) or produced by an infectious microbe.
- **Endogenous: Antibody against self-components** (autoimmunity), e.g. nucleoproteins.

Sites of Antigen-antibody Formation

- **Circulating immune complexes:** They are **formed within the circulation.**
- **In situ immune complex:** Less frequently, the immune complexes may be formed at sites where antigen has been "planted" previously producing in situ immune complexes.

Sites of Immune Complex Deposition

- **Systemic:** Circulating **immune complexes** may be **deposited in many organs.**
- **Localized:** Immune complexes may be **deposited or formed in particular organs/tissues**: **Kidney** (glomerulonephritis), **joints** (arthritis), **small blood vessels of the skin.**

Examples of immune complex disorders are listed in Table 6.3.

T CELL-MEDIATED (TYPE IV) HYPERSENSITIVITY

- Type IV hypersensitivity reaction is **mediated by T-lymphocytes.**
- It develops in response to antigenic exposure in a previously sensitized individual.

Table 6.3: Examples of immune complex-mediated diseases

Disease	Antigen	Manifestations
Exogenous antigen		
Poststreptococcal glomerulonephritis	Streptococcal cell wall antigen(s)	Glomerulonephritis
Endogenous antigen		
Systemic lupus erythematosus (SLE)	Nuclear antigens	Glomerulonephritis, skin lesions, arthritis, others

Box 6.1: Examples of T cell-mediated (type IV) hypersensitivity

Disease
- Type 1 diabetes mellitus
- Rheumatoid arthritis
- Inflammatory bowel disease
- Hashimoto thyroiditis
- Contact sensitivity (dermatitis)

Table 6.4: Examples of autoimmune diseases

Diseases mediated by antibodies	Diseases mediated by T cells
Organ-specific	**Organ-specific**
Autoimmune hemolytic anemia	Type 1 diabetes mellitus
Autoimmune thrombocytopenia	Hashimoto thyroiditis
Goodpasture syndrome	Crohn's disease
Myasthenia gravis	Multiple sclerosis
Graves' disease	
Systemic	**Systemic**
Systemic lupus erythematosus (SLE)	Rheumatoid arthritis

- Reaction is delayed by 48–72 hours after exposure to antigen. Hence, also called as delayed-type hypersensitivity (DTH).
- This hypersensitivity reaction is involved in several **autoimmune diseases** (e.g. rheumatoid arthritis, Hashimoto thyroiditis), pathological **reactions to environmental chemicals** (e.g. poison ivy, nickel) and **persistent microbes (e.g. tuberculosis, leprosy).**

Examples of T cell-mediated (type IV) hypersensitivity are shown in Box 6.1.

AUTOIMMUNE DISEASES

Definition: Autoimmunity is defined as **immune reactions** in which **body produces autoantibodies** and **immunologically competent T- lymphocytes against self-antigens.**

Autoimmunity is an important cause of certain diseases in humans (Table 6.4).

- **Organ-specific disease:** It may be restricted to a single organ or tissue (e.g. type 1 diabetes).
- **Systemic or generalized disease:** For example, systemic lupus erythematosus (SLE).
- **Involving more than one organ:** For example, Goodpasture's syndrome, in which lung and kidney are involved.

General Features of Autoimmune Diseases

- Autoimmune diseases are usually chronic, sometimes with relapses and remissions.

- Damage caused is often progressive.
- Clinical and pathological features of an autoimmune disease depend on the nature of the underlying immune response.

SYSTEMIC LUPUS ERYTHEMATOSUS

Systemic lupus erythematosus (SLE) is a **chronic autoimmune disease** having following characteristics:

1. **Protean manifestation and variable behavior**.
2. **Remission and relapses.**
3. **Multisystemic involvement:** Mainly affects **skin, kidneys, joints, serous membranes and heart**.
4. **Broad spectrum of autoantibodies**, most important is antinuclear antibodies (ANAs).

Etiology

Systemic lupus erythematosus is an **autoimmune disease** in which fundamental defect is **failure of self-tolerance**. It leads to production of **many autoantibodies** that **damages the tissue either directly or indirectly by depositing immune complex deposits**. A combination of genetic and environmental factors plays a role in the pathogenesis of SLE.

Genetic Factors

Evidence to support genetic predisposition are:

- **Familial association: Family members** of SLE patients have an **increased risk** of SLE. About 20% of unaffected first-degree relatives may show autoantibodies. **High rate** of concordance (>25%) in **monozygotic twins** when compared with dizygotic twins (1–3%).
- **HLA association:** Risk is more with HLA-DR2 or HLA-DR3.
- Other genetic factors.

Immunological Abnormalities

Several immunological abnormalities of both **innate** and **adaptive immune** system have been observed in SLE.

Environmental Factors

- **Ultraviolet (UV) radiation:** Exposure to sunlight exacerbates the lesions of the disease.
- **Cigarette smoking:** It is associated with development of SLE.
- **Sex hormones:** SLE is 10 times greater during the reproductive period (17–55 years) **in women** than in men. SLE shows exacerbation during normal menses and pregnancy.
- **Drugs:** Examples include **hydralazine, procainamide, isoniazid, and D-penicillamine** can produce SLE-like disease and disease remits after withdrawal of the drug.

Autoantibodies in SLE

Systemic lupus erythematosus is characterized by the production of **several diverse autoantibodies**. Some antibodies are against different nuclear and cytoplasmic components of the cell that are not organ specific. Other antibodies are directed against specific cell surface antigens of blood cells.

Antinuclear antibodies (ANAs): They are directed against various nuclear antigens including DNA, RNA, and proteins (all together called generic ANAs).

Morphology

SLE is a systemic autoimmune disease and morphologic changes in SLE are **extremely variable**.

The most **characteristic lesions** of SLE are **due to deposition of immune complexes** in **blood vessels, kidneys, connective tissue, and skin**.

Clinical Features

- SLE is a **multisystem** disease with **variable clinical presentation**.
- **Age:** It usually occurs in young woman between **20 to 30 years**, but may manifest at any age.
- **Sex:** It predominantly affects **women**, with female-to-male ratio of 9: 1.
- **Onset:** Acute or insidious with fever.
- **Typical presentation: Butterfly rash over the face, fever, pain** without deformity in one or more **peripheral joints, pleuritic chest pain, and photosensitivity**. SLE patients are **susceptible to infections**, because of immune dysfunction and treatment with immunosuppressive drugs.

ACQUIRED IMMUNODEFICIENCY SYNDROME

Acquired immunodeficiency syndrome (AIDS) is caused by the retrovirus **human immunodeficiency virus** (HIV).

Characteristic Features

- **Infection and depletion of CD4+ T-lymphocytes**.
- **Severe immunosuppression → leads to opportunistic infections, secondary neoplasms, and neurologic manifestations**.

Route of Transmission

Transmission of HIV occurs when there is an exchange of blood or body fluids containing the virus or virus-infected cells. The three major routes of transmission are:

1. **Sexual transmission:** It is the **main route of infection** in more than 75% of cases of HIV.
2. **Parenteral transmission:** Three groups of individuals are at risk.
   - **Intravenous drug abusers:** Transmission occurs by **sharing of needles, and syringes contaminated** with HIV-containing blood.
   - **Hemophiliacs:** Mainly those who received large amount of factor VIII and factor IX concentrates before 1985. Now increasing use of recombinant clotting factors have eliminated this mode of transmission.
   - **Transfusion of blood or blood components:** Recipients of blood transfusion of **HIV-infected whole blood or components** (e.g. platelets, plasma) was one of the modes of transmission.
3. **Perinatal transmission (mother-to-infant transmission):**
   - **Major mode of transmission of AIDS in children.**
   - Transmission of infection can occur by **three routes:**
     - **In utero:** It is transmitted by transplacental spread.
     - **Perinatal spread:** During normal vaginal delivery or child birth (intrapartum) **through an infected birth canal** and in the immediate period (peripartum).
     - **After birth:** It is transmitted by ingestion of breast milk or from the genital secretions.

Transmission of HIV infection to healthcare workers: There is an extremely small risk of transmission to healthcare professionals, after accidental needle-stick injury or exposure of nonintact skin to infected blood.

Etiology

Properties of HIV

AIDS is caused by HIV, which is a **nontransforming human retrovirus** belonging to the lentivirus family. Retroviruses are **RNA viruses having an enzyme called reverse transcriptase**, which **prepares a DNA copy of the RNA genome of the virus in host cell.**

Genetic forms: HIV occurs in two genetically different but related main forms, **HIV-1 and HIV-2**.

- **HIV-1** is most common in the United States, Europe, and Central Africa.
- **HIV-2 is common** in West Africa and India.

Structure of HIV (Fig. 6.1)

- HIV-1 is **spherical enveloped** virus which is about 90–120 nm in diameter.
- It consists of electron-dense, cone-shaped core surrounded by nucleocapsid cell which is covered by lipoprotein envelope.
  - **Viral core** contains:
    - **Major capsid protein p24:** This viral antigen and the antibodies against this are **used for the diagnosis of HIV infection** in enzyme-linked immunosorbent assay (**ELISA**).
    - **Nucleocapsid protein p7/p9.**

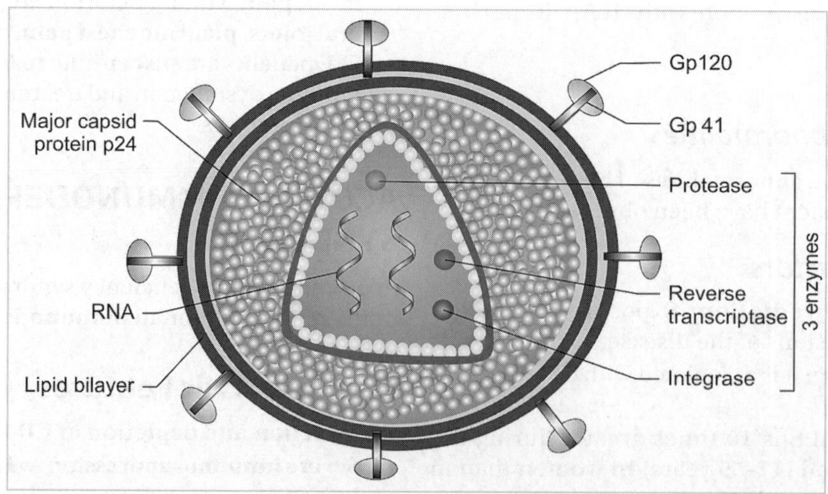

Fig. 6.1: Diagrammatic representation of structure of the human immune deficiency virus (HIV)–1 virion. The viral particle is covered by a lipid bilayer derived from the host cell and studded with viral glycoproteins gp 41 and gp120

- **Two identical copies of single stranded RNA genome.**
- **Three viral enzymes: (1) Protease, (2) reverse transcriptase** (RNA-dependent DNA polymerase), and **(3) integrase.**

- **Nucleocapsid:** The **viral core is surrounded by a matrix protein p24 and p17**, which **lies underneath the lipid envelope** of the virion.
- **Lipid envelope:** The virus contains a lipoprotein envelope, which **consist of lipid derived from the host cell and two viral glycoproteins**. These glycoproteins are: **(1) gp 120** which project as a knob-like spikes on the surface and **(2) gp 41** anchoring transmembrane pedicle. **These glycoproteins are essential for HIV infection of cells.**

Natural History of HIV Infection

Virus usually enters the body through mucosal epithelia and clinical course can be divided into three main phases:

- **Early acute phase:** It may present as an acute, usually **self-limited nonspecific illness**. These symptoms include **sore throat, myalgias, fever, weight loss, and fatigue. Other features, such as rash, cervical adenopathy**, diarrhea, and vomiting, may also occur.
- **Middle chronic phase:** It may have **few or no clinical manifestations**, and is called the clinical latency period. The **symptoms may be due to minor opportunistic infections**, such as oral candidiasis (thrush), vaginal candidiasis, herpes zoster, and perhaps mycobacterial tuberculosis.
- **Final crisis phase:** It is **final phase of HIV with progression to AIDS**. It presents with **fever, weight loss, diarrhea, generalized lymphadenopathy, multiple opportunistic infections, neurologic disease, and secondary neoplasms**. Most of untreated (but not all) patients with HIV infection **progress to AIDS after a chronic phase lasting from 7 to 10 years.**

The opportunistic infections and neoplasms found in patients with HIV infection are presented in Box 6.2.

Diagnosis of HIV Infection or AIDS

- **ELISA:** Detects antibodies against viral proteins. It is the **most sensitive** and best screening test for the diagnosis of AIDS.
- **Western blot: Most specific** or the **confirmatory test** for HIV.
- **Direct detection of viral infection:**
  - **p24 antigen capture assay.**
  - **Reverse transcriptase polymerase chain reaction (RT-PCR).**
  - **DNA-PCR.**
  - **Culture of virus from the monocytes and CD4+T cells.**

Box 6.2: AIDS-defining opportunistic infections and neoplasms found in patients with HIV infection

Opportunistic Infections
Protozoal and helminthic infections Cryptosporidiosis or isosporidiosis Toxoplasmosis
Fungal infections Pneumocystosis Candidiasis Cryptococcosis Coccidioidomycosis Histoplasmosis
Bacterial infections Mycobacteriosis • Atypical, e.g. *Mycobacterium avium*—intracellulare • *M. tuberculosis* Nocardiosis *Salmonella* infections
Viral infections Cytomegalovirus Herpes simplex virus Varicella-zoster virus Progressive multifocal leukoencephalopathy
Neoplasms Kaposi sarcoma (KS) Non-Hodgkin B-cell lymphoma—Primary lymphoma of the brain Cervical cancer in women Anal carcinoma

Prognosis: The prognosis of AIDS is poor.

AMYLOIDOSIS

Definition: Amyloid is a **pathologic fibrillar protein deposited in the extracellular space** in **various tissues and organs** of the body in variety of clinical condition.

General Features

- **Associated with** number of **inherited and inflammatory disorders.**
- **Extracellular deposits** cause structural and functional damage to involved tissue.
- **Basically a disorder of protein misfolding** and is produced by aggregation of misfolded proteins (normal folded proteins are soluble) or protein fragments.
- It also contains abundant charged sugar groups and has staining characteristics that were thought to resemble

starch (amylose) and were called as amyloid. But these deposits are not related to starch.
- **Usually a systemic** (sometimes localized) disease.

Forms of Amyloid

All amyloid have same morphological and staining property but amyloidosis is **not a single disease**. It is a **group of diseases** having **in common the deposition of similar-appearing proteins** in which biochemical structure (more than 20 different proteins) and mechanism of formation are different.

Physical Nature of Amyloid

All types of amyloid are **composed of nonbranching fibrils of 7 to 10 nm diameter**.
- **Each fibril consists of β-pleated sheet polypeptide chains** and is wound around one another.
- **Congo red dye** binds to these fibrils and produces **classic apple-green birefringence** (dichroism). Hence, Congo red stain is used to identify amyloid deposits in tissues.

Chemical Nature of Amyloid

Fibrillar proteins bind with variety of substances:
- **About 95%** of the amyloid material consists of **fibril proteins**.
- **Remaining 5%** consists of **proteoglycans, glycosaminoglycans, serum amyloid P, etc**.

Biochemical forms of amyloid

It consists of three major distinct proteins and more than 20 minor forms.

A. Major forms: These are **AL**, **AA** and **Aβ amyloid**.
1. **Amyloid light (AL) chain protein:**
   - Consists of **complete immunoglobulin** (Ig) **light chains** or the **aminoterminal fragments of light chains, or both**.
   - **Produced by plasma cells** and associated with some monoclonal B cell proliferation (e.g. plasma cell tumors).
2. **Amyloid-associated (AA) protein:**
   - **Non-immunoglobulin**.
   - **Derived from** a larger precursor in the serum called **serum amyloid-associated (SAA)** protein **synthesized by the liver. Increased synthesis of SAA** protein occurs **during inflammation**.
   - Associated with **chronic inflammation** (called as secondary amyloidosis).
3. **Aβ amyloid:**
   - **Derived from** transmembrane glycoprotein called **amyloid precursor protein (APP)**.
   - **Found in the cerebral lesions** of **Alzheimer disease**.

B. Minor types:
1. **Transthyretin (TTR)**
2. **β_2-microglobulin**
3. **Other minor types:** Serum amyloid P component, proteoglycans, and highly sulfated glycosaminoglycans.

Pathogenesis of Amyloidosis (Fig. 6.2)

Misfolding of Proteins

Amyloidosis is a **disorder due to abnormal folding or misfolding of proteins**.
- **Normally, misfolded proteins are degraded either intracellularly** in proteasomes, or **extracellularly** by macrophages.
- **In amyloidosis**, there is **failure of control mechanism** → production of misfolded proteins, which exceeds the degradation → accumulation outside cells. These misfolded proteins are unstable and self-associated → deposited as fibrils in extracellular tissues.

Categories of Proteins

Misfolded proteins that form amyloid may be the result of:
1. Production of abnormal amounts of normal protein
2. Production of normal amount of mutant protein

Pathological Effects

- **Pressure on adjacent normal cells** → leads to **atrophy of cells.**
- **Deposition in the blood vessel wall** causes:
  - Narrowing of the lumen → lead to **ischemic damage**.
  - **Increased permeability** → escape of protein out of vessel.

Classification of Amyloidosis

Amyloidosis is classified **depending on biochemical and clinical characteristics** (Table 6.5).

Systemic (Generalized)

It involves several organ systems.

Primary amyloidosis

Immunocyte dyscrasias with amyloidosis:
- Usually **systemic** and is of **AL type**.

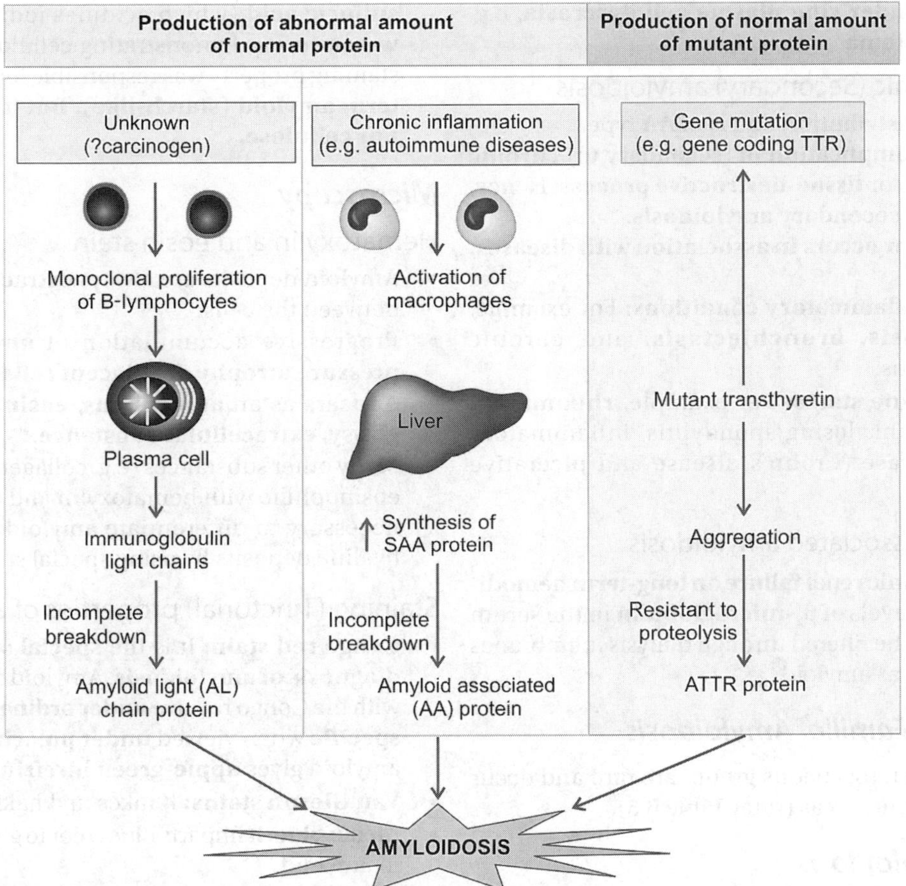

Fig. 6.2: Pathogenesis of amyloidosis. AL protein is seen in association with B-lymphocyte and plasma cell proliferation which secrete immunoglobulin light chains that are amyloidogenic. AA protein is seen in variety of diseases associated with the activation of macrophages, which in turn leads to the synthesis and release of SAA. The SAA is converted to AA protein. ATTR protein is due to mutant proteins which aggregate and deposit as amyloid

Abbreviation: SAA, serum amyloid; ATTR, transthyretin.

Table 6.5: Classification of amyloidosis

Type	Precursor protein	Fibril protein	Associated disease/s
A. Systemic (generalized) amyloidosis			
1. Immunocyte dyscrasias with amyloidosis (primary amyloidosis)	Immunoglobulin light chains (mainly λ)	AL	Multiple myeloma, other plasma cell dyscrasias
2. Reactive systemic amyloidosis (secondary amyloidosis)	Serum amyloid associated (SAA)	AA	Chronic inflammatory process
3. Hemodialysis-associated amyloidosis	β_2-microglobulin	$A\beta_2m$	Chronic renal failure
B. Hereditary or familial amyloidosis			
1. Familial mediterranean fever	SAA	AA	
2. Familial amyloidotic neuropathies 3. Systemic senile amyloidosis	Transthyretin	ATTR	
C. Localized amyloidosis			
1. Senile cerebral	Amyloid precursor protein (APP)	$A\beta$	Alzheimer disease
2. Endocrine			
• Thyroid	Calcitonin	A Cal	Medullary carcinoma
• Islets of Langerhans	Islet amyloid peptide	AIAPP	Type 2 diabetes

- **Many have underlying plasma cell dyscrasia**, e.g. **multiple myeloma.**

Reactive systemic (Secondary) amyloidosis

- **Systemic in distribution** and is of **AA** type.
- Occurs as a **complication of** (secondary to) **chronic inflammatory** or **tissue-destructive process**. Hence, was known as **secondary amyloidosis.**
- **Complicates or occurs in association with diseases,** such as:
  - **Chronic inflammatory conditions:** For example, **tuberculosis, bronchiectasis,** and chronic osteomyelitis.
  - **Autoimmune states:** For example, **rheumatoid arthritis**, ankylosing spondylitis, inflammatory bowel disease (Crohn's disease and ulcerative colitis).

Hemodialysis-associated amyloidosis

Patients with **chronic renal failure on long-term hemodialysis** have high **levels of β_2-microglobulin** in the serum because it cannot be filtered through dialysis membranes → gets deposited as amyloid.

Hereditary or Familial Amyloidosis

It constitutes a heterogeneous group, are rare and occur in certain geographic areas (refer Table 6.5).

Localized Amyloidosis

- Amyloid deposits are **limited to a single organ** (e.g. **heart**) or tissue.
- Either grossly visible as nodular masses or detected only by microscopic examination.
- **Sites:** Lung, larynx, skin, urinary bladder, and tongue.
- **Microscopy:** Amyloid deposits may be surrounded by lymphocytes and plasma cells.

Morphology of Main Organs Involved

- **Secondary amyloidosis:** Kidneys, liver, spleen, lymph nodes, adrenals, and thyroid.
- **Primary amyloidosis:** Heart, GI tract, respiratory tract, peripheral nerves, skin and tongue.

Gross

- May or may not be apparent grossly.
- If large amount accumulates → affected organs are **enlarged, firm and have a waxy appearance**.
- **Cut surface:** If the amyloid deposits are large, **painting** the cut surface **with iodine** gives a **yellow color, which is transformed to blue violet after application of sulfuric acid** (which acidifies iodine). This method was used for demonstrating cellulose or starch. This staining property was responsible for the coining of the **term amyloid (starch-like). But it is neither starch nor cellulose**.

Microscopy

Hematoxylin and eosin stain

- Amyloid deposits are always **extracellular** and begin between the cells.
- Progressive accumulation of **amyloid produces pressure atrophy of adjacent cells**.
- Appears as an **amorphous, eosinophilic, hyaline, glassy, extracellular substance.**
- Many other substances (e.g. collagen, fibrin) also stain eosinophilic with hematoxylin and eosin. Hence, it is necessary to differentiate amyloid from these other hyaline deposits by using special stains.

Staining (Tinctorial) properties of amyloid

- **Congo red stain:** It is the **special stain used for the diagnosis of amyloidosis**. Amyloid **stains pink or red** with the Congo red dye **under ordinary light**. But **more specific** when viewed **under polarizing microscope**; amyloid gives **apple-green birefringence**.
- **Van Gieson stains:** It takes up khaki color.
- **Alcian blue:** It imparts blue color to glycosaminoglycans in amyloid.
- **Periodic acid-Schiff reaction (PAS):** It stains pink.
- **Methyl violet and cresyl violet:** These metachromatic stains give rose pink color.
- **Thioflavin T:** It is not specific for amyloid, but amyloid gives fluorescence when viewed in ultraviolet light.
- **Immunohistochemical staining:** It can distinguish AA, AL, and ATTR types.

Morphology of Major Organs Involved

Kidney

Kidney involvement is the **most common** and the **most serious** form of organ involvement.

- **Gross:** It may be of normal size and color during early stages. In advanced stages, it may be shrunken due to ischemia, which is caused by vascular narrowing induced by the amyloid deposit within arterial and arteriolar walls.
- **Microscopy:** Most commonly renal amyloid is of light-chain (AL) or AA type.
  - **Glomeruli:** It is the main site of amyloid deposition.

- ◆ First, focal deposits within **mesangial matrix**, accompanied by diffuse or nodular thickening of the **glomerular basement membranes**.
- ◆ Later, both the mesangial and basement membranes deposits cause **capillary narrowing**. Progressive accumulation of amyloid results in **obliteration of the capillary lumen** and glomerulus shows broad ribbons of amyloid.

– Amyloid may also be deposited in the **peritubular interstitial tissue**, **arteries**, and **arterioles**.

Spleen

- **Gross:** It may be normal in size or may cause moderate to marked splenomegaly (200–800 g). It may show one of **two patterns of deposition**.
  - **Sago spleen:** Amyloid **deposits are limited to the splenic follicles**, which **grossly appear like tapioca/sago granule**; hence known as **sago spleen**. Microscopically, the **amyloid is deposited in the wall of arterioles in the white pulp**.
  - **Lardaceous spleen: Amyloid is deposited in the walls of the splenic sinuses** and connective tissue framework in the red pulp. This may result in moderate to marked enlargement of spleen. Fusion of the early deposits gives rise to large, maplike areas of reddish color on cut surface. This resembles pig fat (lardaceous) and hence called as **lardaceous spleen**. Microscopically, it shows amyloid deposits in the wall of the sinuses.
- **Light microscopy:** These deposits appear homogenous pink, which when stained with Congo red and viewed under polarizing microscope, give rise to characteristic green birefringence.

Clinical Features

- Amyloidosis may not produce any clinical manifestations, or it may produce symptoms related to the sites or organs affected. Clinical manifestations **initially may be nonspecific** (e.g. weakness, weight loss). Specific symptoms appear later and are related to renal, cardiac, and gastrointestinal involvement.
- **Renal involvement:** It gives rise to **proteinuria** sometime massive enough to cause nephrotic syndrome. In advanced cases, the obliteration of glomeruli causes renal failure and uremia.
- **Cardiac amyloidosis:** It may present as **congestive heart failure**, conduction disturbances and arrhythmias.
- **Gastrointestinal amyloidosis:** It may be asymptomatic, or present as **malabsorption, diarrhea, and digestive disturbances**. Amyloidosis of the tongue may hamper speech and swallowing.

Diagnosis

It depends on the **histologic demonstration of amyloid deposits** in tissues.

- **Biopsy:** The most common sites are the **kidney, rectum or gingival tissues** in systemic amyloidosis.
- **Examination of abdominal fat aspirates** stained with Congo red is quite specific, but has low sensitivity.
- In immunocyte-associated amyloidosis, **serum and urine protein electrophoresis and immunoelectrophoresis** should be done. Bone marrow aspirates may show monoclonal plasmacytosis, even in the absence of multiple myeloma.
- **Scintigraphy with radiolabeled serum amyloid P** (SAP) component is a **rapid and specific test**.

SELF-ASSESSMENT EXERCISE

I. Short Notes

1. Type I/immediate hypersensitivity reactions.
2. Type II hypersensitivity reactions.
3. Type III hypersensitivity reactions.
4. Type IV/delayed hypersensitivity reactions.
5. Mention types of hypersensitivity reactions.
6. Autoimmune diseases.
7. LE cell.
8. Opportunistic infections associated with AIDS.
9. Modes/routes of transmission of AIDS.
10. Etiopathogenesis of AIDS.
11. HIV virus.
12. Classification of amyloidosis.
13. Special stains for amyloid.
14. Spleen in amyloidosis.

CHAPTER 7

Neoplasia

CHAPTER OUTLINE

INTRODUCTION

Neoplasia literally means new growth, and a new growth formed is known as a neoplasm (Greek, *neo* = new + *plasma* = thing formed). The term tumor was originally used for the swelling caused by inflammation, but it is now used synonymously with neoplasm. Oncology (Greek *oncos* = tumor) is the study of tumors or neoplasms.

Willis Definition: "A neoplasm is an **abnormal mass of tissue**, the **growth of which exceeds and is uncoordinated with that of the normal tissues** and **persists in the same excessive manner after cessation of the stimuli which evoked the change.**"

CLASSIFICATION

Tumors are classified as **benign and malignant, depending on** the **biological behavior** of a tumor.

1. **Benign tumors:** They have a relatively innocent microscopic and gross characteristic.
   - **Remain localized without invasion or metastasis.**
   - **Well-differentiated:** Their cells **closely resemble their tissue of origin.**
   - **Prognosis:** It is **very good**, can be cured by surgical removal in most of the patients and the patient generally survives.
2. **Malignant tumors: Cancer is the general term** used for malignant tumors. The term cancer is derived from the Latin word for *crab*, because similar to a crab, malignant tumors adhere to any part that they seize on, in an obstinate manner.
   - **Invasion:** Malignant tumors invade **or infiltrate into the adjacent tissues or structures.**
   - **Metastasis:** Cancers **spread to distant sites** (metastasize), where the malignant cells reside, grow and again invade.
     - **Exception: Basal cell carcinoma** of the skin, which is histologically malignant (i.e. it invades aggressively), but **rarely metastasize** to distant sites, **glioma** (malignant tumor) of CNS also does not metastasize.
   - **Prognosis:** Most malignant tumors cause death.

Microscopic Components of Neoplasms

Tumors (both benign and malignant) consist of two basic components:

1. **Parenchyma:** It is made up of neoplastic cells. The **nomenclature and biologic behavior of tumors** are **based primarily** on the **parenchymal component** of tumor.
2. **Stroma:** It is the **supporting, non-neoplastic tissue** derived **from the host.**
   - **Components: Connective tissue, blood vessels, and inflammatory cells** (e.g. macrophages and lymphocytes). **Parenchymal tumor cells may stimulate the formation of an abundant**

collagenous stroma → referred to as desmoplasia (refer Fig 22.5). For example, some carcinoma in female breast have **stony hard consistency** (or **scirrhous**).

NOMENCLATURE OF NEOPLASMS

Benign Tumors

A tumor is said to be benign when its **gross and microscopic appearances are innocent, remain localized, will not spread to other sites, and can be surgically removed locallly**, the patient usually survives. They are generally **named by attaching the suffix "oma" to the cell of origin.**

Mesenchymal Tumors

They usually follow the above nomenclature (Table 7.1).

Epithelial Tumors (Fig. 7.1)

Their nomenclature is **not uniform but more complex**. They are classified in different ways:

- **Cells of origin.**
- **Microscopic pattern.**
- **Macroscopic architecture.**
  - **Adenoma:** It is a **benign epithelial tumor arising from glandular epithelium**, although they **may or may not form glandular structures** (e.g. follicular adenoma of thyroid) (Fig. 7.1A).
  - **Papilloma:** It is a **benign epithelial neoplasm** that produces microscopically or macroscopically **visible finger-like, exophytic or warty projections** from epithelial surfaces. Example: squamous papilloma (Fig. 7.1B).
  - **Cystadenoma:** It is a tumor forming large cystic masses. Example: Serous cystadenoma of ovary (Fig. 7.1C).
  - **Papillary cystadenoma:** It is a tumor which consists of papillary structures that project into cystic spaces. Example: Papillary serous cystadenoma of ovary (Fig. 7.1D).

Polyp (Fig. 7.2)**:** It is a neoplasm that grossly produces **visible projection above a mucosal surface and projects into the lumen**. It may be either **benign or malignant**. It may have a stalk (**pedunculated** polyp) or may be without a stalk (**sessile** polyp). Example: Polyp of stomach or intestine.

Malignant Tumors

Malignant tumors **can invade the adjacent structures and spread to distant sites (metastasize)** and **can cause death.** They are termed as carcinoma or sarcoma depending on the parenchymal cell of origin.

Table 7.1: Nomenclature of few benign and malignant mesenchymal tumors

Cell of origin	Benign	Malignant
Fibrous tissue	Fibroma	Fibrosarcoma
Fat cell	Lipoma	Liposarcoma
Blood vessel	Hemangioma	Angiosarcoma
Cartilage	Chondroma	Chondrosarcoma
Bone	Osteoma	Osteogenic sarcoma
Smooth muscle	Leiomyoma	Leiomyosarcoma
Skeletal muscle	Rhabdomyoma	Rhabdomyosarcoma

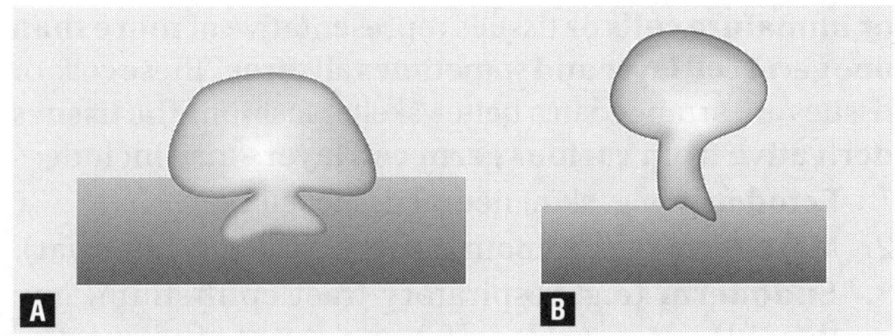

Fig. 7.2: Gross types of polyps. (A) Sessile polyp without a stalk and (B) Pedunculated poly with stalk

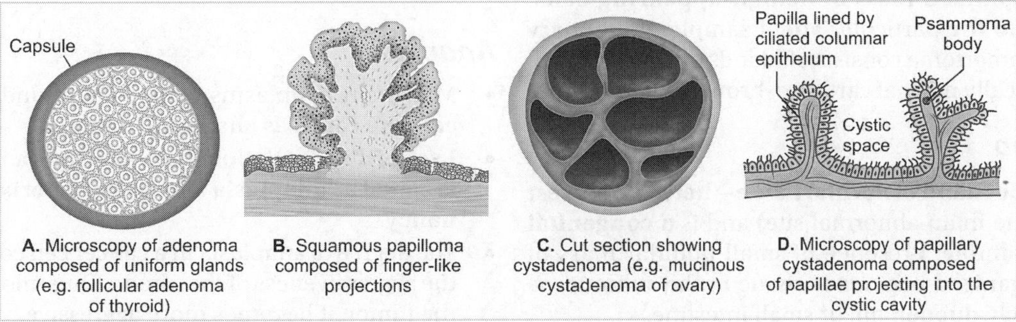

Figs 7.1A to D: Morphological (gross/microscopic) appearance of some benign epithelial tumors

Sarcomas

They are **malignant tumors arising in mesenchymal tissue**. These tumors have little connective tissue stroma and are fleshy (Greek *sar* = **fleshy**). Examples: Fibrosarcoma, liposarcoma, osteosarcoma. Malignant tumors arising from blood-forming cells are called *leukemias* (literally, white blood) or *lymphomas* (tumors of lymphocytes or their precursors).

Carcinomas

They are **malignant neoplasms arising from epithelial cell,** e.g. squamous cell carcinoma, adenocarcinoma.

Mixed Tumors *(refer Fig. 16.4)*

They are **derived from a single germ layer** but show **divergent differentiation** along two lineages. Example: **Mixed tumor of salivary gland** (pleomorphic adenoma) is derived from a single clone (either myoepithelial or ductal reserve cell) and give rise to two components, namely epithelial and myoepithelial cells (refer page 198).

Teratomas

They are special types of mixed tumors **derived from totipotent germ cells** (normally present in **ovary, testis** and sometimes abnormally present in sequestered embryonic rest in midline). These cells have the capacity to **differentiate into any of the cell types** found in the adult body. Thus, teratoma contains recognizable **mature or immature cells** or tissues representative of **more than one germ cell layer and sometimes all three**. These cells or tissues are arranged in a helter-skelter fashion. The **tissues derivative from various germ cell layers** may include:

1. **Ectoderm** (e.g. skin, neural tissue, glia).
2. **Mesoderm** (e.g. smooth muscle, cartilage, bone, fat).
3. **Endoderm** (e.g. respiratory tract epithelium, gut, thyroid).

Hamartomas

It is a **disorganized mass of benign-appearing cells, indigenous to the** particular **site**. Example: Pulmonary chondroid hamartoma consists of islands of disorganized, but histologically normal cartilage, bronchi, and vessels.

Choristoma

It is an **ectopic island of normal tissue—heterotopic rest** (normal tissue in an abnormal site) and is a **congenital** anomaly. Example: Presence of small nodular mass of normally organized pancreatic tissue in the submucosa of the stomach, duodenum, or small intestine.

Nomenclature of the more common forms of neoplasia is listed in Table 7.2.

CHARACTERISTICS OF BENIGN AND MALIGNANT NEOPLASMS

It is **very important to differentiate** benign from malignant tumors mainly because of the different prognostic outcome. In general, benign and malignant tumors can be distinguished on the basis of four fundamental features, namely: (1) differentiation and anaplasia, (2) rate of growth, (3) local invasion, and (4) metastasis.

Differentiation and Anaplasia

Differentiation

Defined as the **extent to which neoplastic parenchymal cells resemble** the corresponding **normal parenchymal cells**. This includes both morphological and functional differentiation. Differentiation **determines the grade of the tumor**.

Benign tumors

- **Well-differentiated:** The neoplastic cell **closely resembles the normal cell of origin** (Fig. 7.3).

Malignant neoplasms

- Show a **wide range of differentiation** of parenchymal cells.
- Cancers are usually graded either as **well, moderately or poorly differentiated** or numerically, often by strict criteria, as grade 1, grade 2 or grade 3.
- **Well-differentiated** tumors**:** Squamous cell carcinomas may show cells which appear similar to normal squamous epithelial cells (refer Fig. 16.1).
- **Poorly differentiated tumors:** They consist of cells that have little resemblance to the cell of origin.
- **Moderately differentiated:** These tumors show differentiation in between the well and poorly differentiated tumors.

Anaplasia

- Malignant neoplasms composed of undifferentiated cells are called as anaplastic tumors.
- **Lack of differentiation** (both structural and functional) **is called as anaplasia** and is **characteristic of malignancy.**
- The degree of anaplasia in a cancer cell correlates with the aggressiveness of the tumor. Thus, more anaplastic the tumor, it becomes more aggressive.

Table 7.2: Nomenclature of common tumors

Tissue of origin	Benign	Malignant
Composed of Single Parenchymal Cell Type		
Tumors of mesenchymal origin		
• Connective tissue and derivatives	Fibroma	Fibrosarcoma
	Lipoma	Liposarcoma
	Chondroma	Chondrosarcoma
	Osteoma	Osteogenic sarcoma
• Endothelial tissues		
• Blood vessels	Hemangioma	Angiosarcoma
• Peripheral nerve		
• Nerve sheath	Neurofibroma, neurilemmoma	Malignant peripheral nerve sheath tumor
Blood cells and lymphoid cells		
• Hematopoietic cells		Leukemia
• Lymphoid tissue		Lymphoma
• Muscle		
– Smooth	Leiomyoma	Leiomyosarcoma
– Striated	Rhabdomyoma	Rhabdomyosarcoma
Tumors of epithelial origin		
• Stratified squamous	Squamous cell papilloma	Squamous cell carcinoma
• Basal cells of skin or adnexa		Basal cell carcinoma
• Epithelial lining of glands or ducts or organs	Adenoma	Adenocarcinoma
	Papilloma	Papillary carcinoma
	Cystadenoma	Cystadenocarcinoma
	Papillary cystadenoma	Papillary cystadenocarcinoma
• Transitional epithelium	Transitional-cell papilloma	Transitional-cell carcinoma
• Tumors of melanocyte	Nevus	Malignant melanoma
More than One Neoplastic Cell Type—Mixed Tumors, Derived from One Germ Cell Layer		
• Salivary glands	Pleomorphic adenoma (mixed tumor) of salivary origin	Malignant mixed tumor of salivary gland origin
More than One Neoplastic Cell Type Derived from More than One Germ Cell Layer		
• Totipotential cells in gonads or in embryonic rests	Mature teratoma, dermoid cyst	Immature teratoma

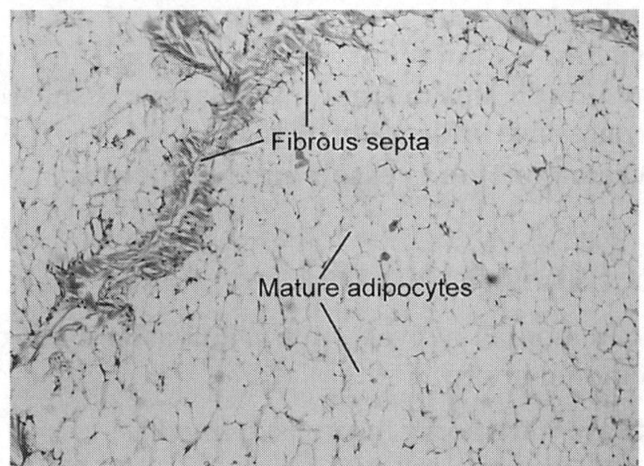

Fig. 7.3: Lipoma is a benign, well-differentiated tumor composed of lobules of fat cells that are identical in appearance to normal fat cells

Microscopic features of anaplasia (Fig. 7.4)

- ***Pleomorphism:*** It is defined as **variation in the size and shape of cells and cell nuclei.**
- ***Abnormal nuclear morphology:***
  - **Extremely hyperchromatic nuclei** of tumor cells compared to that of a normal cell. Microscopically, these **nuclei stain darkly (hyperchromatic nuclei**).
  - **Nuclear shape and size is variable** and may be irregular. **Large prominent nucleoli** are usually seen.
  - **Mitoses:** Presence of mitotic figures **indicates the higher proliferative activity** of the parenchymal cells.
    - **Number of mitotic figures:** Compared to benign and few well-differentiated malignant tumors,

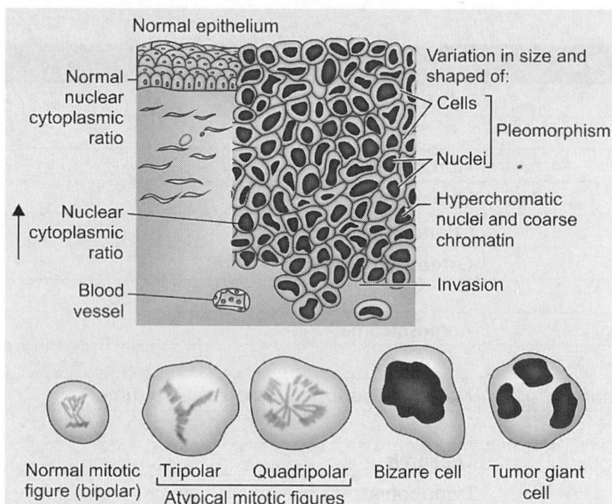

Fig. 7.4: Microscopic features of anaplasia. (Diagrammatic) showing nuclear and cytoplasmic pleomorphism, hyperchromatic nuclei, high nuclear cytoplasmic ratio and loss of polarity

undifferentiated tumors usually show abundant (many) mitotic figures.

- **Atypical mitotic figures:** Normal mitosis produces bipolar spindles, and one cell divides into two. When the mitotic spindles are more than two, it is called as atypical. Presence of atypical bizarre mitotic figures is important morphologic features of malignancy.

- **Nuclear cytoplasmic (N:C) ratio:** In a normal cell N:C ratio is 1:4 or 1:6. In a malignant cell, the nuclei are enlarged, and the nuclear-to-cytoplasm ratio may be **increased** and may reach even up to 1:1.
- **Loss of polarity: Orientation of cells to one another** is known as polarity. The anaplastic cells lose the normal polarity leading to markedly disturbed orientation (architecture) of tumor cells.
- **Bizarre cells, including tumor giant cells:** Some tumors may show **bizarre cells with a single large polymorphic nucleus** and others having **two or more large, hyperchromatic nuclei** (Fig. 7.4).

Rates of Growth

- **Benign tumors** are well-differentiated and **usually grow slowly**.
- **Most malignant tumors grow more rapidly**.

Local Invasion

Benign Tumors

- **Localized:** Most benign tumors **grow as expansile masses** that remain localized to their site of origin.

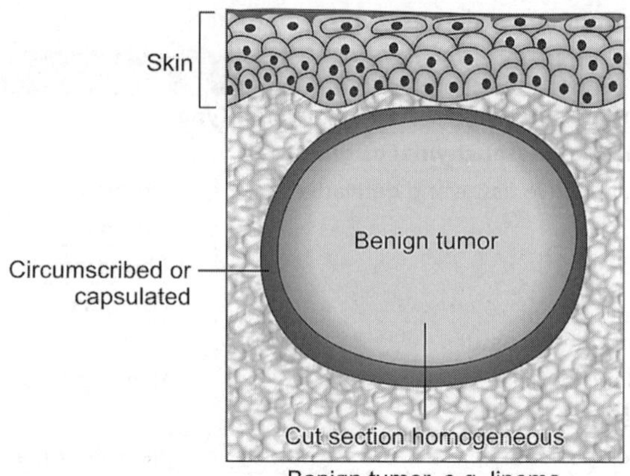

Fig. 7.5: Diagrammatic representation of a capsule in a benign tumor

  - **No infiltration** into adjacent tissue or capsule (if present).
  - **No metastasis**.
- **Capsule** (Fig. 7.5)**:** It is a rim of compressed connective tissue derived mainly from the extracellular matrix of the surrounding normal tissue.
  - **Capsule makes tumor palpable and movable mass** and can be surgically enucleated.
  - **Benign tumors without capsule (unencapsulated)**. Examples: Hemangiomas, uterine leiomyoma.

Malignant Tumors

- **Lack of capsule:** Malignant tumors are poorly demarcated from the surrounding normal tissue and lack true capsule.
- **Invasion** (refer Fig. 22.4)**: Two most reliable features** that differentiate malignant from benign tumors are **local invasion and metastases.**

Local invasion:

- **Invasion of adjacent tissue/organ:** The cancers may invade and destroy the adjacent tissues/organ **(progressive infiltration, invasion).**
- **Invasion of blood vessels and lymphatics.**

CARCINOMA IN SITU

Some carcinomas evolve from a **preinvasive stage** called as carcinoma in situ.

Definition: Carcinoma in situ is defined as:

1. A **preinvasive epithelial neoplasm.**
2. Shows **all the cytological features of malignancy**.
3. **Involves the entire thickness of the epithelium.**
4. Remains **confined within the epithelial basement membrane.**

The tumor cells cannot reach the potential routes of metastasis, such as blood vessels and lymphatics until the basement membrane has been breached or invaded.

Dysplasia

- The term **dysplasia** is used for the **cells that show cytological changes of malignancy** (Fig. 21.2). It literally means disordered growth. The cytological changes of dysplasia include:
  - **Cellular pleomorphism**.
  - **Large hyperchromatic nuclei**.
  - **High nuclear-to-cytoplasmic ratio**.
  - **Loss of polarity (architectural orientation)**.
- **Classification of dysplasia: (1) mild**, **(2) moderate**, and **(3) severe** depending on the thickness of epithelium involved by the dysplastic cells. When severe dysplasia is marked and involve the full thickness of the epithelium, but the lesion does not penetrate the basement membrane, it is a preinvasive neoplasm and is termed as **carcinoma in situ**.
- **Fate:**
  - **Mild to moderate dysplastic changes may be reversible**, if the cause is removed.
  - **Once the tumor cells breach the basement membrane,** the **tumor is said to be invasive** and carcinoma in situ may take years to become invasive. Most in situ tumor, with time penetrate the basement membrane and invade the subepithelial stroma.
- **Sites: Uterine cervix**, **skin**, and breast.
- **Asymptomatic:** In this stage, tumors are usually asymptomatic.

METASTASIS

Definition: Metastases are **tumor deposits discontinuous with the primary** tumor. The process of formation of secondary deposits is known as **metastasis** and the resulting tumor deposits are called **metastases.**

Significance: The presence of metastases clearly **indicates that the tumor is malignant** because benign neoplasms never metastasize.

Pathways (Modes) of Spread

The invasiveness of cancers allow them to penetrate blood vessels, lymphatics, and body cavities, and provide the opportunity for spread. Dissemination of cancers may occur through the following pathways:

- Lymphatic spread
- Hematogenous spread
- Direct seeding of body cavities or surfaces
- Epithelial lined spaces
- Direct transplantation

Lymphatic Spread

Spread of tumors through lymphatics is the **most common pathway** for carcinomas but sarcomas may also spread by this route. Cancers arising in tissues with a rich lymphatic network (e.g. the breast), metastasize through lymphatics. The pattern of lymph node spread in metastases follows the natural routes of lymphatic drainage. **Sentinel lymph node** is the **first node in a regional lymphatic drainage that receives lymph flow** from the primary tumor.

Hematogenous Spread

Sarcomas usually spread through hematogenous/blood route, but carcinomas can also follow this route. Cancer cells easily invade **capillaries and venules**, but thick-walled arterioles and arteries are relatively resistant to invasion by cancer.

Target organ for metastasis

- **Liver and lungs:** These are the most frequently involved organs.
- **Bone metastasis: Vertebral column** is the commonest site.
- **Other common sites:** These include brain, kidney and adrenals.

Seeding of Body Cavities and Surfaces-Transcelomic Spread

Malignant tumor arising in organs adjacent (lying near) to body cavities (e.g. ovaries, gastrointestinal tract, and lung), may seed (deposit) in the body cavities. The malignant cells may be shed (deposit) from their surfaces into these body cavities and cytological examination of this fluid may show malignant cells. Such body cavities include peritoneal, pleural, pericardial, joint space, and subarachnoid space.

Spread Along the Epithelial Lined Spaces

This is not a common mode of spread. For example, carcinoma endometrium may spread to ovary (or vice-versa) through fallopian tube, carcinoma of kidney may spread to lower urinary tract via ureters.

Direct Transplantation

In this very rare method, the tumor cells may be directly transplanted (e.g. by surgical instruments like scalpel, needles, sutures) or implanted by direct contact (e.g. transfer of cancer of lower lip to the corresponding opposite site in the upper lip).

Table 7.3: Differences between benign and malignant tumors

Characteristics	Benign	Malignant
Microscopic features		
• Differentiation/anaplasia	Well-differentiated	Varies from well-differentiation to poor differentiation. Lack of differentiation with anaplasia is characteristic
• Pleomorphism	Usually not seen	Commonly present
• Nuclear morphology	Usually normal	Usually hyperchromatic, irregular outline, and pleomorphic
• Nucleoli	Usually absent	Usual and prominent
• Mitotic activity	Rare and if present they are normal bipolar	High and may be abnormal or atypical (tripolar, quadripolar, multipolar)
• Tumor giant cells	Not seen	May be seen and show nuclear atypia
• Nuclear cytoplasmic (N:C) ratio	Normal (1:4 to 1:6)	Increased (may be as much as 1:1)
• Polarity	Maintained	Usually lost
• Chromosomal abnormality	Not found	Usually seen
Gross features		
• Border/capsule	Mostly circumscribed or encapsulated	Usually poorly defined
• Areas of necrosis and hemorrhage	Rare	Common, often found microscopically
Clinical features		
• Rate of growth	Usually slow	Relatively rapid
• Local invasion	Usually well-demarcated without invasion or infiltration of the surrounding normal tissues	Locally invasive, infiltrate surrounding normal tissue
• Metastasis	Absent	Frequent
• Biological behavior/ prognosis	Usually prognosis is good and produces few local complications if any	Prognosis is poor; usually death due to local invasion or metastatic complications

The various modes of spread of malignant tumors are shown in Figure 15.14.

The differences between benign and malignant tumors are summarized in Table 7.3.

EVENTS IN INVASION AND METASTASIS

Invasion and metastasis are multistep events characteristic of malignant tumors.

Metastatic Cascade (Fig. 7.6)

The sequence of events from the beginning of invasion to the development of metastasis constitute metastatic cascade. It can be mainly divided into **two phases**:
- **Invasion of the extracellular matrix (ECM)**
- **Metastasis.**

Invasion of Extracellular Matrix

Invasion is an active multistep process. Various steps in invasion are:
- **Detachment of tumor cells from each other**
- **Local degradation of ECM and interstitial connective tissue**
- **Attachment of tumor cells to new sites generated in ECM components**
- **Migration of tumor cells through extracellular matrix.**

Metastasis

Following the invasion of surrounding interstitial tissue, malignant cells may spread to distant sites. Metastasis is a multistep process by which tumor produces secondary growth at a distant site or location. Steps in metastasis are:
- **Penetration of vascular or lymphatic channels**
- **Formation of tumor emboli in the blood and/or lymphatic** circulation
- **Arrest at a distant site within circulation**
- **Exit from the circulation into a new tissue site** to form metastasis
- **Local growth at metastatic sites.**

PRECANCEROUS CONDITIONS/LESIONS

Precancerous conditions are **non-neoplastic disorders** in which there is a **well-defined association with an increased risk of cancer.** However, in majority of these lesions no malignant neoplasm develops except that they have an increased risk. For examples:

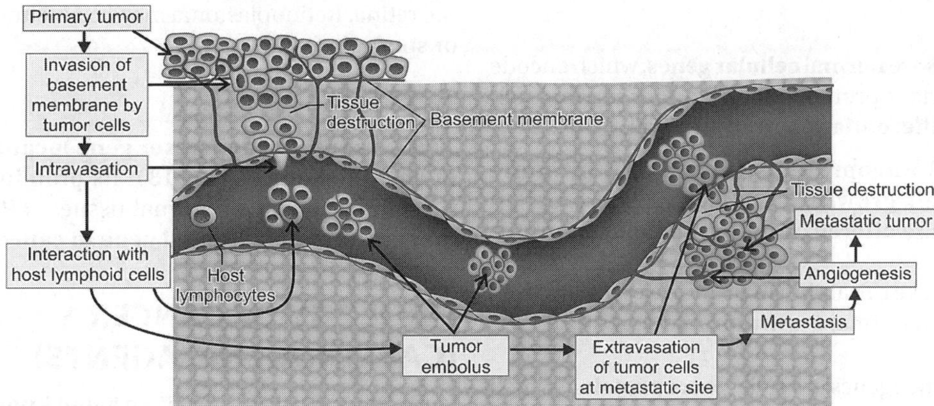

Fig. 7.6: Steps in metastatic cascade

- **Chronic atrophic gastritis** of pernicious anemia may progress to carcinoma of stomach.
- **Solar keratosis of the skin (squamous cell carcinoma).**
- **Chronic ulcerative colitis (carcinoma colon).**
- **Leukoplakia** (erythroplakia) of the oral cavity, vulva, and penis (squamous cell carcinoma).
- Barrett esophagus (adenocarcinoma of esophagus).
- Squamous metaplasia and dysplasia of bronchial mucosa observed in chronic smokers.
- Endometrial hyperplasia and dysplasia in women with unopposed estrogen stimulation.
- **Precancerous benign tumors:** Few forms of benign tumors may transform into malignant. Example: Villous adenoma of the colon, as it increases in size, becomes malignant.
- **Benign develops occasionally into malignant:** Most benign tumors do not become malignant. However, occasionally it may arise from benign tumors. For examples:
  - Leiomyosarcoma beginning in a leiomyoma.
  - Carcinoma developing in long-standing pleomorphic adenomas.
  - Malignant peripheral nerve sheath tumor in patients with neurofibromatosis.
- Congenital abnormalities may predispose to cancer. Example: The undescended testis is more prone to neoplasms than the normally located testis.

MOLECULAR BASIS OF CANCER

Fundamental Principles

- **Cancer is a genetic disease** and arises through a series of somatic alterations in DNA that result in uncontrolled proliferation.
- **Nonlethal genetic damage** (mostly in DNA) **known as mutations is essential for carcinogenesis**, because lethal damage cause death of cells. Mutation may be:
  - **Inherited** in the germline and occurs in certain families.
  - **Acquired** by the action of environmental agents (e.g. chemicals, viruses or radiation) and result in sporadic cancers.
- **Tumors are monoclonal,** i.e. they originate from a clonal proliferation of a **single type of progenitor cell that has undergone genetic damage.**
- **Carcinogenesis is a multistep process.**
- **Four classes of normal regulatory genes** are the **main targets of genetic damage.**
  - **Growth-promoting proto-oncogenes: Mutation of** normal cellular genes known as **proto-oncogenes** produces genes that leads to tumor formation and are known as **oncogenes.** They behave as **dominant genes.**
  - **Growth-inhibiting tumor suppressor genes:** They normally **prevent uncontrolled growth.**
  - **Genes involved in DNA repair:** Normally, they **repair nonlethal damage in other genes,** including proto-oncogenes, tumor suppressor genes, and genes that regulate apoptosis.
  - **Genes that regulate programmed cell death** (apoptosis)**:** They can behave as **proto-oncogenes** (loss of one copy is enough) or **tumor suppressor genes** (loss of both copies required).

HALLMARKS OF CANCER

Normal cell may undergo malignant transformation by corrupting any one of the normal steps involved in cell proliferation.

Oncogenes

Proto-oncogenes are **normal cellular genes**, which encode a number of nuclear proteins that **regulate normal cell proliferation, differentiation, and survival**.

Oncogenes and oncoproteins: Genes that promote autonomous cell growth in cancer cells are called **oncogenes** and are **altered/mutated versions of proto-oncogenes**.

- **Oncogenes** have the ability to **promote cell growth in the absence** of normal growth-promoting/**mitogenic signals**.
- **Products** of oncogenes are called **oncoproteins**, which resemble the normal products of proto-oncogenes.
- **Oncoprotein production** is **not under normal regulatory control** and cells proliferate without the usual requirement for external signals and are freed from checkpoints → **growth becomes autonomous**.

Classification of oncogenes: Oncogenes can be classified according to the function of gene product (oncoprotein).

- Growth factors (e.g. *SIS* coding for platelet-derived growth factor)
- Growth factors receptors (e.g. *ERBB* coding for epidermal growth factor receptor)
- Signal transduction proteins (e.g. *RAS* and GTP)
- Nuclear-regulatory proteins (e.g. *MYC*)
- Cell cycle regulators (e.g. cyclins).

Tumor Suppressor Genes

Normally, the **products of tumor suppressor genes have a negative regulatory control of cell growth**. So, a second mechanism of **carcinogenesis results from** failure of growth inhibition, due to **deficiency of normal tumor suppressor genes** and **their products**.

General Characteristic Features of Tumor Suppressor Genes

1. **Apply brakes to cell proliferation:** Oncoproteins stimulate cell proliferation; whereas the products of tumor suppressor genes apply brakes and prevent uncontrolled cell proliferation. Two important tumor suppressor genes are ***RB*** and ***TP53*** gene.
2. **Mutations of tumor suppressor genes may be hereditary and spontaneous**.

Retinoblastoma Gene (RB gene)

***RB (RB1)* gene** was the **first discovered tumor suppressor gene**, which is present **on chromosome locus 13q14. Inactivation of *RB* gene was found in retinoblastoma**, which is a rare malignant childhood tumor derived from the retina. Retinoblastoma may occur either as a hereditary or sporadic form.

TP53 Gene

TP53 is a **tumor suppressor gene located on small arm of chromosome 17(17p13)**. Its protein product p53 is present in almost all normal tissues. ***TP53*** is one **of the most commonly mutated gene in cancer**.

ETIOLOGY OF CANCER (CARCINOGENIC AGENTS)

Definition: A **carcinogen** is an **agent known or suspected to cause tumors** and such agents are said to be **carcinogenic** (cancer causing).

Carcinogenic agents (Fig. 7.7)**:** (1) chemicals, (2) microbial agents, and (3) radiation.

Chemical Carcinogenesis

Chemical carcinogenesis is a **multistep** process in which normal cells go through multiple stages during the progression to cancer and involves many mutations.

Steps Involved in Chemical Carcinogenesis

Four steps of chemical carcinogenesis

- **Initiation:** Initiation produces **nonlethal permanent alterations or damage to DNA (mutations)** in a cell.
- **Promotion:** Promoters are agents that are **nontumorigenic or noncarcinogenic** by themselves and thus do not directly damage DNA (no mutation). Promoters **stimulate the initiated (mutated) cells** to enter into the cell cycle. For examples, phorbol esters, hormones, phenols and drugs.
- **Progression:** Continuous proliferation of initiated cells leads to secondary genetic abnormalities, and the tumor growth becomes autonomous.
- **Cancer:** Final result is the development of neoplasm which can invade and metastasize.

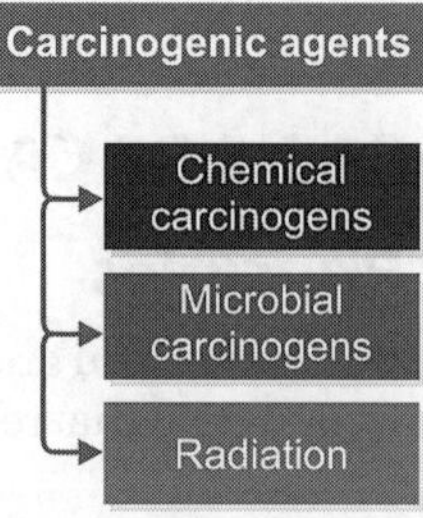

Fig. 7.7: Major types of carcinogenic agents

Box 7.1: Major chemical carcinogens

Direct-acting carcinogens which do not require metabolic conversion to become carcinogenic.
- ***Alkylating agents:*** β-Propiolactone, anticancer drugs (e.g. cyclophosphamide, chlorambucil)
- ***Acylating agents:*** 1-Acetyl-imidazole, dimethylcarbamyl chloride

Procarcinogens that require metabolic activation
- ***Polycyclic and heterocyclic aromatic hydrocarbons:*** Benz[*a*] anthracene, benzo[*a*]pyrene and dibenz[*a,h*]anthracene
- ***Aromatic amines, amides, azo dyes:*** 2-Naphthylamine (β-naphthylamine), benzidine, 2-acetylaminofluorene and dimethylaminoazobenzene (butter yellow)
- ***Natural plant and microbial products:*** Aflatoxin B_1, griseofulvin, betel nuts
- ***Others:*** Nitrosamine and amides, vinyl chloride, nickel, chromium, insecticides

Chemicals carcinogens may be classified into two categories: Direct acting and indirect acting (Box 7.1).

Radiation Carcinogenesis

Radiation is a well-known carcinogen. Extremely long latent period is common in injury by radiant energy and it has a cumulative effect. Radiation also has additive or synergistic effects with other potential carcinogenic agents.

Ultraviolet-rays

UV rays are derived from the sunlight. The tumors produced UV rays are **skin cancer** such as squamous cell carcinoma, basal cell carcinoma and malignant melanoma. UV radiation leads DNA damage which is responsible for carcinogenicity.

Microbial Carcinogenesis

Viruses which can cause tumors are called as **oncogenic viruses**. Many viruses have been proved to be oncogenic in animals, but only a few have been associated with human cancer.

Classification

They are mainly classified depending on the genetic material (in the virus) into oncogenic RNA viruses and oncogenic DNA viruses.

Oncogenic RNA viruses

Human T-Cell Leukemia Virus Type 1 causes adult **T-cell leukemia/lymphoma**, in humans.

Oncogenic DNA viruses

These include:
- Human papillomavirus (HPV)
- Epstein-Barr virus (EBV)
- Hepatitis B virus (HBV)
- Kaposi sarcoma herpesvirus, also called human herpesvirus 8
- Merkel cell polyoma virus causing Merkel cell carcinomas.

Human papillomavirus: Human papilloma viruses (HPV) have marked tropism for epithelial tissues. **Various types of HPV and associated lesions are:**
- **Warts** (benign squamous papillomas) are caused by HPV types 1, 2, 4 and 7
- **Condylomata acuminata** (genital warts) of the vulva, penis, and perianal region
- **Laryngeal papillomas:** Caused by HPV types 6 and 11
- **Squamous cell carcinoma of the cervix and anogenital region:** Caused by high-risk HPVs (e.g. types 16 and 18)
- **Oropharyngeal cancers.**

Epstein-Barr virus (EBV): EBV is a human herpesvirus which infects B lymphocytes. EBV is also associated with the development of few human cancers:
- **African form of Burkitt lymphoma**
- **B-cell lymphomas**
- A subset of **Hodgkin lymphoma**
- **Nasopharyngeal carcinoma**
- **Some gastric carcinomas.**

Hepatitis B and C viruses: HBV is a DNA virus where as HCV is an RNA virus. There is a strong and close association between chronic infection with HBV and HCV (chronic hepatitis and cirrhosis) and the development of primary **hepatocellular carcinoma**.

Bacteria

Helicobacter pylori

It can cause **gastric adenocarcinomas and gastric lymphomas.**

LABORATORY DIAGNOSIS OF CANCER

Confirmation of lesion as neoplastic usually requires cytological and or histopathological examination of the suspected organ or tissue. Different laboratory methods available for the diagnosis of malignant tumors are:

1. **Histopathological examination:** Histopathological diagnosis is based on the microscopic features of neoplasm and by which accurate diagnosis can be made in majority of cases.
2. **Cytological examination:** This is performed on many tissues and usually done for identifying neoplastic cells.

3. **Histochemistry and cytochemistry:** These are stains which identify the chemical nature of cell contents or their products.
4. **Immunohistochemistry:** It is an immunological method of identifying the antigenic component in the cell or one of its components by using specific antibodies. Now, it is widely used in the diagnosis and management of malignant neoplasms.
5. **Electron microscopy:** This helps in the diagnosis of poorly differentiated/undifferentiated cancers, whose origin cannot be identified by light microscopy.
6. **Flow cytometry:** It quantitatively measures various individual cell characteristics, such as membrane antigens and the DNA content of tumor cells. Flow cytometry is useful for identification and classification of tumors of T and B lymphocytes and mononuclear-phagocytic cells.
7. **Molecular diagnosis:** Molecular techniques are used for diagnosis or predicting behavior of tumors. These are helpful in diagnosis of malignant tumors, to determine the prognosis, detect minimal residual disease and diagnosis of hereditary predisposition. The various methods include: routine cytogenetic analysis by FISH technique, PCR, spectral karyotyping, comparative genomic hybridization and DNA microarrays.
8. **Tumor markers:** Tumor markers are products of malignant tumors that can be detected in the cells themselves or in blood and body fluids.

PROGNOSIS

The prognosis of malignant tumors vary and is determined partly by the characteristics of the tumor cells (e.g. growth rate, invasiveness), and partly by the effectiveness of therapy.

Prognostic Indices

Prognosis and the treatment of a malignant tumor depend on:

- **Tumor type:** It is usually identified from the growth pattern of the tumor and its origin by only histopathological examination.
  - **Prognosis depends on the histological type** (e.g. squamous cell carcinoma, melanoma, adenocarcinoma, leiomyosarcoma).
  - **Prognosis depends on cell type:** Some tumors like lymphomas require further subclassification into Hodgkin and non-Hodgkin's lymphoma, each of which is then further subclassified by the cell type.
- **Grading of malignant tumors:** It is done by histological examination and is mainly based on the **degree of differentiation** of the tumor cells.
  - In general, there is a **correlation between histologic grade and biologic behavior**.
  - Most grading systems classify tumors into three or four grades of increasing malignancy. Low-grade tumors are well-differentiated; high-grade ones tend to be anaplastic.
- **Staging of tumors:** It **refers to the extent of spread of a malignant tumor** and is independent of grading. The **mode of treatment is determined by the stage of a cancer** than by its grade.
  - **Criteria:** Staging requires **both histopathological examination** of the resected tumor and **clinical assessment** of the patient [including additional non-invasive techniques like computed tomography (CT), magnetic resonance imaging (MRI) and positron emission tomography (PET)].
  - The **criteria used** for staging **vary with different organs**. Commonly the staging of cancers is based on:
    - **Size and extent of local growth of the primary tumor:** Example: in colorectal cancer, the tumor which has penetrated into the muscularis and serosa of the bowel is associated with a poorer prognosis than with a tumor restricted to superficial mucosa/submucosa.
    - **Extent of spread to regional lymph nodes:** Presence of lymph node metastases indicates poor prognosis than without lymph node involvement.
    - **Presence of or absence of blood-borne (distant) metastases:** The presence of blood-borne distant metastases is bad prognostic sign and is a contraindication to surgical intervention other than for palliative measures.

TNM Staging Systems

It is the cancer staging system widely used and it varies for each specific form of cancer. Its general principles are:

- T refers to the **size of the primary tumor**.
  - It is suffixed by a number which indicates the size of the tumor or local anatomical extent. The number varies according to the organ involved by the tumor. With increasing size, the primary lesion is characterized as T1 to T4. T0 is used to denote an in situ lesion.
- N refers to **lymph node status**.
  - It is suffixed by a number to indicate the number of lymph regional nodes or groups of lymph nodes showing metastases.
  - N0 would mean no nodal involvement, whereas N1 to N3 would denote involvement of an increasing number and range of nodes.

- **M** refers to the presence and anatomical extent of **distant metastases.**
  - M0 signifies no distant metastases, whereas M1 indicates the presence of metastases.

COMMON SPECIFIC EPITHELIAL TUMORS

Squamous Papilloma

Squamous papillomas are benign neoplasms.
Sites: Larynx, vulva and skin.

Laryngeal Squamous Papillomas

Usually located on the true vocal cords.

- **Gross:** Soft, raspberry-like proliferations rarely more than 1 cm in diameter. They are usually single in adults but may be multiple in children (referred to as juvenile laryngeal papillomatosis).
- **Microscopy:** Composed of multiple slender, finger-like projections supported by central fibrovascular cores and covered by an orderly stratified squamous epithelium (Fig. 7.8 and 7.1B).

Vulvar Squamous Papillomas

Located on vulvar surfaces and may be single or numerous (vulvar papillomatosis).

- **Microscopy:** Exophytic lesions covered by nonkeratinized squamous epithelium (Figs 7.8 and 7.1B).

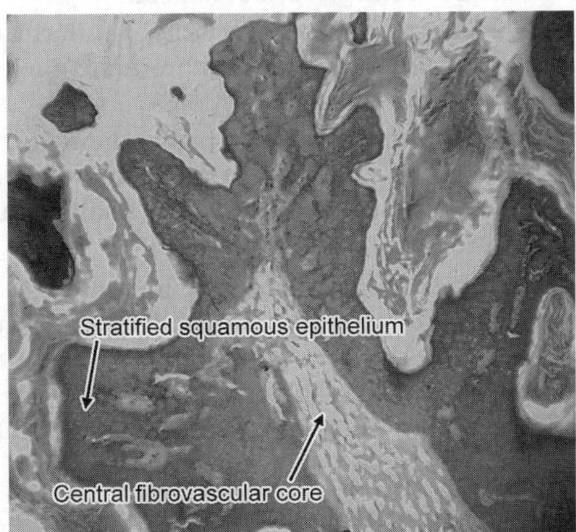

Fig. 7.8: Squamous papilloma composed of finger-like projections supported by central fibrovascular core and covered by an orderly stratified squamous epithelium

MESENCHYMAL TUMORS

Fibroma

A benign tumor arising in fibrous tissue is called a *fibroma.* True fibromas are uncommon in soft tissue. Combination of fibrous and other mesenchymal tissue is more often seen. These include neurofibroma, fibromyoma, dermatofibroma and fibrolipoma.

- **Oral cavity: Fibroma** is common in the oral mucosa. It is a reactive lesion rather than a neoplastic process. It is called as irritation fibroma (traumatic fibroma or focal fibrous hyperplasia).
  - **Gross:** It occurs as a submucosal nodular mass primarily on the buccal mucosa along the bite line or the gingiva.
  - **Microscopy:** It shows fibrous connective tissue stroma. It is thought to be a reactive proliferation caused by repetitive trauma.
- **Ovary:** Fibromas of ovary are relatively common benign tumors composed of fibroblasts. They constitute about 4% of all ovarian tumors.
  - **Gross:** They are predominantly unilateral in about 90% of cases. They are usually solid, spherical, encapsulated, gray-white tumors.
  - **Microscopy:** They consists well-differentiated fibroblasts and a scant interspersed collagenous stroma.
- **Dermis:** Benign fibrous histiocytoma (dermatofibroma) constitutes a heterogeneous family of benign dermal neoplasms of uncertain lineage. They are usually seen in adults and often on the legs of young and middle-aged women. They consist of mixture of both fibrous tissue and histiocytes.

Fibrosarcoma

Fibrosarcomas are very rare tumors because many of the tumors earlier diagnosed as fibrosarcomas presently belong to a group of tumors known as fibrous histiocytomas.

Fibrosarcoma is a slow growing malignant tumor arising from fibrous tissue. It is often found between 4th to 7th decades of life. Most commonly they occur in the lower extremity (thigh and around knee), upper extremity, trunk, head and neck, and retroperitoneum.

- **Gross:** They are circumscribed gray-white, firm and lobulated tumors. Cut section has a **soft, fish flesh-like appearance**. Areas of hemorrhage and necrosis are usually seen.
- **Microscopy:** The tumor consists of spindle-shaped fibroblasts arranged in intersecting fascicles (Fig. 7.9).

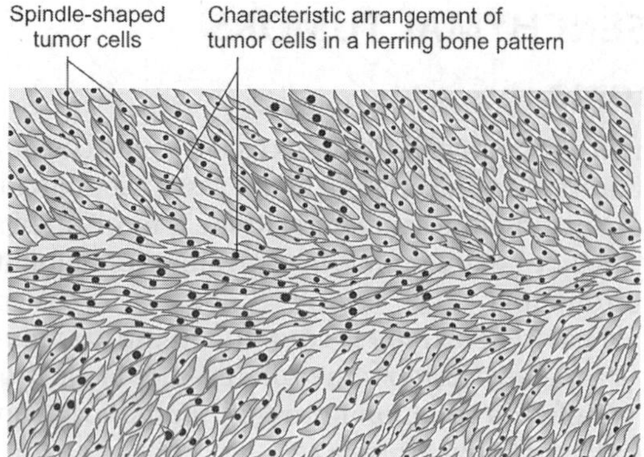

Fig. 7.9: Fibrosarcoma composed of spindle-shaped fibroblasts arranged in intersecting fascicles (characteristic herring-bone pattern)

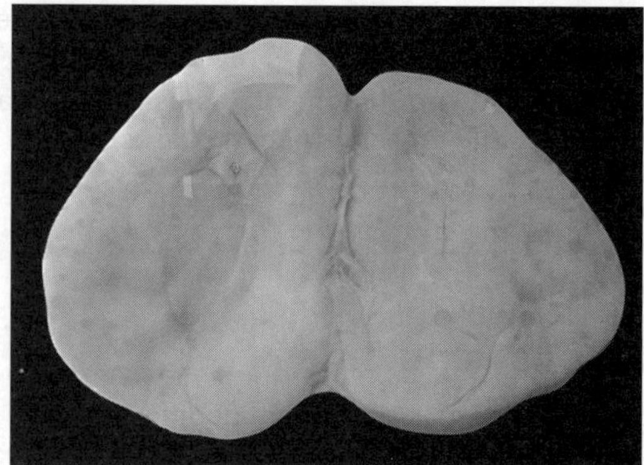

Fig. 7.10: Lipoma: Well-capsulated, lobulated benign tumor of fat

Well-differentiated fibrosarcomas show characteristic **herring-bone pattern (herring = a type of sea-fish)**. Poorly-differentiated fibrosarcomas show pleomorphic fibroblasts with frequent mitotic figures.

Tumors of Adipose Tissue

Lipoma

- Lipoma is the **commonest benign tumor of fat**.
- It is the **most common soft issue tumor of adulthood**.
- Occur most often during 4th to 5th (middle adulthood) decades of life.
- Lipomas are usually single, soft, mobile painless mass.
- **Site:** Usually arises in the subcutaneous tissues of the proximal extremities, neck, back, shoulder and trunk. Infrequently, lipomas are large and intramuscular.
- **Gross** (Fig. 7.10)**:** It is usually a **well-encapsulated** (may be poorly circumscribed), small, round to oval mass. The cut surface is **soft, yellow, greasy and often lobulated**.
- **Microscopy** (Fig. 7.3)**:** It shows **lobules of mature adipocytes** separated by delicate fibrous septa.
- A thin fibrous capsule is usually found surrounding the tumor.

Liposarcoma

- Liposarcoma is one of the most common soft tissue sarcomas of adulthood.
- **Age:** It occurs mainly during 5th to 6th decades of life.
- **Sites: Deep soft tissues** of the proximal extremities and in the retroperitoneum.

Gross

- Liposarcomas appear as nodular masses of 5 cm or more in diameter. Tumors are usually appearing circumscribed but infiltrate into surrounding tissue. Cut section show gray-white to yellow color with myxoid and gelatinous appearance.

Microscopy

The cell required for the diagnosis of liposarcoma is **lipoblast**. These cells may be univacuolated or multivacuolated and uninucleated or multinucleated. Liposarcomas are histologically divided into four morphologic subtypes:

1. **Well-differentiated liposarcoma:** Contains adipocytes with scattered atypical spindle cells and lipoblasts.
2. **Myxoid liposarcoma:** Most common histological subtype. Contains abundant basophilic extracellular matrix, arborizing capillaries (**chicken-wire pattern**) and primitive cells at various stages of adipocyte differentiation reminiscent of fetal fat.
3. **Round cell liposarcoma:** It consists of uniform, round to oval cells with central hyperchromatic nuclei. The cytoplasm shows multiple vacuoles.
4. **Pleomorphic liposarcoma:** It is highly undifferentiated/ anaplastic liposarcoma and consists of sheets of anaplastic cells, bizarre nuclei and variable amounts of immature adipocytes (lipoblasts).

Behavior: All histological types of liposarcoma recur locally and often repeatedly unless adequately excised. Well-differentiated liposarcoma is relatively indolent; the myxoid/round cell liposarcoma is intermediate in its malignant behavior. The pleomorphic variant usually is aggressive and frequently metastasizes.

PERIPHERAL NERVE SHEATH TUMORS

Common types of peripheral nerve sheath tumors are schwannoma, neurofibroma, and malignant peripheral nerve sheath tumor (MPNST).

Schwannoma (Neurilemmoma)

- **Benign** peripheral nerve sheath **tumor that shows Schwann cell differentiation**.
- **Gross:** Schwannomas are well-circumscribed and encapsulated tumors. Firm and gray.
- **Microscopy:** Composed of mixture of dense and loose areas referred to as **Antoni A** and **Antoni B** areas, respectively.
  - **Antoni A** areas: These dense areas contain spindle cells arranged in intersecting fascicles. The cells show palisading of nuclei and "nuclear-free zones" are observed between the regions of nuclear palisading are termed **Verocay bodies.**
  - **Antoni B** areas: These are loose, hypocellular areas in which the spindle cells are widely separated by a prominent myxoid extracellular matrix. Schwann cells are characterized by the presence of a spindled elongated nucleus having a wavy or buckled shape.

Neurofibromas

- **Benign nerve sheath tumor**.
- May be either sporadic or NF1-associated.
- **Localized cutaneous neurofibroma**
  - Small, well-delineated but unencapsulated nodular lesions arise in the dermis and subcutaneous fat.
  - Relatively low cellular containing Schwann cells admixed with stromal cells.
  - Stroma contains loose collagen.
- **Diffuse neurofibroma:** Morphologically similar to those seen in localized cutaneous neurofibromas.
- **Plexiform neurofibroma:** They grow within and expand nerve fascicles entrapping associated axons. The ropy thickening of multiple nerve fascicles produces a "bag of worms" appearance. Morphologically, it is similar to that of other neurofibromas.

SKELETAL MUSCLE TUMORS

Rhabdomyosarcoma

Malignant mesenchymal tumor with skeletal muscle differentiation.

Most common soft tissue sarcoma of childhood and adolescence, usually presents before age 20.

Sites: In children, it arises in the sinuses, head and neck and genitourinary tract.

Morphology

Subtypes

1. **Embryonal** (60%)**:** Presents as soft gray infiltrative mass. The tumor cells mimic skeletal muscle at various stages of embryogenesis. Rhabdomyoblasts with visible cross-striations may be found. **Sarcoma botryoides** is a variant of embryonal rhabdomyosarcoma that develops in the walls of hollow, mucosal-lined structures (e.g. nasopharynx, vagina).
2. **Alveolar** (20%)**:** In these tumors fibrous septae divide the tumor cells into clusters or aggregates producing an alveolar pattern. The tumor cells are uniform round, with little cytoplasm without cross striations.
3. **Pleomorphic** (20%)**:** It is characterized by large, sometimes multinucleated, bizarre eosinophilic tumor cells.

SELF-ASSESSMENT EXERCISES

I. Essay

1. Define and classify neoplasia. Discuss/tabulate the differences between benign and malignant tumor.
2. Define neoplasm. Describe the routes of spread of malignant tumors.
3. Classify carcinogens/enumerate the types of carcinogens and describe in detail chemical carcinogenesis.
4. Discuss the mechanism of invasion and metastasis.

II. Short Notes

1. Nomenclature and classification of tumors.
2. Histological features of malignant cell.
3. Anaplasia.
4. Characteristics of malignant tumors.
5. Morphology of malignant cells.
6. Precancerous lesions/premalignant neoplasms.
7. Dysplasia.
8. Differences between benign and malignant tumors.
9. Mode/routes of spread of malignant tumors.
10. Routes of metastasis.
11. Lymphatic spread of malignant tumors.
12. Hematogenous spread of malignant tumors.
13. Metastasis.
14. Oncogenic virus.
15. Chemical carcinogenesis.
16. Carcinogen.
17. Radiation carcinogenesis.
18. Staging of cancer.
19. Grading and staging of cancer.
20. Papilloma.
21. Teratoma.
22. Neurofibroma.

CHAPTER 8

Nutritional Disorders

CHAPTER OUTLINE

INTRODUCTION

Vitamins are vital organic substances required in limited amounts with key roles in certain metabolic pathways.

Categories

Thirteen vitamins are necessary for health and are categorized as:

- **Fat-soluble vitamins:** These include A, D, E, and K. Fat-soluble vitamins are stored in the body, but their absorption may be poor in fat malabsorption disorders or in disturbances of digestive functions.
- **Water-soluble vitamins:** All other vitamins (vitamins of the B complex group and vitamin C).

FAT-SOLUBLE VITAMINS

Vitamin A (Retinol)

Vitamin A (retinol) is part of the family of retinoids which is present in food and the body as esters combined with long chain fatty acids.

Functions

Vitamin A has several metabolic roles:

- **Maintenance of normal vision.**
- **Regulation of cell growth and differentiation of epithelial cells.** In vitamin A deficiency, mucus-secreting cells are replaced by keratin-producing cells and this process is known as **squamous metaplasia**.
- **Regulation of lipid metabolism.**
- **Host resistance to infections:**
  - **Immune function.**
  - **Antioxidant.**

Causes of Deficiency

Due to general undernutrition or as a secondary deficiency as a consequence of malabsorption of fats.

Pathologic Effects (Clinical Features) of Vitamin A Deficiency (Fig. 8.1)

Effects in the eye

- **Night blindness:** Impaired vision, particularly impaired adaptation to the dark (*night blindness*).
- **Xerophthalmia:** It is characterized by keratinization of the cornea—**xerophthalmia** (dry eye). Initially, there is dryness of the conjunctiva (**xerosis conjunctivae**). Subsequently, there is a opaque plaques gives rise to characteristic **Bitot spots** that progresses to erosion of corneal surface, softening and destruction of the cornea (**keratomalacia**), scarring and **irreversible blindness.**

Effects on other epithelia

The epithelium lining the upper respiratory passage and urinary tract also undergoes **squamous metaplasia**.

Immune deficiency

It is responsible for higher mortality rates from common infections such as measles, pneumonia, and infectious diarrhea.

Vitamin D

Vitamin D is a **fat-soluble vitamin.**

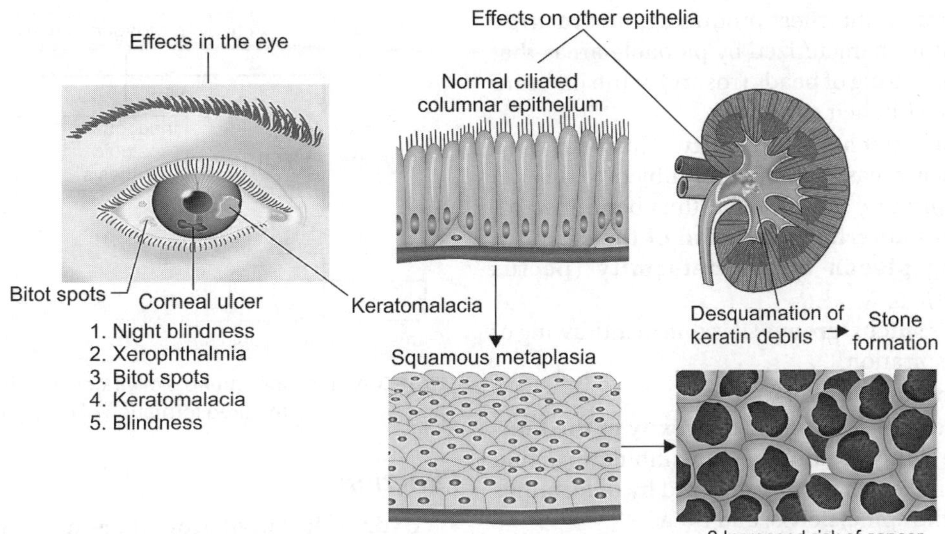

Fig. 8.1: Pathological effects of vitamin A deficiency

Functions

- **Regulation of plasma levels of calcium and phosphorus:**
  - **Stimulates intestinal absorption of calcium.**
  - **Stimulates calcium reabsorption in the kidney.**
  - **Interaction with PTH in the regulation of blood calcium.**
  - **Mineralization of bone.**
- **Antiproliferative effects.**
- **Immunomodulatory:** Vitamin D is involved in the innate and adaptive immune system.

Causes of Deficiency

- Impaired cutaneous production due to **limited exposure to sunlight.**
- **Dietary absence:** Diets deficient in calcium and vitamin D.
- **Malabsorption.**

Skeletal Effects of Vitamin D Deficiency

Milder forms of vitamin D deficiency is also called as **vitamin D insufficiency**, leads to an increased risk of bone loss and hip fractures in older adults.

Rickets in children (Fig. 8.2)

In children, before the closure of epiphyses, vitamin D deficiency causes retardation of growth associated with an expansion of the growth plate known as **rickets.**

Gross skeletal changes in rickets: It depends on the severity and duration of the vitamin D deficiency and also the stresses to which individual bones are subjected.

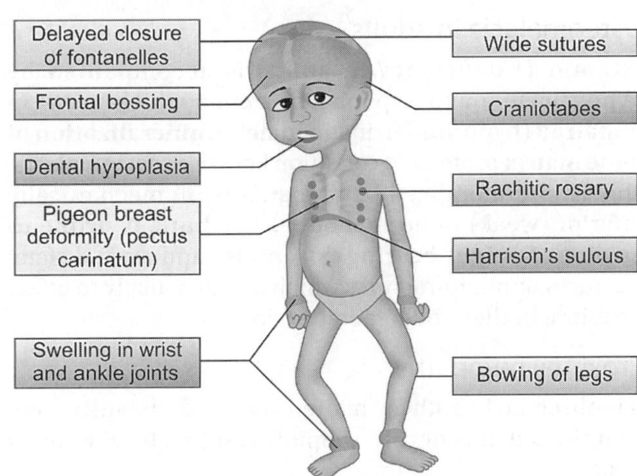

Fig. 8.2: Features of rickets

During the nonambulatory stage of infancy:

- **Head:**
  - **Craniotabes (an abnormal softening of the skull bones):** The head and chest are subjected to the greatest stresses. The softened occipital bones become flattened, and the parietal bones buckle inward by pressure; with the release of the pressure, elastic recoil snaps the bones back into their original positions (craniotabes).
  - **Frontal bossing:** Excess of osteoid produces **frontal bossing**. The skull/head appears square and box-like. It causes delayed closure of anterior fontanelle.
- **Chest:**
  - **Rachitic rosary: Overgrowth of cartilage or osteoid tissue at the costochondral junction** causes

deformation of the chest producing the **"rachitic rosary."** It is characterized by palpable areas that resembles a string of beads (rosary) at the juncture of the ribs with their cartilages.
  - **Pigeon breast/chest deformity:** The weakened metaphyseal areas of the ribs are subject to the pull of the respiratory muscles and thus bend inward. This creates **anterior protrusion of the sternum** producing **pigeon breast deformity** (pectus carinatum).
  - **Harrison's sulcus/groove:** It is due to indrawing of ribs on inspiration.
- **During the nonambulatory stage:**
  - **Lumbar lordosis (anterior convexity of the lumbar spine):** This occurs when an ambulating child develops rickets. It is characterized by deformities affecting the spine, pelvis, and tibia.
  - **Bowing (bending) of the legs:** Due to affection of tibia.

Osteomalacia in adults

Vitamin D deficiency in adults is accompanied by hypocalcemia and hypophosphatemia which result in **impaired** (hypo/under/inadequately) **mineralization of bone matrix** proteins, a condition known as osteomalacia. This hypomineralized bone matrix is biomechanically inferior (weak) to normal bone. This **bone is prone to bowing of weight-bearing extremities** and gross skeletal fractures or microfractures which are most likely to affect vertebral bodies and femoral necks.

Proximal myopathy

It is observed in both in children and in adults with severe vitamin D deficiency. It is rapidly resolves by vitamin D treatment.

Hypocalcemic tetany

Calcium is required for normal neural excitation and the relaxation of muscles. Hypocalcemic tetany is a **convulsive state** caused by an insufficient extracellular concentration of ionized calcium.

Nonskeletal Effects of Vitamin D

Low levels of vitamin D may **increase in the incidence of cancers of colon, prostate and breast cancers**, but whether vitamin D supplement can reduce cancer risk has not known.

Vitamin C (Ascorbic Acid)

It is a **water-soluble vitamin.**

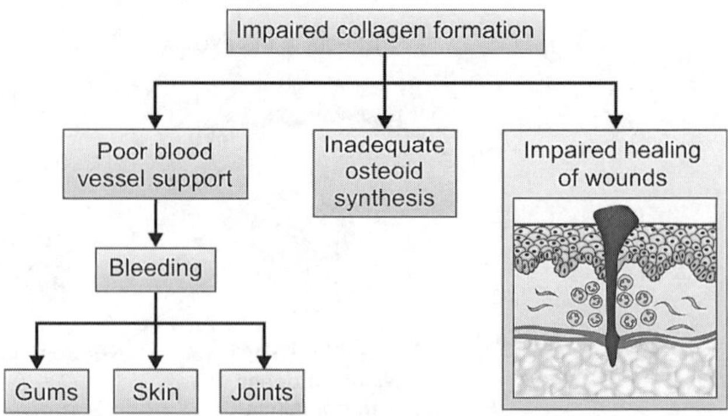

Fig. 8.3: Major consequences of vitamin C deficiency caused by impaired formation of collagen

Functions

- **Hydroxylation of procollagen:** It is necessary for the formation of collagen from procollagen.
- **Antioxidant properties.**
- **Promotion of nonheme iron absorption.**

Causes of Deficiency

- Ascorbic acid is present in abundance in many foods. Hence, its deficiency is rare.
- Rarely, it may occur as a secondary deficiency, particularly among older persons who live alone, and chronic alcoholics.

Effects of Deficiency (Fig. 8.3)

Scurvy: It is characterized by:
- **Bone disease:** Characterized by **deranged formation of osteoid matrix.**
- **Hemorrhages:** Marked tendency to bleed into the skin (petechiae, ecchymoses, perifollicular hemorrhages), bleeding into muscles, joints and underneath peritoneum.
- **Delayed wound healing.**
- **Anemia.**
- **Gums: Inflamed and bleeding** gums.

Vitamin E

Vitamin E is a collective name for 8 stereoisomers of tocopherols and tocotrienols. The most important dietary form is α-tocopherol.

Functions

- **Antioxidant.**
- It **helps to maintain cell membrane structure.**

- It affects DNA synthesis and cell signaling.
- **Anti-inflammatory effect**.
- **Immune systems**.

Causes of Deficiency

- Dietary deficiency of vitamin E is very rare.
- It can cause **mild hemolytic anemias, ataxia and visual scotomas**.

Vitamin K

Forms of vitamin K: There are two natural forms: vitamin K_1 (phylloquinone) derived from vegetable (green leafy vegetables such as kale and spinach) and animal sources (liver), and vitamin K_2 (menaquinone) which is synthesized by bacterial flora in the colon and in hepatic tissue.

Functions

- **Coagulation:** Vitamin K is involved in coagulation process.
- **Others:** It may be involved in **mineralization of bone**.

Causes of Deficiency

- In adults:
  - **Chronic small-intestinal disease:** For example, celiac disease, Crohn's disease.
  - **Obstruction of biliary tracts**.
  - After small-bowel resection.
  - **Broad-spectrum antibiotics:** Can precipitate vitamin K deficiency by reducing gut bacteria.
  - **Warfarin and related anticoagulants:** Warfarin-type drugs prevent the conversion of vitamin K to its active form.
- **Deficiency in newborn:** It is because of (1) low fat stores, (2) low breast milk levels of vitamin K, (3) sterility of the infantile intestinal tract, (4) liver immaturity, and (5) poor placental transport.

Effects of Deficiency

- Vitamin K deficiency leads to **delayed coagulation and bleeding**.
- **Newborn:** In breast-fed newborns, it may cause **hemorrhagic disease of the newborn**. Intracranial, gastrointestinal and skin bleeding, can occur in vitamin K-deficient infants 1–7 days after birth. Thus, vitamin K (1 mg IM) is given routinely to newborn babies to prevent hemorrhagic disease.

WATER-SOLUBLE VITAMINS—VITAMIN B COMPLEX

Thiamine (Vitamin B_1)

Thiamine was the first B complex vitamin identified and is referred to as vitamin B_1.

Functions

- Thiamine functions as a coenzyme
- May have an additional role in neuronal conduction.

Causes of Deficiency

- Most dietary deficiency of thiamine is due to **poor dietary intake**. Alcoholism, chronic renal dialysis and chronic illnesses such as cancer are common precipitant factors.
- Women with **prolonged hyperemesis gravidarum** can develop thiamine deficiency. Maternal thiamine deficiency can lead to infantile beriberi in breast-fed children.
- Anorexia.
- Patients:
  - With overall poor nutritional status on parenteral glucose.
  - On chronic diuretic therapy due to increased urinary thiamine losses.

Effects of Deficiency

- **Mild deficiency:** It is characterized by irritability, decrease in short-term memory, anorexia, fatigue, and headaches.
- **More severe deficiency—beriberi:** It is classically categorized as **wet or dry or combination of two**. It is the classic deficiency syndrome observed **in individuals consuming polished rice** diet. It shows combinations of peripheral neuropathy, cardiovascular dysfunction, and cerebral dysfunction.
  - **Peripheral neuropathy:** Characterized by pain and paresthesia associated with diminished reflexes. The neuropathy affects the legs most markedly.
  - **Cardiovascular dysfunction ("wet beriberi"):** Congestive heart failure and low peripheral vascular resistance.
  - **Cerebrovascular dysfunction:**
    - **Wernicke's encephalopathy:** Acute appearance of nystagmus (involuntary back-and forth or cyclical movements of the eyes), ophthalmoplegia

(paralysis of ocular muscles), ataxia (defective muscular coordination) and psychotic symptoms. The acute symptoms are reversible when treated with thiamine. However, if untreated, they may be followed by a prolonged and largely irreversible condition, called Korsakoff syndrome.
- **Korsakoff syndrome:** Characterized clinically by hallucinations [a dream-like perception occurring while awake disturbances of short-term memory, and confabulation (a behavioral reaction to memory loss in which the patient unconsciously fills in memory gaps with inappropriate words or fabricated ideas, often in great detail)].

- **Wet beriberi** presents primarily with cardiovascular symptoms.
- **Dry beriberi** presents with a symmetric peripheral neuropathy of the motor and sensory systems with diminished reflexes.

Riboflavin (Vitamin B_2)

- It is important for the metabolism of fat, carbohydrate, and protein. It also plays a role in drug and steroid metabolism, including detoxification reactions.
- Serves as a coenzyme.

Causes of Deficiency

Almost always is due to dietary deficiency and is usually seen in conjunction with deficiencies of other B vitamins.

Effects of Deficiency

Nonspecific and mainly manifests as **lesions of the mucocutaneous surfaces of the mouth and skin.** These include **hyperemia (an unusual amount of blood in a part; congestion) and edema of nasopharyngeal mucosa, cheilosis, angular stomatitis (inflammation of the angle of the mouth), glossitis (inflammation of the tongue) and seborrheic dermatitis.** Other lesions include: corneal vascularization, normochromic-normocytic anemia, and personality changes.

Niacin (Vitamin B_3)

The term *niacin* refers to nicotinic acid and the corresponding amide, nicotinamide and their biologically active derivatives.

Nicotinic acid and nicotinamide serve as precursors of two coenzymes, nicotinamide adenine dinucleotide (NAD) and NAD phosphate (NADP), which are important in numerous oxidation and reduction reactions.

NAD and NADP are active in adenine diphosphate-ribose transfer reactions involved in DNA repair and calcium mobilization.

Deficiency

Pellagra

- It is found mostly in populations in which corn is the major source of energy in parts of China, Africa, and India.
- **Early symptoms:** Loss of appetite, generalized weakness and irritability, abdominal pain, and vomiting.
- **Early signs:** Bright red glossitis, stomatitis, vaginitis, esophagitis, vertigo (the sensation of moving around in space), and burning dysesthesia's (an abnormal and unpleasant burning sensation).
- **Advanced stages:** Characteristic skin rash develops that is pigmented and scaling that develops in in skin areas exposed to sunlight. This rash is known as **Casal's necklace** because it forms a ring around the neck.

Four Ds: **D**iarrhea (in part due to proctitis and in part due to malabsorption), **d**epression, seizures, and **d**ementia (or associated symptoms of anxiety or insomnia) leading to **d**eath and **d**ermatitis, are part of the pellagra syndrome.

Pyridoxine (Vitamin B_6)

- *Vitamin B_6* refers to several derivatives of pyridine 5'-Pyridoxal phosphate (PLP) is a cofactor for more than 100 enzymes involved in amino acid metabolism.
- Vitamin B_6 is also involved in synthesis of heme.

Deficiency

- Deficiency usually seen in conjunction with other water-soluble vitamin deficiencies.
- Certain medications, such as isoniazid, ethanol, and theophylline can inhibit B_6 metabolism. Pyridoxine should be given concurrently with isoniazid to avoid neuropathy.

Effects of Deficiency

- **Stomatitis, angular cheilosis (noninflammatory condition of the lips characterized by chapping and fissuring), glossitis, irritability, depression, and confusion** occur in moderate to severe depletion.
- **Microcytic hypochromic** anemia is due to diminished hemoglobin synthesis, since it is the first enzyme involved in heme biosynthesis. It may also produce normochromic-normocytic anemia.

Table 8.1: Vitamins and their principal clinical manifestations

Vitamin	Clinical finding
Thiamine	**Beriberi (dry or wet):** Neuropathy, muscle weakness and wasting, cardiomegaly, edema, ophthalmoplegia, confabulation
Riboflavin	Magenta tongue (glossitis), angular stomatitis, seborrhea, cheilosis, and seborrheic dermatitis
Niacin	**Pellagra:** Pigmented rash of sun-exposed areas, bright red tongue, diarrhea, apathy, memory loss, disorientation
Vitamin B_6	Seborrhea, glossitis, convulsions, neuropathy, depression, confusion, anemia
Folate	Megaloblastic anemia, atrophic glossitis
Vitamin B_{12}	Megaloblastic anemia, loss of vibratory and position sense, abnormal gait, dementia
Vitamin C	**Scurvy:** Petechiae, ecchymosis, inflamed and bleeding gums, joint effusion, poor wound healing, fatigue
Vitamin A	Xerophthalmia, night blindness, Bitot's spots, follicular hyperkeratosis, immune dysfunction
Vitamin D	Rickets in children: Skeletal deformation, rachitic rosary, bowed legs. Osteomalacia in adults
Vitamin E	Peripheral neuropathy, spinocerebellar ataxia, skeletal muscle atrophy, retinopathy
Vitamin K	Elevated prothrombin time, bleeding

- **In infants: Diarrhea, seizures/convulsions, and anemia.**
- **Severe vitamin B_6 deficiency: Peripheral neuropathy** and abnormal electroencephalograms.

Vitamin B_{12}

A group of closely related cobalamine compounds.

Functions

Vitamin B_{12} is indirectly **required for DNA synthesis** in various metabolic steps and its deficiency impairs DNA synthesis.

Causes of Deficiency (Box 13.7)

- Dietary inadequacy is a rare cause of deficiency except in strict vegetarians.
- Mostly due to loss of intestinal absorption. These include pernicious anemia, pancreatic insufficiency, atrophic gastritis, small bowel bacterial overgrowth, or ileal disease.

Effects of Deficiency

- **Hematological changes: Megaloblastic anemia** (refer pages 135–7) and megaloblastic changes in other epithelia.
- **Neurologic complications: Demyelination of peripheral nerves**, posterior and lateral columns of spinal cord, and nerves within the brain.

Folic Acid

Folates are a group of related pterin compounds. The fully oxidized form is called folic acid, which is not found in nature but is the pharmacologic form of the vitamin.

Functions

The active form of folic acid is involved in metabolic processes which synthesize DNA.

Causes of Deficiency (Box 13.7)

Effects of Deficiency

Megaloblastic anemia (refer page 135–7).

Vitamins and their principal clinical manifestations are summarized in Table 8.1.

PROTEIN-ENERGY MALNUTRITION

- **Protein-energy malnutrition (PEM)** or **protein-calorie malnutrition** refers to a group of malnutrition where there is **inadequate calorie or protein intake**.
- Severe PEM is a serious, often lethal disease and usually affects children of low-income countries.
- **PEM include marasmus, kwashiorkor and intermediate states of marasmus–kwashiorkor**.

Marasmus

It develops **due to inadequate intake of protein and calories** and is characterized by emaciation.

Kwashiorkor

- **Inadequate protein intake:** Kwashiorkor develops due to an inadequate protein intake with reasonable caloric (energy) intake.
- **Edema:** In kwashiorkor, marked protein deprivation causes hypoalbuminemia leading to **generalized or dependent edema**. Edema is not a characteristic of marasmus.

Table 8.2: Differences between kwashiorkar and marasmus

Feature	Kwashiorkor	Marasmus
Definition	**Inadequate protein intake with reasonable caloric (energy) intake**	**Inadequate intake of both protein and calories**
Age	Children 6 months to 3 years	Infants under 1 year
Growth failure	Present	Present
Edema	**Localized or generalized**	**Absent**
Liver	Enlarged fatty	Not enlarged

- **Skin lesions:** Children with kwashiorkor have characteristic *skin lesions*. This consists of **alternating zones of hyperpigmentation, and hypopigmentation, producing "flaky paint" appearance**.
- **Hair changes:** These include **loss of color or alternating bands of pale and darker** hair.
- **Other features:** The other features that differentiate kwashiorkor from marasmus are:
  - Presence of enlarged, fatty liver.
  - Development of apathy (lack of emotion), listlessness (having or showing little or no interest in anything), and loss of appetite.
  - Likely presence of vitamin deficiencies.
  - Defects in immunity and secondary infections.

Morphology

- Growth failure.
- Peripheral edema in kwashiorkor.
- Loss of body fat and atrophy of muscle more marked in marasmus.

Differences between kwashiorkar and marasmus are listed in Table 8.2.

Cachexia

- Protein-energy malnutrition is a common complication that develops in patients with AIDS or advanced cancers. In these settings, it is called as cachexia.
- Cachexia occurs most commonly in patients with cancers of gastrointestinal, pancreatic, and lung.
- Characterized by **extreme weight loss, fatigue, muscle atrophy, anemia, anorexia, and edema**.

OBESITY

Definition: Obesity is defined as an accumulation of excess body fat (adipose tissue) that is of sufficient magnitude to impair health.

Prevalence of obesity: Obesity is a major health problem in developed countries and an emerging health problem in developing countries, such as India.

Types of Obesity

The distribution of the stored fat is important in obesity and **according to body fat distribution** obesity is divided into:

- **Central ('abdominal', 'visceral', 'android' or 'apple-shaped') obesity:** This type of obesity shows increased accumulation of fat in the trunk and in the abdominal cavity/intra-abdominal (in the mesentery and around viscera). It is associated with a greater risk for several diseases (e.g. type 2 diabetes, the metabolic syndrome and cardiovascular disease) than generalized obesity.
- **Generalized' ('gynoid' or 'pear-shaped') obesity:** This type is characterized by excess accumulation of fat diffusely in the subcutaneous tissue.

Etiology

Accumulation of fat in obesity can be considered to be the result of caloric imbalance between the energy consumption (intake of calories) in the diet and energy expenditure through exercise and bodily functions. However, the pathogenesis of obesity is complex and incompletely known.

- **Genetic aspects of human obesity:** Obesity is a **polygenic disorder**, with small contributions from a number of different genes.
- **Environmental contributors to human obesity:**
  - **Food:** Many environmental factors can influence food intake. Increased consumption of energy-dense foods, larger food portion size, and increased variety of food, increased availability, reduced cost and increased caloric beverages (soft drinks, juices) promote obesity.
  - **Physical activity:** It can be divided into three categories: (i) exercise (fitness and sports-related activities); (ii) work-related physical activity; and (iii) non-exercise, non-employment (spontaneous) activity. Increased sedentary behavior, reduced activities of daily living and decreased employment physical activity promote obesity.

Pathologic Consequences of Obesity (Complications of Obesity)

- **Morbidity and mortality:** Obesity has many adverse effects on health and is associated with an increase in mortality and morbidity. Obese individuals are at risk of early death, mainly from diabetes, coronary heart disease and cerebrovascular disease.

- **Metabolic complications of obesity:** Central obesity or upper body fat distribution is associated with increased concentration of free fatty acid (FFA) which can produce several metabolic complications of obesity.
  - **Insulin resistance and Type 2 diabetes mellitus: Insulin resistance is the decrease/failure of target (peripheral) tissues to insulin action**. The skeletal muscle is the main site of insulin stimulated glucose uptake, oxidation and storage. The liver is the main site of glucose production. Normally, insulin promotes glucose utilization (i.e. glucose uptake, oxidation and storage) as well as to inhibit the release of glucose into the circulation. Insulin resistance can develop in obesity and may produce type 2 diabetes mellitus. **Central/upper body/visceral obesity are found in more than 80% of patients with type 2 diabetes.**
  - **Dyslipidemia:** Upper body obesity and type 2 diabetes mellitus are associated with an atherogenic lipid profile. Dyslipidemia includes **increased triglycerides, increased low-density lipoprotein (LDL) cholesterol with very-low-density lipoprotein (VLDL) cholesterol, decreased high-density lipoprotein (HDL)** cholesterol, and decreased levels of the vascular protective adipokine adiponectin. Dyslipidemia increases the risk of cardiovascular diseases **(atherosclerosis, cardiomyopathy)** in the metabolic syndrome.
- **Endocrine manifestations of obesity:**
  - **Women: Polycystic ovarian syndrome** (PCOS) and menstrual abnormalities.
  - **Men:** Reduced plasma testosterone and sex hormone-binding globulin (SHBG), increased estrogen levels and gynecomastia.
- **Mechanical complications of obesity:**
  - **Osteoarthritis:** Excessive body weight in obesity predisposes to degenerative joint disease (osteoarthritis) and also gout.
  - **Venous stasis/varicose veins**
  - **Acanthosis nigricans:** It manifests as darkening and thickening of the skinfolds on the neck, elbows and dorsal interphalangeal spaces. It reflects the severity of underlying insulin resistance.
  - **Increased friability of skin:** Especially in skinfolds, thereby increasing the risk of fungal and yeast infections.
  - **Urinary incontinence**.
- **Lung disease:**
  - **Obesity hypoventilation syndrome** (Pickwickian syndrome) may also develop.
  - **Hypersomnolence:** Develops both at night and during the day. It is often associated with apneic pauses during sleep (sleep apnea), polycythemia and right-sided heart failure (*cor pulmonale*).
- **Cancer:**
  - Obesity **in males** is associated with higher mortality from cancer, such as cancer of the **prostate, colon, esophagus, rectum, pancreas** and **liver**.
  - Obesity **in females** is associated with higher mortality from cancer of the **breasts, endometrium, thyroid, gallbladder, bile ducts, cervix,** and **ovaries**.
- **Gastrointestinal disorders**
  - **Gastroesophageal reflux disease**
  - **Gallstones:** Higher incidence of gallstones, especially cholesterol gallstones.
  - **Fatty liver (steatosis) and nonalcoholic steatohepatitis (NAFLD):** Nonalcoholic steatohepatitis can progress to hepatic cirrhosis and rarely to hepatocellular carcinoma.

BULIMIA

Bulimia is an **eating disorder** in which the patient binges on food and then induces vomiting. The average age of onset is at 20 years of age. It occurs primarily in previously healthy young women who have developed an obsession with body image and thinness. The binge eating is the norm in bulimia. Large amounts of food (mainly carbohydrates) are ingested, only to be followed by induced vomiting. There are no specific signs or symptoms and the diagnosis depends on a psychologic assessment of the patient. Menstrual irregularities are common.

Complications

They are due to frequent vomiting and the chronic use of laxatives and diuretics. These include (1) **electrolyte imbalances** (hypokalemia), which may predispose to cardiac arrhythmias; (2) **aspiration** of gastric contents into the lung; and (3) **esophageal and gastric rupture**.

SELF-ASSESSMENT EXERCISE

I. Essay

1. List vitamin A deficiency states.
2. Vitamin A deficiency.
3. Vitamin D deficiency.
4. Rickets.
5. Osteomalacia.
6. Vitamin C deficiency/scurvy.
7. Protein-energy malnutrition.

CHAPTER 9

Genetic Disorders

CHAPTER OUTLINE

- ➢ Genes
- ➢ Classification of Genetic Disorders
- ➢ Mendelian Disorders/Single-Gene or Monogenic Disorders
- ➢ Chromosomal Aberrations
- ➢ Trisomy 21 (Down Syndrome)
- ➢ Klinefelter Syndrome
- ➢ Turner Syndrome

Genetics is the study, which deals with the **science of genes**, heredity and its variation in living organisms.

GENES

Definition: Gene is defined as a **segment of deoxyribonucleic acid (DNA)** which carries the genetic information. Gene is the basic **physical and functional unit of heredity**. DNA has also segments which do not contain genes.

The human genome contains about **21,500 genes** and each gene varies in size.

CLASSIFICATION OF GENETIC DISORDERS

Genetic disorders are classified into three major categories (Box 9.1).

MENDELIAN DISORDERS/SINGLE-GENE OR MONOGENIC DISORDERS

These genetic disorders result from mutations in single gene.

Box 9.1: Classification of genetic disorders

- Single-gene or monogenic disorders/Mendelian disorders
  - Autosomal dominant
  - Autosomal recessive
  - X-linked dominant
  - X-linked recessive
- Cytogenetic disorders-chromosomal disorders (aberrations/abnormalities)
  - Numerical aberrations aneuploidy (trisomy, monosomy), polyploidy, and mosaicism
  - Structural aberrations
    - ◆ Translocations
    - ◆ Inversion
    - ◆ Isochromosome
    - ◆ Ring chromosome
    - ◆ Deletions
    - ◆ Insertions
- Complex/multifactorial multigenic/polygenic disorders
  - Diabetes mellitus
  - Hypertension

Autosomal Dominant Pattern of Inheritance

General Features

- **Location of mutant gene:** It is on **autosomes**.
- **Required number of defective genes:** Only **one copy**.
- **Sex affected:** Both **males and females** are **equally** affected.

Table 9.1 shows common autosomal dominant disorders.

Autosomal Recessive Pattern of Inheritance

Autosomal recessive disorders constitute the **largest group of Mendelian disorders**.

TABLE 9.1: Example of autosomal dominant disorders

System affected	Examples
Nervous system	• Huntington's disease • Neurofibromatosis • Tuberous sclerosis
Musculoskeletal system	• Marfan syndrome • Osteogenesis imperfect • Achondroplasia
Hematopoietic system	• Hereditary spherocytosis • von Willebrand disease
Renal system	• Polycystic kidney disease
Gastrointestinal system	• Familial polyposis coli
Metabolic disorders	• Familial hypercholesterolemia

General Features

- **Location of mutant gene:** It is on **autosome**.
- **Required number of defective gene: Symptoms of the disease appear only when** an individual has **two copies** (both alleles at a given gene locus) of the mutant gene. **When an individual has one mutated gene and one normal gene,** this heterozygous state is called as a **carrier**.
- **Sex affected: Females and males are equally affected.**

Examples of autosomal recessive disorders are shown in Table 9.2.

X-Linked Pattern of Inheritance

Almost all sex-linked Mendelian disorders are X-linked. Males with mutations involving the Y-linked genes are usually infertile and hence there is no Y-linked inheritance. **Expression of an X-linked disorder is different in males and females.**

- **Females:** The **clinical expression** of the X-linked disease is **variable**, depending on whether it is dominant or recessive. **Females are rarely affected by X-linked recessive diseases**; however they are affected by X-linked dominant disease.
- **Males:** Mutation affecting X chromosome is **fully expressed** even with one copy, regardless of whether the disorder is dominant or recessive.

X-linked Recessive Traits

General features

- **Location of mutant gene:** It is on the **X chromosome** and there is **no male-to-male transmission**.
- **Required number of defective gene: One copy** for the manifestation of disease **in males**, but **two copies** are needed **in females**.

TABLE 9.2: Examples of autosomal recessive disorders

System affected	Examples
Inborn errors of metabolism	• Phenylketonuria • Galactosemia • Cystic fibrosis • Homocystinuria • Hemochromatosis • Lysosomal storage diseases • Glycogen storage diseases • Wilson disease • α1-Antitrypsin deficiency
Hematopoietic system	• Sickle cell anemia • Thalassemias
Skeletal system	• Alkaptonuria
Nervous system	• Friedreich ataxia
Endocrine system	• Congenital adrenal hyperplasia

TABLE 9.3: Examples of X-linked recessive disorders

System affected	Examples
Blood	• Hemophilia A and B • Glucose-6-phosphate dehydrogenase deficiency • Chronic granulomatous disease
Musculoskeletal system	• Duchenne muscular dystrophy
Nervous system	• Fragile-X syndrome
Metabolic disorders	• Diabetes insipidus • Lesch-Nyhan syndrome
Immune systems	• Agammaglobulinemia • Wiskott-Aldrich syndrome

- **Sex affected:** Males are more frequently affected than females; daughters of affected male are all asymptomatic carriers. Affected male does not transmit the disorder to his sons.
- **Pattern of inheritance: Transmission is through female carrier** (heterozygous).

Examples of X-linked recessive disorders are shown in Table 9.3.

X-linked Dominant Disorders

General features

They are very rare, e.g. vitamin D resistance rickets.

- **Location of mutant gene:** It is on the X chromosome and there is no transmission from affected male to son.
- **Required number of defective gene:** One copy of mutant gene is required for its effect.
  - Often lethal in males and so may be transmitted only in the female line.

- Often lethal in affected males and they have affected mothers.
- No carrier state.
- More frequent in females than in males.

CHROMOSOMAL ABERRATIONS

Classification (Refer Box 9.1)

1. Numerical chromosomal aberrations.
2. Structural chromosomal aberrations.

Both may involve either the autosomes or the sex chromosomes.

Numerical Chromosomal Aberrations

Total number of chromosomes may be **either increased or decreased**. The deviation from the normal number of chromosomes is called as numerical chromosomal aberrations.

Types of numerical aberrations

- **Aneuploidy:** It is defined as a **chromosome number that is not a multiple of 23** (the normal haploid number-n).
  - **Trisomy:** It is **numerical abnormality with** the presence of **one extra chromosome** (2n + 1). For example, **Down's syndrome** (trisomy 21) have three copies of chromosome 21 (47 XX, +21).
  - **Monosomy:** It is the **numerical abnormality** with the **absence or loss of one chromosome** (2n – 1). For example, **Turner syndrome** 45 XO instead of normal 46 XX.
- **Polyploidy:** This term used when the **chromosome number is a multiple greater than two of the haploid number** (multiples of haploid number 23).
- **Mosaicism:** It is the presence of **two or more populations of cells with different chromosomal complement in an individual.**

Structural Chromosomal Aberration

Aberration of structure of one or more chromosomes may **occur during either mitosis or meiosis**. The various types (Box 9.1) include:

Translocations (Fig. 9.1A and B)**:** It is a structural alteration between two chromosomes in which **segment of one chromosome gets detached and is transferred to another chromosome**.

Inversion (Fig. 9.1C and D)**:** It involves two breaks within a single chromosome, the affected segment inverts with reattachment of the inverted segment. The genetic material is transferred within the same chromosome.

Isochromosome (Fig. 9.1E)**:** They are formed due to faulty centromere division. Normally, centromeres divide in a plane parallel to long axis of the chromosome. If a centromere divides in a plane transverse to the long axis, it results in pair of isochromosomes. One pair consists of two short arms and the other of two long arms.

Ring chromosome (Fig. 9.1F)**:** It is a special form of deletion. Ring chromosomes are formed by a break at both the ends of a chromosome with fusion of the damaged ends.

Deletion (Figs 9.1G and H)**:** It is the loss of a part of a chromosome. It is of two types namely: interstitial (middle) and terminal (rare).

Insertion: It is a form of nonreciprocal translocation in which a fragment of chromosome is transferred and inserted into a nonhomologous chromosome. Two breaks occur in one chromosome, which releases a chromosomal fragment. This fragment is inserted into another chromosome following one break in the receiving chromosome, to insert this fragment.

TRISOMY 21 (DOWN SYNDROME)

- It is a **cytogenetic disorder involving autosome**.
- Most **common chromosomal disorder** and is a **leading cause of mental retardation**.
- About **95%** of these individuals have **trisomy 21** (extra copy of chromosome 21), resulting in **chromosome count of 47** instead of normal 46.
- Parents of children with Down syndrome are normal and have a normal karyotype.

Etiology

- **Maternal age: Older mothers** (above 45 years of age) have much **greater risk**.
- **Other factors:** Increased incidence may be associated with exposure of mother to pesticides, electromagnetic fields, anesthetic drugs, alcohol and caffeine.

Clinical Features

Diagnosis of Down syndrome is **usually apparent at the time of birth** by the infant's **characteristic craniofacial appearance** (Fig. 9.2). The **diagnosis is confirmed by cytogenetic analysis**.

Characteristic features appear as the child grows.

- Mental status: Children are **mentally retarded with low IQ** (25 to 50).
- Craniofacial features: Diagnostic clinical features are:
  - **Flat face and occiput, with a low-bridged nose, reduced interpupillary distance and oblique palpebral fissures.**

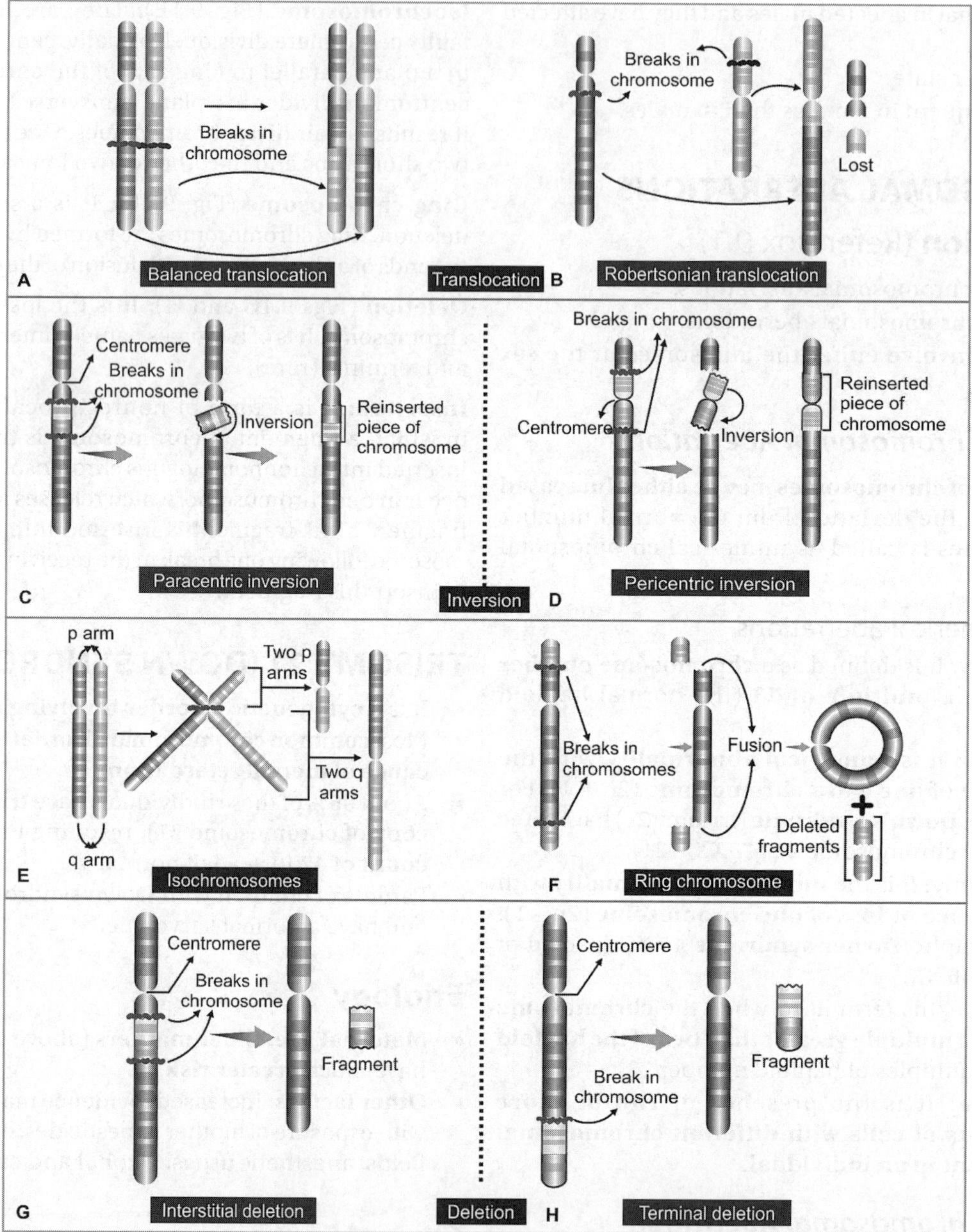

Figs 9.1A to H: Types of chromosomal rearrangements

- Epicanthal folds of the **eyes impart an oriental appearance** (obsolete term Mongolism).
- Speckled appearance of the iris **(Brushfield spots)**.
- **Enlarged and malformed ears.**
- A prominent tongue **(macroglossia)**, which typically **lacks a central fissure** and protrudes through an open mouth.

- Heart: **Congenital cardiac anomalies** are responsible for the majority of the deaths in infancy and early childhood.
- Skeleton: These **children are small** because of shorter bones of the ribs, pelvis, and extremities. The hands are broad and short and show a **Simian crease** (a single transverse crease across the palm). The fifth finger curves inwards.
- Gastrointestinal tract: It may show **esophageal/duodenal stenosis or atresia, imperforate anus and Hirschsprung disease** (megacolon).
- Reproductive system: **Men are sterile** because of spermatogenesis arrest.

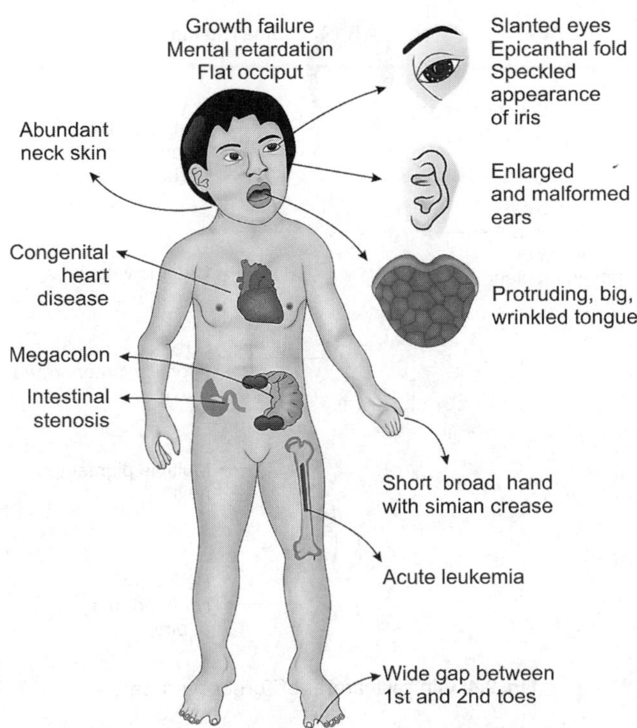

Fig. 9.2: Clinical features of Down syndrome

- Immune system: Affected children are susceptible to serious infections due to defective immunity.
- Endocrine system: **Antithyroid antibodies** may cause hypothyroidism.
- Hematologic disorders: They have increased **risk of** both acute lymphoblastic and acute myeloid **leukemia.** The latter is most commonly acute megakaryoblastic leukemia.
- Atlanto axial instability: It is characterized by excessive movement at the junction of the atlas (C1) and axis (C2) vertebrae, due to laxity of either bone or ligament. Neurological symptoms develop when spinal cord is compressed. Clinically, it may present with easy fatigability, difficulty in walking, abnormal gait, restricted neck mobility, torticollis, etc.

KLINEFELTER SYNDROME

It is a **cytogenetic disorder involving sex chromosomes.**

Definition: Klinefelter syndrome (testicular dysgenesis) is **characterized by two or more X-chromosomes and one or more Y chromosomes.** It is an **important** and **most frequent genetic cause of male hypogonadism**.

It is the most important genetic disease involving **trisomy of sex chromosomes**; it is associated with **reduced spermatogenesis and male infertility**.

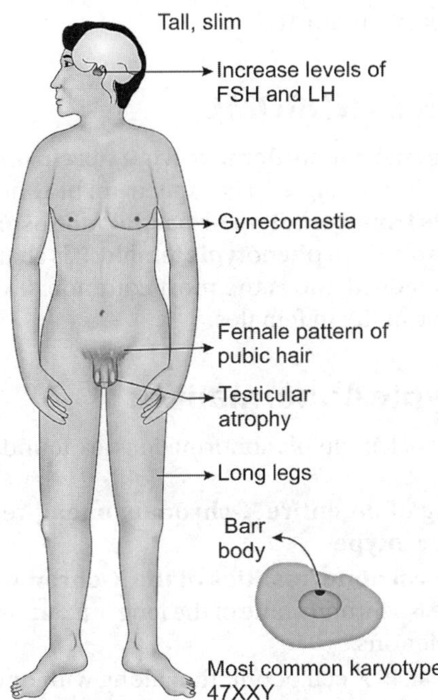

Fig. 9.3: Features of Klinefelter syndrome

Pathogenesis

Most of the patients with Klinefelter syndrome have an extra X-chromosome (47 XXY karyotype). This complement of chromosomes results from **nondisjunction during the meiotic divisions in one of the parents.**

Clinical Features

Klinefelter syndrome (Fig. 9.3) is usually diagnosed after puberty and **hypogonadism is a consistent finding**.

- Most of the patients are **tall and thin** with relatively long legs (eunuchoid body habitus).
- Mental retardation is uncommon, although average IQ is reduced.
- At puberty, **testes and penis remain small** with **lack of secondary male characteristics.**
- Female characteristics include a **high-pitched/deep voice, gynecomastia, and a female pattern of pubic hair.**
- **Hypogonadism, reduced levels of testosterone, remarkably high levels of follicle-stimulating hormone (FSH) and luteinizing hormone (LH).**
- Reduced spermatogenesis → azoospermia → **infertility.**
- **Increased incidence of type 2 diabetes and the metabolic syndrome.** Mitral valve prolapse is seen in about 50% of case.

- **Higher risk for breast cancer, extragonadal germ cell tumors and autoimmune diseases** such as systemic lupus erythematosus.

TURNER SYNDROME

It is a **cytogenetic disorder involving sex chromosomes.** Turner syndrome (Fig. 9.4) is a spectrum of abnormalities that **results from complete or partial monosomy of the X-chromosome** in a **phenotypic female.** It is characterized by hypogonadism and is the most common sex chromosome abnormality in females.

Karyotypic Abnormalities

Three types of karyotypic abnormalities are found in Turner syndrome.

- **Missing of an entire X-chromosome:** It results in a **45 X karyotype.**
- **Structural abnormalities of the X-chromosomes:** It include isochromosome of the long arm, translocations and deletions.
- **Mosaics:** 45 X cell population along with one or more karyotypically normal or abnormal cell types. Examples: (1) 45 X/46 XX; (2) 45 X/46 XY.

Clinical Features

Turner syndrome is usually **not discovered before puberty.** It presents with **failure to develop normal secondary sex characteristics.** Important diagnostic features are:

- **Adult women with short stature** (less than 5 ft tall), **primary amenorrhea and sterility.** At puberty, normal secondary sex characteristics fail to develop.
- **Webbed neck, low posterior hairline, wide carrying angle of the arms** (cubitus valgus), **broad chest** with **widely spaced nipples** and hyperconvex fingernails.
- **Other features: Infantile genitalia, inadequate breast development, and little pubic hair.** The **ovaries** are converted to **fibrous streaks.**
- **Pigmented nevi** become prominent as the age advances.
- **Cardiovascular anomalies** like congenital heart disease particularly coarctation of the aorta.
- **Development of autoantibodies:** About 50% show autoantibodies that react with the thyroid gland and 50% of them may develop **hypothyroidism.**

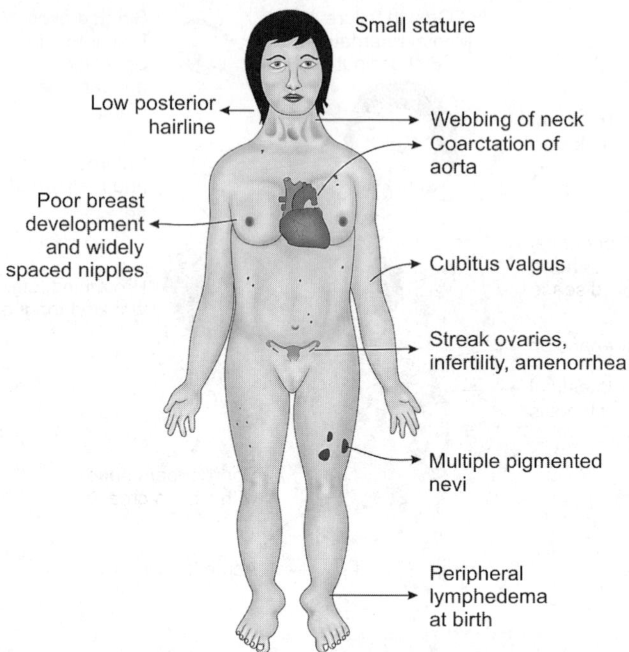

Fig. 9.4: Clinical features of Turner syndrome

SELF-ASSESSMENT EXERCISE

I. Short Notes

1. Down syndrome.
2. Klinefelter syndrome.
3. Turner syndrome.

CHAPTER 10

Radiation

CHAPTER OUTLINE

- Types of Radiation
- Quantitation of Radiation
- Main Determinants of the Biologic Effects of Ionizing Radiation

DEFINITION

Radiation is **energy that travels** in the **form of waves or high-speed particles** through space or through a material medium

TYPES OF RADIATION

They are divided into two types:

Ionizing Radiation

Ionizing radiation is a **double-edged sword**. It is used in medical practice in the treatment of cancer, in diagnostic imaging, and in therapeutic or diagnostic radioisotopes. The main **sources** of ionizing radiation are **X-rays, computed tomography (CT), radionucleotide scans and radiotherapy**. Ionizing radiation has sufficient energy, they interact with atoms and release electrons. This electron release reaction cascade is referred to as ionization. They can cause molecular damage and remove tightly bound electrons. **It can produce short- and long-term effects such as fibrosis, mutagenesis, carcinogenesis, and teratogenesis.**

Penetrating Radiation

It includes uncharged neutrons or high-energy electromagnetic radiations such as **X-rays and gamma (γ) rays**. X-rays and gamma rays dissipate energy over a longer, deeper course, and produce considerably less damage per unit of tissue. They affect the skin and deeper tissues.

Nonpenetrating Radiation

It includes charged subatomic **alpha (α) and beta (β) particles**. Alpha (composed of two protons and two neutrons) and the beta (essentially electrons) particles of elements such as tritium (3H) and carbon 14 (14C) are of immense use scientifically and **has few hazards for humans**. Alpha particles induce heavy damage in a restricted area.

Non-ionizing Radiations

Ultraviolet (UV) rays of sunlight visible light, **laser, infrared, microwave and sound waves.** It can move atoms in a molecule or cause them to vibrate, but is not sufficient to displace bound electrons from atoms. It affects only skin. Non-ionizing UV is **used for therapy in skin diseases and laser therapy for diabetic retinopathy**.

QUANTITATION OF RADIATION

Several terms are used to describe radiation dose. Radiation can be quantified according to the amount of radiation emitted by a source, the amount of radiation that is absorbed by a person, and the biologic effect of the radiation.

- **Roentgen:** It is a measure of the emission of radiant energy from a source. This unit refers to the **amount of ionization produced in air**.
- **Rad (radiation absorbed dose):** It is abbreviated as R. It **measures absorption of radiant energy** and is biologically the more important parameter. A rad defines the energy, expressed as ergs, absorbed **by a tissue**. One rad equals 100 ergs per gram of tissue.
- **Gray (Gy):** It is a unit that expresses the **energy absorbed by the target tissue per unit mass**. One Gray corresponds to absorption of 104 erg/g of tissue. A Centigray (cGy), which is the absorption of 100 erg/g of tissue, is equivalent to 100 Rad. The cGy terminology has replaced the Rad in medical practice.

- **Curie (Ci):** It represents the **disintegrations**/second **of a radionuclide** (radioisotope). One Ci is equal to 3.7 ×1010 disintegrations per second. This is an expression of the amount of radiation emitted by a source.
- **Rem:** It is used to describe the **biological effect caused by a rad of high-energy radiation**, since low energy particles produce more biological damage than gamma or X-rays.
- **Sievert (Sv):** It **is the dose in gray multiplied by an appropriate quality factor Q**, so that 1 Sv of radiation is roughly equivalent in biological effectiveness to 1 Gy of gamma rays. Thus, it depends on the biologic rather than the physical effects of radiation. The relative biologic effectiveness depends on the type of radiation, the type and volume of the exposed tissue, the duration of the exposure, and some other biologic factors. The effective dose of X-rays in radiographs and computed tomography is usually expressed in milliSieverts (mSv). For x-radiation, 1 mSv = 1 mGy.

MAIN DETERMINANTS OF THE BIOLOGIC EFFECTS OF IONIZING RADIATION

Biologic effects depend mainly on the following factors:

- **Rate of delivery:** It has significant role in the biologic effect. The **effect of radiant energy is cumulative**. But in divided doses, the time between exposures give time for cells to repair some of the damage. With radiation therapy of tumors, normal cells have more and rapid capability to repair and recover than tumor cells. The normal cells do not not have much cumulative radiation damage.
- **Field size:** It has a major influence on the consequences of irradiation. The body can withstand relatively high doses of radiation when delivered to small, carefully shielded fields. But if smaller doses is delivered to larger fields it may be lethal.
- **Cell proliferation:** The vulnerability of a tissue to radiation-induced damage depends on its proliferative rate of the constituent cells. Ionizing radiation damages DNA and thus **rapidly dividing cells are more susceptible** to radiation injury than are quiescent cells. Examples of tissues with a high rate of cell division, such as *gonads,* hematopoietic *bone marrow, lymphoid tissue,* and the *mucosa of the gastrointestinal tract*. Example of nondividing cells include neurons (brain) and muscle cells.
- **Oxygen effects and hypoxia:** The **major mechanism of DNA damage** by ionizing radiation is **by the production of reactive oxygen species** from reactions with free radicals generated by radiolysis of water. **Tissues with poor vascularization and low oxygen** such as the central region of rapidly growing tumors, are usually **less sensitive to radiation** therapy than nonhypoxic tissues.
- **Vascular damage:** The **endothelial cells are moderately sensitive to radiation**. Damage to endothelial cells may cause narrowing or occlusion of blood vessels. This may lead to impaired healing, fibrosis, and chronic ischemic atrophy. These changes may be seen months or years after exposure to radiation. The late effects in tissues with a low cell proliferation, such as the brain, kidney, liver, muscle, and subcutaneous tissue, may include cell death, atrophy, and fibrosis.

Pathophysiology

At the cellular level, radiation has two main effects namely:

1. **Somatic effect:** Radiation **causes acute death of cells**. Radiation-induced cell death is caused by the acute effects of the radiolysis of water. It produces activated oxygen species which causes **lipid peroxidation**, injury to cell membrane injury and interact with macromolecules of the cell. Rapid somatic cell death **occurs only with very high doses of radiation** (excess of 10 Gy). Morphologically, it is **coagulative type of necrosis**.
2. **Genetic damage:** It is caused **indirectly by a reaction of DNA with oxygen radicals**. Genetic damage may be either as **mutation or** as **reproductive failure**. Both may lead to delayed cell death, and mutation is responsible for the development of **radiation-induced neoplasia**.

Effects and consequences ionizing radiation on DNA is presented in Figure 10.1.

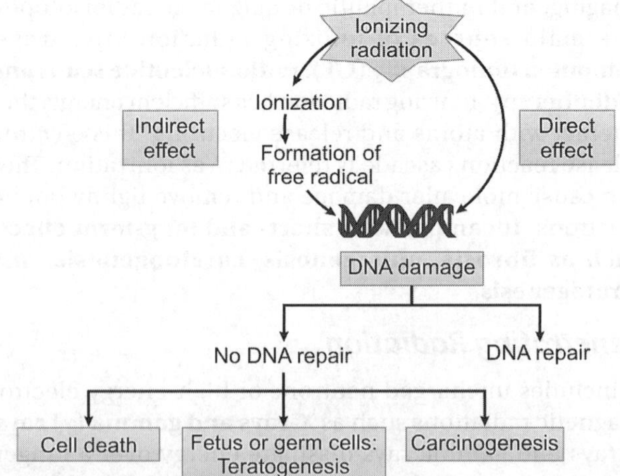

Fig. 10.1: Effects and consequences ionizing radiation on DNA

Morphology

- **Chromosomal changes:** Cells which survive radiant energy damage show a many structural **changes in chromosomes.**
  - **Beak in the double-stranded DNA** including deletions, translocations, and fragmentation. The nucleus often show polyploidy and aneuploidy.
  - **Nuclear swelling** and **condensation, clumping of chromatin** and disruption of the nuclear membrane may be found. **Apoptosis may occur**.
  - **Abnormal nuclear morphology:** There may be giant cells with pleomorphic nuclei or more than one nucleus. At very high doses of radiant energy, nuclear pyknosis and lysis may appear quickly.
- **Cytoplasmic changes:** Radiant energy may produce variety of cytoplasmic changes. These include **cytoplasmic swelling, distortion of mitochondria, degeneration of the endoplasmic reticulum** and focal breaks and defects in plasma membrane.
- **Appear similar to cancer cells:** The above microscopic changes in the radiation-injured cells such as cellular pleomorphism, formation of giant-cell, changes in nuclei, and abnormal mitotic figures produce an appearance similar to cancer cells.
- **Vascular changes and interstitial fibrosis:** May be prominent in irradiated tissues.

Whole-Body Irradiation

- Exposure of large areas of the body to even very small doses of radiation can produce damaging effects. Doses below 1 Sv may cause minimal symptoms. However, exposure to higher doses cause health effects termed *acute radiation syndromes*, which at progressively higher doses involve the hematopoietic, gastrointestinal, and central nervous systems.
- **300 cGy:** At this dose of whole-body radiation, a syndrome of **hematopoietic failure** develops within 2 weeks.
- **10 Gy:** At this dose, the main cause of death is related to the **gastrointestinal system**. The entire epithelium of the gastrointestinal tract is destroyed within 3 days. It may cause severe diarrhea leading to dehydration. Because of loss of epithelial barrier in the intestine, the organisms in intestinal lumen invade and disseminate throughout the body. This can lead to septicemia and shock resulting in death.
- **20 Gy:** Doses of 20 Gy and above may cause damage to CNS and death within hours. With very high doses, necrosis of neurons can develop leading to convulsions, coma and death.

Acute Effects on Hematopoietic and Lymphoid Systems

- **Hematopoietic and lymphoid systems** are **extremely susceptible to radiation injury**.
- **High dose levels (300 cGy)** of radation and large exposure fields, kills lymphocytes directly, both in the circulation and in tissues (nodes, spleen, thymus, gut). It first produces *severe **lymphopenia*** *(*decrease of circulating lymphocytes) within hours of irradiation, along with shrinkage of the lymph nodes and spleen. This is **followed by a progressive decrease in all formed elements of the blood**. This leads to bleeding (due to decreased platelets), anemia (due to decreased RBCs) and infection (due to decreased WBCs). Infection is often the cause of death.
- With sublethal doses of radiation, regeneration from precursors occurs, leading to restoration of a normal blood lymphocyte count within weeks to months.
- Very high doses kill hematopoietic precursors (i.e. marrow stem cells) in the bone marrow and can produce a dose-dependent **marrow aplasia** and permanent aplasia **(*aplastic anemia*)**.

Fibrosis

- Fibrosis in the tissues included in the irradiated field is a common consequence of radiation therapy for cancer. It may occur weeks or months after irradiation due to replacement of dead parenchymal cells by connective tissue. Fibrosis leads to scar formation and adhesions.
- **Common sites of fibrosis** after radiation treatment include **lungs, the salivary glands after radiation therapy for head and neck cancers**, and **colorectal and pelvic areas after treatment for cancer of the prostate, rectum, or cervix**.

Fetal Effects

Pregnant women exposed to 25 cGy or more delivered **infants with reduced head size, diminished overall growth and mental retardation**. If pregnant women is exposed to therapeutic doses of radiation between the 3rd and 20th weeks of gestation, **growth retardation and microcephaly** were found in the fetus. Other effects of irradiation in utero include hydrocephaly, microphthalmia, chorioretinitis, blindness, spina bifida, cleft palate, clubfeet and genital abnormalities.

Effects of Radiation Exposure

Excessive exposure to ionizing radiation may occur **accidently in industry, nuclear power plants and hospitals**. It may be also due to deliberate nuclear explosions designed to eliminate populations and rarely by poisoning, e.g. with polonium.

Radiation sickness

- **Mild acute radiation sickness:** It is characterized by nausea, vomiting and malaise which follow doses of about 1 Gy. Individual develops lymphopenia within several days, followed 2–3 weeks later by a fall in all WBCs and platelets.
- **Acute radiation sickness:** It **involves several systems** and the extent of damage depends on the dose of radiation. Commonly involved systems are **hematopoietic, gastrointestinal, central nervous system and skin.**

Effects on the individual are classified as either deterministic or stochastic.

Deterministic (threshold) effects

Intensity of exposure: Radiation effects depend on the type of radiation, the distribution of dose and the dose rate. The severity of deterministic effects is proportional to the dose of radiation above a threshold level.

Tissue vulnerability

- **Tissue with labile cells:** Tissues with actively dividing cells (labile cells), such as bone marrow and gastrointestinal mucosa, are more sensitive to ionising radiation.
- **Hemopoietic system: Lymphocyte depletion** is the most sensitive indicator of bone marrow injury and after exposure to a fatal dose, **marrow aplasia** is a commonest cause of death.
- **Gastrointestinal mucosal toxicity:** May cause death due to severe **diarrhea, vomiting, dehydration and sepsis.**
- **Gonads:** Highly radiosensitive and may cause **temporary or permanent sterility.**
- **Eye:** Cataracts.
- **Skin:** Radiation **dermatitis** (radiation burns) characterized by skin erythema, purpura, blistering and secondary infection may occur. Complete loss of body hair develops after an exposure > 5 Gy.
- **Lung: Acute inflammatory reactions, pulmonary fibrosis.**
- **Central nervous system syndrome:** Exposures of >30 Gy are followed rapidly by nausea, vomiting, disorientation and coma. Death due to cerebral edema can follow within 36 hours. It may also cause **permanent neurological deficit.**
- **Bone necrosis and lymphatic fibrosis** occur following regional irradiation, particularly for breast cancer.
- **Thyroid gland** due to its capacity to concentrate iodine is responsible for its susceptibility to damage even after exposure to relatively low doses of radioactive.

Stochastic Effects

Stochastic (chance) effect is directly proportional to the dose of radiation.

Cancer Risks from Exposures to Radiation-Carcinogenesis

Radiation is a well-known carcinogen. Carcinogenesis represents a stochastic effect.

- **Latency:** Extremely long latent period is common and it has a cumulative effect. Radiation has also additive or synergistic effects with other potential carcinogenic agents.

Radiation can cause mutation. Any cell which has the capacity to undergo division can develop mutation due to radiation can also become cancerous. The evidence that radiation can lead to cancer came from many sources.

Occupation and cancer

- During early part of the 20th century, **scientists and radiologists** tested their X-ray equipment by placing their hands in the path of the beam. They later developed **basal and squamous cell carcinomas of the exposed skin.** This was rectified with the use of modern shielding and protective equipment.
- An unusual occupational exposure to radiation was found in **workers who painted radium-containing material onto watches to create luminous dials.** These workers used to lick their paint brushes to produce a point, which led to their ingesting the radium. The body handles radium similar to calcium and it subsequently localized in their bones. These individuals had a **high incidence of cancer of the bone and of the paranasal sinuses.**
- A high rate of **lung cancer** was found **in uranium miners** who inhaled radioactive dust and radon gas.

Exposure to radiation

- Any organ after exposure to ionizing radiation has an **increased chance of developing a cancer.** Though the level of radiation needed to increase the risk of cancer development is difficult to determine, an acute or prolonged exposures in doses of greater than 100 mSv may cause cancer.
- **Increased incidence of leukemias and solid tumors in several organs** (e.g. thyroid, breast, and lungs) was

found in survivors of the atomic bombings of Hiroshima and Nagasaki; the high number of thyroid cancers in survivors of the Chernobyl accident.

- Development of "**second cancers**," such as acute myeloid leukemia, myelodysplastic syndrome, and solid tumors, **in individuals who were given radiation therapy for cancers such as Hodgkin lymphoma**. The risk of secondary cancers following irradiation is greatest in children. With acute exposures, leukemias (e.g. acute myeloid leukemia) may develop after a latent period of 2–5 years and solid tumors (e.g. skin, thyroid and salivary glands) after a latent period of about 10–20 years. Thereafter the incidence of cancer increases with time. Cancer risk depends on the amount of radiation received, the time to accumulate the total dose and the interval following exposure.

Ultraviolet Rays

They are derived from the sunlight.

Tumors caused: Skin cancer namely: (1) **squamous cell carcinoma**, (2) **basal cell carcinoma**, and (3) **malignant melanoma**. They are more common on parts of the body regularly exposed to sunlight, and ultraviolet light (UVL).

Risk factors

The amount of damage incurred depends on:

- **Type of UV rays**.
- **Intensity of exposure**.
- **Protective mantle of melanin**.
  - **Melanin** absorbs UV radiation and has a **protective effect**.
  - Skin cancers are more common in fair-skinned people and those living in geographic location receiving a greater amount of sunlight (e.g. Queensland, Australia, close to the equator).

Pathogenesis

- UV radiation leads to **formation of pyrimidine dimers in DNA**, which is a type of DNA damage which is responsible for carcinogenicity.
- **DNA damage is repaired by the nucleotide excision repair pathway**.
- With **excessive sun exposure**, the DNA **damage exceeds the capacity of the nucleotide excision repair pathway** and **genomic injury becomes mutagenic and carcinogenic**.
- **Xeroderma pigmentosum:** It is a rare **hereditary autosomal recessive disorder** characterized by **congenital deficiency of nucleotide excision repair DNA**. These individuals **develop skin cancers** (basal cell carcinoma, squamous cell carcinoma, and melanoma) due to impairment in the excision of UV-damaged DNA.

Ionizing Radiation

Electromagnetic (X-rays, γ rays) and particulate (α particles, β particles, protons, neutrons) radiations are all carcinogenic.

Cancers produced

- **Medical or occupational exposure**, e.g. **leukemia, and skin cancers**.
- **Nuclear plant accidents:** Risk of **lung cancers**.
- **Atomic bomb explosion:** Survivors atomic bomb explosion (dropped on Hiroshima and Nagasaki) had increased incidence of **leukemias** mainly acute and chronic myelogenous leukemia after about 7 years. Subsequently, increased mortality due to **solid tumors** (e.g. breast, colon, thyroid, and lung).
- **Therapeutic radiation:** (1) **papillary carcinoma of the thyroid** follows irradiation of head and neck and (2) **angiosarcoma of liver** due to radioactive thorium dioxide used to visualize the arterial tree.

Mechanism: Hydroxyl free radical injury to DNA.

- **Tissues which are relatively resistant** to radiation-induced neoplasia: Skin, bone, and the gastrointestinal tract.

Teratogenic Effects

Radiation is teratogens and can cause developmental anomalies.

SELF-ASSESSMENT EXERCISE

I. Short Notes

1. Effects of radiation.
2. Radiation carcinogenesis.

SECTION

2

Systemic Pathology

CHAPTER 11

Vascular Disorders

CHAPTER OUTLINE

INTRODUCTION

The blood vessels consist of arteries, arterioles, capillaries, venules, veins and large veins. Depending on the caliber and microscopic features, the arteries are grouped into large elastic arteries, medium and muscular arteries and smaller arterioles.

Layers of blood vessel: Veins and arteries typically have three layers namely tunica intima, tunica media and tunica adventitia.

- **Tunica intima:** The innermost layer is intima which consists of a single layer of endothelial cells.
- **Tunica media:** The middle layer, or tunica media, is composed of layers of smooth-muscle cells.
- **Tunica adventitia:** The outer layer, the adventitia, consists of **connective tissue**.

ARTERIOSCLEROSIS

Arteriosclerosis ("hardening of the arteries") is characterized by arterial wall thickening and may be caused by:

1. **Arteriolosclerosis:** It affects small arteries and arterioles.
2. **Mönckeberg medial sclerosis:** It is characterized by deposition of calcium in muscular arteries seen in old age (above 50 years).
3. **Atherosclerosis:** It is the most frequent and important disease of intima.

Box 11.1: Risk factors for atherosclerosis

- **Modifiable major risk factors**
  - Hyperlipidemia
  - Hypertension
  - Cigarette smoking
  - Diabetes mellitus
- **Nonmodifiable (constitutional) risk factors**
  - Increasing age
  - Male gender
  - Genetic abnormalities
  - Family history
- **Additional risk factors**
  - Metabolic syndrome
  - Inadequate physical activity
  - Stressful lifestyle
  - Obesity
  - Alcohol

ATHEROSCLEROSIS

Definition: Atherosclerosis is primarily a progressive **disease of intima** involving large and medium-sized elastic and muscular arteries. It is characterized by focal lipid-rich intimal lesion called **atheroma** (also known as **atheromatous or atherosclerotic plaque**). Atherosclerosis is a world-wide disease seen in both developed and developing countries.

Risk Factors

Risk factors for atherosclerosis may be broadly classified as **modifiable** and **nonmodifiable** (Box 11.1).

Modifiable Risk Factors in IHD

The **four** major modifiable risk factors are: Hyperlipidemia, hypertension, cigarette smoking, and diabetes.

- **Hyperlipidemia:** Increase in the serum lipids mainly cholesterol (hypercholesterolemia) is a major **modifiable** risk factor. **Low-density lipoprotein (LDL)** is one of the serum lipids known as **"bad cholesterol", because its** high **level** is associated with **increased risk**

of atherosclerosis. High-density lipoprotein (HDL) is called "good cholesterol" and its **higher levels are associated with decreased risk.** Risk of atherosclerosis increases with increasing serum cholesterol concentrations.

- **Hypertension:** It is one of the major risk factors. The risk of atherosclerosis increases as blood pressure rises, and this is related to both systolic and diastolic levels of blood pressure.
- **Cigarette smoking:** It is the most important avoidable cause of atherosclerosis. Atherosclerosis is more severe and extensive among smokers than in nonsmokers. The risk is dose-linked and cessation of smoking reduces the risk.
- **Diabetes mellitus:** It is a potent risk factor for atherosclerosis. It causes hypercholesterolemia and thus increases the risk of atherosclerosis.

Nonmodifiable/Constitutional Risk Factors in IHD

- **Increasing age:** Age is the most significant independent risk factor. Atherosclerosis clinically manifest usually after middle age and the lesions progressively rise with each decade.
- **Sex:** Premenopausal women have lower incidence of atherosclerosis-related diseases compared to males of the same age group.
- **Family history and genetic abnormalities:** Familial predisposition is usually multifactorial, due to genetic, environmental and lifestyle factors.

Pathogenesis of Atherosclerosis

There are several theories for the pathogenesis of atherosclerosis. The most widely accepted is response to injury hypothesis.

Response-to-Injury Hypothesis

According to this theory, **atherosclerosis develops as a chronic** (inflammatory and healing) **response of the arterial wall to the endothelial injury**.

Morphology of Atherosclerotic Plaque

Gross

- **Sites:** In descending order, the most severely involved vessels are: **lower abdominal aorta** (abdominal aorta is involved more than the thoracic aorta), **coronary arteries**, popliteal arteries, internal carotid arteries and vessels of the circle of Willis.
- **Appearance:** These are **yellow** oval (Fig. 11.1) lesions.

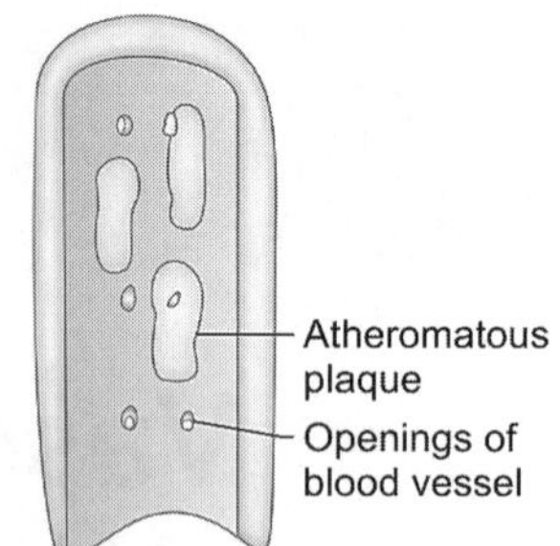

Fig. 11.1: Gross appearance of atheroma

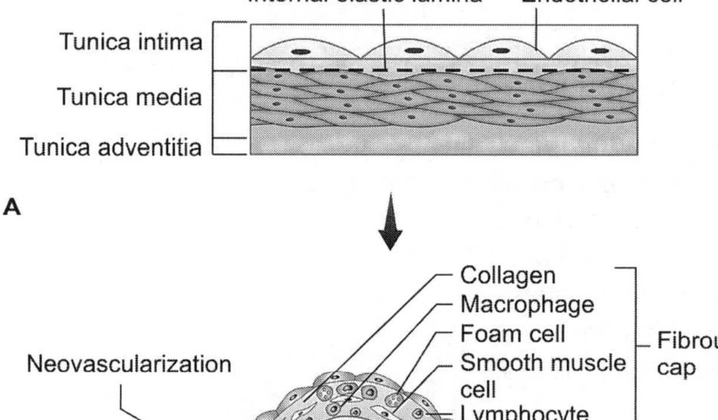

Figs 11.2A to B: (A) Normal blood vessel wall; (B) Diagrammatic appearance of fully developed atheromatous plaque

Microscopy

Atheromatous plaque consists of three regions (Fig. 11.2).

- **Superficial fibrous cap**
- **Necrotic core:** Deep to the fibrous cap is a **necrotic core**, which contains mainly cholesterol and cholesterol esters which appear as needle shaped "cleft" like spaces.
- **Shoulder:** It is the peripheral region beneath and to the side of the superficial fibrous cap.

Complicated Plaques

Atherosclerotic plaques can undergo the following clinically important changes:

- Rupture, ulceration, or erosion
- Thrombosis and embolism
- Hemorrhage into a plaque
- Aneurysm formation
- Calcification of central necrotic core.

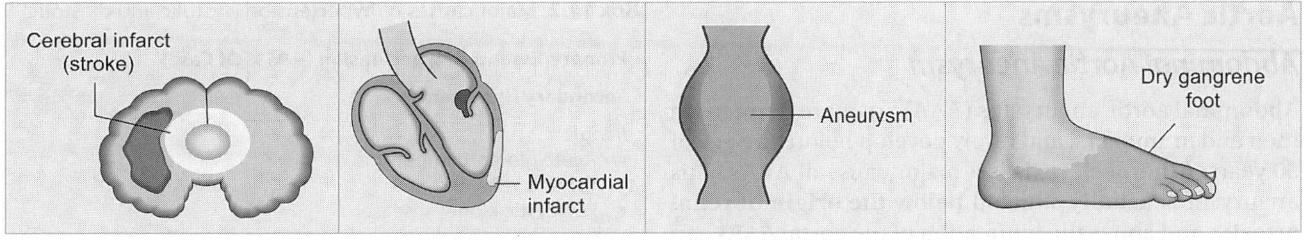

Fig. 11.3: Major clinical consequences of atherosclerosis

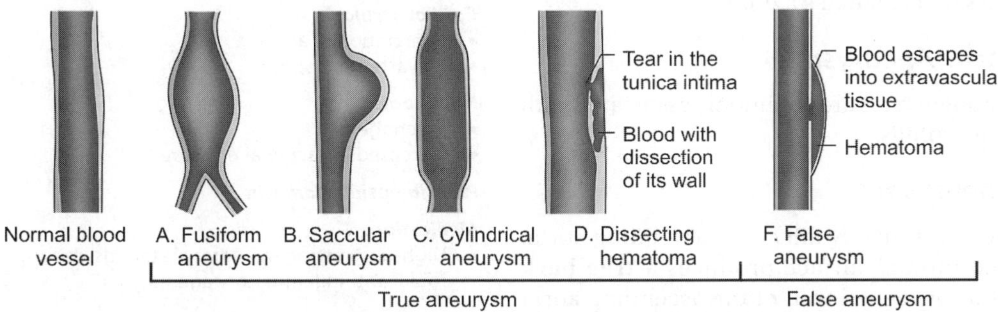

Fig. 11.4: Normal blood vessel and types of aneurysm according to gross appearance

Consequences of Atherosclerotic Disease

Major clinical consequences (Fig. 11.3) of atherosclerosis are: Myocardial infarction (heart attack), cerebral infarction (stroke), aortic aneurysms, and peripheral vascular disease (gangrene of the legs).

ANEURYSM AND DISSECTION

Definition: An aneurysm is defined as a **localized abnormal permanent dilation** of a blood vessel or the heart.

Classification

True aneurysms are classified by origin, gross appearance, composition of vessel wall etiology and location.

Origin

It can be congenital or acquired.

Depending on Gross (Fig. 11.4) Appearance (Shape and Size)

- **Fusiform aneurysm:** It results in an ovoid or fusiform dilation of vessel wall.
- **Saccular aneurysm:** It is a localized (only a portion of the circumference) spherical outpouching from the portion of the vessel wall.
- **Cylindrical aneurysm:** It has parallel dilatation of the vessel wall.
- **Dissecting hematoma:** The blood from the lumen enters into the wall of the blood vessel.
- **Arteriovenous (racemose) aneurysm:** It consists of a direct communication between an artery and a vein.

Depending on the Composition of the Wall of the Aneurysm

- **True aneurysm:** It is composed of all the three layers of thinned arterial wall or ventricular wall of the heart.
- **False aneurysm** (or pseudo-aneurysm)**:** It is a defect in the intimal and medial layer of the vessel wall leading to dilatation which appears like an aneurysm. The dilatation is lined by adventitia with a hematoma (perivascular clot forms around a blood vessel). It differs from a true aneurysm in that its wall does not contain the components of a blood vessel, but consists of fibrous tissue. It usually continues to enlarge, creating a pulsating hematoma.

Depending on the Etiology

They are atherosclerotic aneurysm, syphilitic aneurysm, dissecting hematoma, mycotic aneurysm, berry aneurysm etc.

Location

According to the type of vessel involved it can be **artery, vein or heart**. Aortic aneurysms are also classified according to location, i.e. abdominal versus thoracic.

Aortic Aneurysms

Abdominal Aortic Aneurysm

Abdominal aortic aneurysms (AAA) are more frequent in men and in smokers, and rarely develop before the age of 50 years. **Atherosclerosis** is a major cause of AAAs. This aneurysm is **usually** situated **below the origin of renal arteries** and above the bifurcation of the aorta. AAAs can be **saccular or fusiform**. The aneurysm frequently shows **mural thrombus**. It may present as a palpable pulsating abdominal mass that simulates a tumor.

Thoracic Aortic Aneurysm

Thoracic aortic aneurysms are commonly associated with hypertension or syphilis.

Syphilitic Aneurysm

Syphilitic aneurysms mainly affect the ascending aorta. The roughened intimal surface produces a **tree bark** appearance. The weakened wall of the ascending aorta and aortic arch results in a fusiform aneurysm.

Aortic Dissection

Definition: Aortic dissection develops when **blood** from the aortic lumen **enters into the aortic wall** and travels along the layers of the media to form a blood-filled channel within the aortic wall.

It is fatal, if the dissection ruptures through the adventitia and results in hemorrhages into adjacent spaces.

Etiology: Aortic dissection occurs mainly in association with **hypertension** and **Marfan syndrome**.

Morphology: The aortic dissections show an **intimal tear**. The **dissection** usually **occurs between the middle and outer thirds of the tunica media**. It may rupture out through the tunica adventitia causing massive hemorrhage (e.g. into the thoracic or abdominal cavities) or cardiac tamponade (hemorrhage into the pericardial sac). In few cases, the dissecting hematoma may re-enter the lumen of the aorta through a second distal intimal tear. This creates a new vascular channel and forms a "**double-barreled aorta**". Aortic dissections are generally classified into two types, **type A and type B dissections**.

Classical symptoms: Sudden onset of severe pain, beginning in the anterior chest, radiating to the back between the scapulae, and moving downward as the dissection progresses.

Cause of death: Rupture of the dissection outward into the pericardial, pleural, or peritoneal cavities.

Box 11.2: Major causes of hypertension (systolic and diastolic)

Primary/Essential Hypertension (~ 95% Of Case)
Secondary Hypertension
Renal • Acute glomerulonephritis • Chronic renal disease • Polycystic kidney disease
Endocrine • Adrenal disorders: Cushing's syndrome, primary aldosteronism • Pheochromocytoma
Cardiovascular • Coarctation of aorta • Polyarteritis nodosa
Neurologic • Psychogenic • Increased intracranial pressure
Preeclampsia/eclampsia
Medications • High-dose estrogens, adrenal steroids, decongestants, nonsteroidal anti-inflammatory agents

Prognosis: In the past aortic dissection was fatal, but the prognosis has markedly improved with present day advances in treatment.

HYPERTENSION

WHO definition: Hypertension is defined as **systolic** pressure **above 160 mm Hg and/or diastolic** pressure **above 90**.

Causes of Hypertension (Box 11.2)

- **Primary/essential/idiopathic** hypertension**:** It constitutes about 95% of cases.
- **Secondary** hypertension: It forms about 5% of cases and there is an identifiable cause.

The prevalence and vulnerability to complications of hypertension increase with age.

Consequences of Hypertension

- **Risk factor:** Hypertension is one of the major modifiable risk factors for **atherosclerosis**.
- **Lesions/diseases produced:** Cardiac hypertrophy, congestive heart failure (hypertensive heart disease) and ischemic heart disease (IHD), subarachnoid hemorrhage, hypertensive encephalopathy.
- **Accelerated or malignant hypertension:** It is characterized by **rapid raise in blood pressure** (i.e. systolic pressure over 200 mm Hg, diastolic pressure over 120

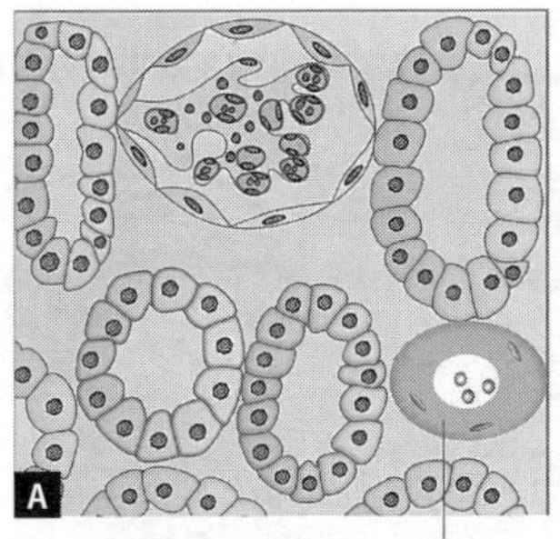

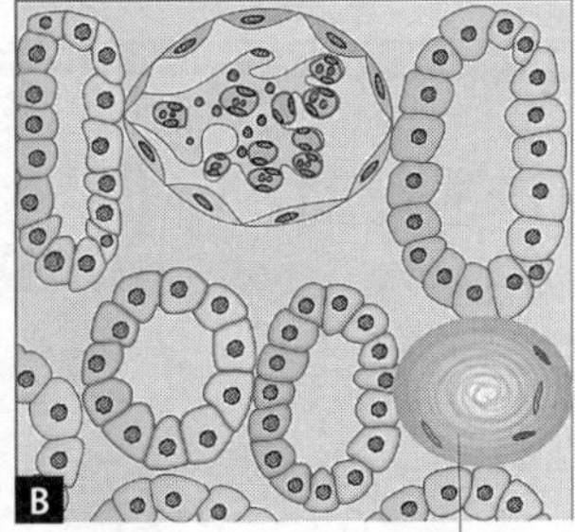

Figs 11.5A and B: Vascular changes (in renal blood vessels) in hypertension. (A) Hyaline arteriolosclerosis in benign hypertension: The arteriolar wall is thickened, hyalinized, and the lumen is narrowed; (B) Hyperplastic arteriolosclerosis in malignant hypertension: Shows onion-skinning with obliteration of arteriolar lumen

mm Hg). It may result in **renal failure, and retinal hemorrhages** and exudates, **with or without papilledema**.

Morphology

Large and Medium Vessel Disease

Hypertension is one of the major risk factor for atheroscleosis.

Small Vessel Diseases

Two forms of small vessel disease can occur in hypertension: (1) hyaline arteriolosclerosis, and (2) hyperplastic arteriolosclerosis.

1. ***Hyaline arteriolosclerosis:*** It is seen in the arterioles in patients with benign hypertension.
   - **Microscopy:** It shows **thickening of the wall due to homogeneous, pink hyaline material** and **narrowing of the lumen** (Fig. 11.5A).
2. ***Hyperplastic arteriolosclerosis:*** It occurs in **severe (malignant) hypertension.**
   - **Microscopy:** The blood vessels show "**onion-skin,**" **concentric, laminated thickening of the arteriolar walls** and narrowing of the arteriolar lumen (Fig. 11.5B). It may be also show **fibrinoid deposits and necrosis** of vessel wall **(necrotizing arteriolitis)**, particularly in the kidney.

Hypertensive Heart Disease

Systemic hypertension can increase the demands on the heart and cause pressure overload and left ventricular hypertrophy. It is termed as hypertensive heart disease (HHD).

Systemic (Left-sided) Hypertensive Heart Disease

Hypertrophy of the heart develops as an adaptive response to the pressure overload produced by chronic hypertension. However, compensatory hypertrophy can ultimately lead to myocardial dysfunction, cardiac dilation, congestive heart failure (CHF).

Morphology of heart

Hypertension produces left ventricular hypertrophy. The left ventricular wall is thickened and may exceed 2.0 cm.

VASCULITIS

Definition: Vasculitis is a **heterogeneous group** of disorders **characterized by inflammation and damage of the blood vessel**. The lumen of the involved vessel is usually narrowed → may lead to ischemia of the tissues supplied. They are classified in different ways.

- **Primary or secondary:** Vasculitis may be primary or secondary component of another primary disease.
- **Vessel involved:** It can involve any type, size, and location of blood vessel. Mostly, involve small vessels (arterioles to capillaries to venules).
- **Organ involved:** Vasculitis may be restricted to one organ (e.g. skin), or may involve many organ systems.

Examples: Giant cell (temporal) arteritis, polyarteritis nodosa, Wegener's granulomatosis.

VASCULAR TUMORS

Tumors of blood vessels are classified as benign and malignant (Box 11.2).

Hemangioma

Hemangiomas are **very common benign tumors of blood vessels** and form about 7% of all benign tumors of infancy and childhood.

Types of hemangioma: Capillary and cavernous.

Box 11.2: Classification of vascular tumors

Benign neoplasms, developmental and acquired conditions
• Hemangioma: Capillary hemangioma, cavernous hemangioma, pyogenic granuloma
Malignant neoplasms
• Angiosarcoma • Hemangiopericytoma

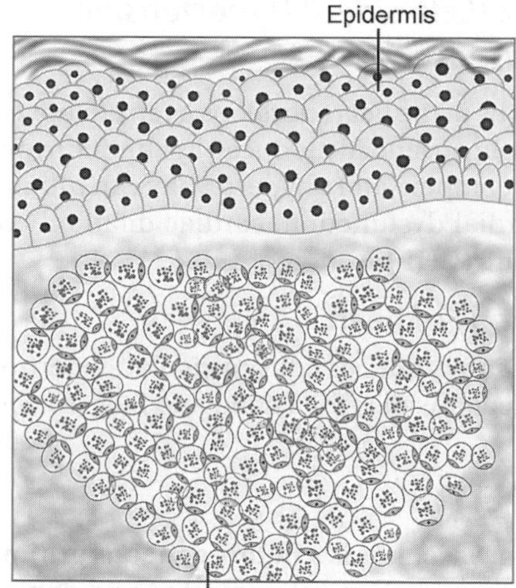

Fig. 11.6: Microscopic appearance of capillary hemangioma (diagrammatic)

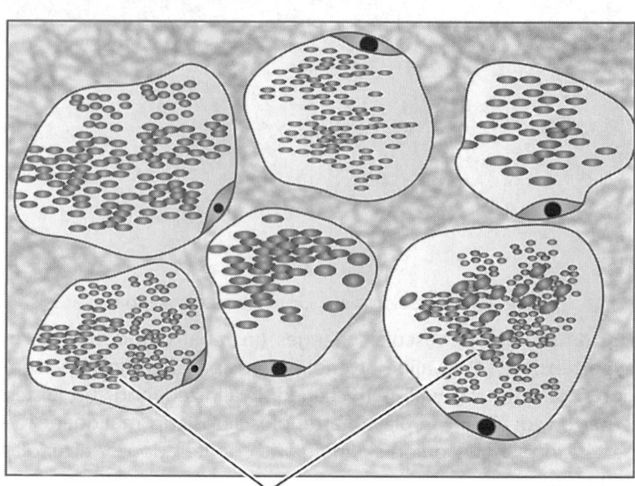

Fig. 11.7: Microscopic appearance of cavernous hemangioma (diagrammatic)

Capillary Hemangioma

- **Most common type of hemangioma.**
- **Sites:**
  - Most commonly in the **skin, subcutaneous tissues**, and mucous membranes of the oral cavities and lips.
  - Internal organs: For example, **liver**, spleen, and kidneys.
- **Microscopy** (Fig. 11.6)**:** Composed of **aggregates of closely packed, thin-walled vascular channels.** The size and structure of these **vascular channels resemble normal capillaries.**

Cavernous Hemangioma

- Consists of **large, dilated vascular channels**; compared with small vascular spaces in capillary hemangiomas.
- **Sites:** More frequently involve **deep structures**. They are found in the skin, on the mucosal surfaces and visceral organs such as the **spleen**, **liver**, and pancreas.
- **Microscopy** (Fig. 11.7)**:** Composed of **large, cavernous blood-filled vascular spaces**, separated by a moderate amount of connective tissue stroma.

SELF-ASSESSMENT EXERCISES

I. Essay

1. Etiopathogenesis and morphological features of atherosclerosis.

II. Short Notes

1. Risk factors for atherosclerosis.
2. Atherosclerosis.
3. Atheromatous plaque/atheroma.
4. Gross and microscopic features of atherosclerosis.
5. Aneurysm.

CHAPTER 12

Heart Disorders

CHAPTER OUTLINE

INTRODUCTION

Cardiovascular system consists of heart and blood vessels. The heart pumps the blood into the arterial tree and receives blood from venous circulation.

Anatomy of Heart

Normal heart weighs about 250–350 g in an adult. It is a two-sided pump having four chambers upper **two atria** (right and left) and the lower **two ventricles** (right and left). The two atria are separated from each other by interatrial septum and the two ventricles are separated by an interventricular septum. The **atria are separated from the ventricles by an atrioventricular valves.** These are **tricuspid on the right side** and **mitral valve on the left side. Blood enters** each side of the heart **into the atrium** and **then enters into the ventricles** across atrioventricular valves, the mitral valve on the left and the tricuspid valve on the right. On the ventricular side, these valves leaflets have strong fibrous cords called chordae tendineae which are attached to the inner surface of the ventricular wall via papillary muscles. The blood flows from ventricles through the semilunar valves namely pulmonary on the right side and aortic on the left side. The direction of blood flow is shown in Figure 12.1. The right ventricle is thinner (<0.5 cm) than the left ventricle (1.3–1.5 cm).

The **heart wall has three layers**: (1) inner **endocardium**, (2) middle **myocardium** and (3) outer **pericardium**. Pericardium has visceral and parietal layer with pericardial cavity in between these layers.

Blood Supply to the Heart

The heart is supplied by the **right and left coronary arteries** which arise directly from the aorta. The **left coronary artery supplies the major part of the heart**. It divides into left anterior descending and left circumflex artery.

The heart contracts at the rate ranging from 60–80 beats per minute. During systole, the heart contracts and relaxes during diastole. The heart sounds are produced during opening and closing of cardiac valves and flow of blood through the cardiac chambers and the valves. These heart sounds can be heard on auscultation.

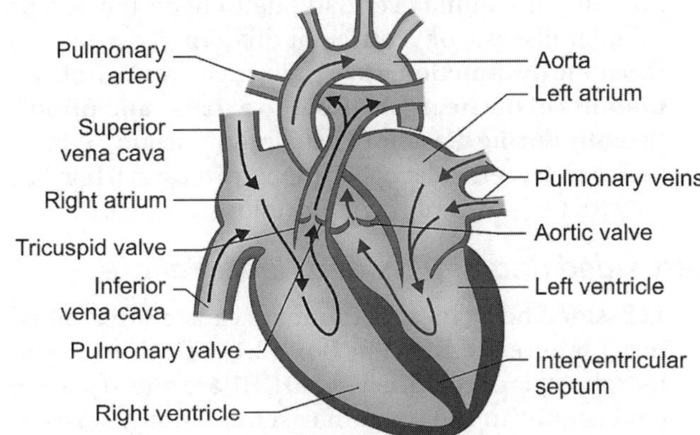

Fig. 12.1: Diagrammatic representation of direction of blood flow through the heart

HEART FAILURE

Heart failure is a common, usually progressive condition with a poor prognosis. **Older term congestive heart failure** (CHF) should be avoided because not all patients with heart failure have volume overload. Heart failure develops when the heart is not able to pump blood at a rate sufficient to meet the metabolic demands of the peripheral tissues or can do so only at an elevated filling pressure. Inadequate cardiac output is usually accompanied by increased congestion of the venous circulation.

Types of Heart Failure

Depending on Onset

- **Chronic heart failure:** Heart failure is the common **end stage of many forms of chronic heart disease.** It is characterized by gradual development of heart failure and systemic arterial pressure is well-maintained, but edema develops. Examples include valvular heart disease, hypertension, ischemic heart disease and dilated cardiomyopathy.
- **Acute heart failure:** It is characterized by **sudden development of heart failure**. Examples include: acute myocardial infarction and rupture of a cardiac valve.

Depending on Output

- **Systolic dysfunction:** Ejection fraction is the percentage of blood volume ejected from the ventricle during systole. Normally during systole, ventricles contract and eject about 45 to 65% of the blood in them at the end of diastole **[ejection fraction (EF)]**. Heart failure can result from **progressive deterioration of myocardial contractile function** (systolic dysfunction). It is characterized by a **decrease in ejection fraction**. Various causes of reduced EF include ischemic injury (myocardial infarction), inadequate adaptation to pressure or volume overload due to hypertension or valvular disease, or ventricular dilation.
- **Diastolic dysfunction:** Heart failure can result from an **inability of the heart chamber to expand and fill sufficiently during diastole** (diastolic dysfunction). Causes include left ventricular hypertrophy, myocardial fibrosis, constrictive pericarditis, or amyloidosis of heart.

Left-sided and Right-sided Heart Failure

- **Left-sided heart failure:** Common causes of left-sided heart failure are listed in Box 12.1. The clinical and morphologic effects of left-sided CHF are due to passive congestion (in the pulmonary circulation), stasis of blood in the left-sided chambers, and inadequate perfusion of tissues.

Box 12.1: Common causes of left-sided heart failure

- Ischemic heart disease (IHD)- most common cause
- Systemic hypertension
- Aortic and mitral valvular diseases
- Primary diseases of the myocardium

- **Right-sided heart failure: Most common cause is left-sided heart failure** (all causes of left-sided heart failure). **Isolated right-sided heart failure** is uncommon and usually develops **in association with disorders of the lungs**; hence it is termed as **cor pulmonale**. Cor pulmonale occurs with diseases of lung parenchyma (e.g. emphysema, chronic bronchitis), secondary to disorders of the pulmonary vasculature (e.g. primary pulmonary hypertension, recurrent pulmonary thromboembolism).

Pathophysiology of Heart Failure (Flowchart 12.1)

In chronic heart diseases compensatory mechanisms maintain cardiac output by increasing diastolic ventricular filling pressure and end-diastolic volume. This produces characteristic signs and symptoms of heart failure. Because of the heart's capacity to compensate, congestive heart failure is usually tolerated for years. Several physiologic mechanisms develop which maintain arterial pressure and organ perfusion. These include:

1. **Frank-Starling mechanism** (also known as **Starling's law**) states that as a larger volume of blood flows into the ventricle (i.e. increased filling volumes), the blood will stretch/dilate the walls of the heart, causing a greater expansion during diastole. This in turn increases the force of the contraction and thus the quantity of blood that is pumped into the aorta also increases during systole.
2. **Myocardial adaptations:** This includes **myocardial hypertrophy** with or without cardiac chamber dilation. Myocardial hypertrophy is a compensatory response to hemodynamic overload and it increases the myocyte contractile strength. In **occurs in association with** many pathological conditions such as **chronic hypertension or valvular stenosis (pressure overload),** myocardial injury, valvular insufficiency **(volume overload)** and other stresses that increase the heart's workload. The molecular, cellular, and structural changes that develops as a response to injury or changes in loading conditions are called ventricular remodeling.
3. **Activation of neurohumoral systems:** This develops to increase heart function and/or regulate filling volumes and pressures.

Flowchart 12.1: Mechanism of heart failure

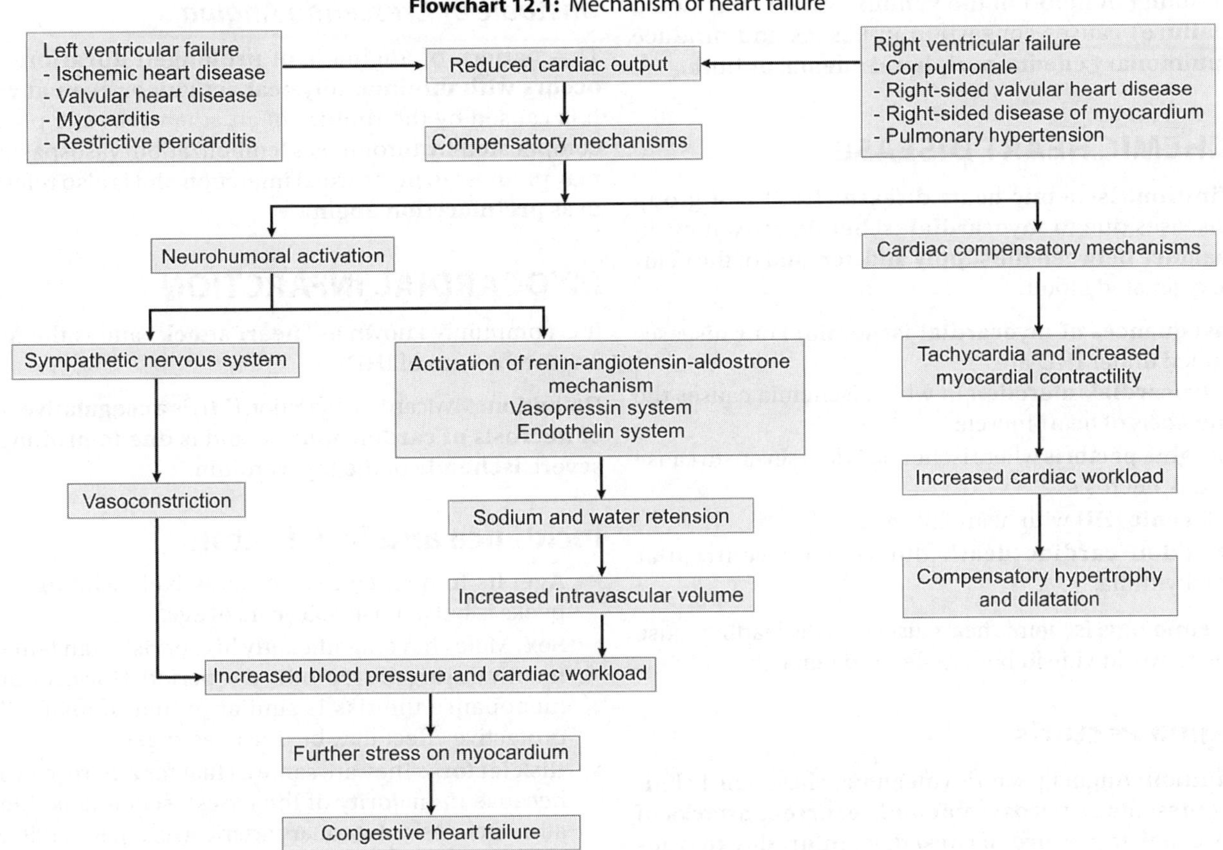

4. **Release of norepinephrine:** It is release by adrenergic cardiac nerves of the autonomic nervous system. Norepinephrine increases heart rate, myocardial contractility and vascular resistance.
5. **Activation of the renin-angiotensin-aldosterone system:** A reduced ejection fraction leads to reduced perfusion of kidney, causing activation of the renin-angiotensin-aldosterone system as a compensatory mechanism. This leads to retention of salt and water, with expansion of the interstitial and intravascular fluid volumes. This turn increases the existing pulmonary edema.
6. **Release of atrial natriuretic peptide:** The last two factors act to adjust filling volumes and pressures. The above mentioned adaptive mechanisms may be adequate to maintain normal cardiac output in the initial phase, but this capacity may be ultimately lost.

Cardiac Hypertrophy

Sustained increase in mechanical work due to pressure or volume overload (e.g. systemic hypertension or aortic stenosis) cause myocytes to increase in size *(hypertrophy)*. This in turn increases the size and weight of the heart.

Causes and patterns of hypertrophy

The pattern of hypertrophy depends the stimulus.

- **Pressure-overload hypertrophy:** It is characterized by a concentric increase in wall thickness (e.g. due to hypertension or aortic stenosis).
- **Volume-overload hypertrophy:** It is characterized by ventricular dilation and the wall thickness may be increased, normal, or less than normal (e.g. myocardial infarction). Hence, heart weight (and not the thickness of wall thickness) is the best measure of hypertrophy in dilated hearts.

Functional changes

Cardiac hypertrophy is associated with increase in oxygen consumption by heart. Hence, the hypertrophied heart is susceptible to ischemia.

Progression of Heart Failure

- Heart failure is characterized by variable degrees of **decreased cardiac output and tissue perfusion** (sometimes called forward failure). This produces hypoxic injury.

- **Pooling of blood in the venous system (backward failure)** causes congestion in tissues and produce **pulmonary edema, peripheral edema, or both.**

ISCHEMIC HEART DISEASE

Definition: Ischemic heart disease (IHD) is a group of diseases due to **myocardial ischemia** caused by an **imbalance between the supply and demand** of the heart for oxygenated blood.

Consequences of myocardial ischemia: Four diseases included under IHD are:

- **Myocardial infarction** in which ischemia causes the necrosis of heart muscle.
- **Angina pectoris** where ischemia is less severe to cause frank necrosis.
- **Chronic IHD** with heart failure.
- **Sudden cardiac death** due to fatal ventricular arrhythmia.

Epidemiology: Ischemic heart disease is the leading cause of death worldwide in both males and females.

Angina Pectoris

Definition: Angina pectoris (meaning, chest pain) clinically presents as **paroxysmal and recurrent attacks of substernal or precordial chest discomfort due to transient myocardial ischemia** which falls short of inducing necrosis of myocardial cell.

Patterns of angina pectoris:

1. Stable or typical angina
2. Prinzmetal variant angina
3. Unstable or crescendo angina.

Stable Angina

It is most common and is also known as **typical angina pectoris**. It is due to **atherosclerosis of coronary artery**. It develops when myocardial oxygen demand increases as with increased physical activity or emotional excitement. Chest pain is **relieved by rest** (which decreases demand) **or by sublingual nitroglycerin** (a strong vasodilator which increases perfusion).

Prinzmetal Variant Angina

It is an uncommon atypical form of angina. This is due to **spasm of coronary artery** having **atherosclerosis**. It **occurs at rest** and responds promptly to vasodilators.

Unstable or Crescendo Angina

This pattern of angina is of **prolonged duration** and **occurs with minimal physical activity or even at rest**. It is caused by the rupture of an atherosclerotic plaque complicated by thrombosis/embolization/vasospasm. It may progress to myocardial infarction and is also referred to as **preinfarction angina.**

MYOCARDIAL INFARCTION

It is commonly known as "**heart attack**" and is the most important form of IHD.

Definition: Myocardial infarction (MI) is a **coagulative type of necrosis of cardiac muscle** and is **due to prolonged severe ischemia** of the myocardium.

Incidence and Risk Factors

- **Age:** Its frequency rises progressively with age and peaks is between 40–65 years of age.
- **Sex:** Males have significantly higher risk than females mainly during the reproductive period. However, after menopause the risk is similar to that of males. The protective effect may be due to estrogen.
- **Risk factors:** They are same as that for atherosclerosis because in majority of the cases ischemia is due to atherosclerosis of coronary arteries (refer pages 109–10).

Etiology and Pathogenesis

Decreased coronary blood flow: In 90% of cases myocardial infarction is due to **narrowing** of one or more **coronary arteries caused by atherosclerosis**. So, IHD is often known as coronary artery disease.

Increased myocardial demand: Some of the etiological factors increase the myocardial demand of oxygen/blood supply. These include:

- Myocardial hypertrophy
- Increased heart rate (tachycardia).

Types of Infarct

Depending on the **thickness of myocardium involved** myocardial infarct can be divided into transmural and subendocardial.

- **Transmural:** This type of ischemic necrosis involves the **full or nearly full thickness** of the ventricular wall in the area supplied by the coronary artery.

- **Subendocardial (nontransmural):** In this type, the area of ischemic necrosis is **limited to the inner one-third to one-half** of the ventricular wall.

Morphology

Gross

- **Within first 12 hours: No** identifiable **gross changes** are seen.
- **Between 12 and 24 hours:** Infarct appears as a **pale reddish-blue area.**
- **Between 1 and 7 days:** It appears as central **pale, yellowish, necrotic region** with well-demarcated border of hyperemic zone (due to granulation tissue).
- **By 1–2 weeks:** The area of infarct appears **soft and rimmed by a hyperemic zone** of highly vascularized granulation tissue.
- **After 2 weeks:** The older, healed infarcts appear **firm, pale gray and contracted,** which develops into a fibrous scar.

Microscopy

The histopathological changes also proceed in a fairly predictable sequence (Fig. 12.2).

- **First 6–12 hours:** The earliest changes can be detected only by electron microscopy during first 6 hours. This is followed by appearance of coagulative necrosis.
- **Between 12 and 24 hours:** The characteristic changes of **coagulation necrosis** appear in the myocardial fibers namely preserved cell outlines, deeply eosinophilic cytoplasm and nuclei show pyknosis.
- **Between 1 and 3 days: Acute inflammatory reaction** with accumulation of **polymorphonuclear leukocytes** at the periphery/borders of infarct.
- **3 to 7 days:** The polymorphonuclear leukocytes are replaced by **macrophages** which phagocytose and remove the necrotic myocytes at the border of infarct. **Granulation tissue** appears at the periphery of infarct, and gradually extends toward the center.
- **1 to 2 weeks:** Process of **healing starts** from its margins toward its center. Fibroblasts proliferate and **collagen deposition** proceeds.
- **More than 2 weeks:** Increased **deposition of collagen and the scar** becomes more solid and less cellular as it matures.

Diagnosis of Myocardial Infarction

It is based on clinical symptoms, laboratory evaluation and electrocardiographic changes.

Clinical Symptoms

Patients with MI usually present with retrosternal chest pain radiating to left jaw or left arm, rapid, weak pulse, profuse sweating and dyspnea.

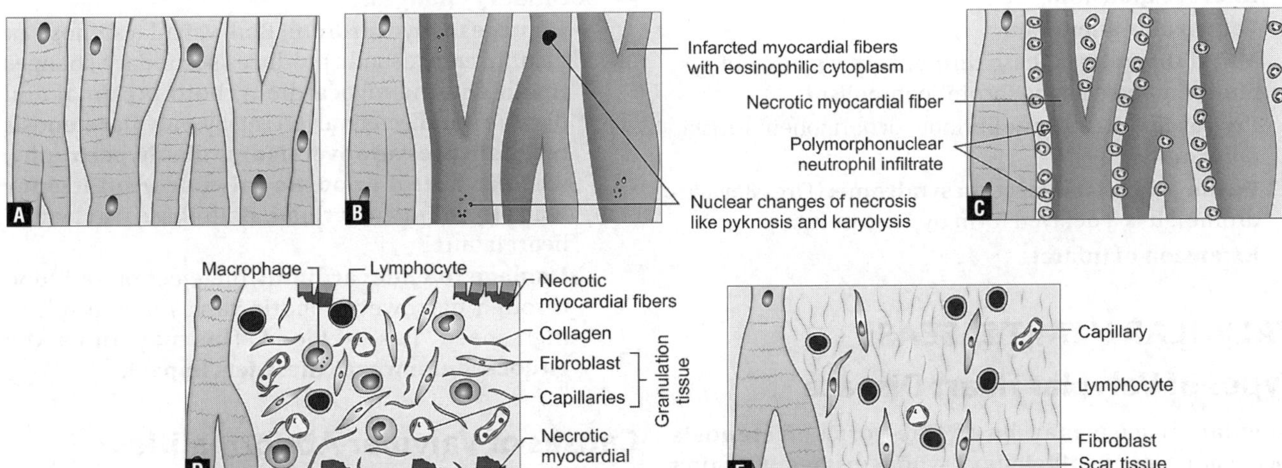

Figs 12.2A to E: Microscopic changes observed during development of a myocardial infarct. (A) Normal myocardium; (B) After about 12–18 hours, the infarcted myocardium shows myocardial fibers with eosinophilia; (C) About 24 hours after the onset of infarction, polymorphonuclear neutrophils infiltrate at the periphery of infarcted area; (D) After about 3 weeks, the infarcted area consists of granulation tissue infiltrated by lymphocytes and macrophages; (E) After 3 months or more, the infarcted region is replaced by collagenous tissue

Laboratory Evaluation

- **Cardiac troponins:** Cardiac-specific proteins are of two types namely *Troponins I and T*. They are released into circulation and the levels begin to **rise at 2–4 hours** and **peak at 48 hours.** The elevated troponin levels may remain for 7–10 days after acute MI.
- **Cardiac creatine phosphokinase (CK):** MB form of creatine kinase (CK-MB) is sensitive but not specific. CK-MB levels rise **within 2–4 hours** of the onset of MI, **peak at 24 hours**, and return to normal within 72 hours.
- **Lactate dehydrogenase (LDH):** This is not a specific marker. It starts rising after 24–48 hours. It remains for many days and returns to normal in 7–14 days.
- **Myoglobin:** It is the earliest marker of MI, the level rises within 1–3 hours. It peaks in about 8–12 hours and returns to normal in about 24–36 hours.

Electrocardiography Changes

Transmural infarct causes elevation of ST segment in ECG, known as "ST elevation infarcts". The subendocardial infarcts are known as "non-ST elevation infarcts."

Complications of Myocardial Infarction

1. **Left ventricular failure and cardiogenic shock**.
2. **Arrhythmias**.
3. **Myocardial rupture:** It is most frequent during 3–7 days after transmural infarcts.
4. **Infarct expansion.**
5. **Ventricular aneurysm.**
6. **Mural thrombus:** These thrombi are a source of systemic emboli causing thromboembolism.
7. **Pericarditis:** It can cause fibrinous or fibrinohemorrhagic pericarditis.
8. **Postmyocardial infarction syndrome:** (Dressler syndrome): It is a delayed form of pericarditis.
9. **Extension of infarct**.

VALVULAR HEART DISEASE

Types of Valvular Heart Disease

Valvular disease may be in the form of **stenosis** (occlusion), **or insufficiency** (synonyms: regurgitation or incompetence), **or both**. Both may be **congenital or acquired**. Acquired aortic and mitral valves stenoses constitute about two-thirds of all valve disease.

- **Stenosis** is the **failure of a valve to open completely** and it obstructs the forward flow of blood.
- **Insufficiency** is due to **failure of a valve to close completely** and it allows the reversed flow of blood.

These abnormalities may be present alone or coexist, and may involve only one valve, or more than one valve.

- **Functional regurgitation** is the **incompetence of a valve resulting from an abnormality in one of its support structures** and **not due to primary valve defect**. E.g. dilation of the right or left ventricle may cause pulling of the ventricular papillary muscles and prevent the proper closure of otherwise normal mitral or tricuspid leaflets. Functional mitral valve regurgitation is common in IHD and dilated cardiomyopathy.

Clinical Consequences of Valve Dysfunction

- It varies **depending on the valve involved, the degree of impairment, mode of onset, and the rate and quality of compensatory mechanisms**. For example, sudden destruction of an aortic valve cusp by infection (infective endocarditis) may produce acute, massive, and rapidly fatal regurgitation. In contrast, rheumatic mitral stenosis which develops slowly and gradually over years and its clinical effects can be minimal for several years.
- **Associated conditions:** Certain conditions may complicate valvular heart disease and increase the demands on the heart. For example, the increased output demands during **pregnancy can worsen the valve disease** and may lead to unfavorable maternal or fetal outcomes.
- **Secondary changes:**
  - **Damage to myocardium:** Both valvular stenosis or insufficiency usually produces secondary changes (mainly in the myocardium) both proximal and distal to the affected valve. Usually, **valvular stenosis results in pressure overload cardiac hypertrophy**, whereas **mitral or aortic valvular insufficiency leads to volume overload**. Both these can lead to heart failure.
  - **Damage to endocardium:** The ejection of blood through narrowed stenotic valves may produce high speed "jets" of blood. This **may injure the endocardium where these jets impact**.

Causes of Valvular Abnormalities (Table 12.1)

It can be congenital or acquired.

- **Acquired valvular stenosis:** It is always due to a remote or chronic injury of the valve cusps and manifest clinically only after many years.
- **Acquired valvular insufficiency:** It can be due to intrinsic disease of the valve cusps or damage to or

Table 12.1: Major causes of acquired heart valve disease

Mitral valve disease	Aortic valve disease
Mitral stenosis	**Aortic stenosis**
• Postinflammatory scarring (rheumatic heart disease)	• Postinflammatory scarring (rheumatic heart disease) • Senile calcific aortic stenosis
Mitral regurgitation	**Aortic regurgitation**
• Postinflammatory scarring • Infective endocarditis • Mitral valve prolapse	• Postinflammatory scarring (rheumatic heart disease) • Syphilitic aortitis • Ankylosing spondylitis

distortion of the supporting structures (e.g. the aorta, mitral annulus, tendinous cords, papillary muscles, ventricular free wall).

The causes of acquired heart valve diseases are listed in Table 12.1. The most frequent causes of the major functional valvular lesions are:

- **Aortic stenosis:** Calcification and sclerosis of anatomically normal/congenital bicuspid aortic valves
- **Aortic insufficiency:** Dilation of the ascending aorta secondary to hypertension and/or aging
- **Mitral stenosis:** Rheumatic heart disease
- **Mitral insufficiency:** Myxomatous degeneration (mitral valve prolapse).

Calcific Valvular Degeneration

Heart valves are delicate structures which are **subjected to high levels of repetitive mechanical stress.** They **can undergo cumulative damage and become calcified.** This may lead to clinically important valvular dysfunction.

Calcific Aortic Stenosis

Calcific aortic stenosis is narrowing of the aortic valve orifice due to deposition of calcium in the valve cusps and ring.

Etiologic factors and pathology

Calcific aortic stenosis is the **most common valvular abnormality.** It usually develops as the consequence of **age-associated "wear and tear"** of either anatomically normal valves or congenitally bicuspid valves.

1. **Degenerative (senile) calcific stenosis:** Aortic stenosis of previously normal valves is called senile calcific aortic stenosis and usually manifests clinically in the 7th to 9th decades of life. Aortic valve calcification occurs probably due to recurrent chronic injury.
2. **Congenital bicuspid aortic stenosis:** Bicuspid aortic valve (BAV) is a developmental abnormality and has a heritability basis. Bicuspid aortic stenosis clinically manifests 1 to 2 decades earlier than normal valves.

Morphology

Grossly, calcific aortic stenosis (involving either tricuspid or bicuspid valves) is characterized by the **presence of calcified masses/nodules** restricted to the base and lower half of the aortic cusps. Later these calcified foci protrude through the outflow surfaces into the sinuses of valsalva, and prevent opening of cusps. Usually, the free margins/edges of the cusps are not involved.

Clinical features

- Calcific aortic stenosis (superimposed on a previously normal or bicuspid aortic valve) produces **obstruction to left ventricular outflow** due to gradual narrowing of the valve orifice.
- **Left ventricular pressures rises** producing concentric **left ventricular** (pressure overload **hypertrophy**). The hypertrophied myocardium is prone to ischemia due to diminished perfusion and often complicated by coronary atherosclerosis. This may produce angina pectoris. Eventually, cardiac decompensation and CHF can develop. Treatment consists of surgical valve replacement.

Mitral Annular Calcification

Calcification of the mitral valve annulus occurs commonly in the elderly. In contrast to calcification in RF (rheumatic fever)—damaged valves, valve leaflets are not deformed and calcification affects the annulus than the leaflets.

Grossly, it appears as irregular, stony hard, occasionally ulcerated nodules (2 to 5 mm in thickness) at the base of the leaflets.

Complications

Mitral annular calcification **usually does not affect valvular function** but **may produce a murmur** and is usually without functional significance.

Mitral Valve Prolapse (Myxomatous Degeneration of the Mitral Valve)

In mitral valve prolapse (MVP), one or both **mitral valve leaflets become enlarged and floppy. Chordae tendineae are thinned and elongated, so that the leaflets prolapse,** or balloon back, into the left atrium during systole. It is also called "floppy mitral valve syndrome". MVP is the most common cause of mitral regurgitation. It is usually an incidental finding on physical examination. MVP needs surgical valve repair or replacement.

Etiopathogenesis of MVP is unknown in majority of cases. Uncommonly, MVP is associated with heritable disorders of connective tissue (e.g. Marfan syndrome).

Morphology

Gross: Mitral valve leaflets are deformed, enlarged, redundant, thick, and rubbery. The characteristic change is interchordal ballooning (hooding) of the mitral leaflets or its portions.

Microscopy: Shows marked thickening with deposition of mucoid (myxomatous) material, called **myxomatous degeneration of the mitral valve.**

Clinical features

- Most patients are asymptomatic and it is detected incidentally by auscultation of mid-systolic clicks, sometimes followed by a mid to late systolic murmur. The diagnosis is confirmed by echocardiography.
- Minority of patients may present with chest pain mimicking angina and dyspnea.

Complications

These include: (1) infective endocarditis, (2) mitral insufficiency (with rupture of chorda tendinae), (3) stroke or other systemic infarct, due to embolism of leaflet thrombi; or (4) arrhythmias (ventricular and atrial); and (5) rarely sudden cardiac death.

Treatment

Valve repair or replacement surgery for symptomatic patients or those with increased risk for significant complications.

RHEUMATIC FEVER AND RHEUMATIC HEART DISEASE

Definition: Rheumatic fever (RF) is an **acute, post-streptococcal, immune mediated, multisystem inflammatory disease**.

Etiology and Pathogenesis

Acute rheumatic fever is a post-streptococcal disease. It develops in a susceptible host after a latent period of 2–6 weeks following pharyngitis by group A β-hemolytic streptococci. It is seen most commonly in **children** between 5–15 years.

Immunologically Mediated Disease (Figs 12.3A and B)

It is an immunological mediated **autoimmune** disease. Specific strains of group A streptococcal infection introduce the streptococcal antigens into the body and produce antibodies. These antibodies cross-react with self-antigens which mimic group A streptococcal antigens. It is believed that both cross-reactive antibodies (humoral immunity) and cross-reactive T cells (cell-mediated immunity) play a role in the disease. The self-antigens that are involved include antigens in the myocardial cells, glycoproteins of the valves in the heart, proteins in other target organs such as synovium, neuronal tissue, subcutaneous, and dermal tissues. The result is **immunological mediated inflammatory damage to the affected tissue**.

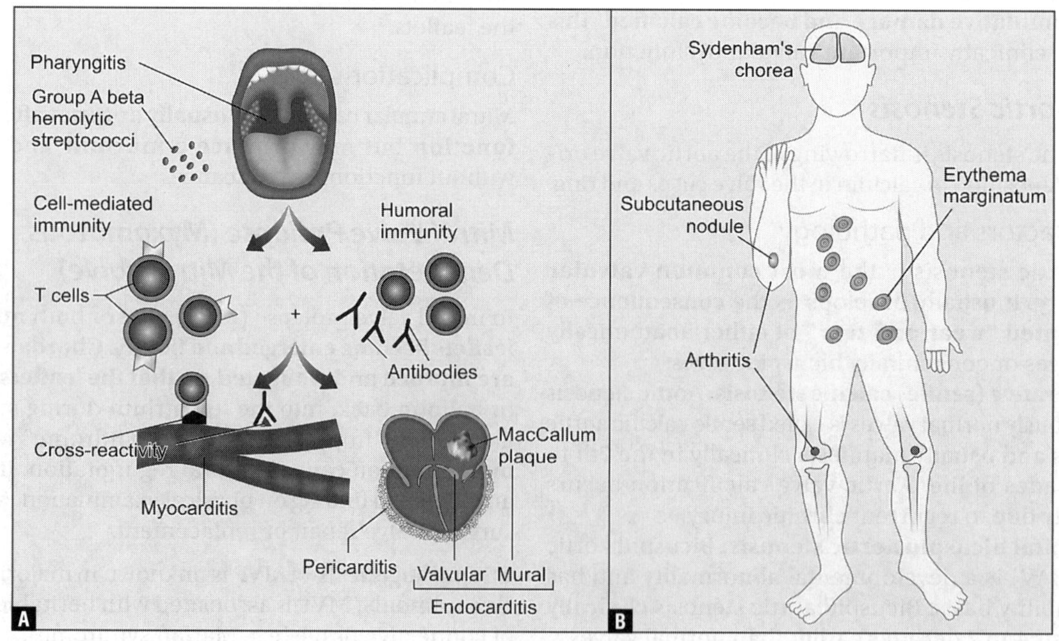

Figs 12.3A and B: Pathogenesis and lesions of rheumatic fever. (A) Cardiac lesions; (B) Extracardiac lesions

Morphology

The lesions of rheumatic fever can be broadly divided into cardiac and extracardiac lesions.

Cardiac Lesions

Acute rheumatic fever manifests usually as **acute rheumatic carditis** which **may progress to chronic rheumatic heart disease (RHD).**

Acute rheumatic carditis

It is characterized by **pancarditis**, involving all three layers of the heart (**endocardium, myocardium, and pericardium**). The characteristic histological lesion of rheumatic heart disease is Aschoff body/nodule.

Aschoff body (Fig. 12.4)

It is the pathognomonic histological lesion of RF having spherical or fusiform shape. It consists of **central fibrinoid degeneration** surrounded by **Anitschkow cells, T-lymphocytes** and **macrophages. Anitschkow cells** are pathognomonic for RF and are activated macrophages having round-to ovoid nuclei. The nuclei of these cells **resemble a caterpillar** when **cut longitudinally** (hence known as **"caterpillar cells"**). On cross-section, the nuclei of these cells have an **owl eye appearance**. Few Anitschkow cells may become **multinucleated** (with 2 to 4 nuclei) and these cells are termed **Aschoff giant cells.**

- **Endocarditis** (Fig. 12.5)**:** Inflammation of the endocardium is known as endocarditis. Inflammation may involve valvular (valvular endocarditis) or mural endocardium (mural endocarditis).
  - **Valvular endocarditis:** Left-sided valves (mitral and aortic) are more commonly involved than right-side. The endocardium shows small (1–2 mm) nodular vegetations, called **verrucae** along the **lines of closure of the valve leaflets.**
  - **Mural endocarditis:** Mural lesion appears as subendocardial thickening in the **posterior wall of the left atrium** and is known as **MacCallum plaque.**
- **Pericarditis:** Rheumatic fever causes **fibrinous pericarditis.** Grossly, this resembles the shaggy surfaces of two slices of buttered bread that have been gently pulled apart. Hence, these lesions are commonly called as **bread-and-butter pericarditis.**
- **Myocarditis:** The myocardium shows nonspecific myocarditis.

Chronic rheumatic heart disease

The myocarditis and pericarditis usually resolve in patients with rheumatic carditis. But the valvular endocarditis may result in structural and functional changes in the valves.

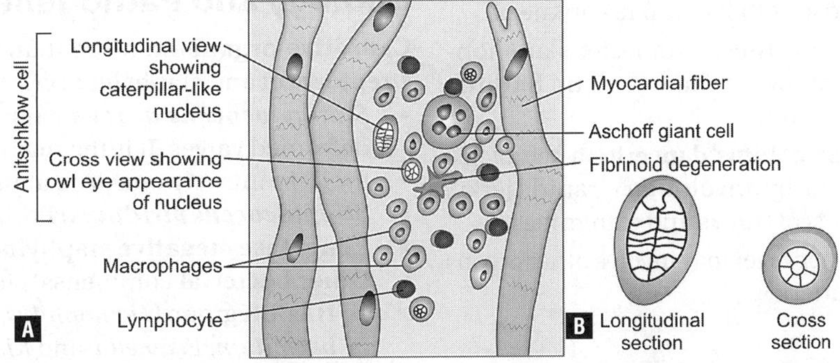

Figs 12.4A and B: (A) Microscopic appearance of Aschoff body; (B) Magnified view of Anitschkow cells

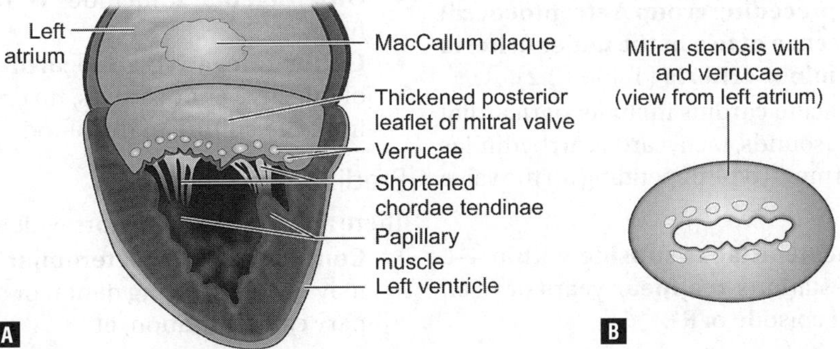

Figs 12.5A and B: Endocardial lesions of rheumatic heart disease. (A) Longitudinal view; (B) View of mitral valve

Valves affected

The **mitral valve** is the most commonly (65–70% of cases) and severely affected valve in chronic rheumatic disease. This is followed by the **aortic valve** in about 25% of cases. The involved mitral/aortic valve may show **stenosis or incompetence.** In rheumatic mitral stenosis, the valve leaflets are diffusely thickened due to fibrosis and become rigid. The mitral commissures fuse, the chordae tendinae fuse and shorten. These changes, in turn, lead to narrowing at the apex of the valve resulting in a funnel shaped ("**fish-mouth**") valve.

Complications of chronic rheumatic heart disease: These include: **Infective endocarditis**, mural thrombi, thromboemboli, congestive heart failure, adhesive pericarditis and arrhythmias.

Extracardiac Lesions (*Fig. 12.3*)

Patients with acute rheumatic fever may show the extracardiac lesions. These include:

- **Migratory polyarthritis:** In migrating polyarthritis, one large joint becomes painful and swollen, which then subsides and another joint gets involved for a period of days.
- **Subcutaneous nodules:** These nodules are oval to spherical and painless. They are usually located at the extensor aspect of wrists, elbows, ankles or knees.
- **Erythema marginatum:** These skin lesions are non-itchy reddish rashes showing characteristic **bathing suit** pattern of distribution.
- **Sydenham chorea or Saint Vitus' dance:** It is a neurologic disorder characterized by involuntary rapid, jerky, purposeless movements of trunks and extremities.
- **Other organs:** Rheumatic fever may involve other organs like lung, pleura and arteries.

Clinical Features

The diagnosis of rheumatic fever is made by using **Jones criteria: Evidence of a preceding group A streptococcal infection**, with the **presence of two of the major criteria or one major and two minor criteria** (Table 12.2).

Clinical findings of acute carditis include: pericardial friction rubs, weak heart sounds, tachycardia, arrhythmias and various cardiac murmurs (type depending on the valve involved).

Course: Most of the **acute attacks subside** within 4–6 weeks. Clinical manifestations **reappear** years or even decades after the initial episode of RF.

Table 12.2: Jones criteria for diagnosis of rheumatic fever

Major criteria	Minor criteria
• Pancarditis • Migratory polyarthritis of the large joints • Sydenham's chorea • Erythema marginatum • Subcutaneous nodules	• Fever • Arthralgia • Elevated blood levels of acute-phase reactants, raised ESR and leukocytosis

Prognosis

Long-term prognosis has improved due to surgical repair or prosthetic replacement of diseased valves.

INFECTIVE ENDOCARDITIS

Definition: Infective endocarditis (IE) is **infection of endocardium** by microbial agents. They usually involve valvular endocardium and produce lesions called vegetations. These **vegetations** are composed of platelets, fibrin, micro colonies of microorganisms, and scant inflammatory cells.

Classification: Infective endocarditis is classified according to its clinical course as **acute or subacute** endocarditis.

Differences between acute and subacute endocarditis are shown in Table 12.3.

Etiology and Pathogenesis

Causative organism: More than 90% of IE is caused by streptococci and staphylococci.

- ***Staphylococcus aureus*** can infect either healthy or deformed valves. It is the major organism responsible for IE in intravenous drug abusers.
- ***Streptococcus viridians:*** Portal of entry is oral cavity.
- **Coagulase-negative staphylococci**.
- **Other bacterial** commensals in the oral cavity:
  - **HACEK** group (*Hemophilus, Actinobacillus, Cardiobacterium, Eikenella*, and *Kingella*). Portal of entry is through the upper respiratory tract.
  - Enterococci.
- **Other agents:** It includes Gram-negative bacilli and fungi.
- **Culture-negative endocarditis:** In 10–15% of cases of infective endocarditis, no organism can be isolated from the culture of the blood.

Predisposing factors

There are three main factors which may predispose to IE.

1. **Conditions with bacteremia: Transient bacteremia** may develop during dental or surgical procedure, urinary catheterization, etc.

Table 12.3: Differences between acute and subacute infective endocarditis

Characteristics	Acute infective endocarditis	Subacute infective endocarditis
Onset	Acute in onset	Insidious in onset
Condition of valve	Infection of normal heart/cardiac valve	Infection of structurally abnormal/deformed valves
Virulence of organisms	Highly virulent (suppurative)	Low virulence
Lesions	Affected valve is rapidly destroyed	Less destructive
Clinical features	Clinical features of acute infection	Clinical features of complications
Course	Death within 6 weeks	Protracted course of weeks to months
Complications	Acute heart failure or overwhelming sepsis	Infectious complications are uncommon

2. **Underlying heart disease:** Infective endocarditis may involve either normal or damaged heart valves. Infective endocarditis on previously normal valves develop usually with high virulence organisms. The damaged heart valve may be due to **congenital heart disease or chronic rheumatic heart disease.**
3. **Impaired host defense mechanism:** These conditions include diabetes, leukemia and lymphomas.

Gross

The pathognomonic lesion of IE is the presence of **vegetations.** They are most commonly found on the aortic and mitral valves. These vegetations are **friable, bulky,** may be **single or multiple** (Fig. 12.6).

Complications of IE

They may be divided into cardiac and extracardiac complications.

Cardiac Complications

- The infection may spread locally from valve and produce an abscess which is known as **ring abscess.**
- **Perforation and rupture of involved** valve leaflets.
- **Myocardial abscess.**
- **Suppurative pericarditis.**
- **Valvular dysfunction** (stenosis or insufficiency).

Extracardiac Complications

- **Septic emboli:** The vegetations are likely to be break, detach and cause embolism. These septic emboli may lead to **septic infarcts** in organs (e.g. spleen, kidney or brain).
- **Immunological phenomena:**
  - **Focal segmental glomerulonephritis**
  - **Osler nodes:** These are small, **tender subcutaneous nodules in the pulp of the digits** and persist for hours to several days.

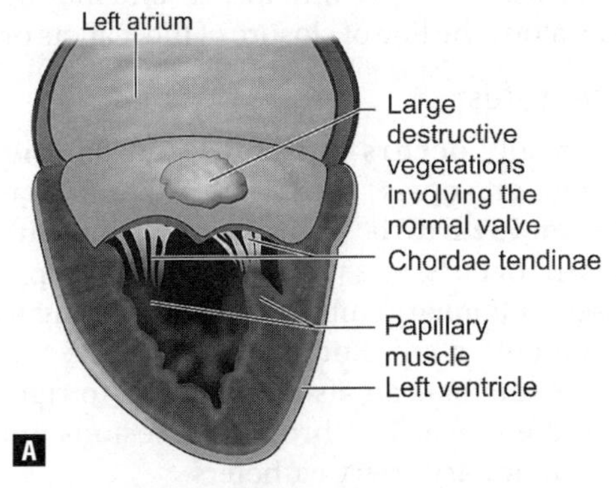

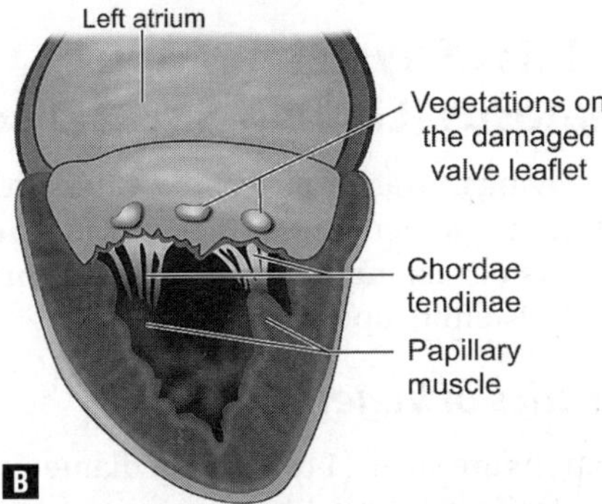

Figs 12.6A to B: (A) Acute bacterial endocarditis showing large vegetations on the normal valves; (B) Subacute bacterial endocarditis showing small vegetations involving the damaged valve

  - **Splinter hemorrhages in the nail.**
  - **Roth spots** are retinal hemorrhages in the eye.

Clinical Features

Fever is the most common symptom of IE. Acute IE develops rapidly and presents with fever, chills, weakness, and lassitude. Murmurs may be heard either due to new valvular defect or a pre-existing cardiac disease.

NONINFECTED VEGETATIONS

Noninfected (sterile) vegetations develop in nonbacterial thrombotic endocarditis and the endocarditis of systemic lupus erythematosus (SLE), called Libman-Sacks endocarditis.

Nonbacterial Thrombotic Endocarditis

Nonbacterial thrombotic endocarditis (NBTE) is characterized by the deposition of small sterile (nonbacterial) thrombi on the leaflets of the heart valves. The thrombi/vegetations measure 1 to 5 mm in size, and may be single or multiple along the line of closure of the leaflets or cusps.

Clinical features

NBTE is usually **occurs in debilitated patients** (e.g. with cancer or sepsis) and was previously termed **marantic endocarditis** (marasmus = malnutrition). It frequently occurs in association with deep venous thromboses, pulmonary emboli, or an underlying systemic hypercoagulable state. Endocardial trauma (e.g. with indwelling catheter) can also predispose to right-sided valvular and endocardial thrombotic lesions along the course of pulmonary artery catheters.

Endocarditis of Systemic Lupus Erythematosus (Libman-Sacks Disease)

Valvulitis involving mitral and tricuspid vales with small, sterile vegetations on them are termed as **Libman-Sacks endocarditis**, is occasionally found in an autoimmune disease called systemic lupus erythematosus.

Characteristics of Vegetations

These vegetations are small (1 to 4 mm in diameter), single or multiple, sterile, pink and have a warty (verrucous) appearance. They are found on the undersurfaces of the atrioventricular valves, on the valvular endocardium, on the chords, or on the mural endocardium of atria or ventricles. The mitral valve is more commonly involved than the aortic valve, and regurgitation is the usual functional abnormality.

CARCINOID HEART DISEASE

Carcinoid **tumors** are **derived from neuroendocrine** cells. **Carcinoid syndrome is a systemic disorder characterized by flushing, diarrhea, dermatitis and bronchoconstriction** which is **caused by bioactive compounds** (e.g. serotonin) released by carcinoid tumors. It usually occurs in patients with carcinoid tumor of the small intestine having massive metastasis to the liver. The liver normally catabolizes circulating mediators before they can affect the heart. Carcinoid heart disease is an unusual condition that refers to the heart manifestations caused by the bioactive compounds and develops in about 50% of the patients with carcinoid syndrome. **Carcinoid heart disease affects the right side of the heart** and **leads to tricuspid regurgitation and pulmonary stenosis.**

Pathogenesis

The **mediators** secreted by carcinoid tumors include **serotonin (5-hydroxytryptamine), kallikrein, bradykinin, histamine, prostaglandins, and tachykinins.** Exact pathogenesis of carcinoid heart disease is not known, but the valvular and endocardial lesions are probably caused by high concentrations of serotonin or other vasoactive amines and peptides secreted by the tumor (metastatic) in the liver. These mediators are metabolized in the lung and hence, carcinoid heart disease exclusively affects the right side of the heart (since right sided cardiac tissues are bathed first by the mediators released by gastrointestinal carcinoid tumors). The left side of the heart may be protected because of the degradation of these mediators by the pulmonary vascular bed. Rarely, left-sided may be involved in patients with atrial or ventricular septal defects (right-to-left flow), or when primary carcinoid tumor of the lung.

COMPLICATIONS OF PROSTHETIC VALVES

Replacement of damaged cardiac valves with prostheses is a common and is usually life-saving mode of therapy.

Types of Valvular Prostheses

- **Mechanical valves:** These consist of rigid nonphysiologic material, such as caged balls, tilting disks, or hinged semicircular flaps (bileaflet tilting disk valves).
- **Tissue valves (bioprostheses):** Porcine aortic valves or bovine pericardium are preserved in a dilute glutaraldehyde and then mounted on a prosthetic frame. Frozen human valves from deceased donors (termed cryopreserved "homografts") may be used. Tissue valves are flexible and function similar to natural semilunar valves.
  - **Drawbacks:** Chemical treatment of the animal valves and freezing and thawing of human homografts renders them largely nonviable.

Complications (Box 12.2)

About 60% of patients with valve recipients develop serious prosthesis-related complications within 10 years of surgery. The complications depend on type of valve used.

- **Thromboembolism:** It is the major complication with mechanical valves. Thrombotic may occlude the pros-

Box 12.2: Complications of cardiac valve prostheses

- Thrombosis or thromboembolism
- Anticoagulant-related hemorrhage
- Infective-prosthetic valve endocarditis
- Structural deterioration (intrinsic) of the prosthetic valve: Wear, fracture, failure, cuspal tear, calcification, etc.
- Others: Inadequate healing (paravalvular leak), obstruction due to overgrowth of fibrous tissue, intravascular hemolysis

thesis or emboli may be released from thrombi formed on the valve.

- **Anticoagulant-related hemorrhage:** Thromboembolism can be prevented by using long-term anticoagulant therapy in all patients with mechanical valves. However, these anticoagulants increase the **risk of hemorrhagic stroke or other forms of serious bleeding.**
- **Infective-prosthetic valve endocarditis:** It is a serious complication of any valve replacement. The major organisms responsible are staphylococcal skin contaminants (e.g. *S. epidermidis*), *S. aureus*, streptococci, and fungi.
- **Structural deterioration: It may rarely cause failure of mechanical valve.** However, almost all bioprosthesis eventually become incompetent due to calcification and/or tearing.
- **Other complications:** These include inadequate healing causing paravalvular leak, obstruction due to overgrowth of fibrous tissue during healing, intravascular hemolysis due to high shear forces, or excessive noise due to hard contacts of moving rigid parts.

CARDIOMYOPATHY

Definition: Cardiomyopathies are a **heterogeneous group of diseases of the myocardium that affect the mechanical or electrical function of the heart.**

- Cardiomyopathy term should be restricted to the conditions which primarily affect the myocardium. It does not include myocardial involvement due to of congenital, acquired valvular, hypertensive, and coronary arterial or pericardial abnormalities.

Etiology

They can be genetic/inherited or have infective, toxic causes or idiopathic.

Classification

Cardiomyopathies may be classified according to a variety of criteria, including the underlying genetic basis of dysfunction. Two fundamental forms of cardiomyopathy are:

1. **Primary cardiomyopathy:** Consists of heart muscle disease predominantly involving the myocardium and/or of unknown cause. Three major forms include **dilated, hypertrophic and restrictive type of cardiomyopathy** (Figs 12.7A to D).
2. **Secondary cardiomyopathy:** Consists of myocardial disease of unknown cause or associated with systemic disease (e.g. chronic alcohol use, amyloidosis).

CONGENITAL HEART DISEASE

Congenital heart disease (CHD) is the **abnormalities of the heart or great vessels** that are **present from birth**.

Etiology and Pathogenesis

Most CHD arise from defective embryogenesis during 3–8 weeks of gestation, when major cardiovascular structures form and begin to function. Factors that are involved in CHD are:

1. **Genetic factors:** The main causes of congenital heart disease are sporadic genetic abnormalities. The most common genetic cause of congenital heart disease is **trisomy 21 (Down syndrome)**.

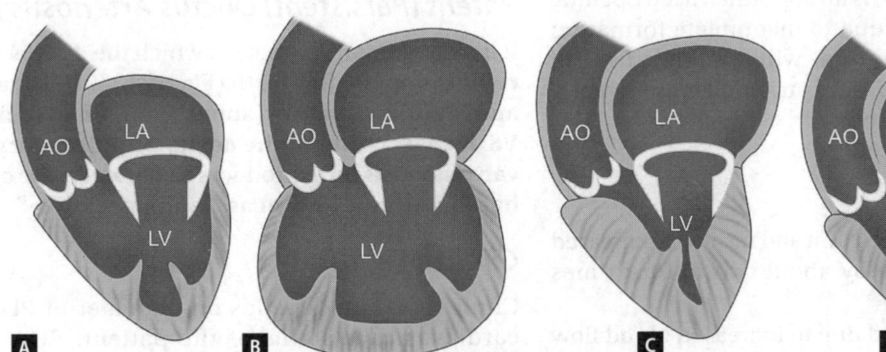

Figs 12.7A to D: Three major morphologic patterns of cardiomyopathy: (A) Normal; (B) Dilated cardiomyopathy; (C) Hypertrophic cardiomyopathy; (D) Restrictive cardiomyopathy

Abbreviations: AO, Aorta; LA, Left atrium; LV, Left ventricle

Box 12.3: Classification of congenital heart diseases

- **Left-to-right shunt**
  - Ventricular septal defect
  - Atrial septal defect
  - Patent ductus arteriosus
- **Right-to-left shunt**
  - Tetralogy of Fallot
  - Transposition of the great arteries
  - Persistent truncus arteriosus
  - Tricuspid atresia
  - Total anomalous pulmonary venous connection
- **Obstructive congenital heart disease**
  - Coarctation of the aorta
  - Aortic stenosis
  - Pulmonary stenosis
- **Malposition of heart**—very rare
  - Dextrocardia

2. **Environmental factors:** These factors may be the primary cause congenital heart disease. **Examples:**
   - **Congenital rubella infection**.
   - **Gestational diabetes.**
   - **Exposure to teratogens** (including drugs).
   - **Nutritional factors: During pregnancy**, consumption of multivitamin containing **folate may reduce the risk**, whereas heavy consumption of **alcohol increases the risk** of congenital heart defects.
3. **Multifactorial:** Majority of CHD may be due to combination of environmental and genetic factors.

Classification (Box 12.3)

The structural anomalies in congenital heart disease may be divided into four major categories: (1) right-to-left shunt, (2) left-to-right shunt, (3) an obstruction, and (4) malposition of heart.

Atrial Septal Defect

An atrial septal defect (ASD) is an abnormal, fixed opening in the atrial septum. It is due to incomplete formation of tissue in the atrial septum, which allows flow of blood between the left and right atria. ASDs are **usually asymptomatic till adulthood**.

Clinical Features

- ASDs cause a left-to-right shunt and results in increased pulmonary blood flow by about two to four times normal.
- A murmur may be heard due to increased blood flow through the pulmonary valve.
- ASDs usually do not produce symptoms before 30 years of age.

Complications: (1) Heart failure, (2) Paradoxical embolization, and (3) Irreversible pulmonary vascular disease.

Prognosis: Mortality is low.

Ventricular Septal Defect

- Incomplete closure of the ventricular septum is known as ventricular septal defect (VSD), is the **most common form of congenital cardiac anomaly**.
- Most (70–80%) VSDs are associated with other congenital cardiac anomalies (e.g. tetralogy of Fallot).
- Cause free blood flow from the left-to-right ventricles.

Clinical Features

The clinical features depend on the size of the defect.

- **Large VSDs:**
  - Usually manifest from birth.
  - Cause **left-to-right shunt** leading to right ventricular hypertrophy and pulmonary hypertension.
  - Irreversible pulmonary vascular disease develops later, in all patients resulting **reversal of shunt, cyanosis, and death.**
- **Small VSDs**
  - May not be recognized until adult life.
  - About 50% of small muscular VSDs may close spontaneously.

Patent Ductus Arteriosus

Normal Function of Ductus Arteriosus

In the fetus, it is an essential structure that carries the blood from the pulmonary artery to the aorta, thus bypasses the flow of blood to lungs (like the patent foramen ovale). After birth, it normally spontaneously closes and the blood from pulmonary artery flows to the lung.

Patent (Persistent) Ductus Arteriosus (PDA)

It is a congenital anomaly in which the **ductus arteriosus remains open after birth** (Fig. 12.8). PDAs may occur as an **isolated anomaly** (about 90%), **or associated with VSD, coarctation of the aorta, or pulmonary or aortic valve stenosis.** PDA produces a **characteristic continuous harsh murmur known as "machinery-like"**.

Clinical Features

Clinical feature depends on diameter of PDA and the cardiovascular status of the patient. PDA is usually asymptomatic at birth, and a narrow PDA may not affect

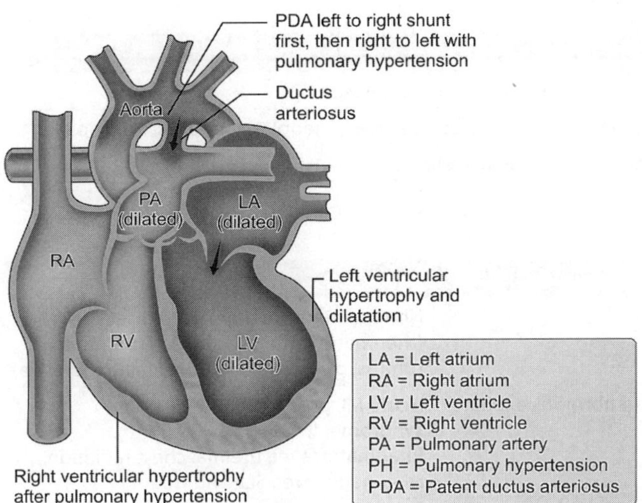

Fig. 12.8: Patent ductus arteriosus

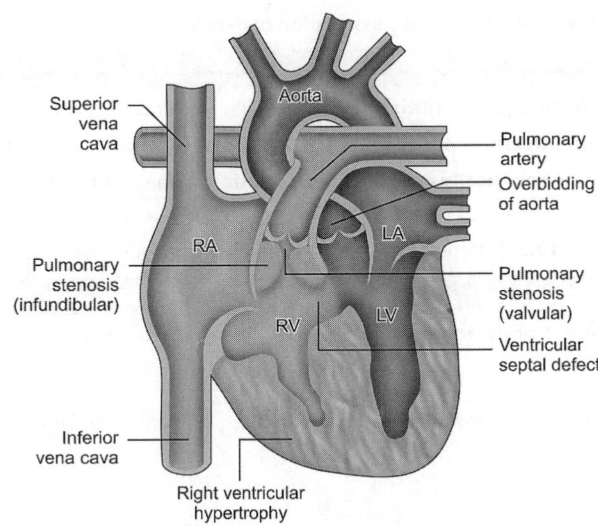

Fig. 12.9: Tetralogy of Fallot

the child's growth and development. First, the shunt is from left-to-right and there is no cyanosis. But additional volume and pressure overload produces obstructive changes in small pulmonary arteries, leading to reversal of flow and its associated consequences.

PDA may be **either life-threatening or life-saving**.

Consequences of patent ductus arteriosus are presented in Figure 12.8.

Tetralogy of Fallot

Components (Fig. 12.9)**:** The **four main features** of the tetralogy of Fallot (TOF) are:

1. **Ventricular septal defect (VSD):** Usually large.
2. **Subpulmonic stenosis/pulmonary valvular stenosis:** It causes obstruction of the right ventricular outflow tract.
3. **Aorta overriding the VSD** and both ventricular chambers.
4. **Right ventricular hypertrophy:** It is due to the obstruction to right ventricular outflow.

Morphology

Heart is enlarged and may be **"boot-shaped"** due to marked right ventricular hypertrophy, particularly of the apical region.

Clinical Features

Clinical features depend mainly on the severity of the subpulmonary stenosis, because this decides the direction of blood flow.

- **Majority of infants with TOF have cyanosis from birth or soon thereafter**.

PATHOLOGY OF PERICARDIUM

The normal pericardium is a two-layered sac which surrounds the heart. It consists of inner serous membrane called **visceral pericardium** and outer fibrous layer called **parietal pericardium.** The space between these two layers is called pericardial sac and contains small quantity (15–50 mL) of thin, clear, straw-colored fluid. This fluid lubricates the surface of the heart.

Pericarditis

Inflammation of pericardium is known as pericarditis. The etiological classification of pericarditis are presented in Table 12.4.

Pericardial Effusion (Table 12.5)

All forms of pericarditis may produce a pericardial effusion characterized by accumulation of fluid in the pericardial sac (Fig. 12.10).

Causes

Pericardial sac may be distended by serous fluid (pericardial effusion), fibrinous exudate (fibrinous pericarditis), blood (hemopericardium), or pus (purulent pericarditis). Different types of pericardial effusion and their causes are shown in Table 12.5.

With chronic effusions, gradual accumulation of less than 500 mL volume of fluid may not manifest clinically. In contrast, sudden/rapid collections of fluid as little as 200–300 mL (e.g. hemopericardium caused by a ruptured MI or aortic dissection) may produce compression of

Table 12.4: Etiological classification of pericarditis

Type	Causes
Infectious pericarditis	Viruses, pyogenic bacteria, tuberculosis, fungi and parasites
Non-infectious pericarditis	Myocardial infarction, uremia, following cardiac surgery, neoplasia, trauma, radiation
Immunologically mediated pericarditis	Rheumatic fever, systemic lupus erythematosus

Table 12.5: Different types of pericardial effusion and their causes

Type	Nature of fluid	Cause
Serous pericarditis	Serous fluid	Noninfectious inflammatory diseases (rheumatic fever, SLE and scleroderma), tumors, cardiac failure, renal failure (uremia)
Fibrinous/serofibrinous pericarditis	Serous fluid mixed with a fibrinous exudate	Acute MI, postinfarction (Dressler) syndrome, Rheumatic fever, uremia, chest radiation, rheumatic fever, SLE and trauma
Purulent or suppurative reaction	Exudate which may range from a thin cloudy fluid to frank pus	Suppurative organisms
Hemorrhagic pericarditis	Blood mixed with a fibrinous or suppurative exudate	Spread of a malignant neoplasm to the pericardial space
Caseous pericarditis	Caseous material	Tuberculosis of pericardium
Chylous	Lymph	Mediastinal lymphatic obstruction

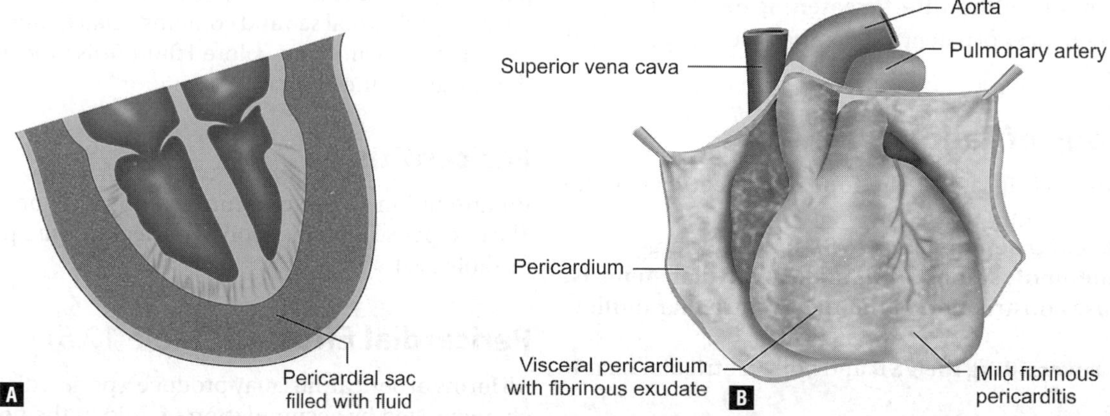

Figs 12.10A and B: (A) Pericardial effusion; (B) Pericarditis in which visceral pericardium shows fibrinous exudate

the thin-walled atria and vena cavae, or the ventricles themselves. This leads to restriction of cardiac filling and produces fatal condition known as cardiac tamponade.

- **Cardiac tamponade:** This term is used to describe acute heart failure due to compression of the heart by a large or rapid accumulation of fluid (effusion) in the pericardial space. This results in obstruction to the inflow of blood to the ventricles.
- **Tuberculous pericarditis:** Tuberculous pericarditis may develop as a complication of tuberculosis of lung, but may also be the first manifestation of the infection.

Chronic Constrictive Pericarditis

Constrictive pericarditis is characterized by progressive thickening, fibrosis and calcification of the pericardium. There is obliteration of the pericardial cavity with the formation of granulation tissue. This results in the heart being encased in a solid shell and cannot fill properly. This often develops as a complication of tuberculous pericarditis, hemopericardium, viral pericarditis, rheumatoid arthritis and purulent pericarditis.

Diagnosis: By aspiration and study of pericardial fluid.

SELF-ASSESSMENT EXERCISE

I. Short Notes

1. Etiopathogenesis of myocardial infarction.
2. Morphology of myocardial infarction.
3. Infective endocarditis.
4. Rheumatic fever.
5. Rheumatic carditis.
6. Rheumatic heart disease.
7. Morphology of heart in rheumatic heart disease.
8. Aschoff bodies (Aschoff nodule).
9. Tetralogy of Fallot.
10. Mitral stenosis.

CHAPTER

13

Hematology

CHAPTER OUTLINE

- Introduction
- Disorders of Red Cells
- Anemia
- Iron Deficiency Anemia
- Megaloblastic Anemia
- Pernicious Anemia
- Anemias of Blood Loss
- Aplastic Anemia
- Hemolytic Anemia
- Hereditary Hemolytic Anemia
- β-Thalassemia Major
- Sickle Cell Anemia
- Acquired Hemolytic Anemias
- Disorders of White Cells
- Normal Differential Leukocyte Count
- Quantitative Disorders of Leukocytes
- Acute Leukemia
- Acute Lymphoblastic Leukemia/Lymphoma
- Acute Myelogenous Leukemia
- Chronic Myelogenous Leukemia
- Chronic Lymphocytic Leukemia
- Disorders of Hemostasis
- Normal Hemostasis
- Classification of Hemostatic Disorders
- Immune Thrombocytopenic Purpura
- Coagulation Disorders
- Hereditary Coagulation Disorders
- Hemophilia
- Acquired Coagulation Disorders
- Laboratory Evaluation of Bleeding Disorders
- Plasma Cell Neoplasms
- Multiple Myeloma (Plasma Cell Myeloma)
- Blood Transfusion
- Spleen

INTRODUCTION

Hematology is defined as the **study of** normal and pathologic aspects of blood and **blood cells**.

Hematopoiesis (hemopoiesis) is the continuous, regulated process of blood cell production or formation.

Hematopoietic (hemopoietic) system: It consists of all organs and tissues involved in hematopoiesis, and these are divided into **myeloid tissue and lymphoid tissue.** The **hematopoietic stem cell (HSC)** is the progenitor of all the cells in blood and gives rise to cells of both myeloid and lymphoid system.

1. **The myeloid tissue** consists of bone marrow (medullary cavity) and the cells derived from it, which include:
   - **Red blood cells** (RBCs/erythrocytes).
   - **White blood cells** (WBCs/leukocytes)**:** WBCs consist of:
     - **Granulocytes: Neutrophils, eosinophils and basophils** are collectively called granulocytes because of their different types of cytoplasmic granules. However, the term granulocyte is often referred to only neutrophils.
     - **Monocytes**.
     - **Lymphocytes** (even though included under WBCs; they are lymphoid derived).
   - **Platelets** (thrombocytes).
2. **The lymphoid tissue** consists of thymus, lymph nodes and spleen.

Functions of Blood Cells

Formed elements of blood are red cells, white cells and platelets. Main functions of blood cells are presented in Table 13.1.

Hematopoiesis

Different stages of hematopoiesis are shown in Figure 13.1.

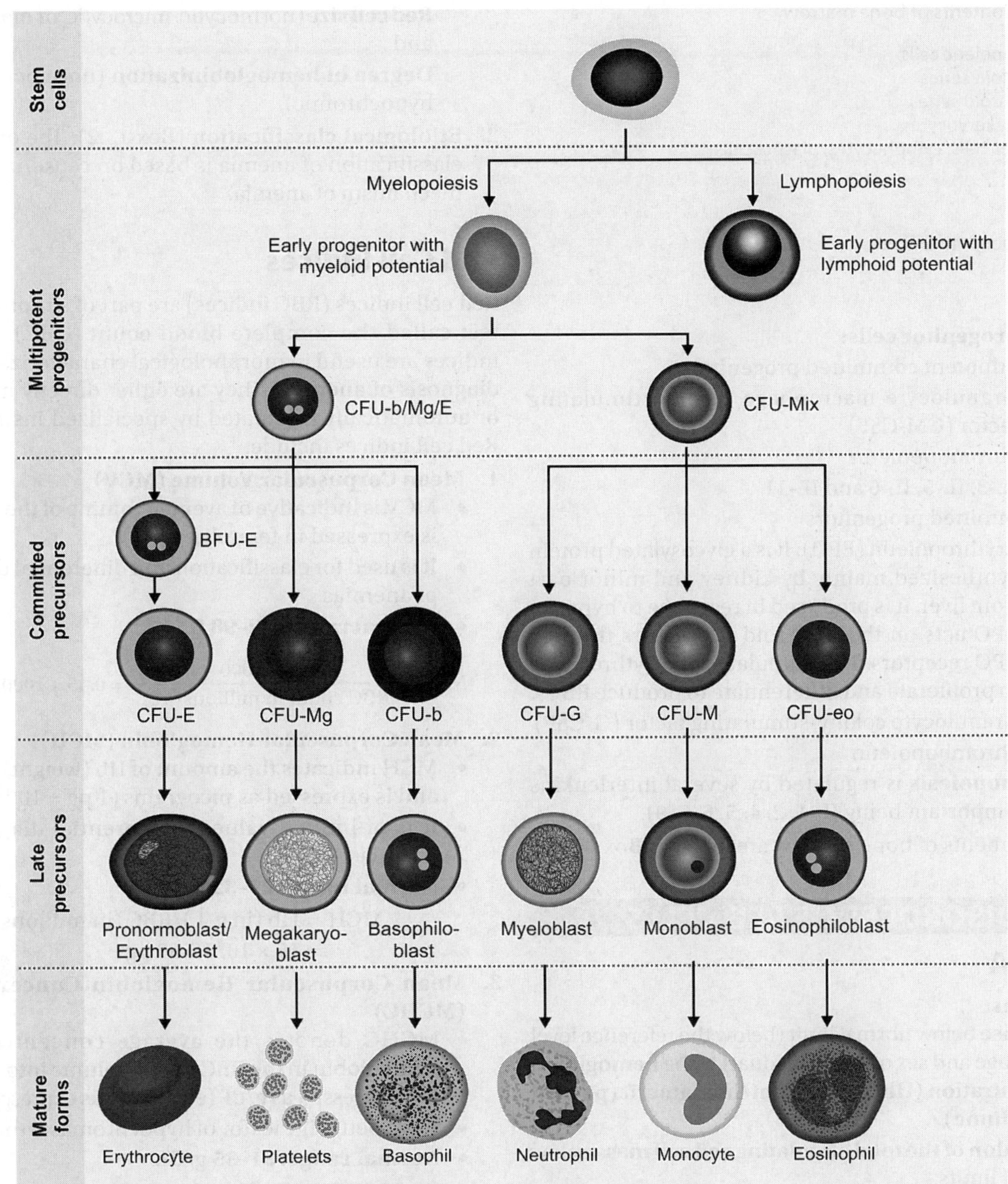

Fig. 13.1: Different stages of hematopoiesis (*Abbreviations:* BFU, burst forming unit; CFU, colony forming unit)

Table 13.1: Main functions of formed elements of blood

Type of blood cell	Main function
Red blood cells	Delivery of oxygen to tissues
White blood cells	Defense against infectious organisms
Lymphocytes	Immune regulation
Platelets	Hemostasis

Regulation of Hematopoiesis

The growth of different hematopoietic cells is regulated by a number of hematopoietic growth factors, which in general are called cytokines.

Most important growth factors acting on various cells are mentioned below.

- **Stem cells:** Stem cell factor (also called c-KIT ligand), IL-6 and FLT3-ligand.

Box 13.1: Contents of bone marrow

- Hematopoietic cells
  - Myeloid series
  - Erythroid series
  - Megakaryocytes
  - Other cells: Lymphocytes, plasma cells
- Fat tissue
- Vessels
- Nerves
- Reticuloendothelial cells
- Stroma

- **CMP progenitor cells:**
  - Multipotent committed progenitors
    - Granulocyte-macrophage colony-stimulating factor (GM-CSF)
    - Thrombopoietin
    - IL-3, IL-5, IL-6 and IL-11
  - Committed progenitors
    - Erythropoietin (EPO): It is a glycosylated protein synthesized mainly by kidney and minor part from liver. It is produced in response to hypoxia. EPO acts on the erythroid precursors through EPO receptors. This stimulates proerythroblasts to proliferate and differentiate to produce RBCs.
    - Granulocyte colony-stimulating factor (G-CSF)
    - Thrombopoietin
- **Lymphopoiesis** is regulated by several interleukins (most important being IL-1, 2, 4, 5, 6, 7, 9).

  Components of bone marrow are listed in Box 13.1.

DISORDERS OF RED CELLS

ANEMIA

Definitions:

- **Decrease** below normal limit (below the reference level for the age and sex of the individual) of the **hemoglobin concentration (Hb)/RBC count/hematocrit (packed cell volume)**.
- **Reduction of the total circulating red cell mass** below normal limits.
- **Decrease in the oxygen-carrying capacity** of the blood, which leads to tissue hypoxia.

Anemia may be **absolute** (decreased RBC mass), or **relative** (associated with a higher plasma volume). Anemia is conventionally used for absolute anemia.

Classification of Anemia

1. **Morphological classification** (Table 13.2)**:** It is based on:
   - **Red cell size** (normocytic, microcytic, or macrocytic), and
   - **Degree of hemoglobinization** (normochromic or hypochromic).
2. **Etiological classification** (Box 13.2)**:** The etiological classification of anemia is based on cause/underlying mechanism of anemia.

Red Cell Indices

Red cell indices (RBC indices) are part of a routine blood test called the complete blood count (CBC). Red cell indices are useful in morphological characterization and diagnosis of anemias. They are either directly measured or automatically calculated by specialized instruments. Red cell indices include:

1. **Mean Corpuscular Volume (MCV)**
   - MCV is indicative of average volume of the RBC and is expressed in femtoliters (fL).
   - It is used for classification and differential diagnosis of anemias.
   - **Normal range: 82–98 fL.**

   $$MCV = \frac{PCV \times 1000}{\text{RBC count in millions}/\mu L} = 0.45 \times 1000/5 = 90 \text{ fL}$$

2. **Mean Corpuscular Hemoglobin (MCH)**
   - MCH indicates the amount of Hb (weight) per RBC and is expressed as picograms (1 pg = 10^{-12} g).
   - It is of limited value in differential diagnosis of anemias.
   - **Normal range: 27–32 pg.**

   $$MCH = \text{Hb (in g/L)/RBC (in millions}/\mu L) = 15 \times 10/5 = 30 \text{ pg}$$

3. **Mean Corpuscular Hemoglobin Concentration (MCHC)**
   - MCHC denotes the average concentration of hemoglobin in the RBC taking volume into account. It is expressed as g/dL (earlier it was expressed as %).
   - It is a better indicator of hypochromasia than MCH.
   - **Normal range: 31–35 g/dL.**

   $$MCHC = \text{Hb (in g/dL)/PCV} = 15/0.45 = 33 \text{ g/dL}$$

4. **Red Cell Distribution Width (RDW)**
   - RDW is a quantitative measure of anisocytosis variaion in size of RBCs.
   - **Normal RDW is 11.5 to 14.5%.**
   - A normal RDW indicates that RBCs are relatively uniform in size. A raised RDW indicates that red cells are heterogeneous in size and/or shape. In early iron deficiency anemia, RDW increases along with

Table 13.2: Morphological classification of anemia

Type of anemia	Microcytic hypochromic	Normocytic normochromic	Macrocytic
Size of RBCs	Smaller than normal	Normal	Larger than normal
Central pallor in RBCs	More than 1/3	Normal	Normal
Mean corpuscular volume (MCV)	Reduced (<80 fL)	Normal (82–98 fL)	Increased (>100 fL)
Mean corpuscular hemoglobin concentration (MCHC)	Reduced (<30 g/dL)	Normal (31–36 g/dL)	Normal (31–36 g/dL)
Examples	Iron deficiency anemia, thalassemia	During blood loss, anemia of chronic diseases	Deficiency of vitamin B_{12} and folic acid
Morphology of RBC			

Box 13.2: Etiological classification of anemia (according to underlying mechanism)

Blood Loss
- **Acute:** Trauma
- **Chronic:** Lesions of gastrointestinal tract (e.g. carcinoma colon), gynecological disorders

Impaired Red Cell Production
- **Nutritional deficiencies**
  - *Deficiencies affecting hemoglobin synthesis:* Iron deficiency
  - *Deficiencies affecting DNA synthesis:* Megaloblastic anemias due to deficiency or impaired utilization of vitamin B_{12} and folic acid
  - *Vitamin C deficiency*
- **Inherited genetic defects**
  - *Defects affecting erythroblast maturation:* Thalassemia syndromes
  - *Defects leading to stem cell depletion:* Fanconi anemia, telomerase defect
- **Erythropoietin deficiency:** Renal failure, anemia of chronic disease
- **Immune-mediated injury of progenitors:** Aplastic anemia, pure red cell aplasia
- **Inflammation-mediated iron sequestration:** Anemia of chronic disease
- **Primary hematopoietic neoplasms:** Acute leukemia, myelodysplastic syndromes, myeloproliferative disorders
- **Space-occupying marrow lesions:** Metastatic tumors, granulomatous disease
- **Infections of red cell progenitors:** Parvovirus B_{19} infection
- **Unknown mechanisms:** Endocrine disorders, liver disease

Increased Red Cell Destruction (Hemolytic Anemias)
- **Inherited genetic defects**
  - *Red cell membrane disorders:* Hereditary spherocytosis, hereditary elliptocytosis
  - *Enzyme deficiencies*
    - Hexose monophosphate shunt enzyme deficiencies: G6PD deficiency
    - Glycolytic enzyme deficiencies: Pyruvate kinase deficiency, hexokinase deficiency
- **Hemoglobin abnormalities**
  - *Deficient globin synthesis:* Thalassemia syndromes
  - *Structurally abnormal globins (hemoglobinopathies):* Sickle cell disease
- **Acquired genetic defects**
  - *Deficiency of phosphatidylinositol-linked glycoproteins:* Paroxysmal nocturnal hemoglobinuria
- **Antibody-mediated destruction**
  - Hemolytic disease (Rh disease) of the newborn, transfusion reactions, drug-associated, autoimmune disorders (e.g. systemic lupus erythematosus)
- **Mechanical trauma**
  - *Microangiopathic hemolytic anemias:* Hemolytic uremic syndrome, disseminated intravascular coagulation, thrombotic thrombocytopenia purpura
  - *Cardiac traumatic hemolysis:* Defective cardiac valves
- **Infections of red cells:** Malaria, babesiosis
- **Toxic or chemical injury:** Clostridial sepsis, snake venom, lead poisoning
- **Sequestration:** Hypersplenism

Abbreviations: G6PD, glucose-6-phosphate dehydrogenase; PK, pyruvate kinase

low MCV while in thalassemia trait, RDW is normal with low MCV.

RDW = (Standard deviation ÷ mean cell volume) × 100

Clinical Features of Anemia

Irrespective of the cause, anemia when severe, presents with certain clinical features. In anemia, the lowered oxygen content of the circulating blood leads to tissue hypoxia. General clinical features are either due to tissue hypoxia or compensatory mechanisms.

- **Due to tissue hypoxia:**
  - **Nonspecific symptoms:** Weakness, malaise and easy fatigability due to hypoxia of muscles.
  - **Dyspnea on mild exertion:** Due to the lowered oxygen content of the circulating blood.
  - **Pallor:** Patients appear pale due to deficiency of red colored hemoglobin which is better appreciated in the conjunctiva, mucous membrane of tongue and nail beds. Pallor associated with icterus is suggestive of a hemolytic anemia.
  - **CNS symptoms:** Patients of severe anemia may complain of headache, vertigo, tinnitus and lack of concentration.
- **Due to compensatory mechanisms:**

Cardiac features: Dyspnea on mild exertion, palpitation, tachycardia and cardiac murmur occur due to compensatory mechanisms. The resulting increase in the cardiac output may cause congestive cardiac failure.

Laboratory Diagnosis of Anemia

General scheme of investigation of anemia are listed in Box 13.3 and classification of severity of anemia according to hemoglobin levels is presented in Box 13.4.

Box 13.3: General scheme of investigation of anemia

- Estimation of hemoglobin and packed cell volume (hematocrit)
- Blood cell counts: RBC, WBC and platelet counts
- Peripheral smear examination
- Red cell indices: MCV, MCH, MCHC, RDW
- Reticulocyte count
- Erythrocyte sedimentation rate
- Bone marrow examination

Box 13.4: Severity of anemia

- Mild anemia: Hb 9.1 to 10.5 g/dL
- Moderate anemia: Hb 6.0 to 9.0 g/dL
- Severe anemia: Hb less than 6.0 g/dL

IRON DEFICIENCY ANEMIA

Iron deficiency anemia (IDA) is the **most common nutritional disorder**.

Etiology (Box 13.5)

IDA is due to deficiency of iron causing **defective heme synthesis**.

Laboratory Findings

Peripheral Blood

- **Hemoglobin and hematocrit (PCV): Decreased.**
- **Red cell indices:**
  - ↓ **MCV:** <80 fL (normal 82–98 fL).
  - ↓ **MCH:** <25 pg (normal 27–32 pg).
  - ↓ **MCHC:** <27 g/dL(31–36 g/dL).
  - **RDW: Increased** and >15%. It is **earliest sign of iron deficiency** (normal 11.5–14.5%).

- **Peripheral smear** (Figs 13.2):
  - *RBCs:* **Microcytic** (small) and **hypochromic** (pale). Severe anemia shows ring/pessary cells. **Moderate anisocytosis** (means **variation in size of RBC**) and **poikilocytosis** (means **variation in shape of RBC**) pencil/cigar-shaped cells are observed.
  - *WBCs:* Normal; eosinophilia in hookworm infestation.
  - *Platelets:* Normal.

Box 13.5: Causes of iron deficiency anemia

- **Dietary deficiency/lack**
  - Milk-fed infants
  - Elderly with improper diet and poor dentition
  - Low socioeconomical sections
  - Vegetarians (contains poorly absorbable inorganic iron)
- **Impaired absorption**
  - Total/partial gastrectomy
  - Intestinal absorption is impaired in sprue, other causes of intestinal steatorrhea and chronic diarrhea
  - Specific items in the diet, like phytates of cereals, tannates, carbonates, oxalates, phosphates and drugs can impair iron absorption
- **Increased demand/requirement**
  - Growing infants, children and adolescents
  - Pregnancy and lactation
- **Chronic blood loss: Due to bleeding from the:**
  - Gastrointestinal tract (e.g. peptic ulcers, gastric carcinoma, colonic carcinoma, hemorrhoids, hookworm infestation or nonsteroidal anti-inflammatory drugs)
  - Urinary tract (e.g. renal or bladder tumors)
  - Genital tract (e.g. menorrhagia, uterine cancer)
  - Respiratory tract (e.g. hemoptysis)

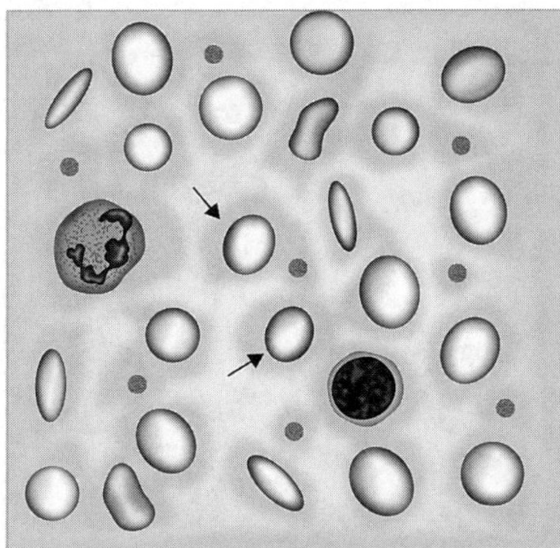

Fig. 13.2: Iron deficiency anemia. Diagrammatic appearance of peripheral blood smear with microcytic hypochromic red blood cells (arrow)

- **Reticulocyte count:** Low for the degree of anemia.

Bone Marrow

- *Cellularity:* Moderately **hypercellular**.
- *M:E (Myeloid:Erythroid) ratio:* Varies from 2:1 to 1:2 (normal 2:1 to 4:1).
- *Erythropoiesis:* Hyperplasia and **micronormoblastic maturation**.
- *Myelopoiesis:* Normal.
- *Megakaryopoiesis:* Normal.
- ***Absence of bone marrow iron:*** "Gold standard" test, demonstrated by **negative Prussian blue reaction**.

Serum Iron Profile (Table 13.3)

Clinical Features of IDA

Nonspecific and related to both severity and the cause of the anemia (e.g. gastrointestinal disease).

- **Onset:** Insidious.
- **Nonspecific symptoms: Fatigue, palpitations, breathlessness**, weakness and irritability.
- **Pharyngeal/esophageal webs** formed cause dysphagia.
- **Patterson-Kelly or Plummer-Vinson syndrome:**
  - Microcytic hypochromic anemia.
  - Atrophic glossitis.
  - Esophageal webs.
- **Congestive heart failure in severe** anemia.
- **Central nervous system: Pica**-unusual craving for substances with no nutritional value like clay or chalk. **Craving for ice** (pagophagia) **specific to iron deficiency**. Pica may be the cause rather than effect of IDA.

Physical Findings

Diminished tissue enzymes cause characteristic epithelial changes of iron deficiency anemia.

- Angular stomatitis and glossitis.
- Chronic atrophic gastritis.
- Koilonychia (spoon nails).

Causes of Microcytic Hypochromic Anemia (Box 13.6)

Box 13.6: Causes of microcytic hypochromic anemia

- **Iron deficiency anemia**
- **Thalassemia major**
- **Anemia of chronic disorders**
- **Others:** Alcohol, lead poisoning and drugs
- Sideroblastic anemia (rare cause)

MEGALOBLASTIC ANEMIA

Anemias characterized by **defective**/impaired **DNA synthesis** and **distinct megaloblasts in the bone marrow.** Megaloblastic anemias are common among anemias due to impaired red cell production.

Etiology of Megaloblastic Anemia (Box 13.7)

Table 13.3: Serum iron profile in IDA

	Normal range	Value in IDA	Observation
Serum ferritin	15–300 µg/L	<15 µg/L	↓
Serum iron	50–150 µg/dL	10–15 µg/dL	↓
Serum transferrin saturation	30–40%	<15%	↓
Total plasma iron-binding capacity (TIBC)	310–340 µg/dL	350–450 µg/dL	↑
Serum transferrin receptor (TFR)	0.57–2.8 µg/L	3.5–7.1 µg/L	↑
Red cell protoporphyrin	30–50 µg/dL	>200 µg/dL	↑

Box 13.7: Causes of megaloblastic anemia

Vitamin B_{12} Deficiency
- **Decreased intake:** Inadequate diet, "pure vegetarians" (vegans).
- **Impaired absorption**
  - Gastric: Deficiency of gastric acid or pepsin or intrinsic factor
    - Pernicious anemia
    - Post-gastrectomy
  - Intestinal
    - Loss of absorptive surface
      - Malabsorption syndromes
      - Diffuse intestinal disease, e.g. lymphoma, systemic sclerosis
      - Ileal resection, Crohn disease
    - Bacterial or parasitic competition for vitamin B_{12}
      - Bacterial overgrowth in blind loops and diverticula of bowel
      - Fish tapeworm infestation
- **Increased demand:** Pregnancy, hyperthyroidism, disseminated cancer

Folic Acid Deficiency
- **Decreased intake:** Inadequate diet—alcoholism, malnutrition
- **Impaired absorption**
  - Malabsorption states: Nontropical and tropical sprue
  - Diffuse infiltrative diseases of the small intestine (e.g. lymphoma)
  - Drugs: Anticonvulsant phenytoin and oral contraceptives
- **Increased loss:** Hemodialysis
- **Increased demand:** Pregnancy, infancy, disseminated cancer, markedly increased hematopoiesis
- **Impaired utilization:** Folic acid antagonists, such as methotrexate

Pathogenesis of Megaloblastic Change

Impaired DNA synthesis: Megaloblastic anemia is commonly due to deficiency of **vitamin B_{12} (cyanocobalamin) or folic acid.** Both vitamins are coenzymes necessary for the synthesis of DNA.

- **Delayed maturation of nucleus**. The **nuclear maturation lags behind the cytoplasmic maturation** and results in **abnormally large** nucleated **erythroid precursors** named as **megaloblasts.**
- Cytoplasm matures normally. RBCs are larger than normal and are called as **macrocytes**.

Laboratory Findings of Megaloblastic Anemia

Blood findings in vitamin B_{12} and/or folic acid deficiency are similar.

Peripheral Blood

- **Hemoglobin and hematocrit (PCV): Reduced.**
- **Red cell indices.**
  - ↑ **MCV:** Above 100 fL (normal 82–98 fL).
  - ↑ **MCH** (normal 27–32 pg).
  - **Normal MCHC** (31–36 g/dL).

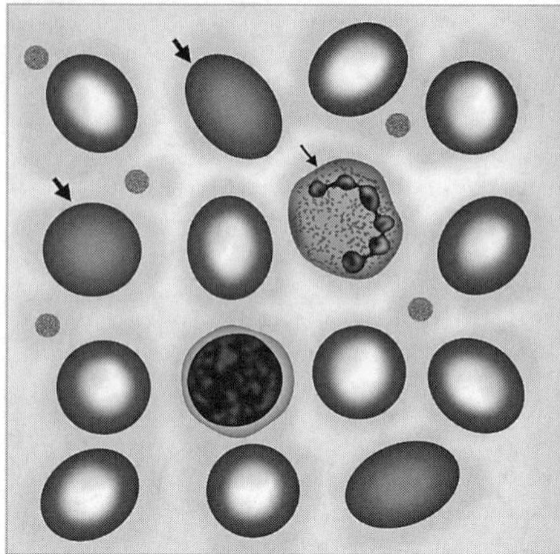

Fig. 13.3: Diagrammatic peripheral blood smear showing macro-ovalocytes (thick arrows) and hypersegmented neutrophil (thin arrow)

Peripheral smear (Fig. 13.3)

Pancytopenia (decreased RBC, WBCs and platelets).

- *RBCs:*
  - Macrocytic and oval (**macro-ovalocytes**)-**diagnostic** of megaloblastic anemia
  - Most macrocytes **lack the central pallor** (Fig. 13.3).
  - **Marked** variation in the size and shape of red cells (**aniso-poikilocytosis**).
  - Evidence of dyserythropoiesis: Basophilic stippling, (precipitated ribosomal RNA). Cabot ring nuclear remnants and Howell Jolly bodies nuclear remnants.
- *WBCs:*
  - **Decreased** WBC count (leukopenia).
  - **Hypersegmented neutrophils** (more than five nuclear lobes): First and specific morphological sign of megaloblastic anemia. These neutrophils are also larger than normal (**macropolys**).
- *Platelets:* **Decreased.**

- **Reticulocyte count:** Normal or low.

Bone marrow

- *Cellularity:* Moderately to **markedly hypercellular.**
- *M: E (Myeloid: Erythroid) ratio:* Due to marked erythroid hyperplasia, M: E ratio is reversed ranging from 1:1 to 1:6 (normal 2:1 to 4:1).
- *Erythropoiesis:* **Megaloblastic type** (Fig. 13.4).
  - **Megaloblasts: Large, abnormal counterparts of normal normoblasts**. Megaloblast shows **asynchrony of nuclear and cytoplasmic maturation.** The cytoplasm shows normal hemoglobinization.
- *Myelopoiesis:*
  - Granulocytic precursors display nuclear-cytoplasmic asynchrony in the form of **giant metamyelocytes and band forms**.
- *Megakaryopoiesis:* Normal or increased in number.
- *Bone marrow iron:* Moderately increased.

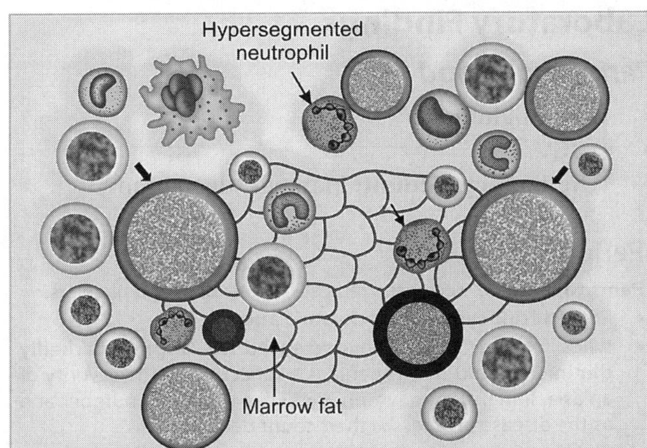

Fig. 13.4: Megaloblastic anemia. Diagrammatic picture of bone-marrow aspirate showing megaloblastic precursors (thick arrows) in varying stages of maturation

Biochemical Tests for Megaloblastic Anemia

Common for both vitamin B_{12} and folic acid deficiency

- ↑ Serum homocysteine.
- ↑ Serum bilirubin: Mild increase causes mild jaundice.
- ↑ Serum iron and ferritin.
- ↑ Plasma lactate dehydrogenase (LDH).
- **Serum vitamin B_{12}/folate decreased.**

Diagnostic tests for vitamin B_{12} deficiency

- **Serum vitamin B_{12} levels:** Decreased.
  - ↑ Serum methylmalonic acid.
  - ↑ Urinary excretion of methylmalonic acid.
- **Schilling test** for vitamin B_{12} absorption (Refer below).

Specific tests for folic acid deficiency

- **Serum folic acid levels:** Decreased.
- **FIGLU in urine: Excessively excreted.**

Dimorphic anemia

- **Combined vitamin B_{12}/folic acid and iron deficiency.**
- Peripheral smear shows two populations of RBCs namely: Macro-ovalocytes and microcytic hypochromic.

PERNICIOUS ANEMIA

Pernicious anemia (PA) is an autoimmune disease due to **deficiency of intrinsic factor** causing **impaired absorption of vitamin B_{12}** and megaloblastic anemia.

Rare in India. A genetic predisposition is suspected.

Age: Older age—**fifth to eighth decades** of life.

Sex: Females are more involved than males (F: M is 1.5: 1).

Etiopathogenesis

- An **autoimmune** disease due to destruction of gastric mucosa.
- Stomach shows **damage to parietal cells**, dense infiltration by lymphocytes and plasma cells causing **chronic atrophic gastritis and failure of production of intrinsic factor**.

Laboratory Findings

Blood, bone marrow and biochemical test findings are similar to those described earlier for megaloblastic anemias (refer pages 138-9).

Specific Diagnostic Tests for Pernicious Anemia

- **Schilling test for vitamin B_{12} absorption: Abnormal.**
  - Radioactive vitamin B_{12} is used to assess the status of intrinsic factor (IF) and vitamin B_{12}.
  - Helps in distinguishing megaloblastic anemia due to IF deficiency (pernicious anemia) from other causes of vitamin B_{12} deficiency.
- **Serum antibodies to intrinsic factor** are highly specific for pernicious anemia.
- **Achlorhydria** with histamine/pentagastrin stimulation.
- Severe **deficiency of intrinsic factor**.

Clinical Features of Megaloblastic Anemia

The clinical features of vitamin B_{12} deficiency anemia and pernicious anemia are:

- **Onset: Insidious** and progresses slowly.
- **Classic triad of presentation:** Weakness, sore throat and paresthesias.
- **Tongue:** Painful red **"beefy"** tongue.
- **Neurological manifestations:**
  - **Bilateral peripheral neuropathy:** Glove and sock distribution of **numbness or paresthesia.**
  - **Demyelination of spinal cord: Subacute combined demyelination/degeneration of dorsal and lateral tracts—ataxia**, uncoordinated gait, impairment of vibration and position sense.

ANEMIAS OF BLOOD LOSS

Acute Blood Loss (hemorrhage)

- Causes loss of intravascular volume and if massive can lead to hypovolemic shock and death.

- Bleeding may be external (e.g. open fracture, knife wound) or internal (e.g. ruptured spleen, ruptured abdominal aneurysm).

Chronic Blood Loss

Produces anemia when the rate of blood loss exceeds the regenerative capacity of the bone marrow or when iron reserves are depleted and results in iron deficiency anemia.

APLASTIC ANEMIA

Hematopoietic stem cell (HSC) disorder characterized by:

- **Pancytopenia** (anemia, neutropenia and thrombocytopenia).
- With **markedly hypocellular bone marrow** (less than 30% cellularity).

Etiology

The most common causes associated with aplastic anemia are shown in Box 13.8.

Clinical Features

- Any age of both sexes.
- Insidious.
  - Progressive weakness, pallor and dyspnea due to anemia.
  - Frequent (mucocutaneous bacterial infections) or fatal infections due to neutropenia.
  - Bleeding manifestations in the form of petechiae, bruises and ecchymoses due to thrombocytopenia.

Box 13.8: Common causes of aplastic anemia

ACQUIRED
Idiopathic
- Acquired defects in stem cell
- Immune mediated

Secondary
Chemical agents
- Cytotoxic drugs: Alkylating agents, antimetabolites
- Inorganic arsenicals

Idiosyncratic
- Chloramphenicol
- Penicillamine
- Carbamazepine
- Methylphenylethyl hydantoin

Physical agents: Whole-body irradiation
Viral infections: Hepatitis virus, Epstein-Barr virus, cytomegalovirus, herpes zoster (Varicella zoster), HIV

INHERITED: Fanconi anemia

Laboratory Findings

Peripheral Blood

↓
- **Hemoglobin.**
- **PCV.**
- **Reticulocyte count:** Markedly decreased.

Peripheral smear

Pancytopenia, i.e. decreased red cells, neutrophils and platelets.
- *RBCs:* **Normocytic normochromic anemia.**
- *WBCs:* Total leukocyte count **decreased. Neutrophils markedly diminished** and neutropenia is a reflection of the severity of aplasia. Initial stages, lymphocytes are normal in number and as the disease progresses their count decreases.
- *Platelets:* Count is **decreased.**

Bone marrow

- **Marrow aplasia**—best appreciated in a **bone marrow (trephine) biopsy.**
  - *Cellularity:* Marked **hypocellularity.**
  - *Hematopoiesis:* **Paucity of all erythroid, myeloid and megakaryocytic precursors.**
  - *Other cells:* **Lymphocytes and plasma cells are prominent.**

No Splenomegaly

Diagnosis: Diagnosis is made with **peripheral blood** and **bone marrow biopsy findings.**

Prognosis: Unpredictable.

Pancytopenia

Definition: Combination of anemia, leukopenia and thrombocytopenia.

Causes of Pancytopenia (Box 13.9)

Box 13.9: Causes of pancytopenia

Decreased bone marrow function
- Aplastic anemia
- Bone marrow infiltration with leukemia, lymphoma, myeloma, tumors (carcinoma), granulomatous diseases (e.g. disseminated tuberculosis)
- Nutritional deficiencies: Megaloblastic anemia (vitamin B_{12} and folic acid deficiency)

Increased peripheral destruction: Hypersplenism

HEMOLYTIC ANEMIA

Definition: Hemolytic anemias are due to **increase in the rate of red cell destruction** (hemolysis).

Classification of Hemolytic Anemias (refer Box 13.2)

Depending on:
- **Location of hemolysis: Intravascular and extravascular.**
- **Source of defect causing hemolysis: Intracorpuscular defect** and **extracorpuscular defect**.
- **Mode of onset: Hereditary and acquired disorders.**

HEREDITARY HEMOLYTIC ANEMIA

Causes: Hereditary hemolytic anemia may be due to:
- **RBC membrane abnormalities:** Spherocytosis, elliptocytosis.
- **RBC enzyme deficiencies:** Glucose-6-phosphate dehydrogenase, pyruvate kinase.
- **Disorders of hemoglobin synthesis.**
  - **Deficient globin synthesis:** Thalassemia syndromes.
  - **Structurally abnormal globin synthesis** (hemoglobinopathies): Sickle cell anemia.

One of the example of hemolytic anemia due to RBC membrane abnormality is hereditary spherocytosis.

Hereditary Spherocytosis

Hereditary spherocytosis (HS) is a rare **inherited hemolytic anemia** resulting from the **defect in the red cell membrane.**

Etiopathogenesis

- **Autosomal dominant** disorder.
- RBC membrane protein defect caused by various **mutations**. Most common mutations involve **ankyrin, band 3, spectrin, or band protein 4.2.**

Laboratory Findings

Peripheral blood

- **Hemoglobin: Decreased.**
- **Red cell indices.**
  - **MCV: Reduced** (normal 82–98 fl).
  - **MCHC: Raised and >35 g/dL** (normal 31–36 g/dL).
- **Peripheral smear: Very important** for diagnosis.
  - **RBCs:**
    - **Spherocytes** are **most distinctive** but **not pathognomonic**. Spherocytosis can also be found in autoimmune hemolytic anemias. Spherocytes are **small, dark-staining** (hyperchromic) **RBCs without any central pallor.**
    - Polychromatophilia due to reticulocytosis.
  - **WBCs:** Total leukocyte count (TLC) increased.
  - **Platelets:** Normal.
- **Reticulocyte count: Increased.**

Biochemical findings

- **Serum bilirubin:** Mildly **raised.**
- **Urine urobilinogen: Increased.**
- **Serum haptoglobin: Decreased.**

Osmotic fragility test

- **Osmotic fragility is increased and there is shift of the curve to the right.**

Clinical Features

- **Age:** Anytime from the neonatal period to adulthood.
- **Family history:** Most (75%) are inherited as autosomal dominant trait.
- **Anemia:** Mild to moderate.
- **Jaundice: Intermittent attacks**, precipitated by pregnancy, fatigue, or infection.
- **Splenomegaly: Moderate** (500 to 1,000 g).
- **Gallstones: Pigment** gallstones.
- **Aplastic crises:** May be triggered by an acute parvovirus infection.

One of the example of hemolytic anemia due to RBC enzyme deficiency is anemia due to Glucose-6-phosphate dehydrogenase deficiency.

Glucose-6-Phosphate Dehydrogenase Deficiency

- Hemolytic disease due to **red cell enzyme defects.**
- In G6PD deficiency, **RBCs are susceptible to oxidative injury** by free radicals.
- It is an **X-linked recessive disorder** and its **full expression is seen only in males.**

Clinical Presentation

G6PD deficiency manifests in several distinct clinical patterns. Usually present as acute self-limited acute intravascular hemolytic anemia following exposure to oxidative stress.

Laboratory Findings

Peripheral blood

- **Hemoglobin: Decreased.**
- **Reticulocyte count: Increased.**
- **Peripheral smear:**
  - **RBCs:** Moderate anisopoikilocytosis with **polychromatophilia, microspherocytes** and **bite cells. Heinz bodies** identified **with a supravital stain** and are best seen during active hemolysis.
  - **WBCs:** Mild leukocytosis.
  - **Platelets: Normal.**

- **Self-limited hemolysis:** Primarily the **old red cells are hemolyzed**, hence hemolysis is self-limited.

Urine

- **Hemoglobinuria** will be found **during hemolysis** and may last for about 1–6 days.

RBC enzyme analysis

- **Tests for G6PD deficiency** are positive and should be assessed a few weeks after the acute hemolytic episode.

Hereditary Defects in Hemoglobin

Classification

Hemoglobin defects may be quantitative (reduced production of normal hemoglobin) or qualitative (production of abnormal hemoglobin).

- ***Quantitative defect:*** Characterized by reduced of α-globin or β-globin chain (e.g. thalassemia). It leads to net reduction of hemoglobin.
- ***Qualitative defect:*** Characterized by production of abnormal hemoglobin (e.g. sickle cell anemia).

Thalassemia Syndrome

- These are group of inherited disorders due to **abnormality of globin production**.
- It is characterized by **decreased or absence of synthesis** of either α **or β-globin** chain of adult hemoglobin, HbA ($\alpha_2\beta_2$).

Classification

They are mainly classified as:

- **β-Thalassemia syndromes: Impaired synthesis of β-chains** of globin.
- **α-Thalassemia syndromes: Impaired synthesis of α-chains** of globin.
- **Miscellaneous thalassemia syndromes**.

β-Thalassemia

- **Autosomal recessive** hereditary disorder. Different types of **mutations in β-globin gene**.
- **Diminished synthesis** of **β-globin chains** and normal synthesis of α-chains. It may be classified as β thalassemia major, intermedia and minor.

β-THALASSEMIA MAJOR

- It is a **hereditary hemolytic anemia** due to **absence of synthesis of β-globin** chain of hemoglobin. The **synthesis of α-globin** chain **is not affected**.
- Most common in Mediterranean countries, parts of Africa and South East Asia.
- **Hemolytic anemia** is of **severe degree**.

Pathophysiology of β-thalassemia Major

Consequence of Defective or Absent β-chains

- **Severe hemolytic anemia** due to:
  - **Absence of β-globin chain.**
  - **Ineffective erythropoiesis**
  - **Extravascular hemolysis**
- **Synthesis of fetal hemoglobin (HbF):** Leading to **increased levels of HbF** ($\alpha_2\Upsilon_2$). The level of HbF varies from 30 to 90%.

Consequences of Ineffective Erythropoiesis

- **Changes in bone marrow: Marked erythroid hyperplasia**.
- **Changes in bone:**
  - **Skull X-ray: Hair on end ("crew-cut") appearance**.
  - **Typical facies: Thalassemic facies**—prominent forehead, cheekbones and upper jaw.
- **Extramedullary hematopoiesis:** In **liver and spleen** → consequent hepatosplenomegaly.
- **Cachexia:** Develops in untreated patients.

Iron Overload and its Consequences

- **Causes of iron overload:**
  - **Increased absorption of dietary iron** from duodenum.
  - **Hemolysis.**
  - **Repeated transfusions** (usual mode of treatment).
- **Consequences:** Iron overload produces **hemosiderosis** and **secondary hemochromatosis** and damages to parenchyma of organs (e.g. **heart, liver** and **pancreas)**.

Clinical Features

- **Age:** Infants develop **moderate to severe anemia** 6–9 months after birth.
- **Growth and development:** Untreated/untransfused children **fail to thrive** and die within 4–5 years of age.
- **Bone changes:** Those who survive longer develop distortion of skull and facial bones. X-ray **skull** shows **hair on end appearance** (Fig. 13.5) and face shows a characteristic **thalassemic facies.**
- **Marked splenomegaly:** Up to 1,500 g due to hyperplasia and extramedullary hematopoiesis.
- **Extramedullary hemopoiesis: Liver and lymph nodes** may show **extramedullary hematopoiesis**.

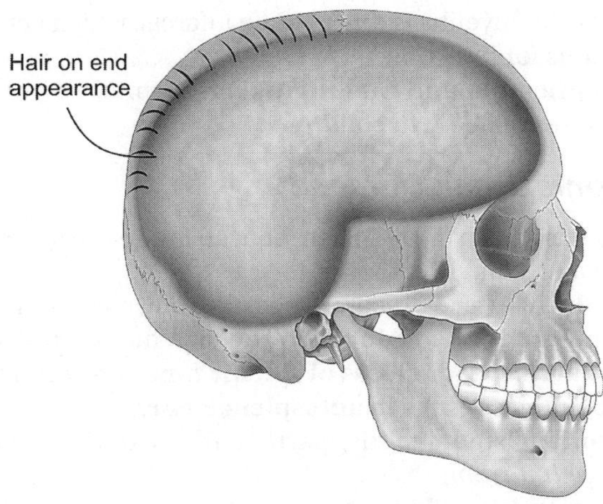

Fig. 13.5: Radiologically thalassemia major patients develop hair on end appearance in skull X-ray

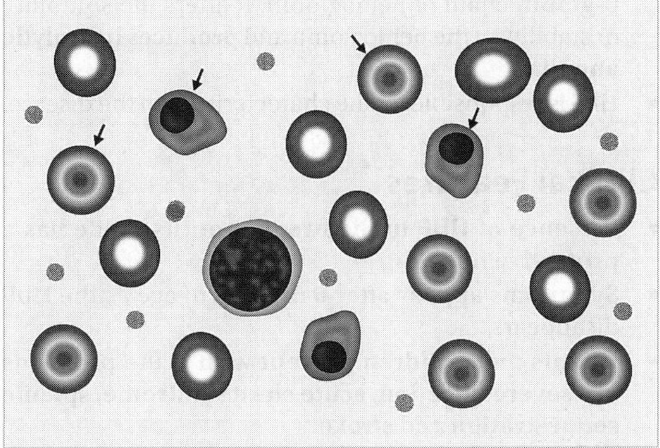

Fig. 13.6: Diagrammatic appearance of peripheral blood smear in β-thalassemia showing target cells (short arrows) and nucleated red cells (long arrows)

- **Iron overload:** Multiple blood transfusions may lead to iron overload and result in **hemosiderosis and secondary hemochromatosis** (heart, liver and pancreas).

Laboratory Findings

Peripheral Blood

- **Hemoglobin** (ranges from 3 to 8 g/dL) **and hematocrit** (ranges from 8 to 23%)**: Markedly reduced.**
- **RBC count increased/normal** (in contrast to iron deficiency anemia where it is decreased).
- **Reticulocyte count increased** and in the range of 5–15%.
- **Red cell indices:**
  - **MCV decreased** and in the range of 45–70 fL (normal range 82–98 fL).
  - **MCHC decreased** and in the range of 22–30 g/dL (normal range 31–35 g/dL).
  - **MCH decreased** and in the range of 20–28 pg (normal range 27–32 pg).
  - **RDW-within normal limits** (in contrast to iron deficiency anemia where it is increased).

Peripheral smear

- *RBCs:*
  - **Microcytic hypochromic** anemia.
  - Moderate to marked anisocytosis and poikilocytosis.
  - Many **target cells** (Fig. 13.6).
  - Basophilic stippling.
  - **Nucleated red cell precursors** (normoblasts) in variable numbers (5–40%).
- *WBCs:* Leukocytosis with mild left shift.
- *Platelets:* Normal.

Bone marrow

- *Cellularity:* **Markedly hypercellular.**
- *M: E ratio:* Reversed to 1:1 to 1:5 depending upon the degree of erythroid hyperplasia.
- *Erythropoiesis:* **Normoblastic with marked erythroid hyperplasia.**
- *Myelopoiesis:* Normal.
- *Megakaryopoiesis:* Normal.
- *Bone marrow iron:* **Markedly increased** due to increased dietary absorption and hemolysis.

SICKLE CELL ANEMIA

Sickle cell anemia is a **hereditary disorder** of hemoglobin characterized by **production of defective hemoglobin** called **sickle hemoglobin (HbS).** On low oxygen tension or deoxygenation, HbS imparts **sickle shape to RBCs.** HbS is produced due to **qualitative defect** in hemoglobin production caused by **mutation in β-globin gene.**

Characteristic Features

- **Autosomal recessive disorder** manifests early in life.
- **Homozygous state** (SS) caused by a **mutation in the β-globin gene.**
- **HbS** constitutes **more than 70% of hemoglobin** in their RBCs with no HbA.

Etiopathogenesis

- **Production of abnormal hemoglobin** called **sickle hemoglobin (HbS).**
- **Missense point mutation:** In HbS, there is **substitution of glutamic acid by valine in the 6th position the**

β-**globin** chain of hemoglobin. It alters the solubility or stability of the hemoglobin and **produces hemolytic anemia**.

- HbS is responsible for the characteristics of the disease.

Clinical Features

- Presence of **HbF in the first 6 months** of life has a **protective** role.
- **Symptoms appear after 6 months** of age as the HbF disappears.
- **Infants and children present with** acute problems like **severe infection, acute chest syndrome, splenic sequestration** and **stroke**.
- **Chronic hypoxia** in children is responsible for generalized **impairment of growth** and development. **Adults manifest with chronic organ damage**.

Chronic Hemolytic Anemia

- **Lifelong hemolysis** (mainly extravascular) and causes **chronic hemolytic anemia**, which is of **moderate degree**. This produces **raised unconjugated (indirect) bilirubin**, and predisposes to **pigment** bilirubin **gallstones** (cholelithiasis) and **cholecystitis**.

Crises

Four types of crises are encountered. These are:

1. **Sickling crisis (vaso-occlusive/pain/painful/ infarctive crisis)**.
   - Most common.
   - **Blockage of microcirculation** by sickled red cells produces **hypoxic injury and infarction**.
   - **Bone:** Manifest as the **hand-foot syndrome, dactylitis** of the bones of the hands or feet or both.
   - **Lung: Acute chest syndrome (dangerous)**.
   - **Spleen: Acute abdominal pain** due to infarcts of abdominal viscera caused by occlusion of vessels. **Recurrent splenic infarction** results in **autosplenectomy**.
2. **Hemolytic crisis:** Rare type and presents with **marked increase in hemolysis**.
3. **Aplastic crisis:** Associated **with parvovirus B19**.
4. **Sequestration crisis: Sudden trapping of blood** in spleen or liver causes rapid enlargement of the organ and **drop in hematocrit** leading to **hypovolemic shock**.

Increased Susceptibility to Infections

- Common infections are **pneumonia** due to ***Pneumococcus***, **meningitis** due to ***S. pneumoniae*** and **osteomyelitis** due to ***Salmonella***. Increased frequency of osteomyelitis is due to bone infarcts, which act as a nidus for infection.
- **Septicemia** and **meningitis** are the most common causes of death in children.

Chronic Organ Damage

Particularly seen in the spleen, bones, kidneys, heart, lungs, brain and skin.

- **Spleen:** After 5–6 years of age, the spleen gets fibrosed and **gradually reduces in the size** due to **multiple infarcts**. Gradual **loss of splenic function** secondary to infarcts results in **autosplenectomy**.
- **Bone:** Osteomyelitis, particularly with *Salmonella typhimurium*.
- **Extremities: Skin ulcers** over the lower extremities.

Laboratory Findings in Sickle Cell Anemia

Peripheral Blood

- **Hemoglobin: Decreased.**
- **Hematocrit (PCV): Decreased.**
- **ESR: Reduced.**
- **Reticulocyte count: Increased** and range from 3 to 10%.

> **Peripheral smear**
> - *RBCs:*
>   - Normocytic normochromic to mildly hypochromic.
>   - Moderate to severe degree of **anisopoikilocytosis.**
>   - **Characteristic cell is** the **sickle cell**—appear as long, curved cells with pointed ends (Fig. 13.7); may also show **target cells** (due to red cell dehydration) **and ovalocytes.**
>   - **Polychromatophilia due to reticulocytosis.**
> - *WBCs:* Mildly increased with shift to left.
> - *Platelets:* Mildly increased.

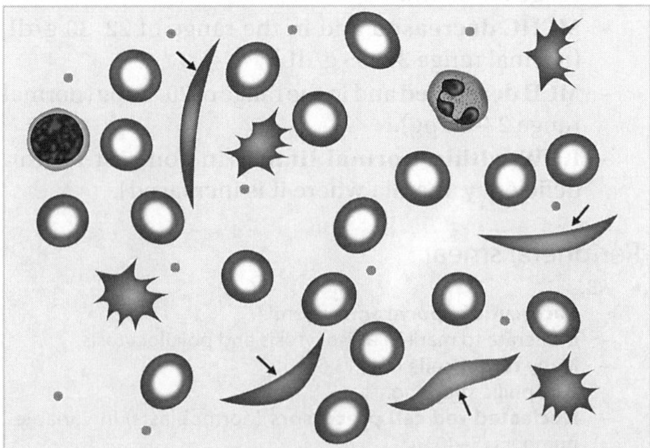

Fig. 13.7: Diagrammatic peripheral blood smear with sickle cells (arrows)

Bone marrow

- *Cellularity:* **Hypercellular.**
- *Erythropoiesis:* **Compensatory normoblastic erythroid hyperplasia**, which expands the marrow and causes resorption of bone and secondary new bone formation.
- *Myelopoiesis:* Normal.
- *Megakaryopoiesis:* Normal.
- *Iron stores:* Usually increased.

Serum Findings

- **Serum bilirubin: Raised** and **predisposes to** pigment **gallstones**.
- **Iron status: Raised** serum iron, serum ferritin and transferrin saturation.
- **Serum haptoglobin: Reduced.**
- **Urine urobilinogen: Increased**.

Diagnostic/Confirmatory Tests

- **Sickling test:**
  - **Sickling** is **induced** by adding a **reducing** (oxygen-consuming) **agent** like 2% sodium metabisulfite or sodium dithionite to blood sample.
  - Red cells with HbS show **sickled and holly leaf** appearance.
  - It is **diagnostic** of sickle cell anemia.
- **Hemoglobin electrophoresis:** HbS is a slow moving compared to HbA and HbF.
- **Estimation of HbF:** In homozygous state constitutes about 10–30% of hemoglobin.
- **High-performance liquid chromatography (HPLC):** Useful for confirmation of diagnosis.
- **Prenatal diagnosis:** By analysis of fetal DNA obtained by amniocentesis or chorionic villous biopsy, to detect the point mutations.

ACQUIRED HEMOLYTIC ANEMIAS

Immunohemolytic Anemias

Anemias due to **premature RBC destruction** (hemolysis) mediated **by antibodies** that bind to RBCs.The antibodies may be either allo or auto type.

Classification

- Alloimmune:
  - Production of antibody against foreign antigen not present on an individual red blood cells (e.g. hemolytic disease of newborn).
  - Alloantibodies are present either in the serum or bound to red cells.
- Autoimmune.

Hemolytic Disease of the Newborn

- Hemolytic disease of the newborn (HDN) is an alloimmune hemolytic anemia developing in the fetus and newborn baby.
- HDN develops when the IgG antibodies against blood group of fetus passes from mother to fetus through the placenta.
- Occurs in two forms:
  - **Rh hemolytic disease of newborn**
    - **Rh incompatibility** in which mother is Rh-ve and fetus is Rh +ve. The anti-D antibodies are responsible for hemolytic anemia.
    - Bilirubin gets deposited in the central nervous system (especially the basal ganglia) of infant producing neurological damage and is known as **kernicterus** (yellow coloration of cerebellum and basal ganglia due to bilirubin deposition). It can cause **death** of the infant.
    - **Antiglobulin test (Coombs test):** Antibodies in the mother and baby are detected by indirect and direct Coombs test respectively.
    - **Prevention of Rh HDN:** By the prophylactic removal of fetal cells entering the maternal circulation before sensitization develops, by **injecting anti-D** into the **Rh D negative mother**.
  - **ABO hemolytic disease of the newborn**
    - **ABO incompatibility** in which mother's blood group is O and fetus is either of A or B blood group. Either anti-A or anti-B antibodies cause hemolysis.
    - It is less severe.

Autoimmune Hemolytic Anemia (AIHA)

- Antibodies against self-antigens on the RBC membrane cause premature destruction of RBCs.
- Anti-RBC antibodies can be divided into three general categories. Interaction of the autoantibody with the red cell antigen is **dependent on the temperature, i.e. warm or cold type**.
  - **Warm antibody type.**
  - **Cold agglutinin type.**
  - **Cold hemolysins type (Donath-Landsteiner antibodies).**

Fragmentation Syndrome

RBCs subjected to trauma (physical or mechanical) in the circulation can undergo fragmentation and result in intravascular hemolysis leading to hemolytic anemias. These are known as fragmentation syndrome.

Classification: According to the site of hemolysis it is classified as:

- **Macroangiopathic** (large vessels) **hemolytic anemia:** red cell trauma from an abnormal vascular surface (e.g. prosthetic heart valve, synthetic vascular graft).
- **Microangiopathic hemolytic anemia (MAHA):** It occurs in capillaries due to abnormal narrowing of the lumen (e.g. disseminated intravascular coagulation).

DISORDERS OF WHITE CELLS

NORMAL DIFFERENTIAL LEUKOCYTE COUNT

The normal range of differential leukocyte count (DLC) in an adult is presented in Table 13.4.

QUANTITATIVE DISORDERS OF LEUKOCYTES

Leukocytosis

An increase in the **total** number of **leukocytes** in the blood **more than 11,000/cu mm** (11×10^9/L).

Causes: Common causes of leukocytosis are shown in Box 13.9.

Leukopenia

Total leukocyte count is less than 4,000/cu mm (4×10^9/L).

Causes: Common causes of leukopenia are shown in Box 13.10.

Disorders of Neutrophils

Neutrophilia

An absolute neutrophil count of more than 8,000/cu mm (8×10^9/L). Differential count shows more than 70% neutrophils and is usually accompanied by leukocytosis ($15–30 \times 10^9$/L).

Table 13.4: Normal range of different leukocytes in an adult

Type of white blood cell	Normal range
Neutrophils	40–70% ($2.0–7.0 \times 10^9$/L)
Lymphocytes	20–40% ($1.0–3.0 \times 10^9$/L)
Monocytes	2–10% ($0.2–1.0 \times 10^9$/L)
Eosinophils	1–6% ($0.02–0.5 \times 10^9$/L)
Basophils	Less than 1% ($0.02–0.1 \times 10^9$/L)

Box 13.9: Common causes of leukocytosis

- Infections
  - Bacterial
  - Viral infections (e.g. infectious mononucleosis)
- Leukemia
  - Acute
  - Chronic: Chronic lymphocytic leukemia and chronic myeloid leukemia
- Leukemoid reactions
- Physiological
  - Pregnancy
  - Exercise

Box 13.10: Common causes of leukopenia

- Typhoid and paratyphoid
- Anemia
  - Aplastic anemia
  - Megaloblastic anemia
- Hypersplenism
- Drugs including cytotoxic drugs
- Radiation
- Rarely leukemia

Box 13.11: Major causes of neutrophilia

- **Pathological:**
  - Acute bacterial and fungal infections:
    - Localized: Pyogenic microorganisms causing infections, e.g. pneumonias, pyogenic meningitis, cellulitis, diphtheria, abscess, tonsillitis, etc.
    - Generalized: Septicemia, acute rheumatic fever.
  - Acute inflammatory processes: Inflammatory conditions (acute appendicitis).
  - Tissue necrosis: Burns, myocardial infarction, gangrene, neoplasms (tumor necrosis).
- **Physiological:**
  - Exercise (shift from marginating pool to circulating pool), newborns, extremes of temperature, pain, emotional stress and during obstetric labor.

Causes of neutrophilia: Major causes of neutrophilia are shown in Box 13.11.

Leukemoid Reaction

Benign leukocytic proliferation characterized by a **total leukocyte count of more than 25 × 10^9/L** with immature white cells (like band forms, metamyelocytes and myelocytes).

It is different from chronic myelocytic/myeloid leukemia (Table 13.5).

Table 13.5: Differences between leukemoid reaction and chronic myeloid leukemia

	Leukemoid reaction	Chronic myeloid leukemia
Clinical features	Features of causative disease	Splenomegaly, and bone pain are common
Peripheral blood findings		
WBC		
Total WBC count	Moderately increased, rarely exceeds 50 × 10^9/L	Markedly increased and usually 50 × 10^9/L
Differential leukocyte count	Shift to the left with few immature forms. Toxic granulation seen	Shift to the left with numerous immature forms. Myelocyte and neutrophil peak
Eosinophilia and basophilia	Variable	Present
Leukocyte alkaline phosphatase (LAP)	Increased	Decreased
RBC		
Anemia	Usually minimal or absent	Severe and progressive
Platelets		
Number	Variable	Normal or increased
Extramedullary myeloid tumors	Absent	Present
Philadelphia chromosome	Absent	Present

Box 13.12: Causes of neutropenia

- **Inadequate production:**
  - ***Suppression of stem cells:*** In these disorders granulocytopenia represents a component of pancytopenia
    - Aplastic anemia
    - Marrow infiltration
    - Metastatic tumors
  - ***Suppression of committed granulocytic precursors***
    - Drugs and chemicals (e.g. sulfonamides, analgesics, arsenicals)
    - Ionizing radiation
  - ***Diseases associated with ineffective hematopoiesis***
    - Megaloblastic anemias: Vitamin B_{12} or folate deficiency
  - ***Severe infections***
    - Bacterial (e.g. typhoid, paratyphoid, septicemia)
    - Viral (e.g. influenza, infectious mononucleosis, hepatitis, measles)
    - Protozoal (e.g. malaria, kala-azar)
- **Increased destruction of neutrophils:**
  - ***Immunologically mediated destruction***
    - Idiopathic
    - Secondary
      - Drugs
      - Autoimmune disorders, e.g. systemic lupus erythematosus
  - ***Splenic sequestration*** may be associated with pancytopenia.

Neutropenia (Agranulocytosis)

Reduction in the absolute neutrophil count (total WBC × % segmented neutrophils and band forms) below 1.5 × 10^9/L (1,500/cu mm).

Etiology

The causes of neutropenia are presented in Box 13.12.

Eosinophilia

Eosinophil count of more than 450/cu mm (0.45 × 10^9/L). Causes of eosinophilia are presented in Box 13.13.

Lymphocytosis

Lymphocyte count more than 4,000/cu mm (4 × 10^9/L) in adults and more than 8,000/cu mm (8 × 10^9/L) in child.

Common causes of lymphocytosis are given in the Box 13.14.

Box 13.13: Causes of eosinophilia

- **Allergic/atopic conditions**
  - Asthma
  - Urticaria
  - Hay fever
  - Drug reactions
  - Allergic rhinitis
- **Parasitic infestations (with tissue invasion)**
  - Roundworm infestation
  - Hookworm infestation
  - Filariasis
- **Fungal infections** (e.g. coccidioidomycosis)
- **Skin diseases**
  - Dermatitis (eczema)
  - Scabies
- **Hematological diseases**
  - Chronic myeloid leukemia
  - Hodgkin lymphoma
  - Eosinophilic leukemia
- **Miscellaneous**
  - Tropical eosinophilia
  - Löeffler's syndrome

Box 13.14: Causes of lymphocytosis

- **Acute infections**
  - Viral infections: Infectious mononucleosis, mumps, measles, chickenpox, infectious hepatitis
  - Toxoplasmosis
- **Chronic infections/inflammatory diseases**
  - Tuberculosis
  - Syphilis
- **Hematologic malignancies**
  - Acute lymphoblastic leukemia
  - Chronic lymphocytic leukemia

ACUTE LEUKEMIA

Definition: Acute leukemia is a malignant disease of the bone marrow stem cell and its characteristic features are:

- **Bone marrow: Diffuse replacement** with proliferating neoplastic blast cells that fail to mature. **Blast cells constitute more than 20%** (WHO criteria) of the nucleated cells in the marrow.
- **Peripheral blood: Abnormal numbers and forms of immature white blood cells.**

Aleukemic/subleukemic leukemia is characterized by very few/no blasts in the peripheral blood.

Classification

Traditional classification depending on microscopic appearance of the involved cell and the course of leukemias is presented in Box 13.15. Acute leukemia are mainly divided into two groups namely acute lymphoblastic leukemia (ALL) and acute myeloblastic leukemia (AML).

FAB Classification of Acute Leukemias

- **First French, American and British (FAB)** classification was **based on the (1) morphological and (2) cytochemical characteristics of blast cells** (Box 13.16).

WHO Classification (2016) of Acute Leukemia (Box 13.17)

Differences between Myeloblast and Lymphoblast (Table 13.6)

ACUTE LYMPHOBLASTIC LEUKEMIA/ LYMPHOMA

- **Acute lymphoblastic leukemia/lymphoma (ALL)** is a group of neoplasms consisting of **lymphoblasts**.

Box 13.15: Traditional classification of leukemia

- **Acute leukemia**
  - Acute myelogenous/myeloblastic/myelocytic/myeloid leukemia (AML)
  - Acute lymphoblastic/lymphocytic leukemia (ALL)
- **Chronic leukemia**
  - Chronic myeloid leukemia (CML)
  - Chronic lymphocytic leukemia (CLL)

Box 13.16: Revised French, American and British (FAB) classification of acute leukemias

Acute lymphoid leukemia	
L_1	Small homogenous cells with inconspicuous nucleoli
L_2	Large cells with variable size and 1–2 nucleoli
L_3	Large, homogeneous cells with finely stippled chromatin and prominent nucleoli. Cytoplasm is basophilic and vacuolated.
Acute myeloid leukemia	
M_0	Minimally differentiated AML
M_1	AML without maturation
M_2	AML with maturation
M_3	Promyelocytic leukemia
M_4	Myelomonocytic leukemia
M_5	Monocytic leukemia
M_6	Erythroleukemia
M_7	Megakaryocytic leukemia

Box 13.17: WHO classification (2016) of acute lymphoblastic and myeloid leukemia

- **Acute lymphoblastic leukemia**
  - **Precursor**-B lymphoblastic leukemia/lymphoma
  - **Precursor** -T lymphoblastic leukemia/lymphoma
- **Acute myeloid leukemia**
  - AML with recurrent genetic abnormalities e.g.:
    - AML with t(8;21)(q22;q22); *RUNX1-RUNX1T1.*
    - AML with inv(16)(p13;1q22); *CBFB-MYH11.*
  - AML with MDS-related changes.
  - Therapy-related myeloid neoplasms.
  - AML not otherwise specified.
  - Myeloid sarcoma.
  - Myeloid proliferation related to Down syndrome.

Abbreviations: AML, acute myeloid leukemia; APL, acute promyelocytic leukemia; MDS, myelodysplastic syndrome

- Lymphoblast is immature, precursor B (pre-B) or T (pre-T) lymphocyte.
- WHO classification (Box 13.17):
  - **Precursor B cells** ALL (about 85%) seen in **childhood** and present as **acute leukemias.**
  - **Precursor T cells** ALL (15%) present in adolescent males as **lymphomas**, often with involvement of mediastinum (thymus).

Table 13.6: Differences between myeloblast and lymphoblast based on morphology and cytochemistry

	Lymphoblast (Fig. 13.8)	Myeloblast (Fig. 13.9)
Size	2–3 times the size of lymphocyte	3–5 times the size of lymphocyte
Cytoplasmic characters		
Amount	Scanty (less cytoplasm than myeloblast)	Scanty to moderate (more cytoplasm than lymphoblast)
Color	Blue	Gray
Cytoplasmic granules	Agranular	May have cytoplasmic granules
Auer rod	Negative	Positive
Nuclear characters		
Nuclear chromatin	Uniform, coarse	Uniform, fine
Nucleoli	Inconspicuous or 1 to 2	3 to 5, prominent
N:C ratio	High	High
Accompanying cells	Lymphocytes	Promyelocytes, myelocytes, metamyelocytes, band forms and neutrophils
Cytochemistry		
Myeloperoxidase	Negative	Positive
Sudan black	Negative	Positive
PAS	Block positivity	Negative
Nonspecific esterase	Negative	Positive in M4 and M5

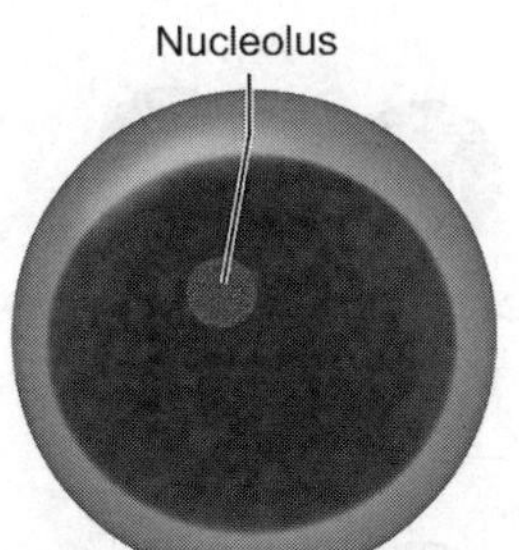

Fig. 13.8: Diagrammatic appearance of lymphoblast

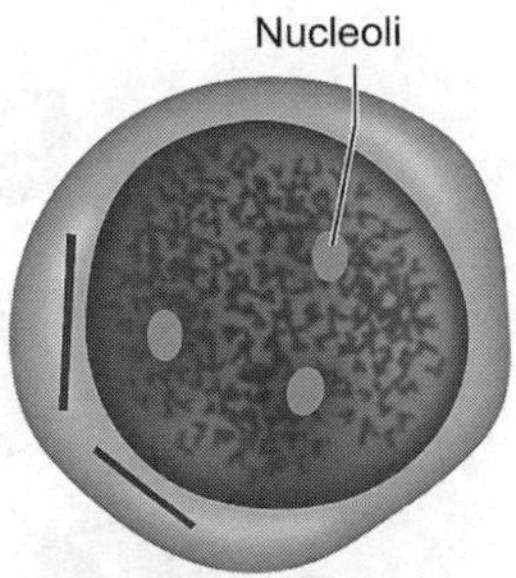

Fig. 13.9: Diagrammatic appearance of myeloblast

Classification of Acute Lymphoblastic Leukemia (Boxes 13.16 and 13.17)

Clinical Features

Age: Most common hematological malignancy of **children**. Most common between **1 and 5 years** of age and between **30 and 40 years**.

Sex: Slight male preponderance.

Onset: **Abrupt**.

Symptoms:

- **Bone marrow failure:**
  - Anemia: Causes **fatigue, weakness**.
  - Neutropenia: **Infections** by bacteria or opportunistic fungi. Develop sore throat and respiratory infections.
  - Thrombocytopenia: **Bleeding** into the skin and mucosa in the form of purpura or ecchymoses.
  - **Bone pain** and **sternal tenderness**.
- **Extramedullary infiltration:**
  - **Lymphadenopathy:** 75% of patients, usually involve **cervical lymph nodes**.
  - **Hepatosplenomegaly:** Splenomegaly is more common than hepatomegaly.
  - **Mediastinal thymic mass:** More common in T-ALL.
- **CNS involvement:** Spread into the meninges causes **leukemic meningitis** ALL (pre-B).
- **Testicular involvement** (ALL).

Laboratory Findings

Peripheral Blood

- **Total WBC count: Markedly raised** ranging from 20 $\times 10^9$/L to 200 $\times 10^9$/L.
- **Platelet count: Reduced** (thrombocytopenia).
- **Hemoglobin: Decreased** and may be as low as 3 g/dL.

Peripheral smear (Fig. 13.10)

- *RBCs:* Normocytic normochromic anemia.
- *WBCs:* Total count **markedly increased** and **20% or more lymphoblasts.**
  - **Morphology of lymphoblasts:**
    - Larger than small lymphocyte.
    - High N:C ratio.
    - Nucleus with condensed chromatin and nucleoli are either absent or inconspicuous.
    - Scant to moderate agranular basophilic cytoplasm.
- *Platelets:* Thrombocytopenia.

Cytochemistry of lymphoblasts

- Periodic acid schiff (PAS): Cytoplasmic aggregates of **PAS positive** material **(block positivity)**.
- **Myeloperoxidase (MPO) negative**.
- **Sudan black B negative**.

Bone marrow

- *Cellularity:* Markedly **hypercellula**r due to proliferation of blasts.
- *Erythropoiesis and myelopoiesis:* Reduced.
- *Megakaryopoiesis:* Megakaryocytes gradually decrease.
- ***Blasts:* Constitute 20–100% of the marrow cells.**

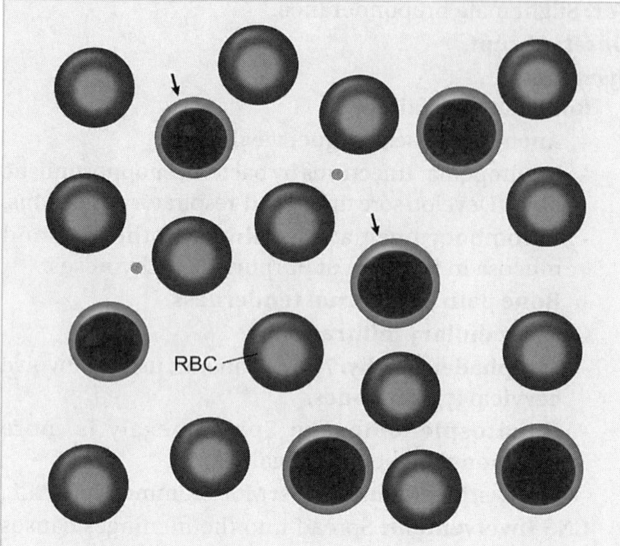

Fig. 13.10: Diagrammatic peripheral blood smear in acute lymphoblastic leukemia showing lymphoblasts (arrows)

Biochemical Findings

- **Serum uric acid: Raised.**
- **LDH: Raised.**

CSF Examination

To know/rule out CNS involvement by ALL.

ACUTE MYELOGENOUS LEUKEMIA

Definition: Neoplasm of hematopoietic progenitors characterized by proliferation resulting in **accumulation of immature myeloblasts in the marrow.**

Classification of acute myelogenous leukemia (AML): Refer Boxes 13.15 to 13.17.

Clinical Features

Age: AML may develop at **any age**, but is more **common in adults.**

Onset: Acute leukemias are **abrupt in onset.**

Symptoms: Related to depressed marrow function.

- ***Bone marrow failure:***
  - **Anemia:** Fatigue and weakness.
  - **Neutropenia:** Life-threatening infections by bacteria or opportunistic fungi.
  - **Thrombocytopenia:** Bleeding, patient may also develop disseminated intravascular coagulation (DIC) in AML M3 and primary fibrinolysis.
  - **Bone pain and tenderness.**
- ***Extramedullary infiltration***
  - Gingival hypertrophy (M4 and M5) and infiltration of skin (leukemia cutis).
  - Hepatosplenomegaly: Usually more than in ALL.

Laboratory Findings

Peripheral Blood

- **Total WBC count: Markedly raised** ranging from 20 × 10^9/L to 100 × 10^9/L.
- **Hemoglobin: Decreased** and ranges from 5 to 9 g/dL.

Peripheral Smear (Fig. 13.11)

- *RBCs:* Normocytic normochromic type of anemia.
- *WBCs:* Total WBC **count markedly increased.**
  - Differential count: **More than 20% myeloid blasts.** May show more than one type of blast or blasts with hybrid features.
  - **Morphology of myeloblasts**
    - 3–5 times larger than the diameter of a small lymphocyte
    - High N:C ratio
    - Fine nuclear chromatin with 2–4 variably prominent nucleoli
    - More cytoplasm than lymphoblasts—azurophilic, peroxidase-positive granules
    - Presence of Auer rods is definitive evidence of myeloid differentiation.
  - **Auer rods** are azurophilic needle-like peroxidase-positive structures in the cytosol of myeloblasts (M_2 and M_3 subtype).
- *Platelets:* Moderate to severe thrombocytopenia and causes bleeding from skin and mucosa.

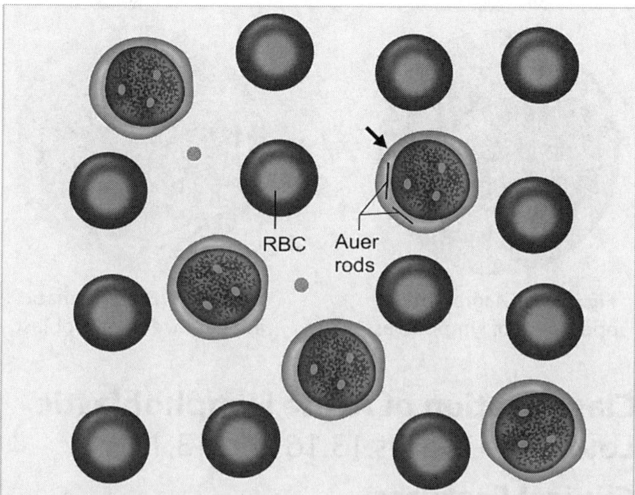

Fig. 13.11: Diagrammatic peripheral blood smear in AML with myeloblasts. One myeloblast with two Auer rods (arrow)

Cytochemistry of Myeloblasts

- **Stain positively** with **myeloperoxidase (MPO) and Sudan black B**
- Monoblasts stain with nonspecific esterases.

> Bone marrow
> - *Cellularity:* Markedly **hypercellular**.
> - *Erythropoiesis:* **Markedly suppressed.**
> - *Myelopoiesis:* Suppression of myeloid maturation and **myeloblasts constitute more than 20% of marrow cells.**
> - *Megakaryopoiesis:* **Gradually decreased.**

CHRONIC MYELOGENOUS LEUKEMIA

Definition: Chronic myelogenous leukemia (CML) is one of the myeloproliferative neoplasm (MPN) of **pluripotent hematopoietic stem cell** characterized by overproduction of cells of the myeloid series which results in marked splenomegaly and leukocytosis.

Distinguished from other myeloproliferative neoplasms by the presence of:

1. **Philadelphia (Ph) chromosome** in more than 90% of cases.
2. **Chimeric fusion BCR-ABL gene**.

Molecular Pathogenesis

Philadelphia (Ph) Chromosome (Fig. 13.12)

- It is an acquired chromosomal abnormality **in all proliferating hematopoietic stem cells** (erythroid, myeloid, monocytic and megakaryocytic precursors).
- **Balanced reciprocal translocation** between long arm of chromosome 9 and 22, i.e. **t (9; 22) (q 34; q 11.2).** It increases the length of chromosome 9 and shortening of 22. This **shortened chromosome 22** is known as Philadelphia chromosome (Fig. 13.12).

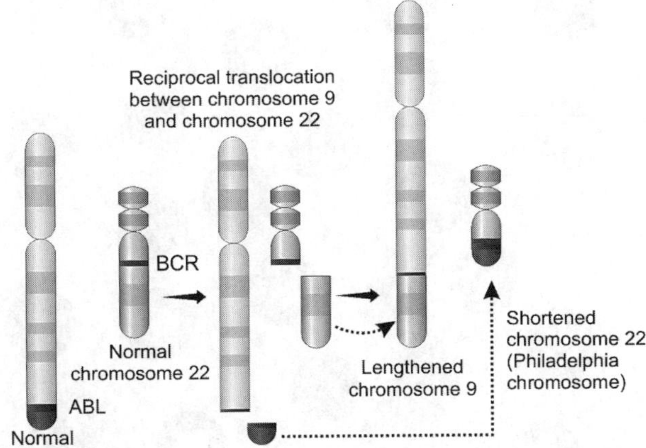

Fig. 13.12: Balanced reciprocal translocation between long arm of chromosome 9 and chromosome 22 resulting in shortened chromosome 22 known as Philadelphia chromosome

BCR-ABL Fusion Gene

- **ABL** proto-oncogene from chromosome 9 **joins** the **BCR** on chromosome 22.
- It produces a new **chimeric (fusion) gene called BCR-ABL, thus converting ABL proto-oncogene into oncogene.** The product of the fusion gene plays a central role in the development of CML.
- The product of this oncogene, i.e. **oncoprotein** (e.g. **p210) causes cell division** and **inhibition of apoptosis.**

Clinical Features

- ***Age*: Usually occurs between 40 and 60 years** of age.
- ***Sex:*** Males slightly more affected than females.
- ***Onset:* Insidious.**

Symptoms:

- **Nonspecific symptoms:** Fatigue, weakness, weight loss, anorexia.
- **Fullness of abdomen due to splenomegaly** (caused by leukemic infiltration and extramedullary hematopoiesis). Splenomegaly is moderate to severe and is characteristic feature in majority (80–90%) of patients.
- **Hepatomegaly:** Mild or moderate seen in 60–70% of cases.

Three different phases of CML are: (1) chronic phase, (2) accelerated phase and (3) blastic phase.

Laboratory Findings

Peripheral Blood

- **Hemoglobin:** Usually less than 11 g/dL.

> Peripheral smear
> - *RBCs:* **Normocytic normochromic anemia**.
> - *WBCs:*
>   - **Marked leukocytosis** (12–600 × 10^9/L) total **leukocyte count** usually **exceeds 100 × 10^9/L (1,00,000/cu mm).**
>   - **Shift to left (shift to immaturity)**—granulocytes at all stages of development (neutrophils, metamyelocytes, myelocytes, promyelocytes and an occasional myeloblasts).
>   - **Predominant cells** are **neutrophils and myelocytes.**
>   - **Blasts** are usually **less than 10%** of the circulating WBCs (Fig. 13.13).
>   - **Basophilia and eosinophilia.**
>   - **Decreased NAP/LAP score:** NAP score in CML is decreased below 20 (normal score range is 40–100). Helpful in differentiating CML from leukemoid reaction.
> - *Platelets:* Platelets range from normal (150–450 × 10^9/L) to greater than 1000 × 10^9/L. Up to 50% have **thrombocytosis.**

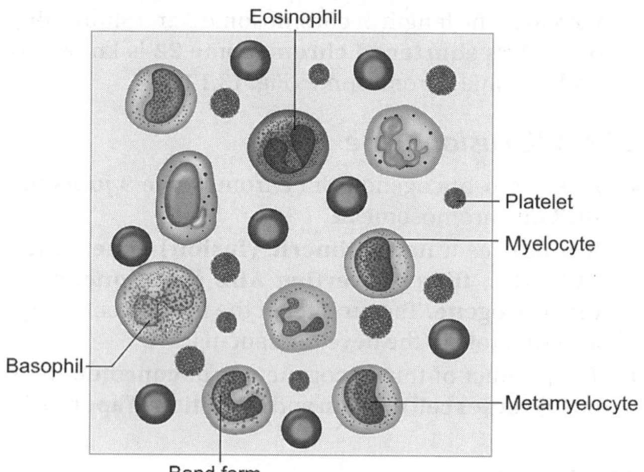

Fig. 13.13: Diagrammatic peripheral blood picture in chronic/stable phase of chronic myeloid leukemia

Bone marrow

- *Cellularity:* Markedly **hypercellular** due to **myeloid hyperplasia**.
- *M: E ratio:* Often exceeds **20:1**.
- *Erythropoiesis:* **Diminished erythropoiesis** as disease progresses.
- *Myelopoiesis:* **Marked hyperplasia. Blast** cells usually **less than 10%.** Basophils, eosinophils and their precursors are usually found.
- *Megakaryopoiesis:* Megakaryocytes are either normal or increased. **Dwarf megakaryocytes.**

Biochemical Findings

- Serum uric acid raised.
- Serum LDH raised.

Philadelphia chromosome **and** ***BCR-ABL fusion gene:*** **Demonstrated** either by chromosomal analysis or **fluorescent in situ hybridization (FISH)** or PCR-based tests.

CHRONIC LYMPHOCYTIC LEUKEMIA

Definition: Chronic lymphocytic leukemia (**CLL**)/small lymphocytic lymphoma (**SLL**) is a **tumor composed of monomorphic small B lymphocytes** in the peripheral blood, bone marrow and lymphoid organs (spleen and lymph nodes).

- Both CLL and SLL is a **single entity with different presentations**.
- **Small lymphocytic lymphoma** (SLL) is tissue equivalent of chronic lymphocytic leukemia (CLL).

Clinical Features

- ***Age:*** Between **50–60 years** of age.
- ***Sex:*** **More in males** than in females (2:1).
- ***Symptoms:***
  - **Asymptomatic** in about 25–30%.
  - **Nonspecific symptoms*:* Fatigue,** loss of weight and anorexia.
  - **Generalized lymphadenopathy.**
  - **Immunological defects** either as **immune deficiency or autoimmunity**.

Laboratory Findings

Peripheral Blood

- **Hemoglobin: Decreased** and usually below 13 g/dL.
- **Total leukocyte count** is **increased (20–50 × 10^9/L)**.

Peripheral smear (Fig. 13.14)

- *RBCs:* Normocytic normochromic anemia.
- *WBCs:*
  - Differential leukocyte count shows **lymphocytosis** and constitutes **more than 50%** of the white cells.
  - **Lymphocytes mature type**—small with scant cytoplasm, **nuclei** round with clumped coarse chromatin **("soccer ball"/block-type chromatin).** Nucleoli absent.
  - **Smudge cells** or basket cells (fragile leukemic cells).
- *Platelets:* Initially **normal** count and later may be decreased.

Bone marrow

- *Cellularity:* **Hypercellular** marrow due to infiltration by mature lymphocytes.
- *Erythropoiesis:* Normal.
- *Myelopoiesis:* Normal.
- *Megakaryopoiesis:* Normal.
- *Lymphocytic infiltrate:* As the disease advances neoplastic lymphocytes replace the normal erythroid, myeloid and megakaryocytic series in the bone marrow resulting in anemia, neutropenia and thrombocytopenia.

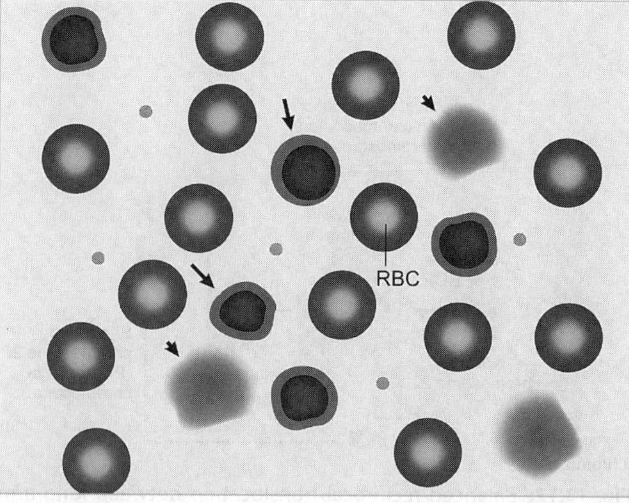

Fig. 13.14: Diagrammatic peripheral blood smears in chronic lymphocytic leukemia showing numerous small lymphocytes (long arrows) and few smudge cells (short arrows)

Lymph Node

- Show loss of normal architecture.
- Diffuse infiltration by monomorphic, small, round lymphocytes.
- Lymphocytes have nuclei with coarse chromatin and scanty cytoplasm.
- Small, nodular aggregates of medium to large-sized lymphocytes known as **proliferation centers or pseudo-follicles or growth centers** and when found are **pathognomonic for CLL/SLL.**

Course and prognosis

Median survival rate is 4–6 years.

DISORDERS OF HEMOSTASIS

NORMAL HEMOSTASIS

- Hemostasis is the **body's response to vascular damage/injury.**
- Includes several sequences of events at the site of vascular injury. First there is formation of primary hemostatic plug followed by secondary hemostatic plug.

Primary Hemostatic Plug

Platelet adhere to subendothelial structures at the site of injury. The **platelets change their shape** and **release granule contents.** The released contents cause platelet **aggregation and form primary hemostatic plug.**

Secondary Hemostatic Plug

Exposure of tissue factor at the site of vascular injury **activates the extrinsic coagulation system. The fibrin formed develops into a secondary hemostatic plug.**

CLASSIFICATION OF HEMOSTATIC DISORDERS (BOX 13.18)

1. **Bleeding disorders (hemorrhagic disorders/hemorrhagic diathesis):** Bleeding disorders have an **abnormal tendency to bleed** (hemorrhage) due to failure of hemostasis.
2. **Thrombotic disorders:** They cause **thrombus formation.**

Bleeding Disorders Caused by Vessel Wall Abnormalities

Vascular purpura (nonthrombocytopenic purpura) is group of **disorders of blood vessels** that results in **bleeding.**

Box 13.18: Classification of disorders of hemostasis

- **Bleeding disorders**
  - **Disorders of primary hemostasis**
    - **Vessel wall abnormalities**
      - ◊ Congenital, e.g. Ehlers-Danlos syndrome
      - ◊ Acquired, e.g. Henoch-Schönlein purpura
    - **Platelet abnormalities**
      - ◊ Quantitative: Thrombocytopenia (e.g. ITP, drug-induced, congenital).
      - ◊ Qualitative: Platelet function disorders.
  - **Disorders of coagulation system (disorders of secondary hemostasis)**
    - **Congenital:** Hemophilia A, B; von Willebrand disease; other coagulation factor deficiencies [XI, VII, II, V, X]
    - **Acquired:** Vitamin K deficiency, liver disease, disseminated intravascular coagulation
- **Thrombotic disorders**
  - **Inherited**
  - **Acquired**

Box 13.19: Classification of bleeding disorders caused by vessel wall abnormalities

- **Acquired disorders**
  - Due to decreased amount of connective tissue
    - Senile purpura
    - Scurvy
    - Cushing syndrome and steroid therapy
  - Due to vasculitis
    - Henoch-Schönlein purpura
    - Infections
    - Drug reactions
  - Associated with plasma cell neoplasms
    - Amyloidosis
  - Miscellaneous
    - Simple easy bruising
- **Congenital/inherited disorders**
  - Hereditary hemorrhagic telangiectasia
  - Ehlers-Danlos syndrome
  - Marfan syndrome

They should be distinguished from bleeding disorders due to abnormalities of platelets.

Classification of bleeding disorders caused by vessel wall abnormalities are presented in Box 13.19.

Bleeding Disorders Due to Abnormalities of Platelet

Classification of Platelet Disorders (Box 13.20)

Thrombocytopenia

- Decrease in the **platelet count below** the lower limit of **150,000/cu mm** (150×10^9/L).

Box 13.20: Classification of platelet disorders

Quantitative Platelet Disorders
• Thrombocytopenia – Increased destruction – Decreased production – Sequestration – Dilutional • Thrombocytosis
Qualitative Platelet Disorders
• **Hereditary** • **Acquired**

Clinical Features of Thrombocytopenia

- Cutaneous bleeding appears as pinpoint hemorrhages (petechiae) and ecchymoses.
- Mucosal bleeding.
- Intracranial bleed (subarachnoid and intracerebral hemorrhage) is rare but serious.

Severity of bleeding

- **Post-traumatic** bleeding—when the platelet **count is 20,000–50,000/cu mm.**
- **Spontaneous** bleeding—when the platelet count falls **below 20,000/cu mm.**
- **Intracranial** bleeding—when platelet count is **<10,000/cu mm.**

Causes of Thrombocytopenia (Box 13.21)

Box 13.21: Causes of thrombocytopenia

• **Increased platelet destruction** – **Immune mediated** ◆ **Autoimmune** ◊ Primary: Immune thrombocytopenic purpura (acute and chronic). ◊ Secondary: Systemic lupus erythematosus, B cell lymphoid neoplasms. ◆ **Alloimmune:** Post-transfusion or pregnancy ◆ **Drug-induced:** Quinidine, heparin, sulfa compounds ◆ **Infections:** HIV infection, infectious mononucleosis, cytomegalovirus – **Nonimmune mediated** ◆ Disseminated intravascular coagulation
• **Decreased production of platelets** – **Generalized primary diseases of bone marrow:** Aplastic anemia (congenital and acquired) – **Bone marrow invasion/infiltration:** Leukemia, disseminated cancer – **Selective impairment of platelet production** – Drug-induced: Alcohol, thiazides, cytotoxic drugs – Infections: Measles, human immunodeficiency virus (HIV) – Ineffective megakaryopoiesis
• **Sequestration** – Hypersplenism
• **Dilutional**

IMMUNE THROMBOCYTOPENIC PURPURA

- Most common form of thrombocytopenia.
- **Due to increased destruction of platelets** by **immune mechanisms**—mainly **autoimmune** mechanism.

Types of Immune Thrombocytopenic Purpura (ITP)

Acute Immune Thrombocytopenic Purpura

- **Self-limited** disease.
- **Children:** 2–4 years and seen equally in both sexes.
- Presents **1–3 weeks after viral** (measles, rubella, EBV) **infection**.
- Platelet destruction by **antiplatelet autoantibodies** (type II hypersensitivity reaction).
- **Platelet count is decreased**, sometimes even below 10,000/cu mm (10×10^9/L).

Clinical features

- **Sudden onset**.
- **Petechiae, gum bleeding, epistaxis** and mild fever.
- Usually **resolve** spontaneously **within 6 months**.
- **Excellent prognosis**.

Chronic Immune Thrombocytopenic Purpura

- Persistent **thrombocytopenia** for **more than 6–12 months.**
- Indolent, females are more affected than males (F:M = 3:1).
- **More common** and usually seen in **adults (20–40 years)**.

Pathogenesis of ITP

- **Autoimmune disorder** characterized by formation of **antiplatelet antibodies**, directed against membrane glycoproteins.
- Antiplatelet antibodies in about 80% of patients and are of the **IgG type.**
- Platelets are destroyed by the mononuclear phagocytes of RE system (mainly spleen) resulting in thrombocytopenia.
- **Splenectomy causes marked improvement** in 75–80% of patients.

Clinical features

Clinical features are due to thrombocytopenia: **Skin bleeding, mucosal bleeding, menorrhagia** in females, etc.

Laboratory Findings

Peripheral Blood

- **Platelet count: Markedly reduced**—below 80,000/cu mm (80 × 10^9/L).
- **Hemoglobin:** Ranges from 7 to 12 g/dL.

Peripheral smear

- *Platelets:* **Markedly reduced** (thrombocytopenia) and **abnormally large sized platelets (mega- thrombocytes/giant platelets).**
- *RBCs:* **Chronic blood loss** (e.g. menorrhagia) due to ITP may **lead to microcytic hypochromic anemia.**
- *WBCs:* Normal.

Bone marrow

- *Cellularity:* **Hypercellular.**
- *Megakaryopoiesis:*
  - **Moderate increase in number** of both **immature and mature** forms of **megakaryocytes.**
  - **Immature megakaryocytes predominate-large nonlobulated single nuclei and basophilic cytoplasm.**
- ***Erythropoiesis:***
  - **Prolonged bleeding** may cause anemia leading to **normoblastic erythroid hyperplasia.**
  - Constant bleeding leads to **iron deficiency** and **micronormoblastic erythroid hyperplasia.**
- **Myelopoiesis:** Normal.
- **Storage iron:** Severe and chronic bleeding causes iron deficiency with reduced iron stores.

- **Bleeding time (BT): Prolonged**, but PT and PTT are normal.
- **Tourniquet test: Positive.**
- **Clotting time (CT): Normal.**
- **Tests for platelet autoantibodies:** May be positive.
- **Spleen:** Normal size.

COAGULATION DISORDERS

Classification of Coagulation Disorders (Box 13.22)

Box 13.22: Classification of coagulation disorders

- **Hereditary coagulation disorders**
  - Hemophilia A
  - Hemophilia B
  - von Willebrand disease
  - Others
- **Acquired (secondary) coagulation disorders**
  - Vitamin K deficiency
  - Liver disease
  - Others

HEREDITARY COAGULATION DISORDERS

Usually, due to deficiency of single coagulation factor.

Factor VIII-vWF Complex

- **Factor VIII-vWF complex** has two components:
  - Plasma **factor VIII.**
  - **von Willebrand factor.**
- **vWF protects factor VIII** and important for its stability. **Subendothelial vWF promotes platelet adhesion.**
- Whenever there is vascular endothelial injury, **plasma vWF** gets **adsorbed to exposed subendothelial matrix** and **augments adhesion of platelets.**

HEMOPHILIA

- Hemophilia **A and B** are **similar in both clinical and pathological features**, the **difference** being **in the deficient factor.**
- Both are **sex-linked recessive disorders** resulting in inherited deficiency of the clotting factor or synthesis of a defective clotting factor.
- **Males are affected** and **females are carriers.**

Hemophilia A (Factor VIII Deficiency)

- **Common hereditary X-linked recessive** disease.
- About 30% of hemophiliacs may be due to acquired mutations.
- **Reduced amount or** activity of **factor VIII** is associated with **life-threatening bleeding.**
- Bleeding is due to both inadequate coagulation and inappropriate clot removal (fibrinolysis).

Mode of Inheritance (Fig. 13.15)

- X-linked recessive disease. **Genes** for factor VIII are located **on the long arm of the X-chromosome.**
- Does not manifest when there is a normal copy of X-chromosome.
- **Males** with a defective/mutant factor VIII gene (hemophiliac gene) on their single X chromosome (X_H) **suffer** from hemophilia.
- **Heterozygous females are carriers** and do not express the full clinical disease because of the paired normal X-chromosome.

Clinical Features

Clinical severity **depends on the level of factor VIII activity with normal range expressed as percentage.** Severe cases have less than 1% residual factor VIII activity.

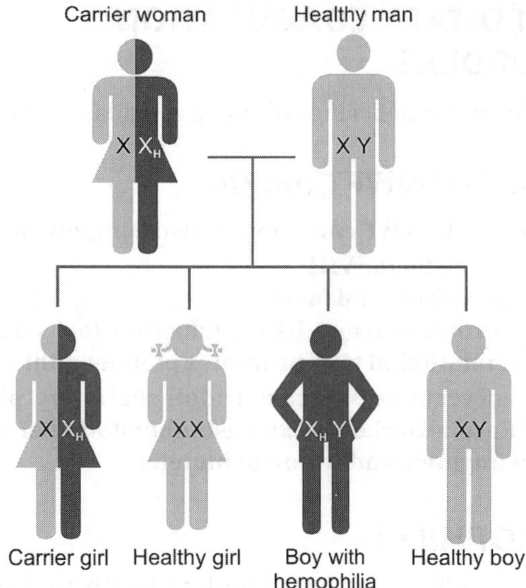

Fig. 13.15: Mode of inheritance in hemophilia

Common clinical presentations include:

- Frequent and spontaneous **hemorrhage into the joints**—hemarthrosis.
- Hemorrhage into **soft tissues**.
- **Prolonged bleeding** following trauma.

Laboratory Findings

- **Bleeding time: Normal.**
- **Clotting time: Prolonged,** but is not a sensitive test.
- **Platelet count: Normal.**
- **Prothrombin time: Normal.**
- **Activated partial thromboplastin time (APTT): Increased** (normal 30–40 seconds).
- **Factor VIII assay: Essential for the diagnosis** and to assess the levels and severity of disease.
- **Fibrinogen assay:** Normal.
- **FDP:** Negative.
- **Detection of carriers:** By DNA markers.
  - To detect female carriers.
  - Prenatal diagnosis of affected fetuses.

Complications

Due to hemophilia

- **Deforming arthritis and contractures:** This is due to repeated bleeding into the joints. Organization and fibrosis of intramuscular hematomas leads to contractures of involved muscles.
- **Anemia:** Excessive, spontaneous or repeated bleeding leads to anemia.

Due to therapy

- **Viral hepatitis: Hepatitis B, C and D** may develop in patients who received multiple transfusions of FFP/cryoprecipitate.
- **AIDS:** This may occur in individuals who received fresh frozen plasma (FFP) or cryoprecipitate, when screening tests for HIV were not available.
- **Factor VIII inhibitors:** Makes further management difficult.

Hemophilia B (Christmas Disease, Factor IX Deficiency)

- **Clinically indistinguishable from hemophilia A.**
- **X-linked recessive** disorder.
- **Variable clinical severity.**
- Assay of factor IX should be done to diagnose Christmas disease (named after the first patient).

Laboratory Findings

Similar to hemophilia A.

- **Bleeding time:** Normal.
- **Clotting time:** Prolonged.
- **Platelet count:** Normal.
- **Prothrombin time:** Normal.
- **Activated partial thromboplastin time (APTT):** Increased (normal 30–40 seconds).
- **Factor IX assay:** Factor IX is decreased.

Von Willebrand Disease (vWD)

- Most common **inherited** bleeding disorders.
- Most cases are **autosomal dominant disorders.**
- Variable clinical picture with more than 20 variants.

Categories

Grouped into two major categories:

- **Quantitative deficiency of vWF:** Decreased circulating vWF.
- **Qualitative defects in vWF.**

Clinical Features

- Most cases are of **mild bleeding.**
- Common symptoms:
  - Spontaneous bleeding from mucous membranes (e.g. epistaxis).
  - Excessive bleeding from wounds or menorrhagia.
- In severe cases, similar to hemophilia A.

Table 13.7: Summary of laboratory tests in hereditary coagulation disorders

	Hemophilia A	Hemophilia B	von Willebrand disease
Bleeding time	N	N	Increased
APTT	Increased	Increased	Increased
Factor VIII	Decreased	N	Low or normal
Factor IX	N	Decreased	N
vWF	N	N	Decreased

Abbreviation: N, normal

Laboratory Findings

- **Platelet count:** Normal.
- **Bleeding time: Prolonged**.
- **Clotting time: Prolonged**.
- **Tourniquet test (Hess test):** Positive due to defect in platelet adhesion.
- **APTT: Prolonged APTT**.
- **PT:** Normal.
- **vWF assay:** Plasma level of active vWF is decreased.
- **Platelet function test:** Defective ristocetin induced platelet aggregation test is diagnostic of vWF.

Laboratory tests in hereditary disorders are summarized in Table 13.7.

ACQUIRED COAGULATION DISORDERS

Coagulation Factor Abnormalities

Usually characterized by multiple clotting abnormalities.

- **Vitamin K deficiency:** In neonates, low levels of vitamin K levels may produce life-threatening hemorrhage during the first week of life known as ***hemorrhagic disease of the newborn.***
- **Liver disease:** Liver synthesizes all the clotting factors and severe liver disease is associated with a hemorrhagic diathesis.
- **Other causes:** Disseminated intravascular coagulation that involves deficiency of several coagulation factors.

Disseminated Intravascular Coagulation

Widespread disorder with **combination of thrombosis and hemorrhage**.

Etiology

Develops as a secondary complication of wide variety of disorders (Box 13.23).

Clinical Features

- **Serious, often fatal**, clinical condition.
- Signs and symptoms are related to:
  - **Hemorrhagic diathesis/bleeding:** Most common, manifest as ecchymoses, petechiae or bleeding from mucous membranes or at the sites of venipuncture.
  - **Microvascular thrombi:** Tissue hypoxia and infarction of the organ leading to multiorgan failure.

Box 13.23: Major disorders associated with disseminated intravascular coagulation

- **Infections**
  - Gram-negative bacterial sepsis
  - Meningococcemia and other bacteria
  - Fungi, viruses, malaria
- **Obstetric complications**
  - Retained dead fetus
  - Septic abortion
  - Abruptio placentae
  - Amniotic fluid embolism
  - Toxemia and pre-eclampsia
- **Neoplasms**
  - Carcinomas of pancreas, prostate, lung and stomach
  - Acute promyelocytic leukemia
- **Massive tissue injury**
  - Traumatic
  - Burns
  - Fat embolism
  - Surgery
- **Vascular disorders**
  - Aortic aneurysm, giant hemangioma
- **Immunologic reactions**
  - Transfusion reactions
  - Transplant rejection
- **Respiratory distress syndrome**
  - Miscellaneous

Snakebite, liver disease, acute intravascular hemolysis, shock, heat stroke, hypersensitivity, vasculitis

Laboratory findings in DIC

Screening Assays

- **Coagulation abnormalities.**
  - **APTT: Increased** as a result of consumption and inhibition of the function of clotting factors.
  - **Prothrombin time: Increased.**
  - **Thrombin time (TT): Increased** because of decreased fibrinogen.
  - **Fibrinogen:** Decreased.
- **Bleeding time: Increased** due to decreased platelet count.
- **Platelet count: Decreased** due to utilization of platelets in microthrombi.
- **Peripheral smear: Microangiopathic hemolytic anemia with schistocytes.**

Confirmatory Tests

- **Fibrinolysis abnormalities.**
- **FDP** (fibrin degradation/split products): Secondary fibrinolysis results in **generation of FDPs**, which can be measured by latex agglutination.
- **D-dimer test:** It is **specific for diagnosing DIC**.

LABORATORY EVALUATION OF BLEEDING DISORDERS

The clinical laboratory evaluation is an integral part of the diagnosis and management of patients with bleeding disorders. Laboratory tests for bleeding disorders depend on the component of hemostasis that is involved (Table 13.8).

Most bleeding disorders are caused by one of three defects: (i) a defect in platelet number or function, (ii) a defect in platelet–vessel wall interactions (i.e. an abnormality in the adhesive interactions between platelets and the vessel wall) or (iii) a defect or deficiency in coagulation factor. The diagnosis of bleeding disorders requires a battery of tests (Table 13.9) which include screening tests done in all patients with history of bleeding, followed by specific tests to identify the exact nature of the disorder.

TABLE 13.8: Laboratory tests for hemostatic disorders depending on the component involved

Platelet component	Plate-vessel wall interaction	Coagulation component
• Platelet count • Platelet aggregation test • Clot retraction test	• Capillary fragility test (Tourniquet test) • Bleeding time	• Clotting time • Prothrombin time (PT) • Activated partial thromboplastin time (APTT) • Thrombin time (TT) • Prothrombin consumption time • Factor assay

TABLE 13.9: Laboratory tests in bleeding disorders

Screening tests	Accessory tests	Others
• Platelet count • Bleeding time • Prothrombin time (PT) • Activated partial thromboplastin time (APTT) • Thrombin time (TT)	• Capillary fragility test (Tourniquet test) • Clotting time • Clot retraction test	• Prothrombin consumption time • Factor assay

Tests for Platelet Component

Platelet Count

It is obtained on anticoagulated blood either manually or by electronic particle counters.

- **Normal range of platelet count:** 1,50,000–4,50,000 platelets/cu mm.
- Causes of thrombocytopenia (refer Box 13.21).

Platelet Aggregation

These tests measure the ability of platelets to aggregate in response to agonists like thrombin and form the basis for qualitative tests of von Willebrand factor. They are used for classification of congenital qualitative disorders of platelets.

Clot Retraction Test

After the coagulation of blood, the clot under the action of thrombasthenin (a substance released from platelets) undergoes contraction and starts retracting within one hour. The clot shows 50% retraction in 2–4 hours. This process is completed in 18–24 hours with separation of serum. Subsequently, the fibrin clot dissolves due to fibrinolysis and the RBCs sink to the bottom. Clot retraction is dependent on normal platelet number, platelet function, concentration of fibrinogen and the activity of the fibrinolytic pathway.

- **Normal value:** Normal clot retraction shows more than 50% of serum separated at the end of 24 hours. A normal clot is firm, rubbery, elastic and not easily broken.
- **Interpretation:** Absent or reduced clot retraction is seen in:
  - Fibrinogen deficiency (congenital or acquired).
  - Thrombocytopenia.
  - Thrombasthenia.

Tests for Platelet and Vascular Component

Capillary Fragility Test (Hess Test/Tourniquet Test)

It measures the ability of capillaries to withstand the increased stress.

Procedure: Sphygmomanometer cuff is tied to the upper arm above the elbow and the cuff is inflated to 80 mm for 5 minutes. Release the pressure after 5 minutes. The number of petechiae present in a circle of 5 cm diameter on the flexor aspect of forearm (below the bend of the elbow) is noted.

- **Normal:** 0–5 petechiae.
- **Interpretation:** Positive test is indicated by more than 10 petechiae and is found in:
  - Vessel wall abnormalities: Vascular purpura, scurvy.
  - Platelet disorders: Thrombocytopenia, defective platelet function.

Bleeding Time

Bleeding time (BT) is used as screening test for disorders of platelet-vessel wall interactions. It measures the time required for bleeding to stop after a standardized superficial cut of the skin capillary bed.

Methods: Duke's method (obsolete), Ivy's method and template method (method of choice). Template method for bleeding time.

Template is a disposable blade fitted on to a holder made of plastic and is used for the test. The blade projects through the bottom so that the incision made through the slit is 9 mm long and 1 mm deep.

Principle: A small skin cut of a standard size and depth is made and the oozing blood is wiped with a filter paper. Bleeding stops when the capillaries contract and platelet plug seals the vessel.

Normal range: 2–9 minutes.

Uses: Tests for bleeding time is prone to problems of reproducibility, sensitivity and specificity. Though, it is one of the screening tests, it is not recommended as routine preoperative screening test. This test evaluates the defects of primary hemostasis. Thus, bleeding time measures the platelet-vessel wall interactions (integrity of capillary and platelet function).

Note: The bleeding time usually is not prolonged in patients with coagulation factor deficiencies.

Interpretation: Causes of prolonged bleeding time is listed in Box 13.24.

Box 13.24: Causes of prolonged bleeding time

Platelet disorders • **Quantitative:** Thrombocytopenia • **Qualitative:** von Willebrand disease, Bernard-Soulier syndrome, Glanzmann's thrombasthenia
Primary vascular disorders: Ehlers–Danlos syndrome
Platelet-vessel wall interactions: von Willebrand disease
Others: Afibrinogenemia, severe hypofibrinogenemia, uremia, aspirin

Tests for Coagulation Component

Coagulation or Clotting Time (Lee–White Method)

- It measures the time taken for the fresh blood to clot.
- **Normal:** 4–11 minutes.
- Disadvantages:
  - **Not a sensitive test:** It is one of the oldest tests and is not sensitive as it fails to detect mild/moderate coagulant defects. Hence, it is obsolete now and not recommended as a screening test. PTT is a more sensitive test for assessment of the coagulation cascade. Clotting time is prolonged only with severe deficiency of factor VIII, IX or fibrinogen (afibrinogenemia) and in heparin therapy.
  - **Misleading:** Normal value may be obtained in mild-to-moderately severe hemophilia A and B and it does not exclude major factor deficiency.

Quick's One Stage Prothrombin Time

- **Principle:** Prothrombin time (PT) is the time taken by citrated plasma to clot after the addition of tissue thromboplastin and calcium. It tests ***extrinsic and common pathway*** of coagulation system.
- **Normal range:** 11–16 seconds.
- **Reporting of prothrombin time:** Prothrombin time may be reported in different ways:
  - Patient PT and control PT in seconds.
  - Ratio of patient PT to control PT.
- Uses of prothrombin time:
  - **Screening test to evaluate coagulation disorders:** It measures coagulation factor I, II, V, VII and X. Deficiency of any one of these factors leads to prolongation of PT. It should be used along with PTT.
  - **To monitor oral anticoagulant therapy**.
  - **To evaluate liver function:** Liver disease can result in deficiency of the coagulation factors. Hence, PT should be performed before a *liver biopsy and prolonged* PT is a contraindication for liver biopsy.
- **Interpretation:** Causes of prolonged PT is listed in Box 13.25.

Box 13.25: Causes of prolonged prothrombin time (PT)

Liver disease
Administration of oral anticoagulants like coumarin
Vitamin K deficiency • Obstructive jaundice • Hemorrhagic disease of the newborn
Deficiency of factors I, II, V, VII and X
Disseminated intravascular coagulation (DIC)

Box 13.26: Common causes of a prolonged APTT

Inherited coagulation disorders • Deficiency of factor II, V, VIII, IX, X, XI, XII (e.g. hemophilia A, hemophilia B) • von Willebrand disease
Disseminated intravascular coagulation
Liver disease
Heparin therapy
Vitamin K deficiency
Oral anticoagulant therapy

Activated Partial Thromboplastin Time (Partial Thromboplastin Time)

- **Principle:** Activated partial thromboplastin time (APTT) is the time taken for citrated plasma to clot in the presence of a surface activator (kaolin), phospholipid and calcium. Partial thromboplastin time (PTT) is a measure of the *intrinsic* and *common coagulation pathways*.
- **Normal range:** 30–40 seconds.
- **Reporting:** The patient's value is always to be reported with the control values in seconds. A prolongation of the patient value more than 8 seconds of the control value is considered as abnormal.
- **Uses:**
  - **Best single screening test for coagulation disorders.** This test is abnormal with deficiencies of II, V, VIII, IX, X, XI and XII.
  - For screening hemophilia A and B.
  - For detecting coagulation inhibitors.
  - For monitoring anticoagulant therapy like heparin.
- **Interpretation:** Common causes of a prolonged APTT are listed in Box 13.26.
  - Inherited coagulation disorders—deficiency of factor II, V, VIII, IX, X, XI, XII (e.g. hemophilia A, hemophilia B).
  - von Willebrand disease.
  - Disseminated intravascular coagulation.
  - Heparin therapy.
  - Vitamin K deficiency.
  - Liver disease.
  - Oral anticoagulant therapy.

Summary of screening tests for bleeding disorders are presented in Table 13.10.

TABLE 13.10: Summary of screening tests for bleeding disorders

Investigation	Normal range	Main causes of abnormal test
Platelet count	150–450 × 10^9/L	Thrombocytopenia
Bleeding time (template method)	2–9 minutes	Thrombocytopenia, abnormal platelet function, deficiency of von Willebrand factor, vascular abnormalities
Coagulation/clotting time (Lee-White method)—not a sensitive test	4–11 minutes	Severe deficiency of factor VIII, IX or fibrinogen (afibrinogenemia) and in heparin therapy
Prothrombin time (PT)	11–16 seconds	Deficiency of factor II, V, VII or X
Activated plasma thromboplastin time (APTT)	30–40 seconds	Deficiency of factor II, V, VIII, IX, X, XI, XII, heparin, antibodies against clotting factors, lupus anticoagulant

PLASMA CELL NEOPLASMS

Definition: Plasma cell neoplasms are group of **B cell neoplasms** associated with the **proliferation of single clone** (monoclonal) **of immunoglobulin-secreting plasma cells** (also known as dyscrasias).

Characteristics of Plasma Cell Neoplasms

Monoclonal neoplastic plasma cells **secrete complete single type of immunoglobulin** (Ig) **or Ig fragment.** Hence, are known as **monoclonal gammopathies.**

- **Serum:** Single Ig proteins detected as **monoclonal spike** [M protein (M for myeloma)] **on electrophoresis.**
- **Urine: Excess of free light chains** is excreted in the urine as **Bence-Jones (BJ) proteins.**

Classification of Plasma Cell Neoplasms (Box 13.27)

Box 13.27: Classification of plasma cell neoplasms (WHO 2008)

- Plasma cell myeloma
- Plasmacytoma
- Immunoglobulin deposition diseases
- Monoclonal gammopathy of undetermined significance (MGUS)
- Osteosclerotic myeloma (POEMS syndrome)

MULTIPLE MYELOMA (PLASMA CELL MYELOMA)

Definition: Multiple myeloma is a **malignant, multifocal plasma cell neoplasm of the bone marrow** associated with **M-protein in the serum and/or urine.**

- **Most common monoclonal gammopathy.**
- Presents as **multiple tumor masses** throughout the **skeletal system.**

Laboratory Findings

Peripheral Blood

- **Hemoglobin: Decreased** and ranges from 6 to 10 g/dL.

Peripheral smear

- *RBCs:* Normocytic normochromic anemia, red blood cells show **rouleaux formation** due to increased immunoglobulins.
- *WBCs:* **normal.**
- *Platelets:* normal.

- **ESR: High** and is due to high gamma globulin (immunoglobulin) and rouleaux formation.
- **Bleeding time: Increased.**

Bone marrow

- *Cellularity:* **Hypercellular** due to **myeloma cells** (neoplastic plasma cells).
- **Myeloma cells: More than 30%** are **diagnostic.**
  - Myeloma cells are neoplastic plasma cells, which are **large oval cells** having **abundant pale blue cytoplasm.**
  - The **nucleus** is round to oval, **eccentric** and shows **perinuclear clearing/hof.**
  - The nuclear **chromatin** appears like a **clock-face/spoke wheel.**
  - These cells are usually uninucleated or may show binucleation.
  - Other cells can also be seen in myeloma.
- *Erythropoiesis:* Diminished and is normoblastic.
- *Myelopoiesis:* Normal.
- *Megakaryopoiesis:* Normal.

Serum Findings

- **Serum β_2 microglobulin: Prognostic marker** and **high values signify poor prognosis.**
- **Hypercalcemia.**
- **Renal function tests: Blood urea, serum creatinine and uric acid levels** are **raised** with renal involvement.
- **Serum albumin:** Decreases in advance stages of the disease.

Electrophoretic Studies on Serum and Urine

- **Monoclonal spikes** in 80 to 90% of cases.
- Raised **monoclonal immunoglobulins** in the blood. Immunoglobulin may be **IgG** (most common)/IgD/IgA/IgE type.
- **Light chains** or **Bence Jones (BJ) proteins** in the urine may be seen in 60 to 80% of cases. BJ protein may be of κ or λ type of light chain.

Morphology of Organs Involved

- **Bone: Destructive—punched-out** lytic lesions.
- **Renal lesions:**
  - **Myeloma kidney:** Light-chain cast of BJ protein **damages renal tubules.**
  - **Amyloidosis** of the AL type and leads to **nephrotic syndrome.**

Clinical Manifestations

Onset: Insidious.

Age and sex: Affects old age between 50 and 60 years with slight male preponderance.

The **clinical features** of multiple myeloma are:

- ***Due to tumor cells causing bone lesions:***
  - **Resorption of bone:** This results in pathologic fractures, chronic bone pain and tenderness.
  - **Compression:** Lesion in the vertebra may compress the spinal cord nerve root.
  - **Hypercalcemia.**
  - **Pallor:** Due to anemia and result in weakness and fatigue.
- ***Production of M-proteins (increased immunoglobulins):***
  - **Bleeding tendency.**
  - **Coagulation abnormalities.**
  - **Amyloidosis** of the AL type.
- ***Humoral immune deficiency:*** Humoral immune deficiency predisposes to recurrent bacterial infections.
- ***Renal disease:*** Renal insufficiency, infections or nephrotic syndrome.

BLOOD TRANSFUSION

Blood transfusion is the process of transferring blood/blood products from donor into the circulating system of recipient. It is important to properly collect the blood from donor, prepare its components (if required) and store blood/components in a proper way and transfuse in such a way to avoid any risks or hazards.

Donor Selection

Donor selection is based on medical history and few routine physical examinations (weight, blood pressure, temperature, hemoglobin) are done to know whether donor is suitable for donating blood.

- Donor should be healthy. There are three types of donors, namely, voluntary (should be encouraged), replacement and professional.
- It is important to know whether the patient has history of diseases like hepatitis, AIDS, syphilis and if so, blood should not be obtained from them. In the blood bank, blood is routinely screen for few common infections.

Anticoagulants used: The different anticoagulants—preservative solutions available (for collecting and storing blood) are:

- Citrate phosphate dextrose (CPD).
- Citrate phosphate dextrose adenine (CPDA-1).
- Acid citrate dextrose (ACD) is not used nowadays.

Storage of blood: Blood is stored in a refrigerator at 2° to 6°C.

Predonation Check-up

Donor blood: The following tests are routinely carried out on donor's blood:

- ABO and Rh grouping.
- Tests for:
  - HBsAg, anti-HCV, anti HIV-1 and HIV-2 and serum alanine aminotransferase (ALT)
  - Malaria and syphilis.

Recipient blood: The recipient's ABO and Rh grouping is also carried out.

Blood Grouping

More **than 400 red blood cell antigens have been identified, most of which are inherite**d in a Mendelian dominant fashion and only few are clinically important. These antigens form more than 20 genetically determined blood group systems.

The two most important blood group systems are ABO and Rh systems. Different methods are available for ABO grouping and Rh typing. These include slide or tile technique, tube technique, microplate method, microtyping system and automated or semi-automated method.

ABO Grouping Technique

ABO grouping is carried out by making a 2% saline suspension of red cells and adding anti-A, anti-B and anti-AB sera. The slide/tile technique is easier to do and is described below.

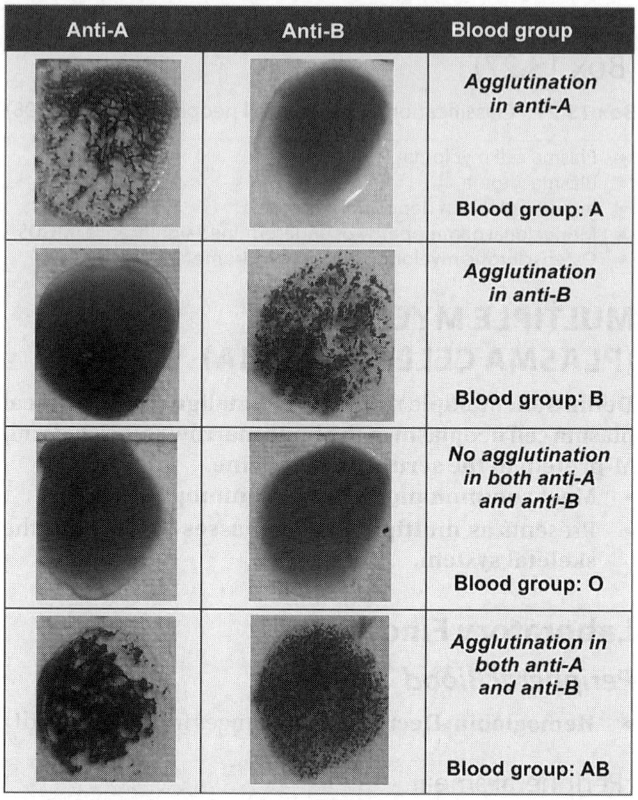

Anti-A	Anti-B	Blood group
		Agglutination in anti-A Blood group: A
		Agglutination in anti-B Blood group: B
		No agglutination in both anti-A and anti-B Blood group: O
		Agglutination in both anti-A and anti-B Blood group: AB

Fig. 13.16: Interpretation of blood group by slide method

- Take a slide/white tile and mark it anti-A, anti-B and anti-AB.
- Put one drop each of anti- A, anti-B and anti-AB sera on the marked slide.
- Add one drop of washed 2% red cell suspension to each anti-sera.
- Mix each one separately with clean applicator stick and spread the mixture over an area of 2 cm.
- Rock the slide gently and look for "agglutination" within 5 minutes.

Interpretation (Fig. 13.16): Blood group A, B, AB or O is interpreted depending on the agglutination in the anti-sera.

Rh (D) Typing Techniques

Slide or tile technique

- Place one drop of anti-Rh (D) reagent (should be monoclonal IgM type) on a slide/white tile.
- Add 1 drop of 2% red cell suspension.
- Mix them using a clean applicator stick.
- Observe for agglutination after 2 minutes.

Interpretation: Presence of agglutination indicates that the blood sample is Rh +ve.

Table 13.11: Types of cross-match

Type of cross-match	Donor's	Recipient's (patient's)
Major cross-match	Red cells	Serum
Minor cross-match	Serum	Red cells

Compatibility Testing (Pretransfusion Testing)

Before transfusion of any blood or its components, it is essential to know whether they are compatible with the recipient's blood. This is achieved by performing a set of procedures known as compatibility testing. Sometimes, the term compatibility test and cross matching are used interchangeably, but cross-match is only a part of compatibility test.

Compatibility tests include:

- Review of patient's past blood bank history and records (if done earlier).
- ABO and Rh typing of the recipient and donor.
- Antibody screening test of recipient's and donor's serum.
- Cross-matching (Table 13.11): Cross-matching is very important before any blood transfusion.

Blood Components (Flowchart 13.2)

It is possible to separate different components of blood from a single unit of whole blood. These components can be used individually to help more than one patient with many purposes. Thus, red cells can be transfused to an anemic patient and plasma for a burns patient. This also ensures that only the required components are transfused.

Transfusion Reactions

Blood transfusion is useful and life-saving when performed with caution and with clear indication. Sometimes (about 2–4% of cases), unfavorable complications occur in spite of precaution and preventive measures, which are known as transfusion reactions. They may be broadly divided into infectious and non-infectious complications (Box 13.27).

Noninfectious Complications

Transfusion reactions may result from immune and nonimmune mechanisms.

Immune mediated (immediate and delayed) reactions

Acute hemolytic transfusion reaction

- ***ABO incompatibility*** between recipient and donor, resulting in destruction of donor cells. This is brought out by the naturally occurring (preformed) antibodies, namely, anti-A and anti-B (depending on the blood group).
  - **Massive intravascular hemolysis:** This is one of the serious complications which develop within 1 to 4 hours and with only a few milliliters of incompatible red cells. The preformed IgM antibodies (anti-A and anti-B) in the recipient coat transfused donor red cells and activate complement system to form membrane attack complex (C5-9). This results in intravascular destruction (hemolysis) of transfused donor red blood cells.

Flowchart 13.2: Blood components

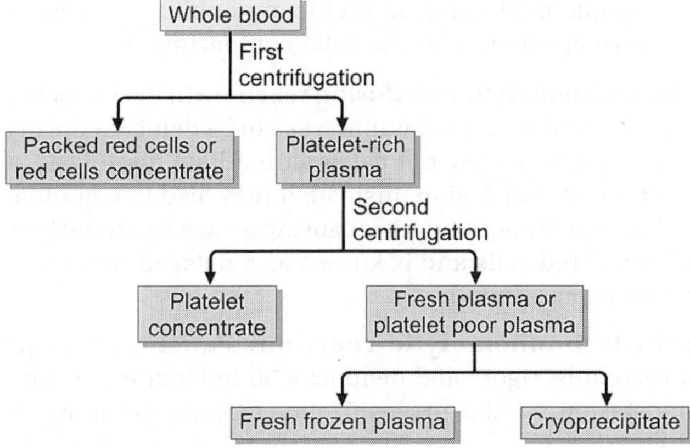

Box 13.27: Complications of blood transfusion

- **Noninfectious complications**
  - Immediate reactions
    - Immunological
      - ◊ Hemolytic transfusion reactions
      - ◊ Febrile nonhemolytic reaction
      - ◊ Allergic reaction
      - ◊ Anaphylactic
      - ◊ Transfusion-related acute lung injury (TRALI)
    - Nonimmunological
      - ◊ Circulatory overload
      - ◊ Air embolism
  - Delayed reactions
    - Immunological
      - ◊ Alloimmunization
      - ◊ Hemolytic transfusion reactions (mostly asymptomatic)
      - ◊ Transfusion associated graft versus host disease
    - Nonimmunological
      - ◊ Iron overload-transfusion hemosiderosis
      - ◊ Thrombophlebitis
- **Infectious complications**

  Few of the diseases transmitted by transfusion are:
  - Hepatitis (HBV, HCV and HDV)
  - HIV (AIDS)
  - Malaria
  - Cytomegalovirus
  - Syphilis

- ***Rh incompatibility:*** Because anti-Rh antibodies are not complement-fixing, in Rh incompatibility, hemolysis develops in the extravascular compartment.

Delayed hemolytic transfusion reaction: In the recipient, if antibody titer is too low and weak to be detected during cross-match, it may not cause immediate hemolysis at the time of transfusion. Instead, it may lead to a gradual increase in the antibody titer causing delayed, gradual lysis of donor red cells and is known as a delayed hemolytic transfusion reaction.

Febrile nonhemolytic reaction: Patient develops fever, chills, rigors and headache 30 to 60 minutes after transfusion. It is due to sensitization to leukocyte antigens.

Allergic reaction: Allergic reaction manifests as urticaria (hives), fever, bronchospasm and rarely anaphylactic shock. It is due to exposure of allergens in donor's plasma to IgE antibodies in recipient's plasma, which activates mast cells and releases histamine/leukotrienes.

Transfusion associated graft versus host disease (TA-GVHD): Transfusion associated GVHD is a rare but potentially fatal complication of blood transfusion. This may develop 10 to 12 days after transfusion.

Transfusion-related acute lung injury (TRALI): It is an uncommon complication of blood transfusion. It results from transfusion of donor plasma containing high levels of anti-HLA antibodies which bind to HLA of leukocytes of the recipient. These leukocytes aggregate in the pulmonary microcirculation and release mediators causing increased vascular permeability. This leads to acute pulmonary edema and signs and symptoms of acute respiratory failure.

Nonimmunological (Immediate and delayed) reactions

Circulatory overload: Following whole blood transfusion, the blood volume and venous pressure also increases. This may be significant in the elderly, pregnant women and those with reduced cardiac function resulting in acute pulmonary edema. This can be avoided using blood components like packed red blood cells.

Air embolism: This was common earlier when transfusion was given from the glass bottle. Presently, due to the use of plastic bags with closed tubing system, this complication does not develop.

Iron overload (transfusion siderosis): This is seen in patients who receive multiple transfusions over a period of few years (e.g. thalassemia). The excess iron gets deposited in reticuloendothelial cells of spleen, bone marrow, liver, heart and endocrine glands.

Box 13.28: Causes of splenomegaly

Infection
• **Acute:** Infectious mononucleosis, viral hepatitis, septicemia, typhoid, cytomegalovirus, toxoplasmosis • **Subacute/chronic:** Miliary tuberculosis, subacute bacterial endocarditis, brucellosis, syphilis, HIV • **Tropical/parasitic:** Malaria, leishmaniasis/kala-azar, schistosomiasis
Hematological disorders
• **Myeloproliferative disorders:** Myelofibrosis, chronic myeloid leukemia (CML), polycythemia vera • **Lymphoma:** Non-Hodgkin lymphoma (NHL), Hodgkin lymphoma • **Leukemia:** Acute leukemia, chronic lymphocytic leukemia (CLL), hairy cell leukemia, prolymphocytic leukemia • **RBC disorders:** Hereditary spherocytosis, thalassemia, megaloblastic anemia
Congestive
• **Portal hypertension:** Cirrhosis, splenic/portal/hepatic vein thrombosis or obstruction • **Cardiac:** Congestive cardiac failure
Inflammatory/granulomatous diseases
• **Granulomatous:** Sarcoidosis • **Collagen diseases:** Systemic lupus erythematosus, rheumatoid arthritis (Felty's)
Other malignancies
• Metastasis rare(lung/breast carcinoma, melanoma
Lysosomal storage diseases
• Gaucher's disease, Niemann–Pick disease
Miscellaneous
• Amyloidosis, cysts

Thrombophlebitis: Inflammation of vein may develop in patients with indwelling catheters.

Infectious Complications

Transfusion of infected blood may transmit few diseases like AIDS, hepatitis (HBV, HCV and HDV), HTLV-I and II, malaria and cytomegalovirus infection. This is prevented by screening the donors for these common and ominous infections.

SPLEEN

The spleen is a hematopoietic organ capable of supporting elements of the erythroid, myeloid, megakaryocytic, lymphoid, and monocyte-macrophage (i.e. reticuloendothelial). Normal weight of the adult spleen is about 50–250 g.

Splenomegaly

Enlargement of spleen can occur in various conditions and is termed splenomegaly. Various causes of splenomegaly are presented in Box 13.28.

SELF-ASSESSMENT EXERCISES

I. Essay

1. Define and classify anaemia. Write laboratory diagnosis of iron deficiency anemia.
2. Classify anemia and describe the peripheral smear findings in megaloblastic anemia.
3. Discuss the etiology and laboratory findings in iron deficiency anemia.
4. Define leukemia. Describe etiology, clinical features and blood picture of chronic myeloid leukemia.

II. Short Notes

1. Define anemia.
2. Classify anemia.
3. Etiological classification of anemia.
4. Etiopathogenesis of iron deficiency anemia.
5. Iron deficiency anemia.
6. Peripheral smear findings in iron deficiency anemia.
7. Megaloblastic anemia.
8. Laboratory findings in megaloblastic anemia.
9. Etiopathogenesis of sickle cell anemia.
10. Laboratory diagnosis of sickle cell anemia.
11. Laboratory investigations in a case of anemia.
12. Leukocytosis.
13. Neutrophilia.
14. Eosinophilia.
15. Define leukemia.
16. Classification of leukemia.
17. Classify acute leukemia.
18. Leukemoid reaction.
19. Acute myeloid leukemia.
20. Laboratory findings/peripheral smear in CML.
21. Chronic lymphocytic leukemia.
22. Immune thrombocytopenic purpura.
23. Hemophilia.
24. von Willebrand disease.
25. Major cross matching.
26. Anticoagulants used in the blood bank for preservation of blood.
27. Blood grouping.
28. Splenomegaly.

CHAPTER 14

Lymph Nodes

CHAPTER OUTLINE

- Structure of lymph node
- Lymphadenopathy
- Lymphadenitis
- Lymphoid neoplasms
- Non-Hodgkin lymphoma
- Hodgkin lymphoma
- Metastatic carcinoma

STRUCTURE OF LYMPH NODE (FIG 14.1)

Lymph nodes are small, bean-shaped glands of the lymphatic system. They are situated along lymphatic vessels throughout the body. Normal lymph nodes are round to bean-shaped, and measure less than 1 cm. Each lymph nodes is surrounded by a thin fibrous capsule. Below the fibrous capsule are the subcapsular sinus, which receives lymph from **afferent lymphatic vessels** that penetrate the node at several points along the. Lymph nodes are composed of an **outer cortex** and an **inner medulla**. The cortex is subdivided into a follicular area (consisting of **follicle germinal centers**) and a paracortical area.

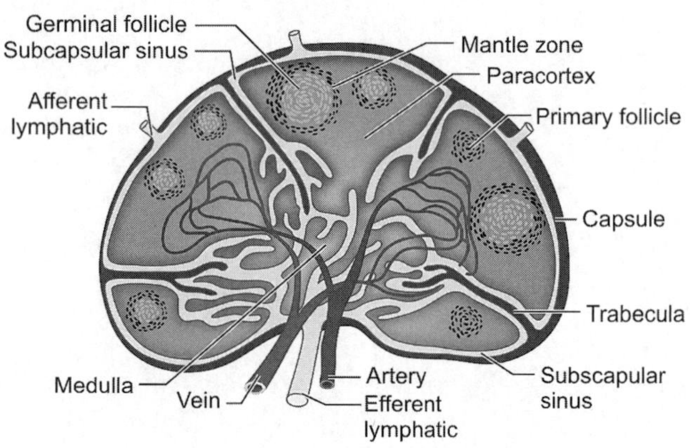

Fig. 14.1: Structure of lymph node

LYMPHADENOPATHY

Lymphadenopathy is clinical enlargement of lymph nodes/ glands. Lymphadenopathy usually develops in reaction to infection or inflammation but may also develop in hematological disease. Lymphadenopathy may develop in response to local infection or inflammation ('reactive nodes'/lymphadenitis) and it usually expands rapidly and are painful. Lymphadenopathy due to hematological disease are more frequently painless.

Causes of Lymphadenopathy (Box 14.1)

Localized vs Generalized

Lymphadenopathy may be localized or generalized.

- **Localized lymphadenopathy:** In these cases, a search should be made for a source of inflammation or cancer in the appropriate drainage area (e.g. the scalp, ear, mouth, face or teeth for neck nodes, the breast for axillary nodes). Staging of cancers depends on identifying lymph node draining the cancer.

Box 14.1: Causes of lymphadenopathy

Infective
- Bacterial: Streptococcal, tuberculosis
- Viral: Epstein–Barr virus (EBV), human immunodeficiency virus (HIV)
- Protozoal: Toxoplasmosis
- Fungal: Histoplasmosis, coccidioidomycosis

Neoplastic
- Primary: Lymphomas (Hodgkin and Non-Hodgkin), leukemias
- Secondary: Lung, breast, thyroid, stomach

Autoimmune connective tissue disorders
- Rheumatoid arthritis
- Systemic lupus erythematosus (SLE)

Drugs
- Phenytoin

Sarcoidosis

Amyloidosis

- **Generalized lymphadenopathy:** It may be secondary to infection, connective tissue disease or extensive skin disease, but is more often signify underlying hematological malignancy. Weight loss and night sweats are usually associated with hematological malignancies, particularly lymphoma.

Investigations

- Complete blood count (to detect neutrophilia in infection or evidence of hematological disease)
- Erythrocyte sedimentation rate (ESR)
- Chest X-ray (to detect mediastinal lymphadenopathy).
- Fine needle aspiration cytology (FNAC)
- Excision biopsy of a representative node is indicated especially if the findings suggest malignancy.

LYMPHADENITIS

Lymphadenitis is the inflammation of a lymph node which may be acute or chronic. It may be specific due to a known cause (e.g. granulomatous/tuberculous lymphadenitis due to Mycobacteria) or non-specific where there is no known cause. Histological features of tuberculous lymphadenitis consists of lymph node with granulomas as in other sites (refer Fig. 4.2)

Acute Nonspecific Lymphadenitis

Acute inflammation of lymph node is termed as acute lymphadenitis. Acute lymphadenitis in the region of neck (cervical lymph node) is most commonly due to drainage of microbes or microbial products from infections of the teeth or tonsils. Axillary or inguinal lymphadenitis is most commonly caused by infections in the extremities. Acute mesenteric lymphadenitis occurs draining acute appendicitis. Systemic viral infections (especially in children) and bacteremia may produce acute generalized lymphadenopathy.

Morphology

The involved nodes are swollen and gray-red in color. Microscopically, it shows prominent large reactive germinal centers containing numerous mitotic figures. When caused due to pyogenic organisms, neutrophils are prominent and the centers of the follicles may undergo necrosis.

Clinical Features

Lymph nodes involved by acute lymphadenitis are enlarged and painful. Pus may be formed and track to the skin to produce draining sinuses.

Chronic Nonspecific Lymphadenitis

Chronic immunological stimuli produce several different patterns of lymph node reaction.

Morphology

- **Follicular hyperplasia:** It is characterized by the presence of **large germinal centers**. Causes of follicular hyperplasia include: rheumatoid arthritis, toxoplasmosis, and early stages of infection with HIV.
- **Paracortical hyperplasia:** It is **characterized by involvement of paracortical region of lymph node.** It is caused by acute viral infections such as infectious mononucleosis.
- **Sinus histiocytosis:** It refers to an increase in the number and size of the cells that line lymphatic sinusoids (subcapsular sinus). It is usually nonspecific, but may be particularly prominent in lymph nodes draining cancers such as carcinoma of the breast.

Clinical Features

Chronic lymphadenitis usually produces nontender, enlargement that occurs slowly over time. Chronic lymphadenitis is particularly common in inguinal and axillary nodes, which drain relatively large areas of the body.

LYMPHOID NEOPLASMS

Definition

- **Lymphomas** are **malignant lymphoid neoplasms** due to lymphoid tissue proliferations that arise as **discrete (separate or distinct) tissue masses**. Lymphomas are mainly subdivided into **Hodgkin lymphoma (HL)** and **non-Hodgkin lymphomas (NHLs)**.
- **Leukemias** are neoplasms that present with widespread **involvement of the bone marrow and** (usually, but not always) the **peripheral blood.**

Many "lymphoma" occasionally have leukemic presentations, and evolution to "leukemia" is not unusual during the progression of incurable "lymphomas." Conversely, few "leukemias" may sometimes arise as soft tissue masses without detectable bone marrow disease. Therefore, the terms leukemia and lymphoma reflect the usual tissue distribution of the disease at presentation.

Classification of Lymphoid Neoplasms

(Box 14.2)

Box 14.2: WHO (abridged) classification of the lymphoid neoplasms (2016)

- **Precursor lymphoid neoplasms**
  - B lymphoblastic leukemia/lymphoma
  - T lymphoblastic leukemia/lymphoma
- **Mature B cell neoplasms**
  - Chronic lymphocytic leukemia/small lymphocytic lymphoma
  - B-cell prolymphocytic leukemia
  - Splenic B cell marginal zone lymphoma
  - Hairy cell leukemia
  - Lymphoplasmacytic lymphoma
  - Heavy chain disease
  - Plasma cell neoplasm
  - Follicular lymphoma
  - Mantle cell lymphoma
  - Diffuse large B cell lymphoma
  - Burkitt lymphoma
- **Mature T and NK cell neoplasms**
  - T-cell prolymphocytic leukemia
  - T-cell large granular lymphocytic leukemia
  - Mycosis fungoides
  - Sézary syndrome
  - Peripheral T-cell lymphoma, NOS
  - Angioimmunoblastic T-cell lymphoma
  - Anaplastic large cell lymphoma
  - Adult T-cell leukemia/lymphoma
- **Hodgkin lymphoma**
  - Classical Hodgkin lymphoma
    - Nodular sclerosis classical Hodgkin lymphoma
    - Mixed cellularity classical Hodgkin lymphoma
    - Lymphocyte-rich classical Hodgkin lymphoma
    - Lymphocyte depleted classical Hodgkin lymphoma
  - Nodular lymphocyte predominance Hodgkin lymphoma

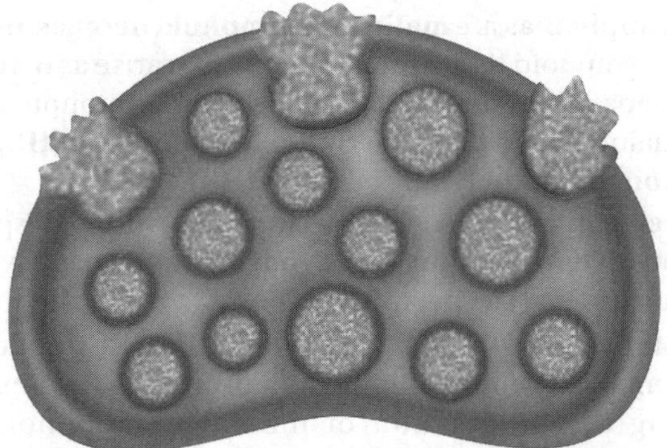

Fig. 14.2: Diagrammatic appearance of follicular lymphoma. Neoplastic follicles are seen in both the cortex and medulla and infiltration of the perinodal tissue

NON-HODGKIN LYMPHOMA

Follicular Lymphoma (FL)

Composed of follicle center (germinal center) **B cells** of lymphoid follicles (centrocytes and centroblasts).

Morphology

Gross

- Involves **lymph nodes**, spleen and bone marrow.
- **Architecture** of lymph node is **lost**; frequently infiltrate the perinodal tissue (Fig. 14.2).

Microscopy

- **Follicular** (nodular) growth pattern, **neoplastic follicles** are **poorly defined**.
- **Two types of B-cells.**
  - **Centrocytes** (small cleaved cells).
    - Cleaved nuclei.
    - Inconspicuous nucleoli.
  - **Centroblasts** (large non-cleaved cells).
    - Round or oval nuclei with open nuclear (vesicular) chromatin.
    - Multiple (1 to 3) nucleoli.
    - Usually 3 times the size of lymphocyte.

Clinical Features

- Peak in **sixth and seventh decades**.
- **Generalized lymphadenopathy**.

Diffuse Large B-Cell Lymphoma (DLBCL)

Heterogeneous group of **aggressive**, neoplasm of large B cell with **diffuse** growth pattern.

Constitutes about 20 to 30% of NHL and 60 to 70% of aggressive lymphoid neoplasms.

Microscopy

- **Loss of** lymph node **architecture** with **diffuse growth pattern.**
- **Neoplastic cells:**
  - **Large** round or oval cells, **4 to 5 times** of a **small lymphocyte.**
  - Moderate pale or basophilic cytoplasm.
  - **Nucleus** equals or larger than the **nucleus of a macrophage** with different appearances.

Clinical Features

- More common between **65 and 70 years** of age.
- Slight **male** preponderance.
- **Rapidly enlarging** mass at a single or multiple **nodal or extranodal sites.**

Burkitt Lymphoma

- **Highly aggressive B-cell** neoplasm, often presents as **extranodal** lymphoma or as an acute leukemia.

- Composed of **medium-sized, monomorphic lymphoid cells** with basophilic **vacuolated cytoplasm.**

Clinical Variants

- **Endemic (African) Burkitt lymphoma (BL):**
  - Occurs in Africa, affects **children and adolescents.**
  - **Associated with Epstein-Barr virus infection and malaria.**
  - Usually involves the **jaw** and present as a mandibular mass.
- **Sporadic (nonendemic) BL:**
  - Occurs in **children or young adults.**
  - **Abdominal mass** and involves **ileocecum** and **peritoneum.**
- **Immunodeficiency-associated (HIV) BL:**
  - Involves lymph nodes and bone marrow.

Microscopy

- Burkitt lymphomas, **irrespective of the categories**, are **histologically similar.**
- Lymph node shows **loss of architecture.**
- Involved tissues show **diffuse** infiltrate of **monotonous medium-sized lymphoid cells** (Fig. 14.3).
- **Appearance of neoplastic lymphoid cells:**
  - **Medium-sized cells.**
  - **Round or oval nuclei** having clumped **coarse chromatin** with **several (2 to 5) nucleoli.**
  - **Moderate** amount of deeply **basophilic cytoplasm, multiple, small, round lipoid** (clear) **vacuoles** which stain positive with oil red O.
  - Numerous mitotic figures.
- **Starry sky pattern:** Tumor cells undergo **apoptosis** and nuclear remnants of these apoptotic cells are phagocytosed and cleared by benign macrophages. These macrophages in the background of lymphoid cells creates **"starry sky"** appearance (Fig. 14.3).

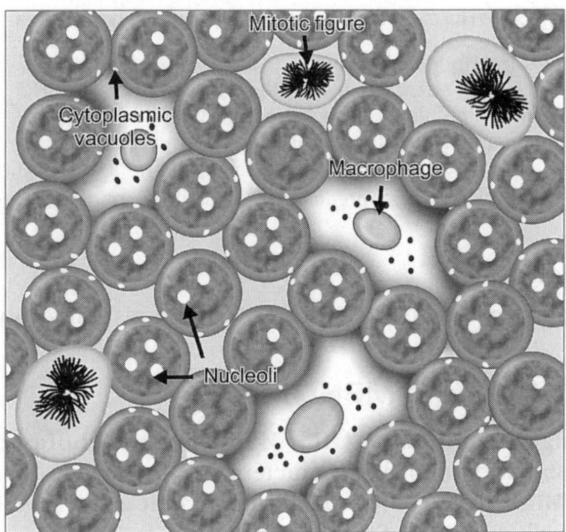

Fig. 14.3: Diagrammatic appearance of Burkitt lymphoma composed of medium-sized lymphoid cells admixed with benign macrophages giving a "starry-sky" appearance

Mature T-Cell and NK Cell Neoplasms

Peripheral T-Cell Lymphoma (PTCL), NOS

Mainly involves lymph node.

Microscopy

- **Lymph node** with **effacement of the normal architecture.**
- **Paracortical or diffuse infiltration** by neoplastic T-cells.
- **Neoplastic T-cells.**
  - **Small, intermediate to large cells** with sparse or abundant; clear, eosinophilic or basophilic.
  - **Vesicular or hyperchromatic nuclei, prominent nucleoli.**

Mycosis Fungoides

- **Cutaneous T-cell lymphoma.**
- Lymphoid cells with **irregular nuclear outlines.**
- Limited to **skin.**

Age: Most are adults or elderly.

Microscopy

- **Epidermis (epidermotropism) and upper dermis** is infiltrated by neoplastic T-cells.
- Groups of neoplastic cells in the epidermis—**Pautrier's microabscess.**
- Tumor cells have **convoluted (cerebriform) nuclear contours.**

Sézary Syndrome

Rare disease and is defined by the triad namely:

1. **Widespread exfoliative erythroderma.**
2. **Generalized lymphadenopathy.**
3. **Presence of characteristic Sézary cells** in the skin, lymph nodes and peripheral blood.

Box 14.3: WHO classification (2008) of Hodgkin lymphoma

- Classical Hodgkin lymphoma (CHL)
  - Nodular sclerosis classical Hodgkin lymphoma (NSCHL)
  - Mixed cellularity classical Hodgkin lymphoma (MCCHL)
  - Lymphocyte-rich classical Hodgkin lymphoma (LRCHL)
  - Lymphocyte depleted classical Hodgkin lymphoma (LDCHL)
- Nodular lymphocyte predominant Hodgkin lymphoma (NLPHL)

Prognosis

Aggressive disease and most die of opportunistic infections.

HODGKIN LYMPHOMA

Hodgkin lymphoma (HL): Malignant lymphoid neoplasms with following characteristics:

- **Minority** (1–3%) **of specific neoplastic cells** (Hodgkin cells and **Reed-Sternberg cells**).
- **Majority background of** reactive **non-neoplastic cells.**
- Usually involves **lymph nodes.**
- Majority occurs in **young** adults.

Classification (Box 14.3)

Hodgkin lymphoma (HL) is broadly divided into **two types,** which differ in clinical features, behavior, morphology and immunophenotype.

Cell of Origin and Immunophenotype

- **Classical Hodgkin lymphoma.**
  - Cell of origin: **Germinal center or post-germinal center B-cell.**
  - Immunophenotype: **CD15** and **CD30 positive.**
- **Nodular lymphocyte predominant Hodgkin lymphoma.**
  - Cell of origin: **Germinal center B cell at the centroblastic stage** of differentiation.
  - Immunophenotype: **CD15** and **CD30 negative.**

Morphology of Neoplastic Cells

Reed-Sternberg (RS) cells are neoplastic cells **pathognomonic** of Hodgkin lymphoma. Appearance and description of diagnostic Reed-Sternberg cells and its variants are shown in Figure 14.4. Various types of cells found in Hodgkin lymphoma are listed in Table 14.1.

Classical Hodgkin Lymphoma

Classical Hodgkin lymphoma (CHL) account for **95%** of Hodgkin lymphomas and has 4 subtypes.

Description	Appearance
Large cells (20 to 60 µm in diameter) Abundant eosinophilic cytoplasm Nucleus: Typically two large nuclei -"mirror image" Prominent eosinophilic nucleolus surrounded by a halo	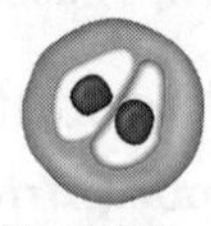 Classic RS cell
Single, large, round nucleus with a large eosinophilic inclusion-like nucleolus May be seen in any subtypes of CHL	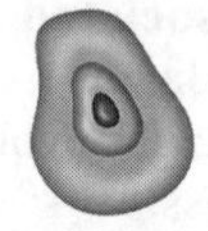 Mononuclear cell variant (Hodgkin cell)
Abundant, lightly acidophilic or water-clear cytoplasm Large folded or multilobed nucleus One or more prominent eosinophilic nucleoli Seen in nodular sclerosis of CHL	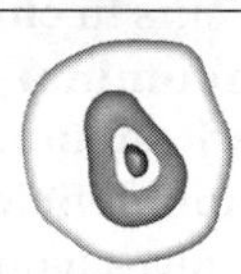 Lacunar cell variant
Dark eosinophilic cytoplasm with pyknotic nuclei Strongly indicate HL but not diagnostic	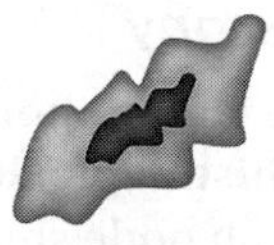 Mummified cell variant
Highly pleomorphic cells Large bizarre hyperchromatic nuclei Commonly found in lymphocyte-depleted CHL	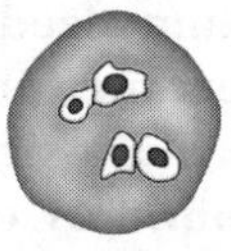 Anaplastic/pleomorphic variant
Abundant pale cytoplasm with popcorn nucleus Specific to the nodular lymphocyte predominance type of HL	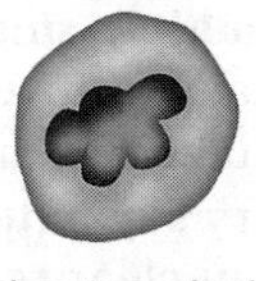 Lymphocyte predominant cell (LP cell)/popcorn cell

Fig. 14.4: Diagrammatic appearances and characteristic features of Reed-Sternberg cells and its variants

Table 14.1: Types of cells found in Hodgkin lymphoma

Non-neoplastic cells	Neoplastic cells
• Reactive lymphocytes	• Reed-Sternberg cells (classical)
• Macrophages/histiocytes – Granulocytes – Eosinophils – Neutrophils	• Variants – Mononuclear – Lacunar – Mummified – Anaplastic/pleomorphic – Lymphocyte predominant (LP) cell/popcorn
• Plasma cells	

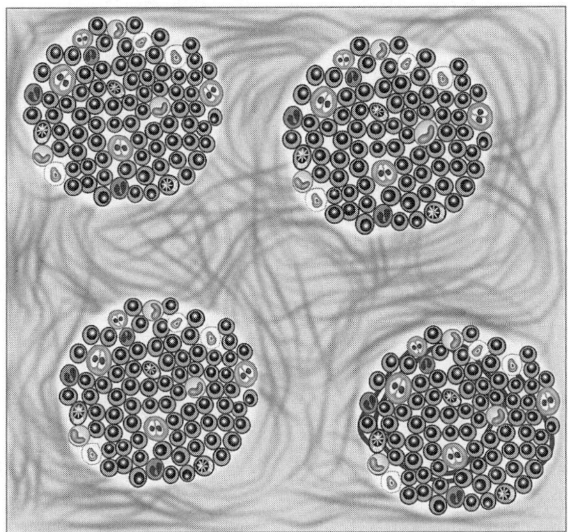

Fig. 14.5: Nodular sclerosis classical Hodgkin lymphoma with nodules separated by bands of collagen. Also seen are lacunar cells and RS cells in each nodule within the background of lymphocytes, eosinophils, plasma cells and macrophages

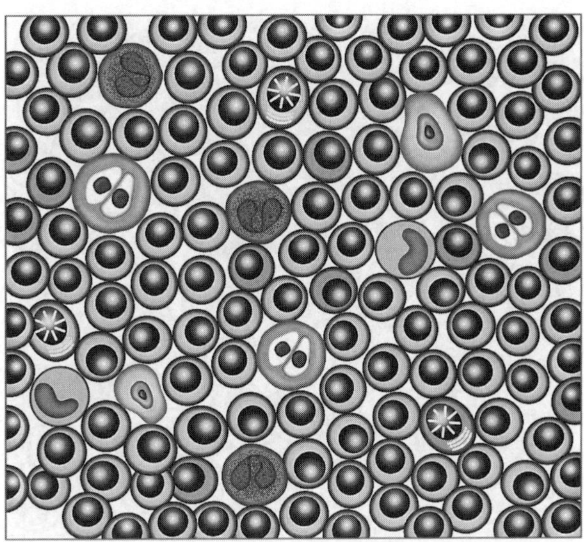

Fig. 14.6: Mixed cellularity classical Hodgkin lymphoma with classical RS cells, Hodgkin cells in the background of mixed cellular population consisting of lymphocytes, eosinophils, plasma cells and macrophages

Nodular Sclerosis Classical Hodgkin Lymphoma (NSCHL)

Subtype of CHL characterized by **collagen bands** that surround **nodules** and have **lacunar cell variant of Reed-Sternberg cells.**

- Most common: **40–70%** of cases.
- Most between **20 and 30 years of age** with **equal** frequency in **males and females.**
- **Rarely associated with EBV.**
- Involves **mediastinal lymph nodes.**

Microscopy of NSCHL (Fig. 14.5)

- Loss of lymphnode architecture.
- **Sclerosis and nodules: Broad collagen** bands (sclerosis) divide the lymphoid tissue into **nodules of varying sizes and shapes.**
- **Presence of lacunar cell.**
- **Background: Small T lymphocytes, eosinophils, plasma cells, and macrophages.**

Mixed Cellularity Classical Hodgkin Lymphoma (MCCHL)

- **Second common subtype:** 20 to 25% of cases.
- **More common in males.**
- **Strongly associated with EBV.**
- **Older age**, with **systemic symptoms** (such as night sweats and weight loss) and **advanced tumor stage.**
- Involves **peripheral lymph nodes.**

Microscopy of MCCHL (Fig. 14.6)

- Lymph node architecture obliterated.
- **Plenty of Reed-Sternberg cells** and Hodgkin cells.
- **Back ground:** Small lymphocytes, eosinophils (sometimes numerous), neutrophils, plasma cells and benign macrophages (histiocytes).

Lymphocyte-rich Classical Hodgkin Lymphoma (LRCHL)

- Subtype of classical Hodgkin lymphoma with **scattered Hodgkin and RS cells.**
- **Uncommon**—about 5% of classical HL.
- More in **elderly** patients, associated with **EBV in 40%** of cases.
- Involves **peripheral lymph nodes.**

Microscopy of LRCHL (Fig. 14.7)

- **Growth patterns:** May show two patterns.
  - **Nodular**—common.
  - **Diffuse**—rare.
- **Only few Reed-Sternberg cells and Hodgkin cells.**
- **Background:** abundant reactive small lymphocytes.

Lymphocyte-depleted Classical Hodgkin Lymphoma (LDCHL)

Subtype of classical Hodgkin lymphoma **rich in Hodgkin and RS cells** in a background depleted in non-neoplastic lymphocytes.

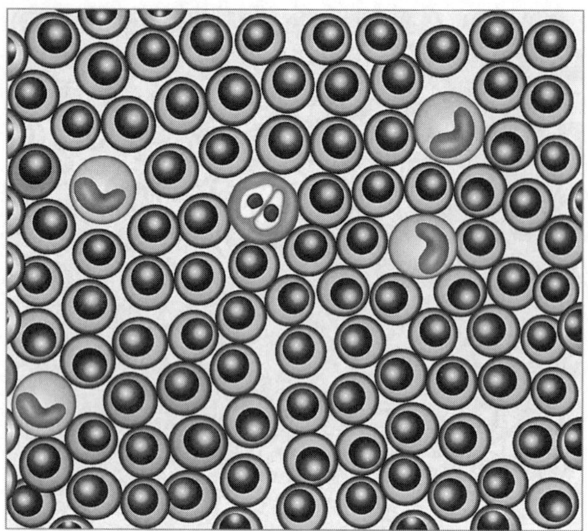

Fig. 14.7: Lymphocyte-rich classical Hodgkin lymphoma. One RS cell is seen in a background of many small lymphocytes and few histiocytes

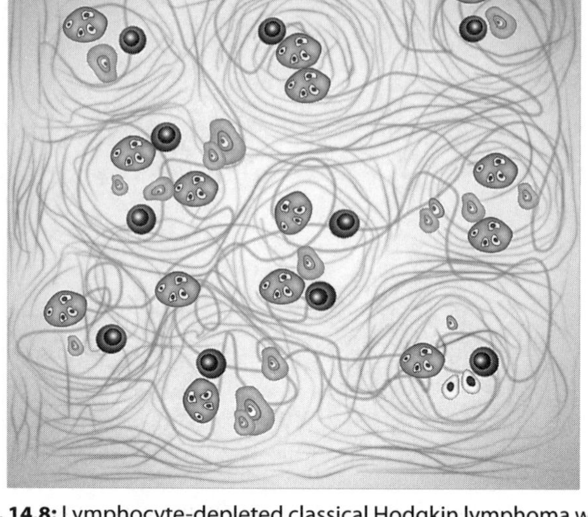

Fig. 14.8: Lymphocyte-depleted classical Hodgkin lymphoma with the pleomorphic variant of RS cells surrounded by fibrous tissue

- **Rarest**—less than 5% of cases.
- Predominantly in **older, HIV-positive patients**, often **EBV-associated** (over 90%).
- Predominantly **retroperitoneal lymph nodes, abdominal organs and bone marrow**.

Microscopy of LDCHL (Fig. 14.8)

- **Paucity of lymphocytes**.
- **Plenty of RS cells** or their **anaplastic/pleomorphic variants**.
- Histological types.
    - **Reticular: Numerous Hodgkin and RS cells** with depletion of lymphocytes.
    - **Diffuse sclerosis/fibrosis:** Hypocellular infiltrate containing bizarre RS cells with fine fibrosis.

Nodular Lymphocyte Predominant Hodgkin Lymphoma (NLPHL)

- **Uncommon—**5% of all Hodgkin lymphomas.
- **Not associated** with **EBV**.
- Majority males, usually **30–50 year** of age.
- Involves mainly **cervical or axillary lymph nodes**.

Microscopy of NLPHL (Fig. 14.10)

- Loss of lymph node architecture.
- Nodular and/or diffuse infiltrate of **abundant small lymphocytes** with histiocytes and **scattered LP cells**.

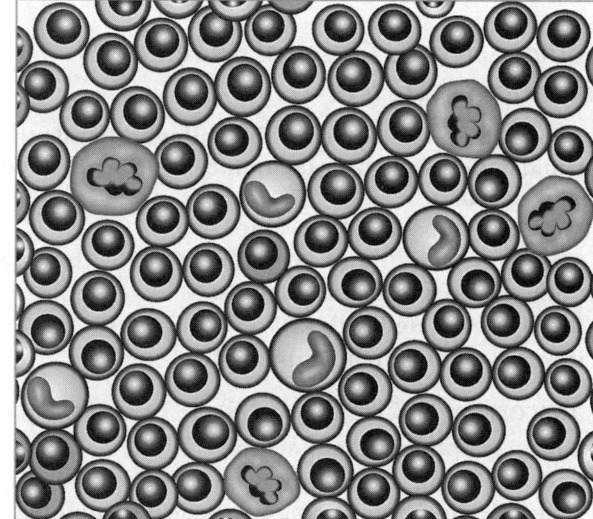

Fig. 14.9: Nodular lymphocyte predominant Hodgkin lymphoma with 'popcorn' cells in a background of reactive lymphocytes and few macrophages

- **Lymphocyte predominant cells** (LP cells)/"popcorn" cells (Fig. 14.9).
    - Specific to NLPHL.
    - Large with relatively abundant, pale cytoplasm.
    - Single large delicate **multilobulated** nucleus **or folded nuclei** resembling bubbly outlines of popcorn kernels.
    - One or more **inconspicuous nucleoli**.
- **Hodgkin and RS cell**s are not found.

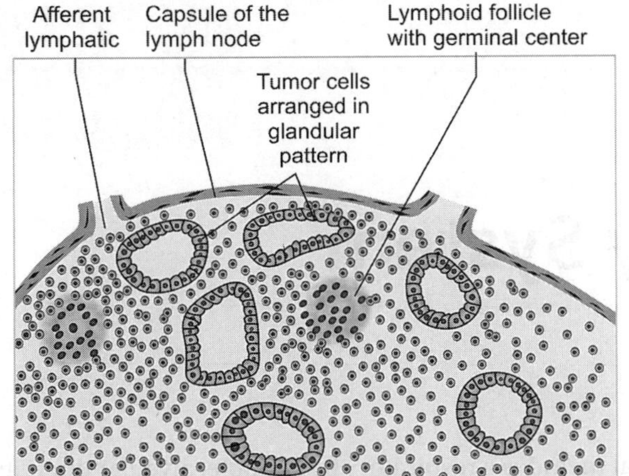

Fig. 14.10: Lymph node with secondaries from adenocarcinoma (diagrammatic)

Spread of Hodgkin Lymphoma

- Mainly **by contiguity**.
- First nodal disease, then splenic disease, hepatic disease and finally marrow involvement and extranodal disease.

METASTATIC CARCINOMA (FIG. 14.10)

Most common pathway of spread for carcinomas is spread through lymphatics. Once the tumor cells gain access into the lymphatic vessels, they are carried to the regional draining lymph nodes.

Pattern of lymph node involvement follows the natural routes of lymphatic drainage.

- **Sentinel lymph node** (refer page 77) biopsy is done to know the presence or absence of metastatic lesions.
- **Skip metastasis:** When **local lymph nodes are bypassed** and **lymphatic metastases develop in lymph nodes distant from the site of the primary tumor**; these are called "skip metastasis". Example: **Abdominal cancers** may be **first detected by an enlarged supraclavicular node**.
- **Retrograde metastasis: Tumors spreading against the flow of lymphatics** may cause metastases at unusual sites. Example: Carcinoma prostate metastasizing to supraclavicular lymph node.

Microscopic pattern of deposits:

- Initially, **tumor cells** are deposited in the **marginal (subcapsular) sinus and later extend throughout the node.**
- **Micrometastases consist of single tumor cells or very small clusters.**

Significance of lymph node metastases: Prognostic value—e.g. in breast cancer, involvement of axillary lymph nodes is very important for assessing prognosis and for type of therapy.

SELF-ASSESSMENT EXERCISE

I. Short Notes

1. Non-Hodgkin lymphoma.
2. Burkitt lymphoma.
3. RS cell and its variants.
4. Classify Hodgkin lymphoma.
5. Hodgkin lymphoma.
6. Causes of lymphadenopathy.

CHAPTER 15

Respiratory System

CHAPTER OUTLINE

- Normal Structure and Function
- Pulmonary Infections—Pneumonia
- Tuberculosis
- Chronic Obstructive Pulmonary Diseases
- Bronchial Asthma
- Bronchiectasis
- Lung Abscess
- Chronic Restrictive Pulmonary Disease
- Pneumoconioses
- Passive Congestion of Lung and Pulmonary Edema
- Lung Cancer
- Pleura

NORMAL STRUCTURE AND FUNCTION

Respiratory tract can be divided into upper respiratory tract and lower respiratory tract (Fig. 15.1).

The **upper respiratory tract** (URT) consists of nose with its adjacent sinuses, the nasopharynx, the larynx and the trachea. The main function of upper respiratory tract is to provide entry for the inhaled air. It prevents the entry of bacteria and foreign bodies.

The **lower respiratory tract** consists of left and right bronchi with its branches and lungs. Lungs are paired organs; right and left. Right lung consists of 3 lobes and the left lung has 2 lobes. A **respiratory lobule** (Fig. 15.1) is the smallest anatomic subunit of lung parenchyma that includes a respiratory bronchiole, alveolar ducts and alveoli. The functional unit of the lung is the acinus where gas transfer takes place. The acinus consists of respiratory bronchiole, alveolar duct and alveoli. The alveoli are lined by two types of pneumocytes (type 1 and type 2).

PULMONARY INFECTIONS—PNEUMONIA

Respiratory tract infections are the most common infections.

Definition: Pneumonia is defined as any **infection of the lung parenchyma**. It causes the alveoli to be filled with inflammatory exudates and **usually results in consolidation ("solidification") of lung**.

Portal of entry of causative agent: Pneumonias may be caused by bacteria or virus. The etiological agent may enter the lung parenchyma **through respiratory tract, blood or locally**.

Classification: Pneumonia can be classified depending on the:

- Specific etiologic agent (Table 15.1)
- Clinical setting in which the infection occurs (if no pathogen can be isolated).

Morphological Classification

Bacterial pneumonia can be classified into two, depending on patterns of anatomic distribution: **lobular bronchopneumonia and lobar pneumonia** (Fig. 15.2).

Table 15.1: Common microorganism causing pneumonia

Microorganism	Predisposing factors/characteristics
Streptococcus pneumoniae or *Pneumococcus*	Most common cause
Haemophilus influenzae	Most common bacterial cause in COPD
Staphylococcus aureus	Important cause of bacterial pneumonia and follows viral respiratory illnesses

Abbreviation: COPD, chronic obstructive pulmonary disease

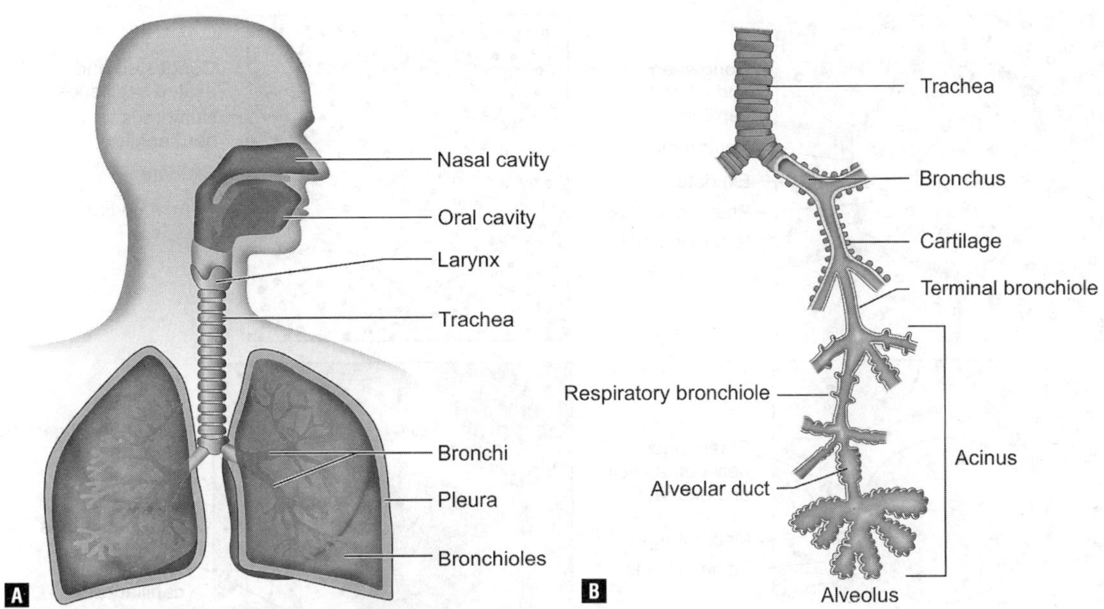

Fig. 15.1: (A) Anatomic components of respiratory tract. (B) The different parts of the airway

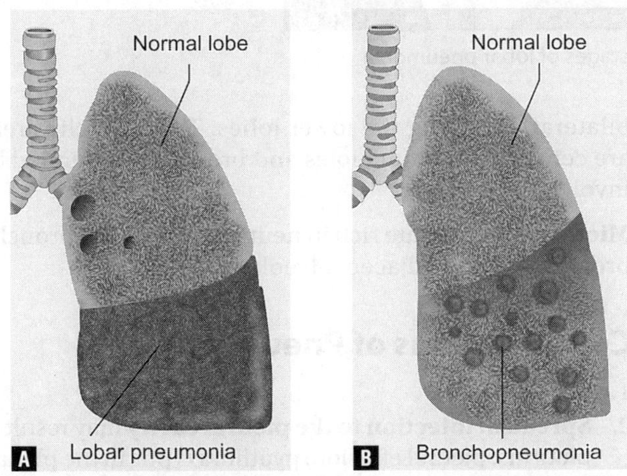

Figs 15.2A and B: Gross involvement of lung in lobar versus bronchopneumonia. (A) Lobar pneumonia affects the entire or part of the lobe; (B) Bronchopneumonia is characterized by focal inflammation centered on the airways and usually multiple

The same organisms may produce either pattern depending on susceptibility of patient. It is **important to identify the causative agent and determine the extent of disease**.

Lobar Pneumonia

It is characterized by fibrinosuppurative **consolidation** of a large portion/**part of a lobe or of a whole lobe**, usually the lower lobes. The common microorganisms causing lobar pneumonia are listed in Table 15.1.

Stages

The inflammatory response of lobar pneumonia can be classified into **four stages** (Fig. 15.3): Congestion, red hepatization, gray hepatization, and resolution.

- **Congestion:** It lasts for less than 24 hours. Pneumococci multiply in the alveolar spaces and produce extensive edema.
  - **Gross:** The **lung is heavy, boggy, and red**. On cut section blood-stained frothy fluid oozes from the cut surface.
  - **Microscopy:** It is characterized by dilatation and congestion of capillaries in the alveolar walls. The **alveoli** are **filled with pale eosinophilic fluid** with few neutrophils, red cells and numerous bacteria.
- **Red hepatization:** It lasts for 2–3 days. Pneumococci incite an acute inflammatory response.
  - **Gross:** The lobe is red, firm and airless. Cut section shows **red, dry and granular** appearance. The affected part of the lung is firm and **resembles the consistency of the liver**. Hence, this stage has been named as red **hepatization.**
  - **Microscopy:** The **inflammatory exudates,** composed of **numerous neutrophils** and **red cells** are seen in the alveolar space.
- **Gray hepatization**
  - **Gross:** The affected lobe appears grayish-brown color. Cut section shows **gray, moist and granular** appearance.
  - **Microscopy:** In this stage, there is progressive disintegration of red cells. The neutrophils are

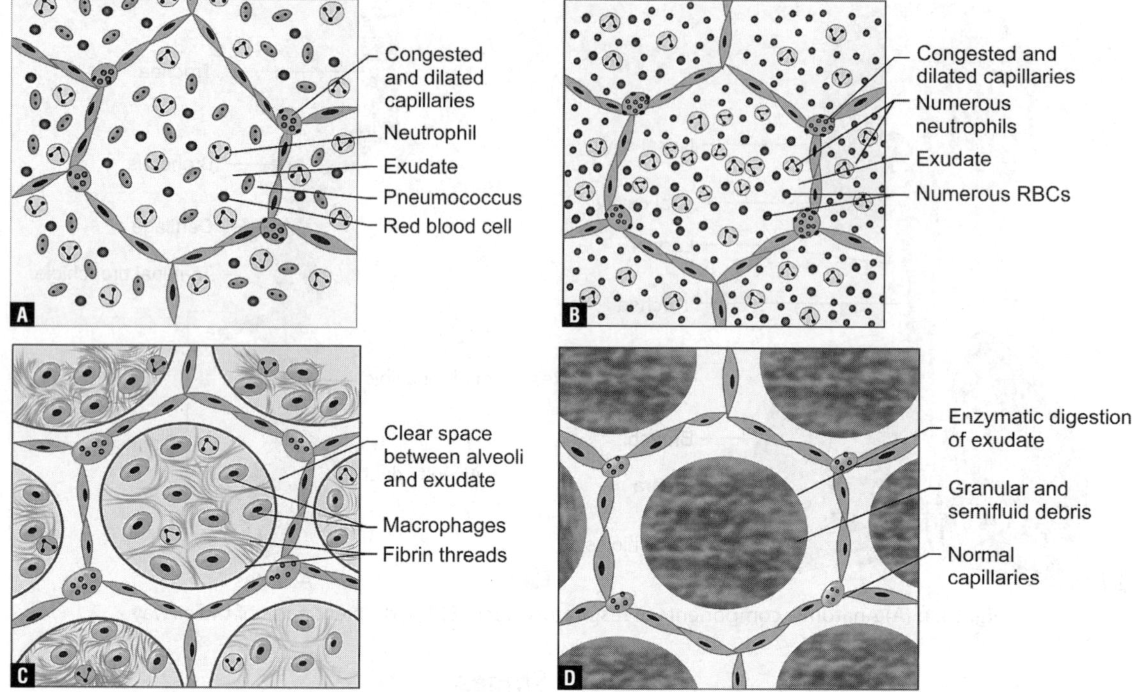

Figs 15.3A to D: Four different stages of lobar pneumonia

replaced by **macrophages**. The alveoli contain fibrinosuppurative exudates. There is a **clear space between the alveoli and the exudate** due to contraction of the exudate (fibrinogen in the exudate is converted into fibrin thread).

- **Resolution**
  - **Gross:** During resolution, the **contents of alveoli undergo liquefaction** and on cut section, lung is frothy.
  - **Microscopy:** The **exudate within the alveolar spaces undergoes progressive enzymatic digestion**. This exudate is resorbed, ingested by macrophages, expectorated, or organized by fibroblasts growing into it.

Pleura may be involved by inflammation **(pleuritis)**. This may resolve or undergo organization.

Bronchopneumonia

It is characterized by **patchy areas of consolidation** in the same or several lobes of the lung (Fig. 15.2).

Morphology

Gross: It has a characteristic patchy distribution of acute suppurative inflammation. The **patchy consolidation** may be found in **one lobe or several lobes**. It is frequently bilateral, involving the lower lobes. These patchy areas are centered on bronchioles and bronchi surrounded by involved alveoli.

Microscopy: Exudate rich in neutrophils fills the bronchi, bronchioles and adjacent alveolar spaces.

Complications of Pneumonia

1. **Lung abscess.**
2. **Spread of infection to the pleural cavity** may result in pleuritis, pleural effusion, pyothorax (pus in the pleural cavity), empyema (loculated collection of pus).
3. **Bacteremic dissemination:** It may result in endocarditis (heart valves), pericarditis (pericardium), meningitis, suppurative arthritis and metastatic abscesses in kidneys or spleen.
4. **Organization:** Ingrowth of granulation tissue can result in organizing pneumonia.

Clinical Features

It presents with abrupt onset of **high fever, chills**, and **cough** with **mucopurulent sputum**. When pleuritis is present, patient may have pleuritic pain and pleural friction rubs. The whole lobe is radiopaque in lobar pneumonia, whereas there are focal opacities in bronchopneumonia.

TUBERCULOSIS

Refer Chapter 4 (pages 33–6).

CHRONIC OBSTRUCTIVE PULMONARY DISEASES

Chronic obstructive pulmonary disease (COPD) is defined as a disease **characterized by airflow limitation** that is not fully reversible. It includes **mainly two diseases namely, emphysema and chronic bronchitis**. In emphysema and chronic bronchitis cigarette smoking is one common extrinsic trigger.

Chronic Bronchitis

Definition: Chronic bronchitis is defined clinically as **persistent cough with sputum production** (chronic productive cough) **for at least 3 months** in at least 2 consecutive years.

Etiology

Following etiological factors have been incriminated in its etiology and progression.

- **Cigarette smoking:** It is the most important risk factor.
- **Air pollutants:** Sulfur dioxide, Nitrogen dioxide.
- **Toxic industrial inhalants:** Occupational dust exposure.
- **Respiratory tract infection:** It may initiate and promote chronic bronchitis.

Pathogenesis

- **Irritation by inhaled air pollutants:** The initiating factor is irritation of large airways mucosa by inhaled air pollutants, such as **tobacco smoke** (90% of patients are smokers), **dust, cotton, sulfur dioxide, nitrogen dioxide** and **silica**. Irritants cause inflammation and infiltration by inflammatory cells (e.g. lymphocytes, macrophages and neutrophils).
- **Hypersecretion of mucus:**
  - **Hyperplasia/hypertrophy of the submucosal glands** in **large airways (trachea and bronchi)**: Develops in response to inhaled **environmental irritants** and **proteases released from neutrophils**. This leads to **hypersecretion of mucus.**
  - **Marked increase of goblet cells in small airways (small bronchi and bronchioles):** They **produce excessive mucus** and **leads to airway obstruction**.

Morphology

Gross: Bronchi and bronchioles show thickening of the mucous membranes with excessive mucinous or mucopurulent secretions in the lumen.

Microscopy: The major characteristic histological features are:

- **Chronic inflammation of the airways** (predominantly lymphocytes).
- **Mucus hypersecretion:** This is due to **hyperplasia** (increase in number) **and hypertrophy** (increase in size) **of the mucus-secreting glands of the trachea and bronchi.** There is also increase in the number of goblet cells.
- The bronchial epithelium may show **squamous metaplasia**.

Clinical Features

Chronic bronchitis is usually seen in middle-aged men who are heavy smokers. The cardinal symptom of chronic bronchitis is persistent cough with expectoration (sputum) for many years.

Complications

Long-standing severe chronic bronchitis leads to cor pulmonale (alteration in the right ventricle of the heart caused by a primary disorder of the respiratory system) and heart failure.

Emphysema

Definition: Emphysema is a chronic lung disease characterized by **abnormal irreversible** (permanent) **enlargement of the airspaces distal to the terminal bronchiole**, associated with destruction of their walls.

Types of Emphysema/Classification

Emphysema is classified into **four major types** (Fig. 15.4) according to location of the lesions within the lobule. These are: **centriacinar, panacinar, paraseptal and irregular**.

- **Centriacinar (centrilobular) emphysema:** In this type of emphysema, the **central or proximal** parts of the acini are affected. It is more common and severe in the **upper lobes**. It occurs in **heavy smokers,** and in association **with chronic bronchitis.**
- **Panacinar (panlobular) emphysema:** This type involves all the air spaces beyond terminal bronchiole. Thus, the **acini are uniformly enlarged**. It is more common in the **lower zones**. This type of emphysema is associated with **α_1-antitrypsin (α_1-AT) deficiency**.
- **Distal acinar (paraseptal) emphysema:** In this type **distal part** of the acinus is predominantly involved. It is more prominent **adjacent to the pleura**. This type of emphysema is the common cause of spontaneous pneumothorax.
- **Irregular (scar or cicatricial) emphysema:** This **irregularly** involves the acini and is associated with scarring.

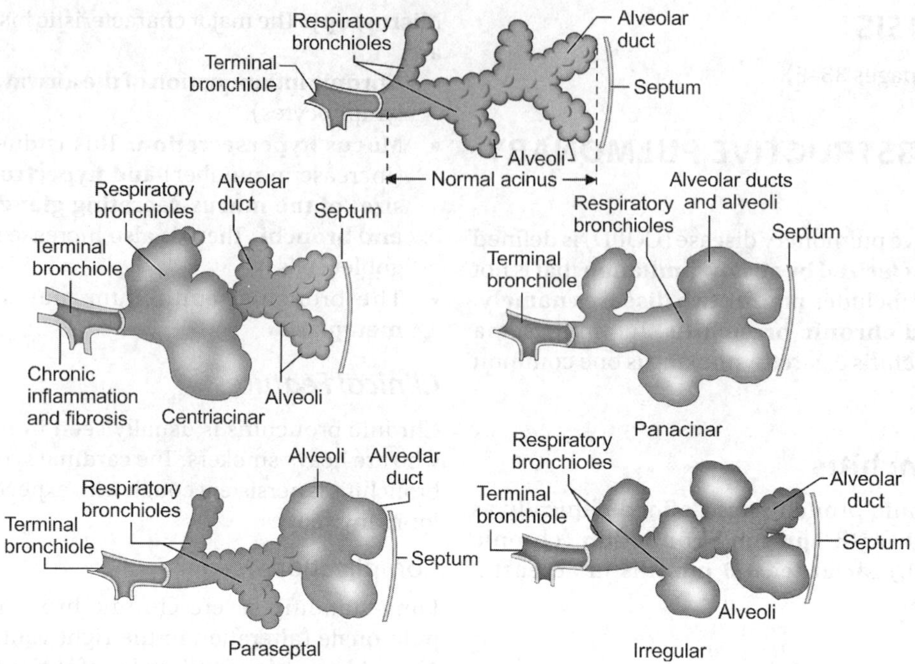

Fig. 15.4: Four major types of emphysema

Etiology and Pathogenesis

Clear-cut association between **heavy cigarette smoking** and development of emphysema is observed. Inhaled cigarette smoke and other toxic substances produce damage to the lung and produces inflammation. This leads to destruction of the lung parenchymal (emphysema) and disease of the airway (bronchiolitis and chronic bronchitis). The major event in emphysema is destruction of alveolar wall. Factors involved in the pathogenesis of emphysema are as follows:

- **Inflammatory mediators and leukocytes:** Mediators are resident epithelial cells and produce structural changes.
- **Protease-antiprotease imbalance:** Inflammatory cells and damaged epithelial cells release proteases which can damage the connective tissue. Normally, the damage by proteases is prevented by antiprotease (e.g. α_1-antitrypsin is a major inhibitor of proteases). About 1% of patients with emphysema have deficiency of protective antiproteases.
  - **Genetic deficiency of α_1-antitrypsin:** Normally, a balance is maintained between protease and antiproteases. α_1-antitrypsin deficiency is inherited as autosomal recessive disorder and in these patients there is excessive digestion of elastic tissue which lead to emphysema. The damage is aggravated by smoking.

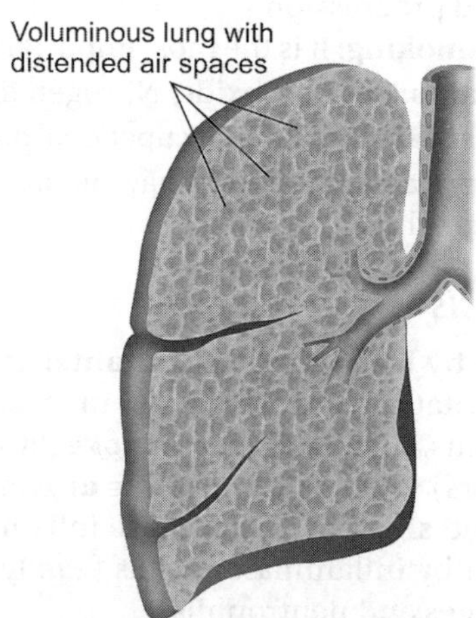

Fig. 15.5: Voluminous lung in emphysema

- **Oxidative stress:** Contents of tobacco smoke produce oxidants. They cause further damage to the tissues and aggravate inflammation.
- **Infection:** may exacerbate the existing inflammatory process and chronic bronchitis.

Morphology

Gross: Advanced emphysema produces **voluminous lungs** (Fig. 15.5).

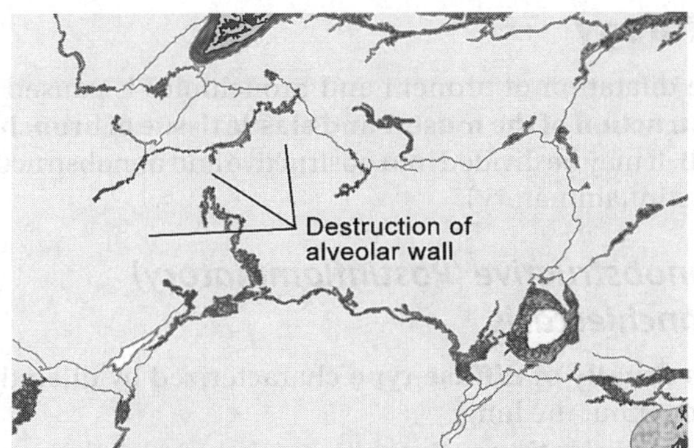

Fig. 15.6: Microscopy of emphysema with extensive destruction of alveolar walls forming large alveoli

Microscopy: Shows abnormally large alveoli separated by thin septa (Fig. 15.6). Inflammatory changes may be seen in small airways.

Clinical features: The clinical manifestations are: **steadily progressive dyspnea, cough and expectoration**. The patient develops a barrel-chest.

Complications: Development of cor pulmonale and congestive heart failure.

Cause of death: Death in most of the patients with emphysema is due to respiratory acidosis, right-sided heart failure or massive collapse of the lungs secondary to pneumothorax.

BRONCHIAL ASTHMA

Definition: Asthma is a chronic inflammatory disorder of the bronchial airways. It is characterized by **airflow obstruction and recurrent episodes of wheezing, breathlessness and cough.**

Classification

It is **classified according to the type of antigen** as **atopic** (allergic) and **non-atopic** (without evidence of allergen sensitization).

- **Atopic asthma:** It is the most common type of asthma which usually begins in **childhood.** Atopy is the major risk factor and is due to the genetically determined production of specific IgE antibody. **Atopic asthma** is mediated by **type I IgE-mediated hypersensitivity reaction**. It is triggered by environmental allergens, such as **dusts, pollens**, cockroach or animal dander, and foods. Many patients with asthma have a positive family history of asthma or allergic diseases (e.g. allergic rhinitis, eczema/atopic dermatitis, urticaria, or hay fever).
- **Non-atopic asthma:** It does not show allergen sensitization. They have normal serum concentrations of IgE. These patients, with nonatopic or intrinsic asthma, usually show later onset of disease (adult-onset asthma).

Etiology

Asthma is a disease developing due to interplay between genetic (endogenous) and environmental (exogenous) factors.

Risk Factors

1. **Endogenous risk factors:** These include:
   - Usually in atopic asthma, there is strong familial association suggesting a **genetic predisposition** to the disease.
   - **Atopy** (refer page 63) is the major risk factor.
   - **Airway hyper responsiveness** to undergo constriction in response to multiple inhaled triggers than normal individuals.
2. **Environmental risk factors:**
   - **Allergens:** Indoor allergens or outdoor allergens especially in atopic individuals.
   - **Occupational sensitizers:** For example, agents like chemicals or small animal allergens.
   - **Passive smoking:** Exposure to passive cigarette smoke may trigger asthma.
   - **Respiratory infections:** It is uncertain whether they play a role in etiology.

Pathogenesis (refer Flowchart 6.1)

The major etiological factors in atopic asthma (refer pages 62–3) are a **genetic predisposition** to type I hypersensitivity ("atopy") and exposure to environmental antigens (allergens).

- **Sensitization:** Individuals who are genetically predisposed to asthma have susceptibility genes. These individuals are **sensitized against many allergens.** The allergen stimulates bronchial submucosal glands to secrete mucus and **B cells to produce IgE**. These **IgE coats bronchial submucosal mast cells.**
- **On re-exposure:** When the individual is re-exposed to the allergen, **the allergens bind to IgE coated on the bronchial submucosal mast cells**. The mast cells get activated and immediately **release bronchoconstrictor mediators** from their granules. Mast cells release preformed mediators and produce cytokines. These **mediators are responsible** for the early-phase (immediate hypersensitivity) reaction and the late-phase **reaction.**

- **Early reaction:** It is characterized by **bronchoconstriction, increased mucus production**, and vasodilatation with increased vascular permeability. Bronchoconstriction is triggered by direct stimulation of vagal receptors in the subepithelium.
- **Late-phase reaction:** It consists of **inflammation** with **recruitment of leukocytes, notably eosinophils, neutrophils and T-cells.**

Morphology

Gross: Bronchial asthma may show occlusion of bronchi and bronchioles by thick, tenacious mucus plugs.

Microscopy

- Bronchial asthma is characterized by edema of the mucosa of bronchi and bronchioles. The **mucosa is infiltrated by mast cells, eosinophils and lymphocytes.**
- Mucus plug is composed of mucus secreted from goblet cells and plasma proteins from leaky bronchial vessels and may form spiral-shaped cast of the airways which are called **Curschmann spirals.**
- **Charcot-Leyden crystals** which are crystallized eosinophil lysophospholipase may also be seen in the lumen of airways.
- There is an increase in size and number (**hypertrophy/hyperplasia**) of the **submucosal glands** in the large airways and increased numbers of epithelial goblet cells. There is also **hypertrophy and/or hyperplasia of the bronchial wall smooth muscle.**

Clinical Features

Acute asthmatic attack usually lasts up to several hours. It presents with dyspnea, wheezing, and cough with or without sputum production. Patients may be asymptomatic between the asthmatic attacks.

Status asthmaticus: Severe acute asthma unresponsive to therapy in which the severe acute paroxysm persists for days and even weeks is termed status asthmaticus. It may lead to severe cyanosis and even death.

BRONCHIECTASIS

Definition: Bronchiectasis is **abnormal permanent dilation of bronchi and bronchioles** caused by destruction of the bronchial wall.

Bronchiectasis may be the result of or associated with chronic necrotizing infections.

Etiology

The dilatation of bronchi and bronchioles is caused by **destruction of the muscle and elastic tissue of bronchial wall.** It may be divided into obstructive and nonobstructive (postinflammatory).

Nonobstructive (Postinflammatory) Bronchiectasis

It is **usually of diffuse type** characterized by dilatation throughout the lung.

- **Postinfectious:** Bronchiectasis may be the result or associated with **chronic necrotizing infections**. The infections include bacterial (e.g. *Mycobacterium tuberculosis, Staphylococcus aureus*), viral [e.g. adenovirus, influenza virus, human immunodeficiency virus (HIV)] or fungal (e.g. *Aspergillus* species).
- **Focal nonobstructive bronchiectasis** usually develops as a **complication of childhood infections, such as measles and pertussis.**
- **Genetic causes:** For example, **Kartagener or immotile cilia syndrome.**
- **Immunodeficiency:** Patients with hypogammaglobulinemia, HIV infection have increased susceptibility to infections and may predispose to localized or diffuse bronchiectasis.
- **Autoimmune and immune-mediated diseases:** For example, rheumatoid arthritis, systemic lupus erythematosus.

Obstructive Bronchiectasis

It is **localized** to the obstructed segment of the lung.

- **Airway/bronchial obstruction: Partial or total obstruction of the bronchial lumen** may be caused by tumor, foreign body aspiration and mucus plugs. It may also develop in patients with atopic asthma and chronic bronchitis.
- **Cystic fibrosis:** Major respiratory diseases in cystic fibrosis (CF) are sinusitis and bronchiectasis.
- **Acquired conditions:**
  - **Postinfectious conditions:** Nonobstructive bronchiectasis may **complicate pneumonia** caused by bacteria, viruses and fungi. It may be localized or generalized.
  - **Bronchial obstruction:** Obstructive bronchiectasis may be obstruction by a **tumor, inhaled foreign bodies**, and mucous plugs. This type of bronchiectasis is localized type.

- **Congenital or hereditary conditions:**
  - This includes cystic fibrosis and **Kartagener syndromes**.

Pathogenesis

Obstruction and infection are the major conditions associated with bronchiectasis.

- **Obstruction:** When bronchi are obstructed, the normal clearing mechanisms will be impaired. This results in collection of secretions distal to the obstruction, and inflammation of the airway.
- **Infection:** Severe infections of the bronchi lead to inflammation, necrosis, fibrosis, and consequent permanent dilation of airways.

Morphology

Gross: Depending on the gross appearance, bronchiectasis may be classified as **cylindrical, fusiform, saccular or varicose** (Fig. 15.7).

Bronchiectasis may be **generalized or localized**. Generalized bronchiectasis is usually bilateral and commonly affects the lower lobes. In localized bronchiectasis, the involvement may be sharply localized to a single segment of the lung.

The **airways are dilated**, sometimes even four times than the normal size. The dilated bronchi and bronchioles are so much dilated that they **can be followed or traced almost to the pleural surfaces** (Normally, they can be traced upto 2 cm away from pleural surface).

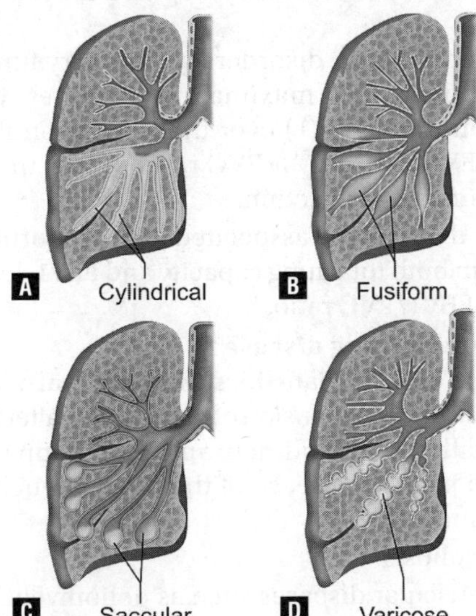

Figs 15.7A to D: Morphological types of bronchiectasis. (A) Cylindrical; (B) Fusiform; (C) Saccular; (D) Varicose

Microscopy

- It shows **dilatation of bronchi and bronchioles** and these dilated airways frequently contain pools of thick, purulent material.
- **Desquamation of the lining epithelium** and extensive areas of necrotizing ulceration. There may be **pseudostratification** of the columnar cells and squamous **metaplasia** in the remaining epithelium.
- The bronchial wall shows **intense acute and chronic inflammatory infiltrate**.

Complications

These include pneumonia (inflammation of the lungs), empyema (collection of pus in the pleural space), septicemia (presence of pathogenic microorganisms in the blood), meningitis (inflammation of the meningeal membranes of the spinal cord or brain), metastatic abscesses (e.g. in brain), cor pulmonale and amyloid formation.

Clinical Features

Bronchiectasis presents with **severe, persistent cough with expectoration.** The sputum is usually foul-smelling. The cough is more prominent when the patient rises in the morning or with changes in position.

LUNG ABSCESS

Definition: Lung abscess is defined as a **local suppurative process within the lung parenchyma**. It is characterized by **accumulation of pus and cavitations** accompanied by the destruction of lung tissue.

Etiology and Pathogenesis

Causative organisms: Any pathogen can produce an abscess. These include **aerobic and anaerobic organisms** normally found in the oral cavity or Gram-negative organisms. Mixed infections can occur due to inhalation of foreign material.

Mechanism: Lung abscess may be primary or secondary.

- **Secondary lung abscess:** Abscesses develop in the lung as a complication of many conditions.
  - **Complication of necrotizing pneumonia:** Lung abscess may develop as a complication of primary lung infection causing pneumonia.
  - **Septic embolism:** Infected emboli from anywhere in the systemic venous circulation or from infective bacterial endocarditis.

- **Bronchial obstruction due to neoplasia:** Secondary infection develops when there is bronchial obstruction by a tumor (post-obstructive pneumonia).
- **Miscellaneous:** Direct penetrating trauma to the lungs; spread of infections from a neighboring organ, and seeding of the lung by pyogenic organisms through blood.

- **Primary lung abscesses**. Lung abscesses without any apparent cause are termed as primary. But most frequently they are due to **aspiration of infected material**. This occurs following unconsciousness during acute alcoholism, coma, anesthesia, oropharyngeal surgical procedures, sinusitis and dental sepsis.

Morphology

Gross: Lung abscess may develop in any part of the lung and may be **single or multiple**.

- Lung abscesses due to **aspiration** are more common on the **right** (because of the more vertical right main bronchus) and are most often **single** (Fig. 15.8).
- Abscesses that develop as a **complication of pneumonia or bronchiectasis** are usually **multiple, and diffusely scattered.**
- **Septic emboli** and pyemic abscesses are **multiple** and may affect **any area** of the lung.

Abscesses vary in diameter from few millimeters to large cavities of 5–6 cm. The abscess cavity shows pus.

Microscopy: Lung abscess shows **suppurative destruction of the lung parenchyma and a central area of cavitation.** The abscess shows necrotic material, numerous polymorphonuclear leukocytes and, variable numbers of macrophages.

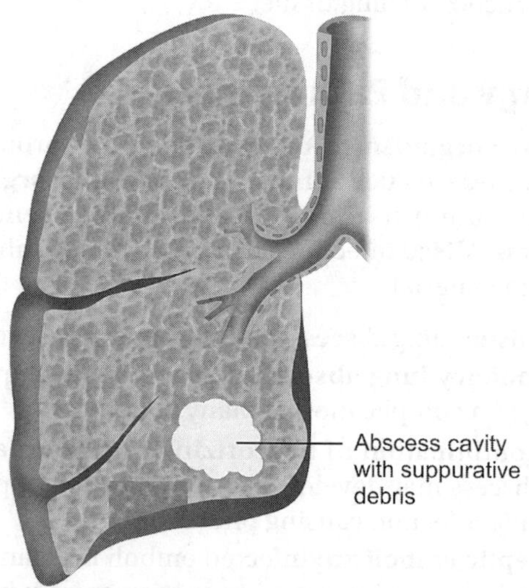

Fig. 15.8: Lung abscess in the lower lobe of lung

Clinical Features

It presents as **cough, fever and copious amounts of foul-smelling purulent sputum**. Fever, chest pain, and weight loss are common. Clubbing of the fingers and toes may also be seen.

Complications

These include: extension of the infection into the pleural cavity resulting in **empyema, hemorrhage, development of brain abscesses or meningitis** from septic emboli and **secondary amyloidosis**.

CHRONIC RESTRICTIVE PULMONARY DISEASE

- **Obstructive lung diseases** (or airway diseases) are characterized by an increase in resistance to airflow due to partial or complete obstruction at any level from the trachea and to the terminal and respiratory bronchioles. These include emphysema, chronic bronchitis, bronchial asthma and bronchiectasis.
- **Restrictive lung diseases** are characterized by reduced expansion of lung parenchyma and decreased total lung capacity.

Differences between obstructive and restrictive pulmonary disease (Table 15.2).

The distinction is based mainly on pulmonary function tests.

- In diffuse obstructive disorders, pulmonary function tests show decreased maximal airflow rates during forced expiration (FEV1) over the forced ventilatory capacity (FVC). An FEV1/FVC ratio of less than 0.7 indicates airway obstruction.
- Restrictive diseases are associated with proportionate decreases in both total lung capacity and FEV1, leading to normal FEV1/FVC ratio.

Types of restrictive lung disease

- **Restriction due to disorders of chest wall:** These diseases restrict the expansion of lungs due to alterations in chest wall, pleura and neuromuscular apparatus. There is no primary disease of the lung parenchyma. Examples include:
  - Kyphoscoliosis
  - Neuromuscular diseases such as poliomyelitis
  - Pleural diseases
  - Severe obesity

Table 15.2: Differences between chronic obstructive and chronic restrictive pulmonary disease

Feature	Obstructive pulmonary disease	Restrictive pulmonary disease
Nature of airway disease	Obstruction at any level from trachea to respiratory bronchiole	Reduced expansion of lung parenchyma
Pulmonary function test	Increased pulmonary resistance and obstruction of maximal expiratory airflow. FEV1/FVC ratio of less than 0.7	Decreased total lung capacity. Normal FEV1/FVC ratio
Chest X-ray	Depends on the cause	Bilateral infiltrates showing ground-glass shadows
Examples	• Chronic bronchitis • Emphysema • Bronchial asthma • Bronchiectasis	• Disorders of chest cage: (For example, kyphoscoliosis, poliomyelitis and pleural disease • Interstitial lung diseases (ILDs): For example, pneumoconioses

Table 15.3: Lung diseases caused by mineral dusts (pneumoconiosis)

Mineral dust	Disease	Exposure
Coal dust	Anthracosis and progressive massive fibrosis	Coal mining (particularly hard coal)
Silica	Silicosis	Foundry work, sandblasting, hard rock mining, stone cutting, others
Asbestos	• Asbestosis • Pleural plaques • Mesothelioma • Carcinoma of the lung, larynx, stomach, colon	Mining, milling, fabrication, and installation and removal of insulation

- **Chronic interstitial and infiltrative diseases:** These diseases are characterized by non-infectious diffuse parenchymal involvement of the lung namely the alveoli, capillary basement membrane, the intervening interstitial space, perivascular tissue and lymphatic tissue. Diffuse involvement of lung parenchyma may be primary, or secondarily to other multiorgan disease process. The term 'infiltrative' is used to denote the radiologic appearance of lungs in chest X-ray which show characteristic diffuse interstitial ground-glass opacities. Most important diseases included under this category are **pneumoconiosis** and interstitial fibrosis.

Major common clinical manifestations: Include exertional dyspnea, non-persistent productive cough, tachypnea, cyanosis and sometimes hemoptysis. There usually no wheezing which is characteristic of COPD.

PNEUMOCONIOSES

Definition: The pneumoconioses are diseases of the lung produced by organic as well as inorganic dust particles, chemical fumes and vapors.

Important lung diseases caused by mineral dusts are shown in Table 15.3.

Coal Workers' Pneumoconiosis

Coal Workers' Pneumoconiosis (CWP) results due to inhalation of **carbon particles**.

Morphology

The lung findings can be divided into three stages.

1. **Asymptomatic anthracosis:** It is the most harmless coal-induced pulmonary lesion in coal miners. Inhaled carbon pigment is engulfed by alveolar or interstitial macrophages. These carbon laden macrophages accumulate in the connective tissue along the lymphatics and in the regional lymph nodes.
2. **Simple CWP:** It may produce little to no pulmonary dysfunction.

   Gross: It is characterized by **coal macules** (1–2 mm in diameter) and **coal nodules**. These are mainly seen in the upper lobes and upper zones of the lower lobes. Later dilation of alveoli may lead to **centrilobular emphysema**.
3. **Complicated CWP** (progressive massive fibrosis): These patients may have significant respiratory impairment. CWP develops in a background of simple CWP.

   Gross: The lession shows **multiple, dark black scars** larger than 2 cm in greatest diameter (Fig. 15.9).

Clinical Features

CWP is usually a benign disease with minimal loss of lung function. When PMF develops, it results in pulmonary dysfunction, pulmonary hypertension and cor pulmonale.

Silicosis

Silicosis is the most prevalent chronic occupational **lung disease caused by inhalation of silica**. It usually presents after decades of exposure as a slowly progressing pneumoconiosis.

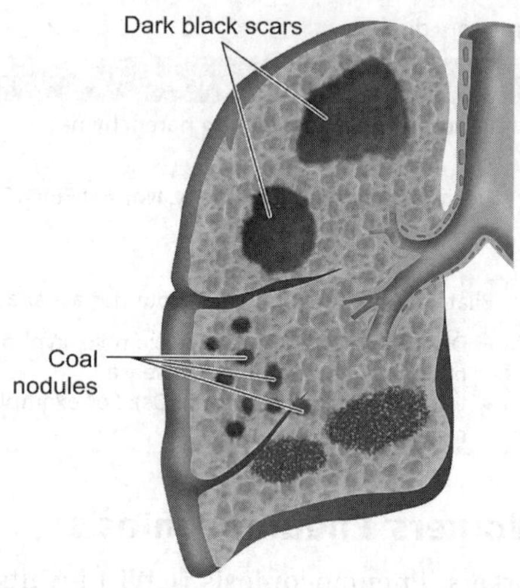

Fig. 15.9: Complicated Coal Worker's Pneumoconiosis showing two large black scars in the upper part of the lung

Susceptible Individuals

Sandblasters, stone cutting, polishing and sharpening of metals, ceramic manufacturing, foundry work, and the cleaning of boilers.

Pathogenesis

After inhalation, the particles interact with epithelial cells and are ingested by alveolar macrophages. Within the macrophages, **silica causes activation and release of mediators** which are **fibrogenic**.

Morphology

Silicosis produces simple nodular silicosis which may progress to progressive massive fibrosis.

- **Simple nodular silicosis:** In this early stage, **small** (usually 2–4 mm) pale to black (if coal dust is also present) silicotic **nodules** are seen in the upper zones of the lungs (Fig. 15.10A). Hilar nodes may become enlarged and calcified, radiographically appear as **eggshell** calcification.
- **Progressive massive fibrosis:** If the disease continues to progress, expansion and coalescence of lesions may produce progressive massive fibrosis. It consists of 5–10 cm sized **hard, collagenous scars** (Fig. 15.10B). Radiologically, they appear as nodular masses in a background of simple silicosis.

Clinical Features

The lung functions are either normal or only moderately affected. Chest radiographs of the lung show a fine nodularity in the upper zones. Patients develop shortness of breath only after progressive massive fibrosis. Silicosis is associated with an increased susceptibility to tuberculosis. The crystalline silica is carcinogenic in humans.

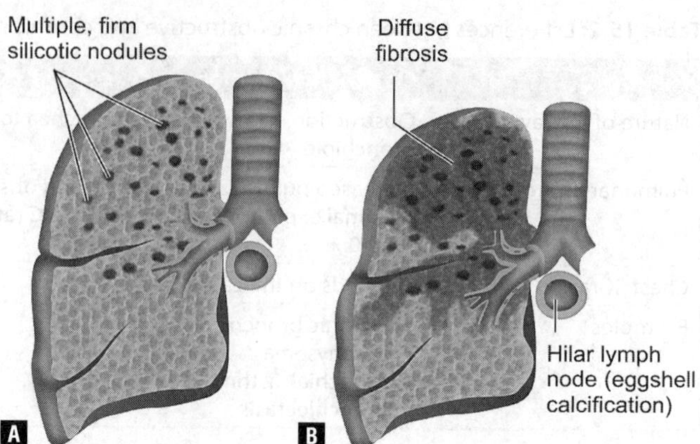

Figs 15.10A and B: (A) Simple nodular silicosis; (B) Silicosis leading to progressive massive fibrosis

Box 15.1: Disease caused by occupational exposure to asbestos

• Localized fibrous plaques
• Pleural effusions
• Parenchymal interstitial fibrosis *(asbestosis)*
• Lung carcinoma
• Mesotheliomas
• Laryngeal and perhaps other extrapulmonary neoplasms, including colon carcinomas

Asbestos-related Diseases

Asbestos is a family of crystalline hydrated silicates that form fibers. Diseases caused by occupational exposure to asbestos are listed in Box 15.1.

Pathogenesis

Fibrogenic effect

Asbestos fibers are fibrogenic. Chronic deposition of fibers and persistent lead to generalized **interstitial pulmonary inflammation and interstitial fibrosis.**

Oncogenic effect

Asbestos can act as a tumor initiator and promoter. The adsorption of carcinogens in tobacco smoke onto asbestos fibers may be responsible for the synergy between tobacco smoking and the development of **lung carcinoma** in asbestos workers.

Morphology

Gross: Lung shows **diffuse interstitial fibrosis** (Fig. 15.11A). In contrast to CWP and silicosis, asbestosis begins

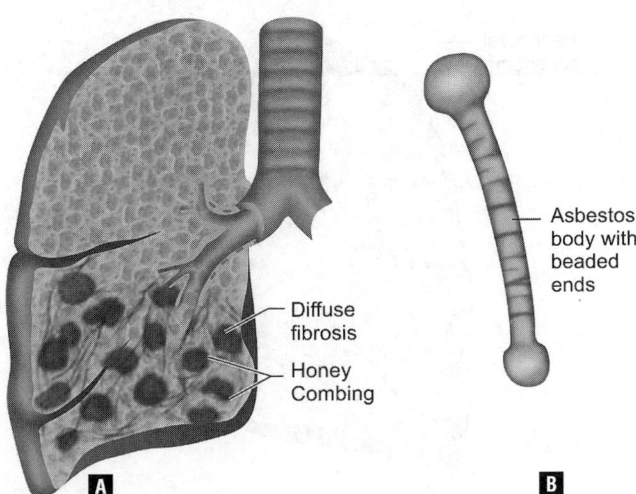

Figs 15.11A and B: Asbestosis of lung (A) involving the lower lobe showing diffuse fibrosis and honey combing; (B) Asbestos body

in the lower lobes and subpleural region. As the fibrosis progresses, the middle and upper lobes of the lungs become involved.

Microscopy

- **Asbestos bodies** (Fig. 15.11B): Asbestos bodies appear as **golden brown, fusiform or beaded rods with a translucent center. They consist of asbestos fibers coated with an iron-containing proteinaceous material**.
- **Ferruginous bodies:** Other inorganic particulates may become coated with similar iron-protein complexes and are called **ferruginous bodies**.
- **Fibrosis: Distorts the architecture,** creating dilated airspaces and the affected regions appear like a **honeycomb**.
- **Pleural plaques:** Appear as pearly white, well-circumscribed plaques on the pleura.
- **Both lung cancers and mesotheliomas (pleural and peritoneal) develop in workers exposed to asbestos.** Concomitant cigarette smoking greatly increases the risk of lung cancer.

Clinical Features

Initially, presents as dyspnea on exertion, but later it is present even at rest. The dyspnea is usually accompanied by a cough with production of sputum. Chest X-ray shows irregular linear densities and as the disease progresses, a honeycomb pattern develops. The disease may progress to respiratory failure, cor pulmonale, and death.

PASSIVE CONGESTION OF LUNG AND PULMONARY EDEMA

Passive Hyperemia or Congestion of Lung

Passive hyperemia or congestion of lung is lung engorgement with venous blood. It may be acute or chronic.

- **Acute passive congestion:** It develops in acute left or right ventricular failure. The venous engorgement of the lungs leads to accumulation of a transudate in the alveoli, which is called **pulmonary edema**.
- **Chronic passive pulmonary congestion:** It is seen mainly in chronic left ventricular failure which impedes blood flow out of the lungs.

Pulmonary Edema

Definition: Pulmonary edema occurs due to leakage of excessive interstitial fluid which accumulates in alveolar spaces.

Classification and Causes of Pulmonary Edema (Box 15.2)

Whatever the clinical setting, pulmonary congestion and edema (perivascular, interstitial and alveolar spaces) in the lung produce heavy, wet lungs.

- **Hemodynamic or cardiogenic pulmonary edema:** It can be **produced as a result of hemodynamic disturbances** and is **due to increased hydrostatic**

Box 15.2: Classification and causes of pulmonary edema

Hemodynamic edema
- Increased hydrostatic pressure (increased pulmonary venous pressure): Left-sided heart failure (common)
- Volume overload: Pulmonary vein obstruction
- Decreased oncotic pressure (less common): Hypoalbuminemia, nephrotic syndrome, liver disease

Edema due to alveolar wall injury (Microvascular or epithelial injury)
- Direct injury
  - Infections: Bacterial pneumonia
  - Inhaled gases: High concentration oxygen, smoke
  - Liquid aspiration: Gastric contents, near-drowning
  - Radiation
- Indirect injury
  - Septicemia
  - Blood transfusion related
  - Burns
  - Drugs and chemicals
  - Shock, trauma

pressure. It **occurs most commonly in left-sided congestive heart failure** which impedes blood flow out of the lungs. It increases the pressure of alveolar capillaries and these vessels become engorged with blood. Increased pressure in the alveolar capillaries has four major consequences:

- **Microhemorrhages** occur with release of red blood cells into alveolar spaces, where they are phagocytosed and degraded by alveolar macrophages. The released iron, in the form of hemosiderin is seen in these macrophages. These **hemosiderin laden macrophages** are termed "**heart failure cells**".
- Fluid is forced from the blood vessels into the alveolar airspaces, resulting in pulmonary edema. Pulmonary edema interferes with gas exchange in the lung.
- When pulmonary congestion (refer pages 50-1) is of long-duration (e.g. in mitral stenosis) increased fibrosis and thickening of the alveolar walls (interstitium of the lung). Grossly, the presence of fibrosis and iron gives rise to a firm, brown coloration of the lung **(brown induration)**.
- **Pulmonary hypertension** occurs when the pressure is transmitted from pulmonary venous system to the pulmonary arterial system. This may lead to right-sided heart failure and consequent generalized systemic venous congestion

• **Due to alveolar wall injury (microvascular or epithelial injury)**.

LUNG CANCER

Carcinoma of the lung is the most common cause of death due to cancer. This is mainly due to the carcinogenic effects of **cigarette smoke**.

Age group

Usually seen in patients between 50 and 80 years.

Sex

More common in males.

Etiology and Pathogenesis

The well-known lung carcinogen is cigarette smoke.

- **Tobacco smoking:** The cigarette smoke contains many carcinogens. These include both initiators **(polycyclic aromatic hydrocarbons such as benzo[a]pyrene)** and promoters (e.g. phenol derivatives).
- **Industrial hazards: Exposure to ionizing radiation, uranium** and **asbestos** increase the risk of lung cancer.
- **Air pollution:** Indoor air pollution by radon is associated with increased lung cancer.

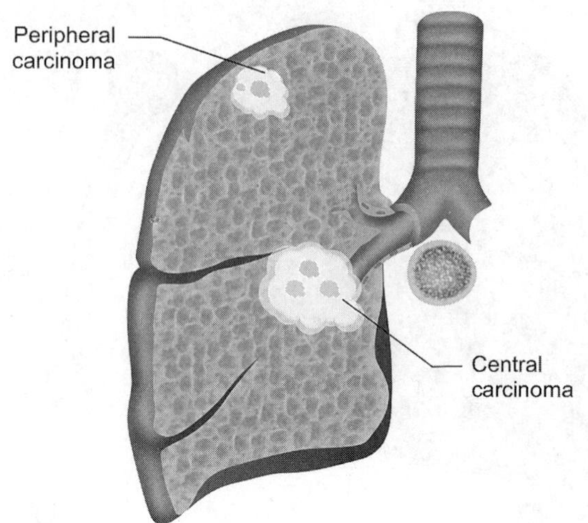

Fig. 15.12: Carcinoma lung arising in the hilar region are called as central and those at the periphery of the lung are known as peripheral

Box 15.3: World Health Organization classification

Primary tumors
• Squamous cell carcinoma • Adenocarcinoma • Large cell carcinoma
Neuroendocrine tumors
• Small cell carcinoma, carcinoid tumor
Metastatic tumors

- **Genetic factors:** Exposure to various carcinogens cause genetic alterations and result in mutations.

WHO classification of lung tumors (abridged) is shown in Box 15.3.

Morphology

Most of the lung tumors arise in the **hilus** of the lung **(central)**. The adenocarcinomas, arise in the periphery **(peripheral)** of the lung (Fig. 15.12).

Squamous Cell Carcinoma

It is most commonly seen in men and is **closely related to a smoking**.

- **Gross:** Mainly arises arise in the hilar region of the lung as nodular growth. Cut section may show focal areas of hemorrhage or necrosis.
- **Microscopy:** It is characterized by tumor cells showing keratinization. This may be seen as epithelial keratin pearls or individual cell keratinization. They are graded as well-differentiated, moderately differentiated or poorly differentiated (Fig. 15.13). Tumor cells may be detected by exfoliative cytology of the sputum.

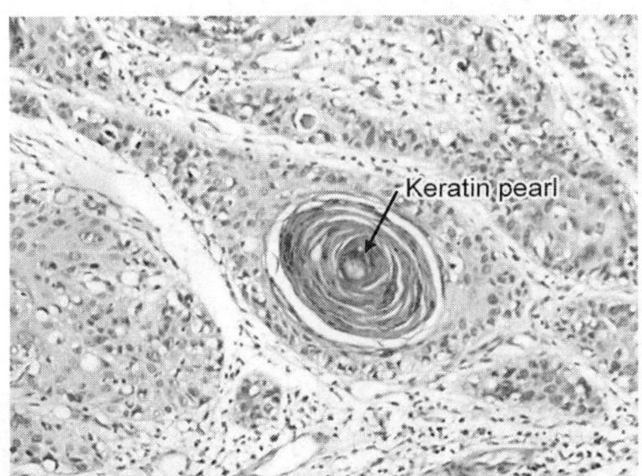

Fig. 15.13: Squamous cell carcinoma showing malignant tumor cells with keratin pearls

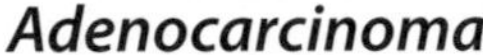

Adenocarcinoma

It is most commonly seen in women and nonsmokers. They appear as irregular masses in the **peripheral area**. Cut section is grayish white. Microscopically, they show glandular differentiation.

Neuroendocrine Tumors

Small cell carcinoma (previously oat cell carcinoma): It is a highly malignant/aggressive epithelial tumor and is strongly associated with cigarette smoking. The male-to-female ratio is 2:1.

- **Gross:** These tumors may arise in major bronchi or in the periphery of the lung. Cut section shows **soft** and **white tumor** with hemorrhage and necrosis.
- **Microscopy:** It consists of **small round, oval, or spindle-shaped cells** having scanty cytoplasm. The **nucleus** has finely granular chromatin (**salt and pepper pattern**), and nuclear molding is prominent. **Necrosis** is common and extensive.

Secondary Changes Due to Tumor

The tumor may result in following changes:

- **Obstruction:** The tumor may grow and obstruct the lumen of a major bronchus.
- **Suppuration:** The impaired drainage of the airways can cause **bronchiectasis or lung abscesses**.
- **Compression or invasion** of the superior vena cava causes edema of the head and upper arm.

Spread of tumor (Fig. 15.14):

- **Local spread:** Extension to the pleural surface, pleural cavity or into the pericardium may cause **pericarditis** or **pleuritis** associated with effusions.
- **Lymphatic spread:** It may spread to the tracheal, bronchial, hilar and mediastinal nodes.

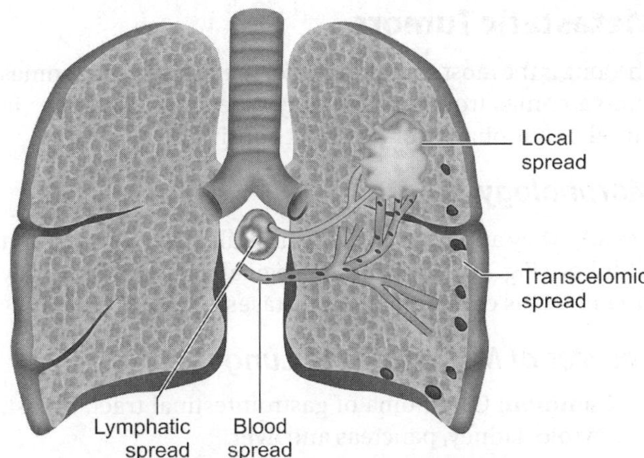

Fig. 15.14: Various routes of spread of lung cancer

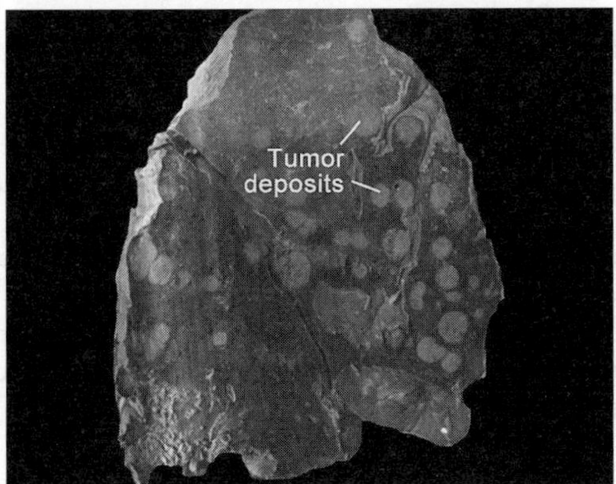

Fig. 15.15: Lung showing numerous metastatic deposits

- **Hematogenous spread:** Common sites of metastases are to adrenals, liver, brain and bone.

Clinical Features

Lung cancer is insidious in onset. It may present with cough, weight loss, chest pain and dyspnea. The tumor may present with symptoms due to secondary spread.

Investigations

- Radiologic examination of the chest
- Cytological examination of sputum, and bronchial washings or brushings
- Histopathological examination
- Immunohistochemistry
- Molecular genetics.

Prognosis: Poor.

Metastatic Tumors

The lung is the most common site for metastasis. Carcinomas and sarcomas from any site may spread to the lungs via blood or lymphatics or by direct continuity.

Morphology

Usually, they appear as multiple nodules seen throughout all lobes (Fig. 15.15). On radiological examination, they are known as cannon ball metastases.

Sources of Metastases to Lung

- **Common:** Carcinoma of gastrointestinal tract, breast, thyroid, kidney, pancreas and liver.
- **Other tumors:** Osteogenic sarcoma, neuroblastoma, Wilms tumor, melanoma, lymphomas and leukemias.

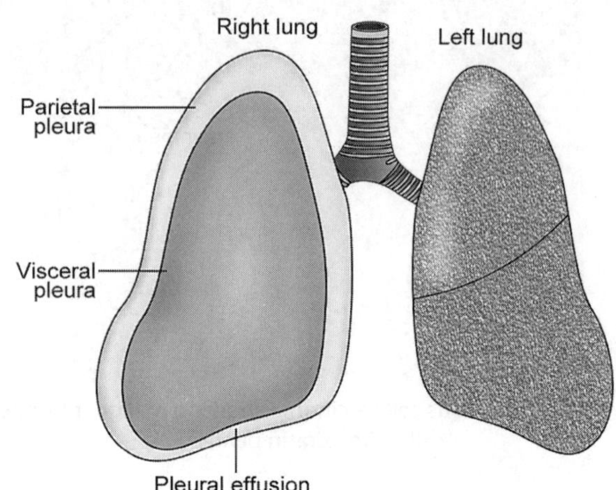

Fig. 15.16: Pleural effusion of right lung characterized by accumulation of fluid in the pleural cavity

PLEURA

The outer aspect of the lungs is covered by pleura. The pleura are serous membranes that have inner visceral layer which covers the lung and the outer parietal layer which covers the inner aspect of thoracic cage. The space between the visceral and parietal layer of the pleura is called pleural cavity. Normally, it contains less than 15 mL of serous, relatively acellular, clear fluid which lubricates the pleural surface. Inflammation of the pleura is known as pleuritis.

Pleural Effusion (Fig. 15.16)

Definition: Accumulation of fluid in the pleural cavity is known as pleural effusion. Pleural effusion is a common feature of both primary and secondary pleural diseases. The disease may be inflammatory or noninflammatory.

Causes of Pleural Effusion

Accumulation of pleural fluid occurs in the following settings:

- Increased hydrostatic pressure: For example, congestive heart failure
- Increased vascular permeability: For example, pneumonia
- Decreased osmotic pressure: For example, nephrotic syndrome, cirrhosis of liver.
- Decreased lymphatic drainage: For example, mediastinal carcinomatosis.

Inflammatory Pleural Effusions

- **Serous, serofibrinous, and fibrinous pleuritis:** The common causes of pleuritis are inflammatory diseases within the lungs. These include tuberculosis, pneumonia, lung abscess, and bronchiectasis. In most of the cases, the fluid is resorbed with either resolution or organization of the fibrinous component.
- A **purulent pleural exudate (empyema):** It is usually due to bacterial or fungal infection of the pleural space. Most commonly, it is due to spread of organisms from lung infection. Empyema is creamy pus composed of numerous neutrophils admixed with other leukocytes. Empyema may resolve, but usually it undergoes organization and forms dense, tough fibrous adhesions between parietal and visceral pleura.
- **True hemorrhagic pleuritis:** It is found in hemorrhagic diatheses, rickettsial diseases, and neoplastic involvement of the pleural cavity.

Noninflammatory Pleural Effusions

- **Hydrothorax: Noninflammatory collections of serous fluid** within the pleural cavities are called hydrothorax. The fluid is clear and straw colored. Hydrothorax may be unilateral or bilateral. The most common cause of hydrothorax is cardiac failure. It may develop with generalized edema and is therefore found in renal failure and cirrhosis of the liver.
- **Hemothorax:** The escape of blood into the pleural cavity is known as hemothorax. The causes include rupture of aortic aneurysm or vascular trauma or may occur postoperatively.
- **Chylothorax:** It is an accumulation of milky fluid, usually of lymphatic origin, in the pleural cavity. Chylothorax is caused by thoracic duct trauma or obstruction that secondarily causes rupture of major lymphatic ducts.

Pleural Tumor

Malignant Mesothelioma

Malignant mesothelioma is a rare malignant tumor of mesothelial cells.

Sites: Mesotheliomas can arise in the **pleura** (most common), **peritoneum, pericardium,** tunica vaginalis of the testis and genital tract (benign adenomatoid tumor). **Thoracic mesotheliom** arises from either the visceral or the parietal pleura.

Etiology: Exposure to **asbestos**.

Gross: Malignant pleural mesothelioma is a **diffuse lesion** that arises either from the visceral or parietal pleura. It usually **spreads widely in the pleural space** and is associated with extensive pleural effusion and direct invasion of thoracic structures.

Microscopy—types

1. **Epithelioid type (60%)**.
2. **Mesenchymal (sarcomatoid) type (20%)**.
3. **Mixed (biphasic) type (20%)**.

Clinical course

- Average age is 60 years.
- Chest pain, dyspnea, recurrent pleural effusions and nonspecific symptoms, such as weightloss and malaise.

Spread

- Direct local invasion of the lung.
- Lymphatic spread to the hilar lymph nodes.
- Hematogenous spread to the liver bones, peritoneum and adrenals.

Prognosis is poor and 50% die within 12 months of diagnosis.

SELF-ASSESSMENT EXERCISES

I. Essay

1. Describe the etiopathogenesis and complications of tuberculosis.
2. Define bronchiectasis. Discuss the etiopathogenesis, gross and microscopic pathology and complications of bronchiectasis.
3. Discuss etiopathogenesis and morphology of lung cancer.

II. Short Notes

1. Primary tuberculosis (Ghon complex) and its fate.
2. Secondary tuberculosis.
3. Lobar pneumonia.
4. Bronchopneumonia.
5. Pneumonia.
6. Lung abscess.
7. Emphysema.
8. Silicosis.
9. Asbestosis related diseases.
10. Bronchogenic carcinoma.
11. Chronic bronchitis.
12. Bronchiectasis.
13. Type of chronic obstructive pulmonary disease.

CHAPTER 16

Head and Neck

CHAPTER OUTLINE

- Oral Cavity
- Upper Airways
- Larynx
- Ears
- Salivary Gland

ORAL CAVITY

Oral Candidiasis (Thrush)

- ***Candida albicans*** is a normal component of the oral flora in about 50% of the population. Candidiasis is the most common fungal infection of the oral cavity.
- **Predisposing factors:** Several factors predispose to Candidiasis. These include the immune status of the individual, the strain of *C. albicans* present, and the composition of an individual's oral flora. It develops in patients on **immunosuppression**, such as in individuals with organ or bone marrow transplants, neutropenia, chemotherapy-induced immunosuppression, AIDS, and diabetes mellitus. It also develops in individuals on broad-spectrum antibiotics which eliminate or alter the normal bacterial flora of the mouth.
- **Clinical forms:** Three major clinical forms of oral candidiasis: **Pseudomembranous** (most common and is also known as ***thrush****)*, **erythematous**, and **hyperplastic**. The pseudomembranous form is characterized by a superficial, gray to white inflammatory membrane. It consists of matted organisms enmeshed in a fibrinosuppurative exudate. It can be easily scraped off.

Precancerous Lesions of Oral Cavity

Leukoplakia and Erythroplakia

Leukoplakia

Definition: It is defined as a **white patch or plaque, not less than 5 mm in diameter**, that cannot be removed (scraped off) by rubbing and cannot be classified as any other diagnosable disease.

If any white patches in the oral cavity can be given a specific diagnosis, it is not a leukoplakia.

- **Sites:** May be seen **anywhere in the oral cavity**. Most common sites are buccal mucosa, floor of the mouth, ventral surface of the tongue, palate, and gingiva.
- **Number:** It may be **single or multiple**.
- **Appearance: White patches or plaques** having **sharply defined borders**. Surface may be smooth or wrinkled.

Erythroplakia

- **Less common** and appears as a **red, velvety area within the oral cavity**.
- It remains level with or slightly depressed in relation to the surrounding mucosa.
- **Microscopically**, the **epithelium is atypical** and has an **increased risk of malignant transformation** than leukoplakia.

Intermediate forms, which have the characteristics of both leukoplakia and erythroplakia, are termed **speckled leukoerythroplakia**.

Features of leukoplakia and erythroplakia

Age and gender: Both leukoplakia and erythroplakia may be found in adults of any age, but they are usually seen between **40 and 70 years**. Male to female ratio is 2:1.

Etiology

Both have **multifactorial** origin and are associated with use of **tobacco** (cigarettes, pipes, cigars, and chewing tobacco).

Microscopy

Leukoplakia

- **Surface stratified squamous epithelium** show a spectrum of changes ranging from **hyperkeratosis and acanthosis** to lesions with **variable degree of dysplastic changes** (including carcinoma in situ).

- **Subepithelial region** shows **inflammatory infiltrate of lymphocytes and macrophages**, the intensity of which is proportional to the degree of dysplasia.

Erythroplakia

- **Epithelium shows erosions with dysplasia, carcinoma in situ, or frank carcinoma.**
- **Subepithelial region** shows **intense inflammatory reaction** and **vascular dilatation,** which is **responsible for the reddish clinical appearance**.

Squamous Cell Carcinoma

In India, oral cavity cancer is the most common malignant tumor.

Etiology

Squamous cell carcinoma (SCC) of oral cavity is **multifactorial disease** usually seen in middle-aged men.

Risk factors

1. **Tobacco products and smoking:** Any irritating smoked product increases the risk for tumors of the oral cavity. Nicotine in tobacco and other tobacco leaf components cause cancer. **Carcinogens in tobacco can act as initiators, as well as promoters.** Risk increases with amount and duration of tobacco use. Tobacco may be used either for **smoking** or as **smokeless tobacco**.
   - **Smoking:** It may be in the form of cigarette, beedi, cigar, or pipe smoking, or reverse smoking (smoking a cheroot with the burning end inside the mouth is practiced in certain regions of India). Regular marijuana use has also been associated with oropharyngeal cancer.
   - **Smokeless tobacco:** It is in the form of **betel quid**/pan that contains several ingredients such as areca nut, slaked lime, and tobacco, which are wrapped in a betel leaf. It is commonly used in India and Southeast Asia, and is associated with marked increase in oral cancer. **Betel quid appears to be the major carcinogen**. However, it may also be related to slaked lime and the areca nut. Other methods of tobacco consumption include snuff dipping and tobacco chewing.

   Oral cancers are found on the **buccal and gingival** surfaces in the sites **where tobacco products** are held in **contact** with the mucosa for long periods.
2. **Alcohol consumption:** It is another important etiologic factor and act synergistically with tobacco as either a cocarcinogen (increasing the risk) or a promoter (decreasing the lag time). The risk of oral SCC is magnified in individuals who smoke as well as consume alcohol.
3. **Other risk factors:**
   - Radiation exposure and solar actinic radiation (sunlight).
   - Welding, metal refining, diesel exhaust, wood stove, and asbestos exposure.
   - **Chronic irritation of the mucosa:** It may be due to ill-fitting dentures, jagged teeth, or chronic infections.
   - Vitamin A deficiency and immunosuppression.
   - Poor nutrition.

Role of oncogenic HPV virus infection

High-risk HPV types 16 and 18 and, less commonly low-risk HPV types 6 and 11 have been found in oral carcinomas.

Morphology

Site

Anywhere in the oral cavity. Common sites are lower lip, the ventral surface of the tongue, floor of the mouth, buccal mucosa, soft palate, and gingiva.

Gross

- **Early stages:** It appears either as raised, firm, pearly plaques or as irregular, roughened, or verrucous areas of mucosal thickening. May be superimposed on a leukoplakia or erythroplakia.
- **Later:** It may appear as **ulcerated and protruding gray white** masses with **irregular and indurated** (rolled) **borders.**

Microscopy

Squamous cell carcinomas (Figs 16.1A and B) range from **well-differentiated keratinizing neoplasms to poorly differentiated/anaplastic tumors**. However, the histological grading does not correlate with behavior.

Spread

1. **Local:** Tissue involved depends on the primary site.
2. **Lymph node:** The involved site of lymph node depends on the location of the primary tumor. The more anterior the tumor, more is the spread to the cervical nodes. Carcinomas of the base of the tongue and oropharynx metastasize to the deep retropharyngeal lymph nodes.
3. **Blood spread:** It spreads to lungs, liver, and bones.

UPPER AIRWAYS

Upper airways include the nose, pharynx, and larynx and their related parts.

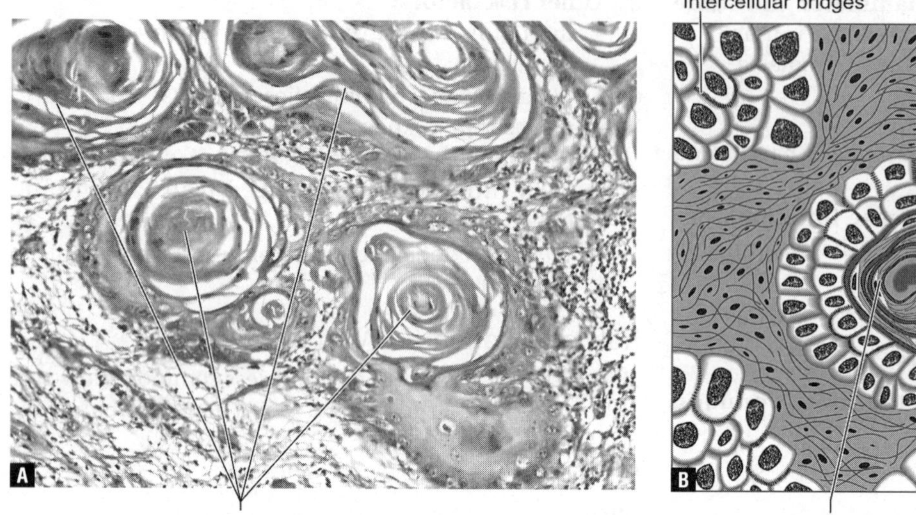

Figs 16.1A and B: Well-differentiated squamous cell carcinoma microscopic appearance. (A) H and E staining; (B) Diagrammatic

Nose and Paranasal Sinuses

Infectious Rhinitis

- Common cold is the most common cause of infectious rhinitis and accessory air sinuses. Most of them are caused by virus (adenoviruses, echoviruses, and rhinoviruses), but can be complicated by superimposed bacterial infections.
- Initial acute stages: The nasal mucosa is thickened, edematous, and red. The nasal cavities are narrowed and the turbinates are enlarged.
- Secondary bacterial infection produces a mucopurulent or sometimes frankly suppurative exudate.

Allergic Rhinitis

- Allergic rhinitis (hay fever) is initiated by hypersensitivity reactions to allergens. These allergens include the plant pollens, fungi, animal allergens, and dust mites.
- The nasal mucosal shows edema, redness, and increased mucus secretion.

Nasal Polyps

- Recurrent attacks of rhinitis can lead to focal protrusions of the mucosa. This can produce nasal polyps.
- Microscopically, these polyps consist of edematous mucosa with a loose stroma, and inflammatory cells (neutrophils, eosinophils, and plasma cells).
- When multiple or large, the polyps may impair sinus drainage.

Chronic Rhinitis

Chronic rhinitis is a sequel to repeated attacks of acute rhinitis (either microbial or allergic). A deviated nasal septum or nasal polyps with impaired drainage of secretions can predispose to microbial infection. Microscopically, it shows inflammatory infiltrate of neutrophils, lymphocytes, and plasma cells.

Sinusitis

Inflammation of sinuses is termed sinusitis.

Acute sinusitis: Most commonly develops following acute or chronic rhinitis, but maxillary sinusitis may occasionally occurs due to extension of a periapical infection through the bony floor of the sinus. The causative agents are usually inhabitants of the oral cavity, and the inflammatory reaction is entirely nonspecific. Impairment of drainage of the sinus may produce empyema (pus) of the sinus.

Chronic sinusitis: Acute sinusitis may give rise to chronic sinusitis. Causative agents include microbial agents that are largely of normal inhabitants of the oral cavity. Chronic sinusitis may also be caused by fungi (e.g. mucormycosis), especially in patients with diabetes.

Rhinoscleroma (Scleroma)

- Rhinoscleroma is a **chronic destructive inflammatory disease** caused by a Gram-negative diplobacillus, *Klebsiella rhinoscleromatis.*

- It begins in the nose and remains localized. But it may extend slowly into the nasopharynx, larynx and trachea. It is endemic in parts of the Mediterranean basin, Asia, Africa and Latin America.
- It can affect both males and females and any age. It is often associated with poor personal hygiene.
- **Microscopically,** it shows granulation tissue infiltrated by numerous plasma cells, lymphocytes and foamy macrophages. Characteristic large macrophages or **Mikulicz cells**, contain masses of phagocytosed bacilli. The disease is treatable with antibiotics.

Rhinosporidiosis

It is caused by *Rhinosporidium seeberi*. Usually, it occurs in nasopharynx but may also be observed in larynx and conjunctiva.

Microscopy

- Structure of nasal mucosa
- A number of spherical sporangia (with chitinous wall) containing small basophilic round spores.
- Chronic inflammatory infiltrate in the subepithelial layer.

Necrotizing Lesions of the Nose and Upper Airways

Causes of necrotizing ulcerating lesions of the nose and upper respiratory tract include:

- **Acute fungal infections** (including **mucormycosis, aspergillosis**), particularly in patients with diabetes and immunosuppressed patients. **Candidiasis** is the **most common** fungus infection of the nasal mucosa.
- **Chronic granulomatous lesions: Tuberculosis** of the nose (uncommon and occurs secondary to pulmonary tuberculosis), **leprosy, syphilis.**
- **Granulomatosis with polyangiitis**, previously called Wegener granulomatosis is a form of necrotizing vasculitis with granuloma formation affecting the upper respiratory tract, lungs and kidneys.
- Extranodal NK/T-cell lymphoma, nasal type, is a lymphoma in which the tumor cells contain EBV.

Nasopharynx

Inflammations

Pharyngitis and tonsillitis

Etiology

- **Viruses:** They are frequent caused by viruses. Most common are the rhinoviruses, echoviruses, and adenoviruses, and, less frequently, various strains of influenza virus.
- **Bacterial infections:** It may be superimposed on viral infections (mentioned above), or may be primary agent. The most common are the β-hemolytic streptococci, but sometimes *Staphylococcus aureus* or others.

It produces reddening and edema of the nasopharyngeal mucosa, with reactive enlargement of nearby tonsils and lymph nodes. If due to bacteria, the inflamed nasopharyngeal mucosa may be covered by an exudative membrane (pseudomembrane). Tonsils may be red and enlarged due to reactive lymphoid hyperplasia (**follicular tonsillitis**). The sore throat caused by streptococci may give rise to late sequelae, such as rheumatic fever and acute diffuse proliferative glomerulonephritis.

Tumors of the Nose, Sinuses, and Nasopharynx

Tumors in the nose, sinuses, and nasopharynx are infrequent. These include a wide variety of mesenchymal and epithelial neoplasms. Few distinctive types are described below.

Benign Tumors

Capillary hemangioma

It occurs in the septum of nose and is a common benign lesion. Morphologically, it is similar to its counterparts elsewhere (refer page 114).

Nasopharyngeal angiofibroma

Nasopharyngeal angiofibroma is a benign, locally aggressive, **highly vascular tumor that occurs almost exclusively in adolescent males.**

Sinonasal papilloma

Sinonasal papilloma is a **benign neoplasm** arising from the respiratory mucosa lining the nasal cavity and paranasal sinuses.

Sites: They may occur in the nasal vestibule, nasal cavity and paranasal sinuses.

Age and gender: Most common in adult males between the ages of 30 and 60 years.

Types: Three forms include:

- **Exophytic** (most common)
- **Endophytic (inverted):** It is biologically aggressive and most important because its downward growth (invaginates into the underlying stroma) must not be mistaken for carcinoma. It has a high rate of recurrence if not adequately excised.
- **Cylindrical.**

Etiology: HPV DNA, often types 6 and 11 may be etiological factor for exophytic and endophytic lesions, but not the cylindrical type.

Malignant Tumors

Olfactory neuroblastoma (Esthesioneuroblastoma)

Olfactory neuroblastomas highly malignant tumor that **arise from the neuroectodermal olfactory cells** present within the olfactory mucosa (particularly in the superior aspect of the nasal cavity).

Age: It has a bimodal age distribution with peaks at 15 and 50 years of age.

Microscopy: Olfactory neuroblastomas consists of nests and lobules of small, blue, round cells separated by a fibrovascular stroma. These tumors may be indistinguishable from other small cell malignancies (e.g. lymphoma, small cell carcinoma, Ewing sarcoma/ peripheral neuroectodermal tumor). They may show pseudorosettes (Homer Wright rosettes) or true neural rosettes (Flexner-Wintersteiner rosettes).

Clinical presentation: Usually present with nasal obstruction and/or epistaxis. It appears as a polypoid mass on the mucosa which may invade the paranasal sinuses or skull.

Spread: They spread through lymphatics to regional and distant lymph nodes. Hematogenous spread is less common.

Prognosis: Depends on tumor grade and stage.

Nasopharyngeal carcinoma

- Nasopharyngeal carcinoma **is malignant tumor** characterized a close anatomic relationship to lymphoid tissue, and an association with EBV infection.
- **Patterns:** It may be of three patterns: (1) **keratinizing squamous cell carcinomas**, (2) **nonkeratinizing squamous cell carcinomas**, and (3) **undifferentiated/ basaloid carcinomas** that have an numerous non-neoplastic, lymphocytic infiltrate. The undifferentiated/ basaloid carcinomas is also termed as *lymphoepithelioma*.
- **Etiological factors:** Three factors play a role namely (1) heredity, (2) age, and (3) infection with EBV. Nasopharyngeal carcinomas are common in some regions of Africa and are the most frequent childhood cancer. In contrast, in southern China, they are very common in adults but rarely occur in children. Apart from EBV infection, diets rich in nitrosamines (e.g. fermented foods and salted fish) and environmental factors (e.g. smoking and chemical fumes) play a role. Nonkeratinizing type is usually associated with anti-EBV antibodies against early antigens or viral capsid antigens.
- **Morphology**
  - **Keratinizing and nonkeratinizing** squamous cell lesions resemble usual well-differentiated and poorly differentiated squamous cell carcinomas arising in other sites.
  - **Undifferentiated/basaloid variant:** It consists of large epithelial cells with oval or round vesicular nuclei, prominent nucleoli, and indistinct cell borders arranged in in a syncytial pattern. These neoplastic epithelial cells are admixed with abundant, mature, normal-appearing lymphocytes.
- **Clinical features:** Primary nasopharyngeal carcinomas are usually silent for long periods, and present with nasal obstruction, epistaxis, and usually metastases to the cervical lymph nodes in as many as 70% of the cases.
- **Treatment:** Radiotherapy is the standard treatment. Overall 5-year survival of about 60% for all subtypes. Depending on stage, the 5-year survival for the nonkeratinizing type is 70–98%, while the 5-year survival for the keratinizing form is about 20%. The undifferentiated carcinoma is the most radiosensitive, whereas the keratinizing squamous cell carcinoma is the least radiosensitive.

LARYNX

The most common disorders of the larynx are inflammatory. Tumors of larynx are not common but are amenable to resection at the cost of loss of natural voice.

Laryngitis

Definition: Inflammation of larynx is termed laryngitis. It may be acute or chronic.

Etiology

- Laryngitis may be caused by **virus, bacteria, chemical or as an allergic response**.
- It is more commonly develops as part of a generalized upper respiratory tract infection or the result of heavy exposure to environmental toxins (e.g. tobacco smoke).
- It may also develop in association with gastroesophageal reflux due to the irritating effect of gastric contents.
- The larynx may also be involved in systemic infections (e.g. tuberculosis and diphtheria).

Consequences

- Most infections are **self-limited**.
- **Sometimes it may be serious** (especially in infancy or childhood) and constitute a medical emergency

when mucosal edema may cause laryngeal obstruction. This may occur in infants and young children with laryngoepiglottitis, caused by respiratory syncytial virus, *Haemophilus influenzae*, or β-hemolytic streptococci.

- **Croup** is the term used for laryngotracheobronchitis in young children, in which the inflammatory laryngeal obstruction/narrowing produces the symptoms of **inspiratory stridor cough and hoarseness**. This was a deadly complication of diphtheria.
- Laryngitis due to heavy smoking can predisposes to squamous epithelial metaplasia and sometimes overt carcinoma.

Reactive Nodules (Vocal Cord Nodules and Polyps)

- Reactive nodules (polyps) **develop on the vocal cords, most often in heavy smokers or in individuals who impose great strain on their vocal cords** *(Singer's nodules).*
- **Etiology:** They represent stromal reactions related to inflammation and/or trauma. It develops after voice abuse, infection (laryngitis), excessive alcohol consumption, or smoking.
- **Age:** Usually found in adults but may be seen in all age groups.
- **Gross:** The nodules are smooth, rounded, sessile or pedunculated excrescences, usually only a few millimeters in diameter, located on the true vocal cords (Fig. 16.2).
- **Microscopy:** They are covered by squamous epithelium and the core of the nodule consists of loose edematous, myxoid connective tissue.

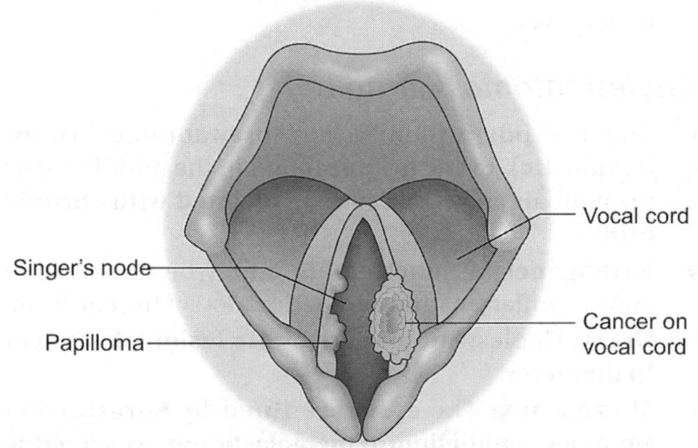

Fig. 16.2: Diagrammatic appearance of Singer's nodule, papilloma and carcinoma of larynx

- **Clinical features:** They may change the character of the voice and hoarseness. They virtually never give rise to cancers.

Tumors of the Larynx

Squamous Papilloma and Papillomatosis

- Laryngeal squamous papillomas are **benign neoplasms, usually located on the true vocal cords.**
- **Etiology:** They may be caused by HPV types 6 and 11.
- **Gross:** They are **usually single** in adults **but may be multiple** in children or adolescents (**juvenile laryngeal papillomatosis).** They form **soft, raspberry-like proliferations rarely more than 1 cm in diameter** on the true vocal cords or epiglottis (Fig. 16.2).
- **Microscopy:** They consist of multiple slender, finger-like projections with central fibrovascular cores and covered by an orderly mature stratified squamous epithelium.
- **Behavior:** They do not become malignant, but may recur.

Carcinoma of the Larynx

Carcinoma of the larynx is usually squamous cell carcinoma and **seen in male chronic smokers.**

Etiology: Risk factors include **tobacco smoking, alcohol,** nutritional factors, exposure to asbestos, irradiation, and infection with HPV.

Morphology

- About 95% of laryngeal carcinomas are **squamous cell tumors**.
- **Sites:** The tumor usually occurs on the vocal cords, but it may also arise above or below the cords, on the epiglottis or aryepiglottic folds, or in the pyriform sinuses.
- Squamous cell carcinomas of the larynx follow the growth pattern of other squamous cell carcinomas. They may be ulcerative or fungating type.
- Microscopically, they are similar to squamous cell carcinoma in other sites.

Clinical features: Carcinoma of the larynx is most commonly seen during the sixth decade of life. It present with persistent hoarseness, dysphagia, and dysphonia.

Prognosis: Depends on clinical staging.

Treatment:

- During early stage: Organ preservation techniques (laser surgery, microsurgery, and radiation therapy).
- Advanced or recurrent disease: Combined chemotherapy and radiation therapy, with or without salvage laryngectomy may be required.

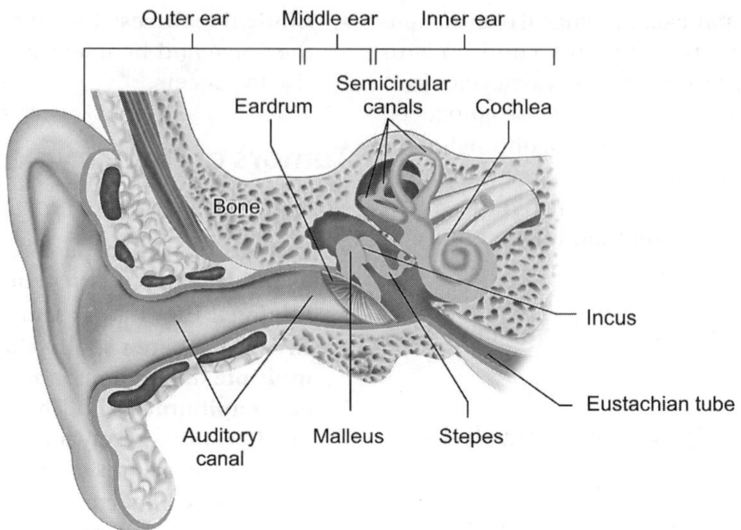

Fig. 16.3: Structure of ear (diagrammatic)

EARS

Normal Structure (Fig. 16.3)

The ear is divided into three parts: (1) the external, (2) middle and (3) inner ear.

- **External ear:** It consists of the auricle or pinna composed of cartilage, the external cartilaginous meatus and the external bony meatus.
- **Middle ear:** The middle ear has an opening, eustachian tube and the three ossicles (the malleus, incus and stapes).
- **Inner ear or labyrinth:** It consists of bony capsule embedded in the petrous bone and contains the membranous labyrinth. The bony capsule consists of 3 parts: (1) posteriorly three semicircular canals, (2) in the middle is the vestibule, and (3) anteriorly contains snail-like cochlea.

Most common ear disorders include: (1) acute and chronic otitis (mostly involving the middle ear and mastoid), (2) otosclerosis, (3) aural polyps, (4) labyrinthitis, (5) carcinomas of the external ear and (6) paragangliomas (in the middle ear).

Diseases of Middle Ear

Otitis Media

- **Inflammations of the middle ear** termed as *otitis media*. It may be acute or chronic and usually occur in infants and children.
- **Acute otitis media:** Usually due to viral infection. It produces a serous exudate but may become suppurative (pus) with superimposed bacterial infection. The most common bacteria causing acute otitis media are *Streptococcus pneumoniae,* non-typeable *H. influenzae,* and *Moraxella catarrhalis.*
- **Chronic otitis media:** Repeated bouts of acute otitis media which fail to resolve lead to chronic otitis media. The causative agents include *Pseudomonas aeruginosa, Staphylococcus aureus,* or a fungus. Chronic infection may cause perforation of the eardrum and spread of infection into the mastoid spaces. Otitis media in the diabetic person, when caused by *P. aeruginosa* may cause destructive necrotizing otitis media.
- **Serous or mucoid otitis media:** It is a nonsuppurative process characterized by accumulation of serous or thick viscid fluid in the middle ear. It develops as a consequence of Eustachian tube obstruction. It is an important cause of hearing difficulties in children causing hearing problems and can be relieved by removing the obstruction (e.g. in patients with tonsillar hyperplasia).

Cholesteatoma (Keratoma)

- This is **a postinflammatory** 'pseudotumor' (**non-neoplastic), cystic lesions** found in the middle ear or mastoid air cells. These are **associated with chronic otitis.**
- **Pathogenesis:** Not clear, but it may be the result of chronic inflammation and perforation of the eardrum.
- **Gross:** Cholesteatomas are **cystic lesions 1 to 4 cm in diameter.**
- **Microscopy:** The **cysts are lined by keratinizing squamous epithelium or metaplastic mucus-secreting epithelium.** The cyst is **filled with amorphous keratin material admixed with cholesterol crystals** and large number of histiocytes.

Diseases of Inner Ear

Ménière's Disease

- Ménière's disease is clinically characterized by attacks of nausea, vertigo, nystagmus, tinnitus and hearing loss.
- **Etiology:** Uncertain, but similar symptoms may develop in postinfectious labyrinthitis following upper respiratory tract viral infections.
- **Pathogenesis:** Unknown. It results in distension of the endolymphatic system in the cochlear duct and saccule.

Labyrinthitis

- Infections of the labyrinth is termed labyrinthitis. It usually caused by virus (e.g. mumps, cytomegalovirus and rubella). The inflammatory process usually subsides spontaneously.

Otosclerosis

- The term **otosclerosis refers to abnormal deposition of bone in the middle ear** around the stapes footplate. It is one of the **commonest causes of hearing loss in young adults**. Both ears are usually affected.
- In most instances, it is inherited as an autosomal dominant trait with variable penetrance.
- Treatment: Surgically by stapedectomy.

Tumors of Ear

Epithelial and mesenchymal tumors in the ear (external, middle, internal) are **rare** except **basal cell or squamous cell carcinomas** of the pinna (external ear). These carcinomas are observed in elderly men and are associated with sun exposure. By contrast, squamous cell carcinomas of the auditory canal are seen mostly in middle-aged to elderly women and are not associated with sun exposure. They morphologically appear similar to their counterparts in other skin locations. Basal cell and squamous cell lesions of the pinna usually invade locally but rarely spread. Squamous cell carcinomas arising in the external canal may invade the cranial cavity or metastasize to regional nodes.

Jugular Paraganglioma (Glomus Jugulare Tumor, Non-Chromaffin Paraganglioma)

- Tumors arising from parasympathetic ganglia are called 'paraganglioma' and are named according to the location of the tissue of origin. Tumor arising from glomus jugulare bodies of the middle ear (jugulotympanic bodies) is called jugular paraganglioma or chemodectoma or non-chromaffin paraganglioma.
- It is the most common benign tumor of the middle ear. **Microscopically**, the tumor cells are arranged in organoid pattern or nests.

Acoustic Neuroma (Acoustic Schwannoma)

- It is a benign tumor of Schwann cells of 8th cranial nerve.
- Site: Usually located in the internal auditory canal and cerebellopontine angle.
- It is similar to other schwannomas. However, because of its location and large size, may produce compression of the important neighboring tissues leading to deafness, tinnitus, paralysis of 5th and 7th cranial nerves, compression of the brainstem and hydrocephalus.
- It may be associated with long-term use of mobile phone.

SALIVARY GLANDS

Salivary glands consists of two main groups namely major and minor. Major salivary glands are three paired glands: parotid, submandibular and sublingual. There are numerous minor salivary glands widely distributed in the mucosa of oral cavity.

Tumors of the Salivary Gland

Salivary gland neoplasms are relatively uncommon.

Incidence

- Parotid gland—65–80% and ~15–30% parotid tumors are malignant
- Submandibular gland—10% and ~40% are malignant
- Minor salivary glands including the sublingual glands—10%. About 50% of minor salivary gland and 70–90% of sublingual tumors are malignant
- Malignancy in salivary gland is inversely proportional to the size of the gland.

Classification of Salivary Glands Tumors (Table 16.1)

Table 16.1: Classification of tumors of the salivary glands

Benign	Malignant
Pleomorphic adenoma (mixed tumor)	Mucoepidermoid carcinoma
Warthin tumor	Adenocarcinoma
Oncocytoma	Acinic cell carcinoma
Basal cell adenoma	Adenoid cystic carcinoma
	Malignant mixed tumor

Clinical Presentation

- **Age:** Benign tumors occur in the fifth to seventh decades of life. The malignant tumors appear later
- **Sex: Slight female predominance**, except **Warthin tumor, which occur often in males than in females**.
- Parotid gland neoplasms produce swellings in front of and below the ear.
- Both benign and malignant tumors range in size from 4–6 cm in diameter.
- Most tumors are mobile except advanced malignant tumor.

Pleomorphic Adenoma

Pleomorphic adenoma is a **most common benign tumor of the salivary glands,** characterized by an **admixture of epithelial and stromal elements**, and is also called **mixed tumors**. In pathology, the term "pleomorphic" is used to indicate nuclear variation (size and shape of nuclei) in neoplasm. However, the term pleomorphic adenoma is used because of variable cell type seen in this lesion.

Age: It occurs usually during **third to fifth decade** of life (middle-age).

Sex: It is most frequent in **females**.

Site

- **Major salivary gland:** Common site and constitute about 60% of tumors in the parotid. Usually arise in the **superficial lobe of the parotid**. Less common in the submandibular glands and very rare in the sub-lingual gland.
- **Minor salivary gland:** Its involvement is relatively rare.

Etiology

Not known. Exposure to radiation increases the risk.

- **Nature:** It is a benign tumor.
- **Cell of origin:** Histogenesis uncertain. **It was called as mixed tumor**, because of the mixture of epithelial and mesenchymal components. However, it is now considered that the tumor neoplastic cells (epithelial and those which appear mesenchymal), are of either **myoepithelial or ductal reserve cell origin.**

Morphology

Gross

- **Size:** Ranges from **2.5 to 6 cm in diameter**.
- **Consistency: Usually rubbery**, resilient mass with a **bosselated surface**.
- **Well-circumscribed/capsulated:** In some, the capsule is not fully developed, and small extensions can be seen protruding into the surrounding salivary gland. This makes enucleation of the tumor difficult.
- **Cut surface:** It shows **gray-white** with **myxoid and blue glistening, translucent chondroid** (cartilage-like).

Microscopy (Fig. 16.4)

Characteristic feature is the **pleomorphic appearance**. Neoplastic cells show varying **mixture of epithelial tissue** component intermingled with **cells showing mesenchymal differentiation.**

- **Epithelial element:** This component consists of **ductal cells and myoepithelial cells**. **Epithelial elements** are arranged in the form of **ducts, acini and irregular tubules**. The ducts are lined by both epithelial (cuboidal to columnar) cells and **surrounded by myoepithelial components** (a layer of deeply chromatic, small myoepithelial cells).
- **Mesenchymal-like elements:** The epithelial elements are dispersed within a varying amount of mesenchyme-like background of loose **myxoid tissue, islands of hyaline, chondroid (cartilaginous), and mucoid matrix.**

Clinical Features

- Pleomorphic adenomas present as **painless, slow-growing, mobile, discrete** tumors in the **parotid or submandibular** areas or in the buccal cavity.

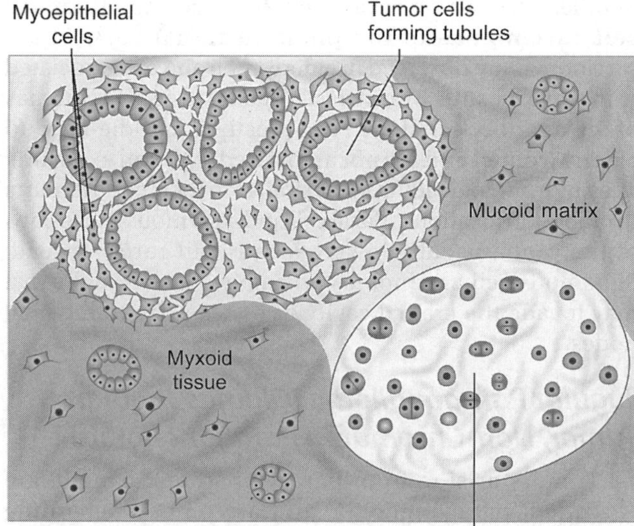

Fig. 16.4: Microscopic features of pleomorphic adenoma of salivary gland (diagrammatic)

- The tumors tend to protrude focally from the main tumor into adjacent tissues.

Warthin Tumor

Warthin tumor (**papillary cystadenoma lymphomatosum, adenolymphoma**) is a **benign** and the **second most common** salivary gland neoplasm.

- **Site:** It almost **exclusively** arises in the **parotid gland**.
- **Sex:** It is the only salivary glands tumor that is more **common in males** than in females.
- **Age:** It usually occur between **fifth to seventh** decades of life.
- **Predisposing factor: Smokers** have eight times the risk of nonsmokers.

Morphology

Gross

- **Shape:** It is round to oval, **encapsulated masses**.
- **Size:** It ranges from **2 to 5 cm** in diameter.
- Usually arises in the **superficial parotid gland** and are readily palpable.
- About 10% are multifocal and 10% bilateral.
- **Cut section:** It is **pale gray** tumor punctuated by narrow cystic or cleft-like spaces filled with a mucinous or serous secretion or even resemble used (dark) motor oil.

Microscopy (Fig. 16.5)

Tumors consist of cystic glandular spaces embedded in dense lymphoid stromal tissue.

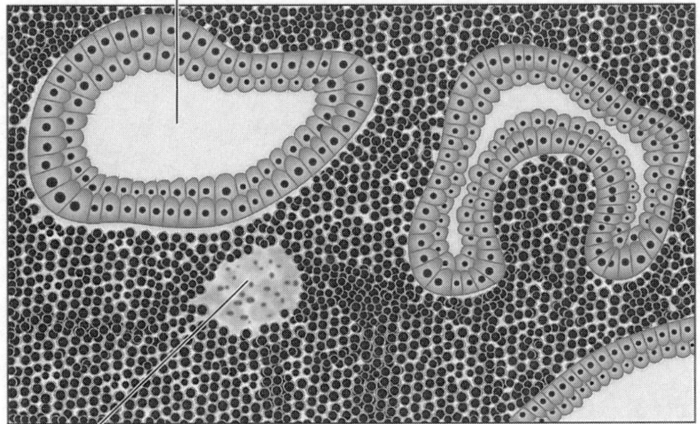

Fig. 16.5: Warthin tumor showing epithelial and lymphoid elements (diagrammatic)

- **Cystic spaces**
  - Cystic glandular spaces show **papillary or polypoid projections**
  - **Cystic spaces** are lined by a distinctive **double layer of neoplastic epithelial cells** consisting of:
    - **Surface superficial layer of columnar cells** with **abundant, finely granular, eosinophilic cytoplasm** (oncocytes).
    - **Second layer** below the superficial layer consisting of **cuboidal to polygonal cells.**
- **Lymphoid stromal tissue:** Cystic spaces are embedded in a dense lymphoid stroma which **closely resembles a normal lymph node.**

Behavior: It is **benign**, and about 2% may recur.

Mucoepidermoid Carcinoma

Most common primary malignant tumor of the salivary glands.

Incidence

- Constitute about 15% of all salivary gland tumors.
- Occur mainly (60–70%) in the parotids.
- Account for a major fraction of the minor salivary gland tumors.

Morphology

Gross

- **Size:** It can grow as large as 8 cm in diameter.
- **Appear circumscribed**, but do not show well-defined capsules and are often infiltrative at the margins.
- **Cut section:** It is **pale and gray-white** and frequently contain small, mucin-containing **cysts.**

Microscopy

Composed of variable mixtures of:

1. Squamous cells
2. Mucus-secreting cells
3. Intermediate cells.

These tumor cells are arranged in cords, sheets, or cystic structures. The intermediate cells have squamous features, with small to large mucus-filled vacuoles. The mucus stains positive with mucin stains. The tumor cells may appear regular and benign or highly anaplastic and malignant.

Grading: These tumors are graded as low, intermediate or high-grade. Clinical features and prognosis depends on the grade of the neoplasm.

Adenoid Cystic Carcinoma

It is relatively uncommon malignant tumor.

Sites

- About 50% of cases is found in the minor salivary glands (mainly in the palate). Among the major salivary glands, the parotid and submandibular glands are the most common locations.
- **Other sites:** Nose, sinuses, upper airways, breast, etc.

Morphology

- **Gross:** Usually small, poorly encapsulated, infiltrative, gray-pink lesions.
- **Microscopy:** Composed of small cells having dark, compact nuclei and scant cytoplasm. These cells are arranged in tubular, solid, or cribriform patterns. The spaces between the tumor cells are often filled with a hyaline material.

Behavior

- Slow growing, unpredictable tumors with a tendency to invade perineural spaces.
- About 50% of tumor spread to distant sites such as bone, liver, and brain. Neoplasms arising in the minor salivary glands have a poorer prognosis than those that arise in the parotid glands.

Treatment of Malignant Salivary Gland Tumors

- Most patients with invasive salivary gland tumors are treated with surgery and radiation therapy. These tumors may recur regionally; adenoid cystic carcinoma has a tendency to recur along the nerve tracks. Distant metastases may occur as late as 10–20 years after the initial diagnosis.
- For metastatic disease, treatment is palliative usually chemotherapy.

SELF-ASSESSMENT EXERCISE

I. **Short Note**
1. Leukoplakia.
2. Squamous cell carcinoma of oral cavity.
3. Rhinosporidiosis.
4. Otitis media.
5. Pleomorphic adenoma.
6. Warthin tumor.

CHAPTER 17

Gastrointestinal Tract Disorders

CHAPTER OUTLINE

- Normal Anatomy
- Esophageal Cancer
- Stomach
- Intestine
- Tumors of Intestine
- Polyps of Colon
- Colorectal Cancer: Adenocarcinoma
- Malabsorption Syndrome
- Inflammatory Bowel Disease
- Peritoneum

NORMAL ANATOMY

Gastrointestinal (GI) tract (Fig. 17.1) is a hollow tube that extends from oral cavity to anus and is divided into upper GI tract and lower GI tract. The major parts of upper GI tract include oral cavity, esophagus, stomach and duodenum. The major components of lower GI tracts are: small intestine, large intestine, appendix, rectum and anus. The organs associated with gastrointestinal tract are salivary glands, liver, gallbladder and pancreas. The wall of the GI tract has four layers and from inside to outside; these layers are mucosa, submucosa, muscle layer and serosa. The main functions of GI tract are ingestion, mastication of food, deglutition, digestion, absorption and excretion of undigested food material as feces.

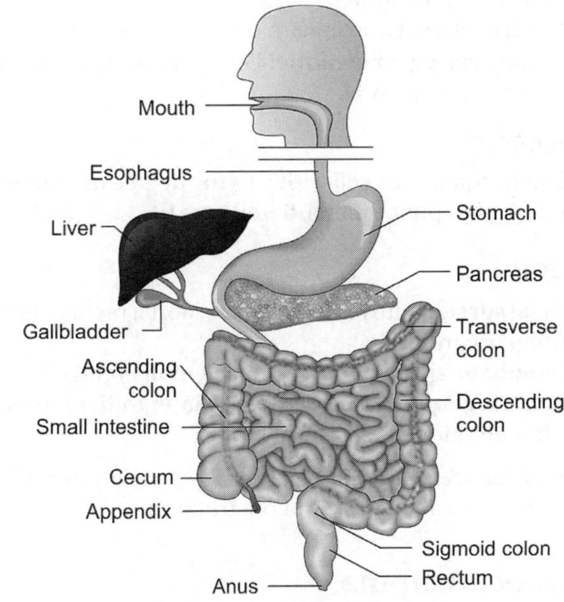

Fig. 17.1: Different anatomical components of gastrointestinal tract

ESOPHAGEAL CANCER

Morphologic types: Squamous cell carcinoma and adenocarcinoma.

Squamous Cell Carcinoma

Malignant neoplasm of the esophagus showing squamous differentiation.

Age and gender: Adults over age 45, M: F = 4:1.

Etiology

Risk factors

- High **alcohol** intake.
- **Tobacco smoking**.
- **Nutrition:** Poverty, **diet deficient in vitamins** and certain trace elements, **polycyclic hydrocarbons**, **nitrosamines**, fungal toxins in pickled vegetables foods, etc.
- **Hot beverages:** Frequent consumption of burning-hot beverages, which causes thermal injury.

Morphology

Gross

- **Location:** Most common in the **middle third of esophagus**.

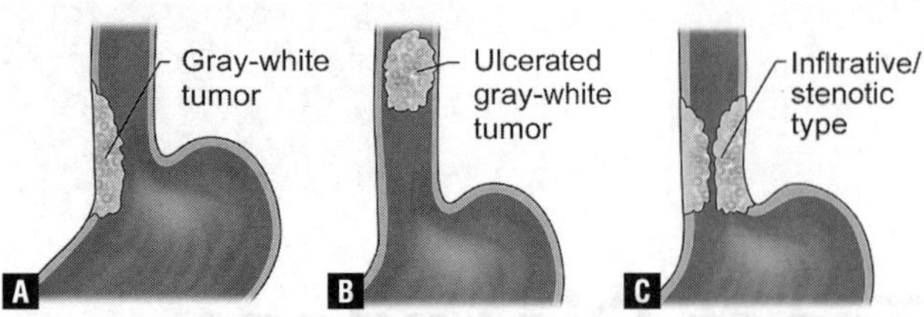

Figs 17.2A to C: Gross types of carcinoma esophagus. (A) Polypoid type; (B) Ulcerative type; (C) Infiltrative/stenotic type

- **Patterns of growth** (Fig. 17.2):
  1. **Fungating or exophytic:** Tumor protrude into and obstruct the lumen.
  2. **Ulcerative:** Growth with elevated ulcer edges.
  3. **Infiltrating, or stenotic:** Least common, predominantly intramural.

Microscopy

Malignant squamous cell with varying degree of differentiation (well to poor differentiated type).

Spread

- **Local spread:** Into respiratory tree, aorta, mediastinum and pericardium.
- **Lymphatic spread:** Into regional lymph nodes.
- **Hematogenous spread:** Occurs late; to liver, lungs, adrenals, kidneys and bones.

Clinical features: Insidious in onset. Dysphagia, odynophagia (pain on swallowing), and obstruction.

Adenocarcinoma

Carcinoma displaying glandular differentiation and usually arises in a **background of Barrett esophagus and long-standing gastroesophageal reflux diseases (GERD).**

Etiology

Risk factors include dysplasia, tobacco use, obesity and prior radiation therapy. Risk is reduced by diets rich in fresh fruits and vegetables.

Morphology

Gross

- **Site:** Usually in the distal third of the esophagus.
- **Appearance: Early lesions—flat or raised** patches, later **infiltrate diffusely or ulcerate**.

Microscopy

- It consists of malignant tumor with **intestinal-type morphology of cells forming glands**.
- Tumors most commonly produce mucin.

Clinical features: Pain or difficulty in swallowing, chest pain, progressive weight loss, hematemesis, or vomiting.

STOMACH

Normal Structure and Function

The stomach is continuous with the esophagus superiorly and the duodenum inferiorly. The convex part of the stomach, extending leftward from the gastroesophageal junction, is termed the greater curvature. The concave right side of the stomach is called the lesser curvature. Lesser curvature is about one-fourth the length of the greater curvature. The entire stomach is covered by peritoneum, which descends from the greater curvature as the greater omentum.

Regions of stomach: The stomach is divided into five regions (Fig. 17.3).

- **Cardia:** It is a small, grossly indistinct zone that extends a short distance from the gastroesophageal junction.
- **Fundus:** It is the dome-shaped part of the stomach located to the left of the cardia. It projects superiorly above the level of the gastroesophageal junction.
- **Body or corpus:** It is two-thirds of the stomach and descends from the fundus to the most inferior region.
- **Antrum:** It is the distal third of the stomach. It is positioned horizontally and extends from the body to the pyloric sphincter.
- **Pyloric sphincter:** It is the most distal tubular segment of the stomach. It is surrounded by a thick muscular layer which controls passage of food into the duodenum.

The lining of the fundus and body has prominent folds, the gastric rugae.

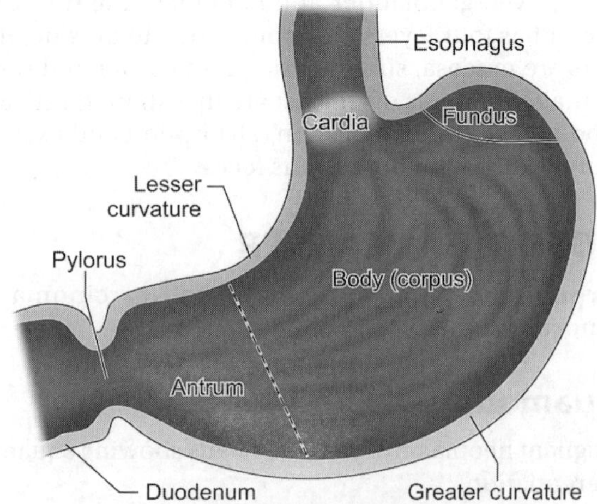

Fig. 17.3: Anatomical regions of the stomach

Definitions

- **Erosion:** Loss of the superficial epithelium which produces a small defect in the mucosa that is limited to the lamina propria (do not penetrate the muscularis mucosae).
- **Ulcer:** Break in the mucosal surface more than 5 mm in size, with depth to the submucosa (i.e. they penetrate the muscularis mucosae). It leads to a local defect or excavation due to active inflammation. **Gastric ulcers (GUs) and duodenal ulcers** (DUs) may be acute or chronic.
- **Gastritis: Inflammation of the gastric mucosa** and is usually a histological diagnosis. It may be acute or chronic.

Acute Gastritis

- Acute gastritis is a **transient inflammation of gastric mucosa**.
- **Etiology:** Drugs (e.g. aspirin, NSAIDs and other drugs), *H. pylori,* alcohol, chemicals, etc.
- **Morphology: Mild acute gastritis may not show** significant changes. **Severe gastritis produces s**evere mucosal damage, erosions and hemorrhage (termed as **acute erosive hemorrhagic gastritis)**.
- **Clinical features:** May be asymptomatic or cause variable degrees of epigastric pain, nausea, and vomiting. When severe, it causes mucosal erosion, ulceration, hemorrhage, hematemesis and melena.

Peptic Ulcer Disease

Definition: Peptic ulcer disease (PUD) is defined as a **mucosal defect** that is **at least 0.5 cm in diameter** and **penetrates the muscularis mucosae**.

PUD is **most often associated with** colonization with ***H. pylori*** and *H. pylori*-induced chronic gastritis (with hyperchlorhydria).

Normal Process in the Stomach

Two opposing sets of forces keep stomach in a normal state: (1) damaging forces and (2) defensive forces (Fig. 17.4).

Damaging forces

These forces are capable of inducing mucosal injury and consists of two gastric secretory products: (1) hydrochloric acid and (2) pepsinogen.

1. **Gastric acidity:** Hydrochloric acid **plays main role in digestion** but also **can damage the gastric mucosa**.

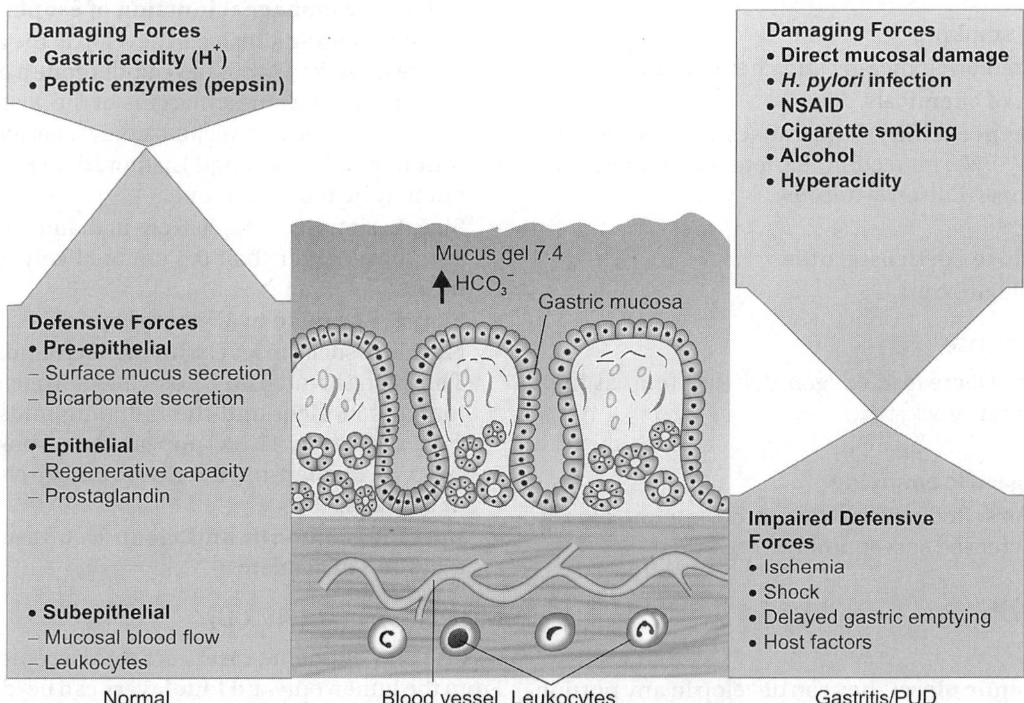

Fig. 17.4: Components involved in mucosal defense and repair in normal (left side) and in acute or chronic gastritis (right side)

2. **Peptic enzymes (pepsinogens):** They **can also damage** the gastric mucosa.

Defensive forces

These are a three-level barrier composed of (1) pre-epithelial, (2) epithelial, and (3) subepithelial elements.

1. **Pre-epithelial barrier:** It is a mucus-bicarbonate layer of the stomach.
2. **Epithelial barrier:** It consists of surface epithelial cells.
3. **Subepithelial barrier:** Rich gastric mucosal blood flow.

Pathogenesis of PUD/Acute or Chronic Gastritis

The imbalances between mucosal defenses and damaging forces cause chronic gastritis and also **PUD**.

Acute or chronic gastritis or PUD can occur due to direct mucosal injury or disruption of any of protective mechanisms.

Direct mucosal injury/increased damage

1. ***H. pylori* infection** is one of the **most important, common, primary cause** of PUD. *H. pylori* is a Gram-negative spiral bacteria with multiple flagella at one end. It is associated with ~ **85–90% of duodenal and ~65% of gastric ulcers**.
2. **Nonsteroidal anti-inflammatory drugs (NSAIDs) and aspirin**.
3. **Cigarette smoking**
4. **Alcohol,** radiation therapy and chemotherapy.
5. **Ingestion of chemicals**.
6. **Gastric hyperacidity:** The causes of hyperacidity include *H. pylori* infection, parietal cell hyperplasia and Zollinger-Ellison syndrome.
7. **Others**
   - **High-dose corticosteroids**.
   - Psychologic stress.

Impaired defense

- **Ischemia:** Decreased oxygen delivery (e.g. at high altitudes and shock).
- **Shock**.
- **Delayed gastric emptying**.
- **Host factors:** Reduced mucin synthesis in the elderly causes increased susceptibility to gastritis.

Morphology

Gross

- **Sites of peptic ulcer:** They can develop in any portion of the GI tract exposed to acidic gastric juices.

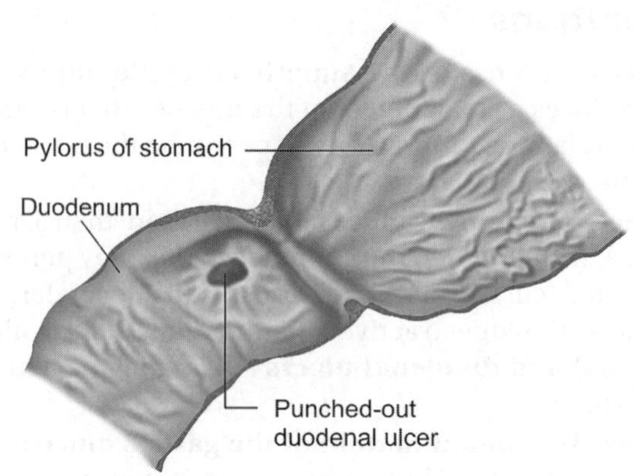

Fig. 17.5: Duodenal ulcer in the first part of duodenum showing characteristic sharp demarcation from the surrounding mucosa

  - **Duodenum** (Fig. 17.5)**: More common in the first portion of the duodenum** (anterior or posterior wall) **than in the stomach**.
  - **Stomach** (Fig. 17.6A)**: Lesser curvature** near the junction (transitional zone) of the body and antrum:
    - Proximal ulcers: Located in the body of the stomach.
    - Distal ulcers: Located in the antrum and angulus of the stomach.
  - **Gastroesophageal junction of esophagus**.
  - **Anastomotic site:** It can develop at the anastomotic site in patients who have undergone a distal gastric resection. Occur at margins of the gastroduodenal anastomosis/gastrojejunostomy (anastomotic ulcer).
- **Number: Solitary** (single) in more than 80% of patients, but may be more than one.
- **Size:** Lesions less than 0.6 cm in diameter are shallow and those larger than 0.6 cm are likely to be deeper ulcers.
- **Shape: Round to oval, sharply punched-out defect**.
- **Margin:** Usually **in level with the surrounding mucosa**. The gastric mucosal folds can be traced up to the margins of ulcer and the radiating folds of mucosa from ulcer (Fig. 17.6A) appear like a spoke wheel. In contrast, **heaped-up margins are more characteristic of cancers**.
- **Base:** It is **smooth and clean** as a result of peptic digestion of exudate.

Microscopy (Fig. 17.6B)

Gastric and duodenal ulcers are microscopically similar. From the lumen outward **four layers** can be identified and are known as **Askanazy zones**.

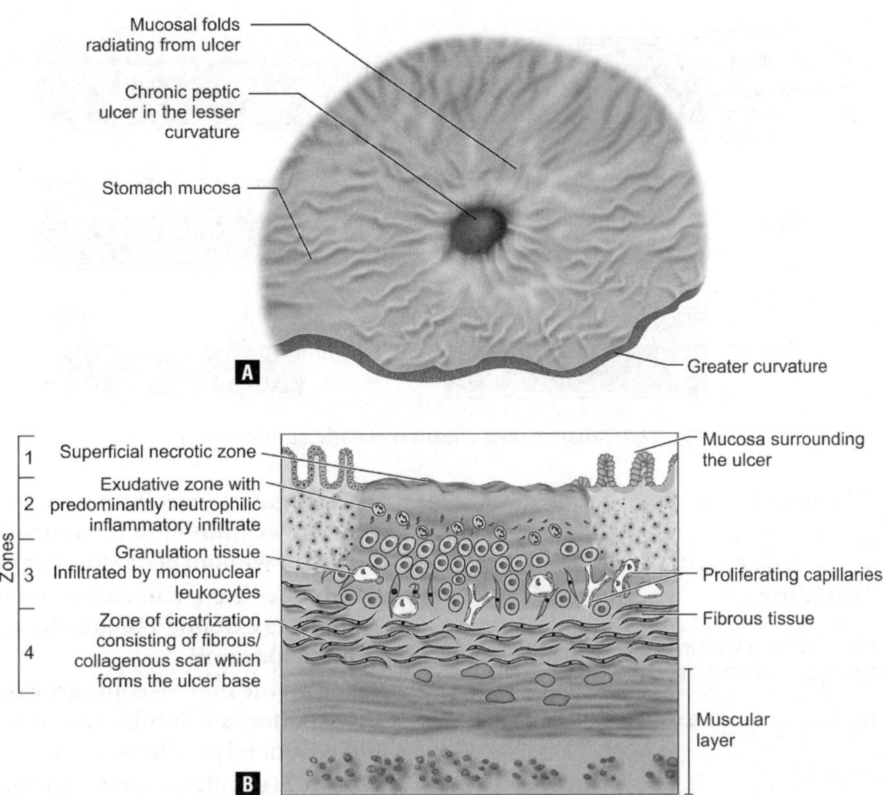

Figs 17.6A and B: (A) Peptic ulcer of stomach (Diagrammatic) showing characteristic sharp demarcation from the surrounding mucosa; (B) Microscopic features of a peptic ulcer (Diagrammatic) showing four layers of chronic gastric ulcer

1. **Necrotic zone.**
2. **Superficial exudative zone.**
3. **Granulation tissue zone.**
4. **Zone of cicatrization.**

Clinical Features

- Peptic ulcers are **chronic, recurring lesions with more morbidity than mortality.**
- **Age: Young adults** but are most often diagnosed in middle-aged to older adults.
- **Periodicity:** After a period of weeks to months of active disease, healing may occur with or without treatment.
- **Pain:** Epigastric burning or aching pain exacerbated by fasting and improved with alkali or food.
- **Other symptoms:** These include nausea, vomiting, bloating, belching, and significant weight loss.

Complications of Gastric Ulcers

- **Bleeding: Most common complication of peptic ulcer.** Chronic blood loss may lead to iron deficiency anemia. Severe bleeding may cause "coffee ground" vomitus or melena and may be life-threatening.
- **Perforation:** Develops in ~ 5% of patients and is the **most common complication of gastric ulcer.**
- **Pyloric obstruction (gastric outlet obstruction):** It is associated with ulcers in the pyloric region and occurs in ~ 10% of ulcer patients.
- **Rarely malignant transformation.**
- **Development of combined ulcers:** In the stomach and duodenum in the same patient.

Gastric Adenocarcinoma

Adenocarcinoma is the most **common malignancy of the stomach**. It comprises ~ 90% of all gastric cancers.

Etiology and Pathogenesis

Gastric cancer is a multifactorial disease.

Risk factors *(Box 17.1)*

Risk factors include: (A) environmental, (B) host and (C) genetic factors.

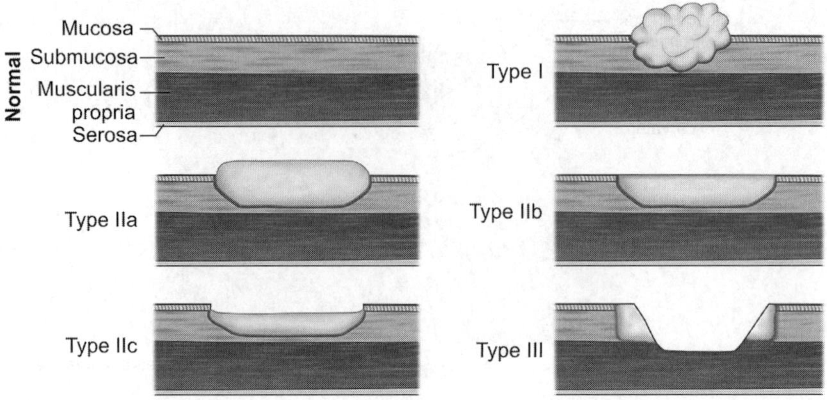

Fig. 17.7: Japanese classification of early gastric cancer

Box 17.1: Risk factors of gastric carcinoma

Environmental factors
- *H. pylori* infection (intestinal-type carcinoma)
- Epstein-Barr virus (EBV) infection
- Dietary/nutritional
  - Nitrites derived from nitrates (water, preserved food)
  - Smoked foods and excess of salt (salted pickled vegetables, chili peppers)
  - Deficiency of fresh fruit, vegetables, vitamins A and C, refrigeration
- Low socioeconomic status

Host factors/predisposing conditions
- Chronic gastritis (especially atrophic gastritis), pernicious anemia
  - Hypochlorhydria: Favors colonization with *H. pylori*
  - Intestinal metaplasia is a precursor lesion
- Partial gastrectomy: Favors reflux of bilious, alkaline intestinal fluid
- Gastric adenomas more than 2 cm

Genetic factors
- Blood group A
- Family history of gastric cancer

Morphology

Site

- **Pylorus and antrum (50–60%)**.
- Cardia (25%).
- Body and fundus (15–25%).

Lesser curvature is involved more often (in ~ 40%) than the greater curvature (~12%). Most favored site is the lesser curvature of the **antropyloric region.**

Classification of gastric carcinoma

There are several classifications of carcinoma of stomach.

- **WHO classification gastric tumors:** It is **based on the histological features.**
- **Based on depth of invasion:** According to this, gastric cancer can be divided into early gastric cancer and advanced gastric cancer.
  - **Early gastric carcinoma** (Fig. 17.7)**:** It is defined as a **cancer limited to the mucosa and submucosa, with or without** perigastric **lymph node metastases.**
  - **Advanced gastric carcinoma:** It is a neoplasm that has **extended below the submucosa into the muscular wall.**
- **Based on the macroscopic growth pattern** (Fig. 17.7)**: Three patterns** are observed and are used for both early and advanced gastric cancers.
  - **Type I (exophytic**/polypoid/fungating**):** It is a solid tumor **which projects/protrudes into the lumen** as a polypoid or nodular mass.
  - **Type II (flat or depressed):** It is a **superficial, flat lesion** with no obvious tumor mass within the mucosa and may be slightly elevated or depressed. Three patterns are: (1) elevated (type IIa) (2) flat (type IIb), and (3) depressed (type IIc).
  - **Type III (excavated):** It is characterized by a **shallow or deeply erosive crater** in the wall of the stomach. Characteristically, the **margins** of the ulcer are **heaped-up, beaded,** shaggy, and irregular and the **base is ragged and necrotic**. This is in contrast to that of the benign peptic ulcer, which shows punched-out margins and a smooth base.
- **Lauren classification depending on the histologic subtype:** According to this, there are two important types: Intestinal type and diffuse type.
  - **Intestinal type:**
    - **Gross:** It forms **polypoid bulky tumors or** may be **ulcerated.**
    - **Microscopy** (Fig. 17.8A)**:** It consists of cohesive tumor cells that **form gland-like tubular structures**, resembling adenocarcinoma of colon.
  - **Diffuse or infiltrating gastric adenocarcinoma** (Fig. 17.9)**:**

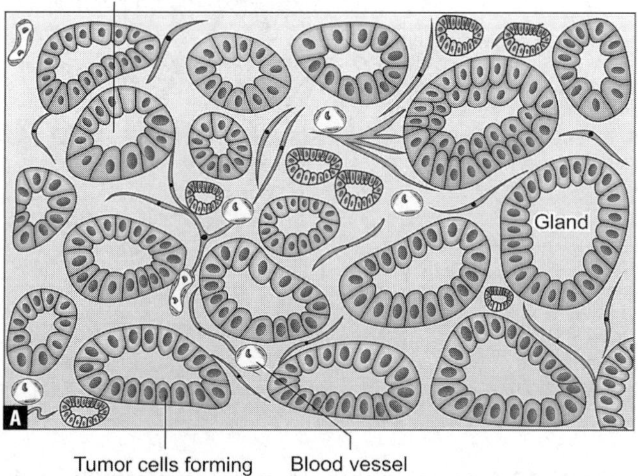

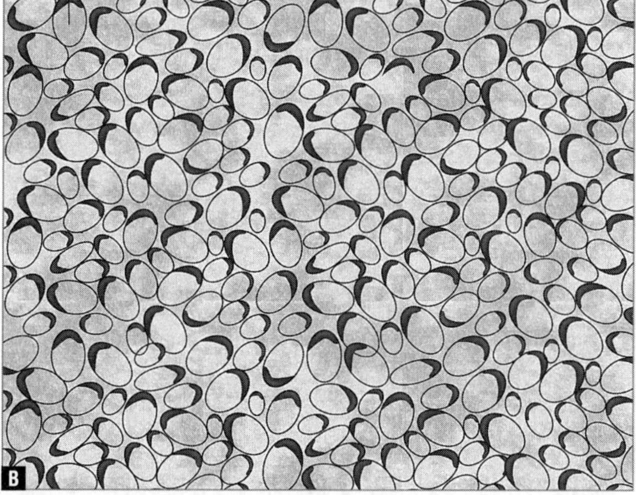

Figs 17.8A and B: (A) Microscopic appearance of intestinal type of gastric carcinoma (diagrammatic); (B) Microscopic appearance of diffuse type of gastric carcinoma predominantly consisting of Signet-ring cells (Signet-ring carcinoma)

- **Gross:** Diffuse gastric cancer **infiltrates deeply into the stomach without forming obvious mass** lesions. It involves broad region or entire stomach with local rigidity of the wall. They produce diffuse **flattening of rugal folds** in the mucosa and rigid, widespread **thickening of the wall.** The stomach may become nondistensible and lumen is narrowed producing **leather bottle appearance** termed **linitis plastic.**
- **Microscopy:** It is composed of **discohesive** (cohesion is absent) **tumor cells** which **do not form glands.** The tumor cells infiltrate and thicken the stomach wall without forming a discrete mass.
  - ◊ The **tumor cells contain abundant mucin** which expand the cytoplasm and push the nucleus to the periphery creating **signet-ring** (Fig. 17.8B) appearance.
    - If the signet-ring cells constitute **more than 50%** of the tumor, it is classified as **signet-ring cell carcinoma.**

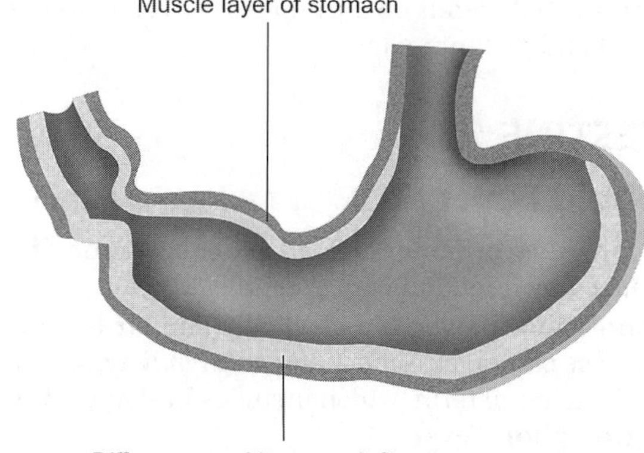

Fig. 17.9: Diffuse type of carcinoma stomach with leather bottle appearance

Spread of Carcinoma Stomach

- **Local/direct spread:** It spreads into the muscularis, and serosa of the stomach. It can invade into the duodenum, pancreas, liver, colon and retroperitoneum.
- **Lymphatic spread:** It spreads via to both regional and distant lymph nodes.
  - Frequently metastasize to the **supraclavicular sentinel (Virchow) node.**
  - Metastasize to the **periumbilical region:** This forms a subcutaneous nodule and is called Sister **Mary Joseph nodule** (after the nurse who noted this lesion as a marker of metastatic carcinoma).
  - Metastasis to the **ovaries** is called **Krukenberg tumor.**
- **Blood spread:** It can spread via the portal vein into **liver**. Other sites **lungs** and **bones**.

Clinical Features

- **Early curable gastric cancer:** It may present with nonspecific features.
- **Advanced cancer:** It presents with **early satiety, bloating, distension and vomiting. The tumor frequently bleeds causing iron-deficiency anemia**. Tumor in the pyloric region may present with **gastric outlet obstruction**.

Prognosis: It depends on the depth of invasion, the extent of nodal and distant metastasis.

INTESTINE

Typhoid Fever

- Typhoid fever (enteric) is an **acute systemic disease** caused by infection with *Salmonella typhi.*
- Paratyphoid fever is a clinically similar but milder disease caused by *Salmonella paratyphi.* **Enteric fever** is the general term, which includes **both typhoid and paratyphoid** fever.

Etiology

Causative agent: Enteric fevers are caused by ***Salmonella typhi* and *Salmonella paratyphi*.** *Salmonella* are Gram-negative, motile bacilli (rods). Boiling or chlorination of water and pasteurization of milk destroy the bacilli.

Source of infection: Humans are the only natural reservoir and includes:

1. **Patient suffering from disease:** Infected urine, feces, or other secretions from patients.
2. **Chronic carriers of typhoid fever:** *S. typhi* or *S. paratyphi* **colonizes in the gallbladder** or biliary tree may be associated with gallstones and the chronic carrier state.

Mode of transmission: From person-to-person contact.

- **Ingestion** of **contaminated food** (especially dairy products) and shellfish or **contaminated water**.
- **Direct spread:** Rare by **finger-to-mouth contact** with feces, urine, or other secretions is rare.

Incubation period: Usually 7–14 days.

Pathogenesis

- The typhoid bacilli (*Salmonella*) are **ingested through contaminated food or water**. They are able to **survive in gastric acid of the stomach** and reach mucosa of small intestine.
- They produce longitudinal ulcers in the Peyer's patches of small intestine.

Morphology

Intestinal lesions (Fig. 17.10)

- **Site:** Most commonly involved is **terminal ileum.**
- **Appearance:** Peyer's patches in the terminal ileum enlarge into sharply delineated, plateau-like elevations. The shedding of surface mucosa produces typhoid ulcers.

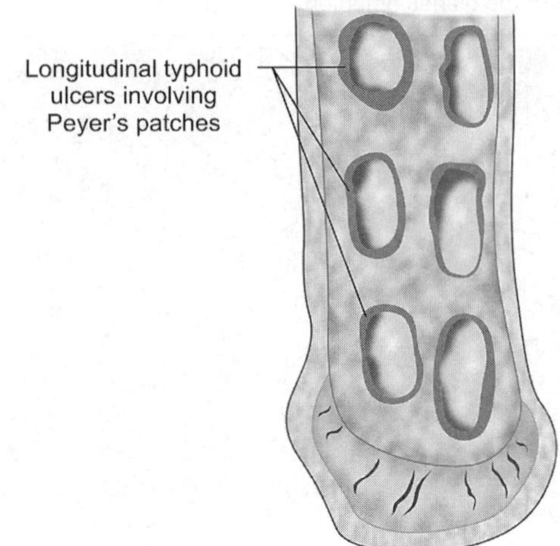

Fig. 17.10: Gross appearance of typhoid ulcers in the ileum of small intestine (diagrammatic)

- **Characteristics of typhoid ulcer: Number varies. Ulcers are oval oriented along the long axis of the bowel** (tuberculous ulcers of small intestine are transverse).

Gallbladder: Typhoid cholecystitis.

Clinical Features

- Onset is gradual and patients present with anorexia, abdominal pain, bloating, nausea, vomiting, and diarrhea.
- **Fever: Continuous rise in temperature** (step-ladder fever).
- **Rose spots:** These are small erythematous maculopapular lesions on the skin that fade on pressure appear on the chest and abdomen, which occur during second or third week.
- **Spleen:** It is soft and palpable may be accompanied by hepatomegaly.

Complications

- **Intestinal complications:** It can be fatal.
  - **Perforations of ulcer**
  - **Hemorrhage from the ulcer**.
- **Extraintestinal complications:** Encephalopathy, meningitis, seizures, endocarditis, myocarditis, pneumonia, and cholecystitis. Sickle cell disease patients are susceptible to salmonella osteomyelitis.
- **Carrier state:** Persistence of bacilli in the **gallbladder or urinary tract** may result in passage of bacilli in the feces or urine. It causes a '**carrier state**' and represent a source of infection to others.

Laboratory Diagnosis

Isolation of bacilli

- **Blood culture:** It is positive in **first week** of fever in 90% of patients.
- **Stool cultures:** It is almost as valuable as blood culture and become positive in the **second and third** weeks.
- **Urine culture:** It reveal is the organism in approximately 25% of patients by **third week**.

Other tests

- **Widal reaction:** Classic Widal test **measures antibodies against O and H antigens** of *S. typhi* but **lacks sensitivity and specificity**. Widal test (immunological reactions) become positive from end of the first week till fourth week. There are many false-positive and occasional false-negative Widal reactions.
- **Other serologic tests:** They are available for the rapid diagnosis of typhoid fever with a higher sensitivity.
- **Total leukocyte count:** It shows **leukopenia with relative lymphocytosis**. Eosinophils are usually absent.

DYSENTERY

Definition: Dysentery is defined as an acute inflammation of the large intestine (colitis) characterized by diarrhea with blood and mucus in the stools. Two causes are bacillary and amebic infections.

Shigellosis-Bacillary Dysentery

Bacillary dysentery is **a necrotizing infection** of the **distal small bowel and colon** caused by ***Shigella.***

Etiology

- *Shigella* causes bacillary dysentery and is one of the **most common causes of bloody diarrhea**.

Source of infection: Humans are the only natural reservoir.

Mode of transmission: By **ingestion** through fecal-oral route or via fecally contaminated water and food. It can be acquired by oral contact with any contaminated surface (e.g. clothing, towels, or skin surfaces).

Incubation period: It ranges from **1 to 3 days**.

Pathogenesis

- *Shigella* is the **most virulent** enteropathogens and ingestion of few (10–100 organisms) produces disease.
- **In the colon**, the bacteria penetrate the intestinal mucous epithelium and damages surface epithelium leading to superficial ulcers.

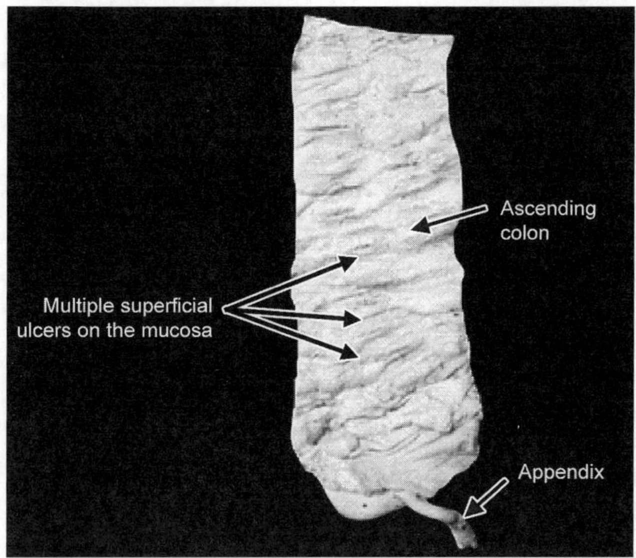

Fig. 17.11: Bacillary dysentery. Specimen of cecum and ascending colon (with appendix). Mucosa shows multiple superficial ulceration with intervening normal mucosa

- *Shigella* **produces a toxin** that has cytotoxic, neurotoxic, and enterotoxic effects.

Morphology

Gross (Fig. 17.11)

- **Site of lesions:** Most prominent in the **left colon** mainly in the **rectosigmoid area**. Mostly, the **lesions are continuous and diffuse**.
- **Characteristics of ulcer:** The ulcers are superficial. Mucosa shows **edema, ulceration** and appears **friable granular and hemorrhagic**. In severe infections, a gray mucopurulent exudate covers the mucosa. **Ulcers** appear first on the edges of mucosal folds, **perpendicular to the long axis of the colon**.

Clinical Features

- Presents as diarrhea, fever, and abdominal pain.
- The initial watery diarrhea progresses to a dysenteric phase.
- Stool culture is required for confirmation of *Shigella* infection.

Amebiasis

Amebiasis is an **infection caused by protozoan *Entamoeba histolytica*** (named so because of its lytic actions on involved tissue).

Etiology

E. histolytica has three distinct stages:

1. **Trophozoite stage**.
2. **Precyst stage**.
3. **Cyst stage**.

Source of infection: Humans are the only known reservoir for *E. histolytica*. It is reproduced in the colon of infected individual and passes in the feces.

Mode of infection: It is **acquired by fecal-oral route** through ingestion of materials contaminated with human feces containing *E. histolytica*.

Incubation period: About 8–10 days.

Morphology

E. histolytica can produce intestinal or extraintestinal disease.

- **Intestinal disease:** It mainly involves the **colon** and ranges from **asymptomatic colonization to severe invasive infections** causing bloody dysentery.
- **Extraintestinal disease:** It can produce **amebic liver abscesses**.

Colon (Fig. 17.12)

- Amebic lesions start as small **foci of necrosis,** which progress to **ulcers**. The floor ulcer **is gray and necrotic**. The **chronic amebic ulcers** described as **flask-shaped ulcer** with a narrow/bottle neck and broad base resembling a **flask**.

Clinical Features

Intestinal amebiasis: It may be asymptomatic or to produce dysentery of varying severity. Amebic dysentery may present with **abdominal pain, bloody diarrhea, or weight loss**. Liquid stools (up to 25 a day) contain blood and mucus.

Amebic Liver Abscess (Fig. 17.13)

It is a **major complication of intestinal amebiasis**.

- *E. histolytica* trophozoites **from the colon** may reach liver **through the portal circulation**.
- **Trophozoites kill hepatocytes** and produce **abscess**.
- Abscess cavity is filled with a dark brown, odorless, semi-solid necrotic material, which resembles **anchovy paste (sauce) in color and consistency**. The size of amebic liver abscess may vary and can exceed 10 cm in diameter.
- **Spread of amebic liver abscess.**
  - **Local spread:** It may expand and rupture through the capsule of the liver. It may directly **spread into the peritoneum, diaphragm, pleural cavity, lungs, or pericardium**.
  - **Hematogenous spread:** Rare and may spread to the **brain** and kidneys and produce necrotic lesions.

Clinical features of amebic liver abscess: It may present with severe right upper quadrant pain, low-grade fever, and weight loss. The diagnosis is usually made by radiologic or ultrasound demonstration of the abscess, in conjunction with serologic testing for antibodies to *E. histolytica*.

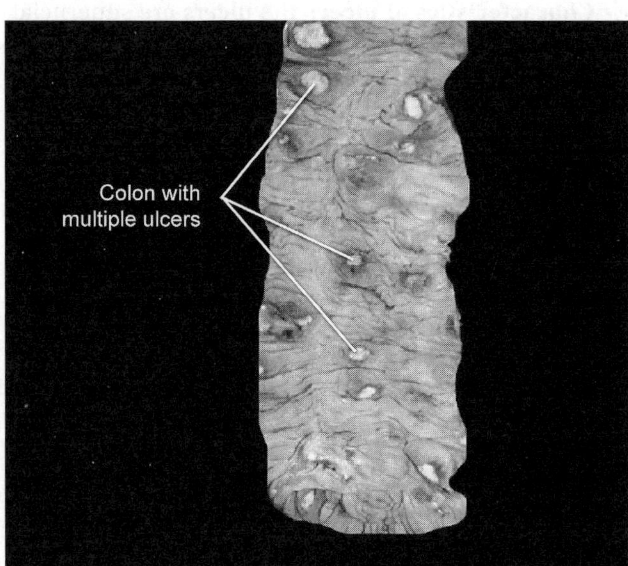

Fig. 17.12: Gross appearance of multiple amebic ulcers in the colon

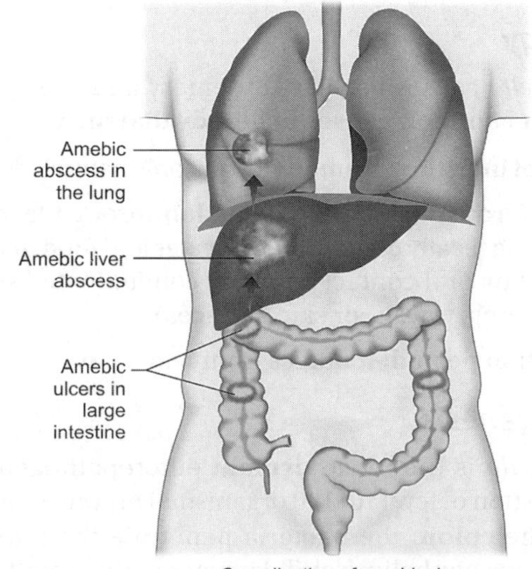

Fig. 17.13: Complications of amebiasis (diagrammatic)

TUMORS OF INTESTINE

Lymphoma

Extranodal lymphomas can occur in any tissue and most common in the GI tract, especially the stomach.

In the gastrointestinal tract, these tumors are called as lymphomas of mucosa-associated lymphoid tissue (MALT), or **MALTomas**.

Pathogenesis: In the GI tract, lymphomas arise at sites of pre-existing MALT, such as the Peyer patches of the small intestine, but more commonly arise within tissues that are normally does not contain organized lymphoid tissue. In the stomach, MALT is induced as a result of chronic gastritis. *H. pylori* infection is the most common inducer of gastric MALToma.

Morphology: Gastric MALToma shows a dense lymphocytic infiltrate in the lamina propria. These the neoplastic lymphocytes infiltrate the glands of stomach focally to produce **diagnostic lymphoepithelial lesions**. The lymphocytes are of B cell type.

Clinical features: These include dyspepsia, epigastric pain, hematemesis, melena, and constitutional symptoms (e.g. weight loss).

Carcinoid Tumor

Origin: Carcinoid tumors **arise from neuroendocrine organs** (e.g. endocrine pancreas) **and neuroendocrine-differentiated epithelial cells** of GI tract (e.g. **G-cells**).

High-grade neuroendocrine tumors are known as **well-differentiated neuroendocrine carcinomas**.

Sites of Carcinoid Tumors

- **GI tract:** Major site.
  - **Small intestine** (more than 40%) mostly in **appendix**.
  - **Stomach:** Gastric carcinoids may be associated with endocrine cell hyperplasia, chronic atrophic gastritis and Zollinger-Ellison syndrome.
- **Tracheobronchial tree and lungs**.

Morphology (Fig. 17.14)

Gross

- Carcinoids are **intramural or submucosal masses** and form small polypoid lesions.
- Mucosa covering the tumor may be intact or ulcerated.
- **Yellow or tan color**.
- **Very firm in consistency** due to intense desmoplastic reaction.
- May invade the wall deeply to involve the mesentery.

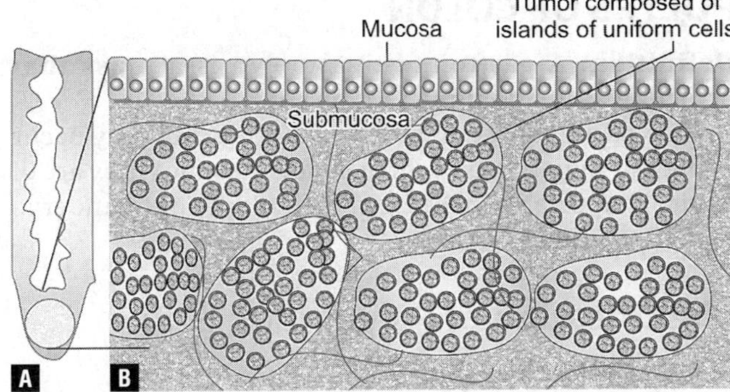

Figs 17.14A to B: Carcinoid tumor of appendix. (A) Longitudinal section of appendix with carcinoid tumor at the tip; (B) Microscopically shows uniform cells with round to oval stippled nuclei

Microscopy

- Composed of **uniform cells** forming **islands, trabeculae, strands, glands, or sheets**.
- Cells have **scant, pink granular cytoplasm** and a **round to oval stippled nucleus**.
- Most tumors show **minimal pleomorphism**.

Immunohistochemical stains:

- Tumor cells are positive for endocrine granule markers, such as **synaptophysin** and **chromogranin A**.

Clinical Features

Age: Peak incidence in the **sixth decade**, but can occur at any age.

Symptoms depend on the hormones produced. For example, if the tumors produce **gastrin it may cause Zollinger–Ellison syndrome. Ileal tumors may produce carcinoid syndrome**.

Carcinoid syndrome

- Develops in less than **10% of patients.**
- Symptoms are **due to vasoactive substances** secreted by the tumor.
- **Carcinoid tumors confined to the intestine, secrete vasoactive substances, which are metabolized to inactive forms by the liver**.
- **Carcinoid syndrome develops when tumors secrete hormones into a non-portal venous circulation**. Therefore, it is **strongly associated with metastatic disease**.
- **Clinical features: Flushing of skin, sweating, bronchospasm, colicky abdominal pain, diarrhea, and right-sided cardiac valvular fibrosis**.

POLYPS OF COLON

Definition: A gastrointestinal polyp is a **mass that protrudes into the lumen of the gut**.

Polyps are most common in the colon but may occur in the esophagus, stomach, or small intestine. They are of clinical importance because of their tendency to undergo malignant transformation.

Classification of Polyps (Box 17.2)

Neoplastic Polyps

The most **common and important** neoplastic polyps are **colonic adenomas** (benign neoplasms of intestinal epithelium) with the **potential for transformation** to **colorectal adenocarcinomas**.

Classification of Neoplastic Polyps

They are classified depending on:

1. **Growth pattern:** (a) pedunculated, (b) sessile, or (c) flat or depressed. Pedunculated adenomas have thin fibromuscular stalks containing prominent blood vessels derived from the submucosa.
2. **Architecture:** Adenomas can be classified as **tubular, tubulovillous**, or **villous**.

Box 17.2: Classification of gastrointestinal polyps

According to gross appearance
- Sessile: Polyps do not have a stalk
- Pedunculated: Polyps have a well-defined stalk

According to histopathological appearance
- Non-neoplastic
  - Inflammatory
  - Hamartomatous
  - Hyperplastic
- Neoplastic
  - Benign: Adenoma (Tubular, tubulovillous and villous)
  - Malignant

Morphology

Tubular adenomas (Adenomatous polyps)

They constitute two-thirds of the adenomas of large intestine.

- **Gross:** Appear as **small, smooth-surfaced, pedunculated polyps** usually **less than 2 cm** in diameter (Figs 17.15A and B). Tubular adenoma over 2 cm have higher risk of invasive carcinoma.
- **Microscopy:** Consists of **closely packed** small **rounded or tubular glands** (Fig. 17.15C) embedded in a **stroma** (increase in the number of glands and cells per unit area compared to the normal mucosa). The cells lining the glands are crowded and contain enlarged hyperchromatic nuclei. May show variable degree of epithelial dysplasia.

Villous adenomas (Villous papilloma)

- They constitute one tenth of colonic adenomas and are **predominantly** found **in the rectosigmoid region**.
- **Gross: Large, broad-based, sessile**, elevated lesions with **cauliflower-like surface** (Figs 17.16A and B). **Most are over 2 cm**, but may be as large as 10 to 15 cm in diameter.
- **Microscopy:** Composed of **thin, long, finger-like projections,** (papillary, crown-like growth) which superficially **resemble the villi of the small intestine** (Fig. 17.16C). The lining epithelium shows dysplasia similar to tubular adenomas. However, **villous adenomas** (larger than 2 cm) likely **contain foci of carcinoma more commonly than tubular adenomas**.

Tubulovillous adenomas

- They show a **mixture of both tubular and villous elements. Polyps with more than 25% and less than 75% villous component** are called as tubulovillous.

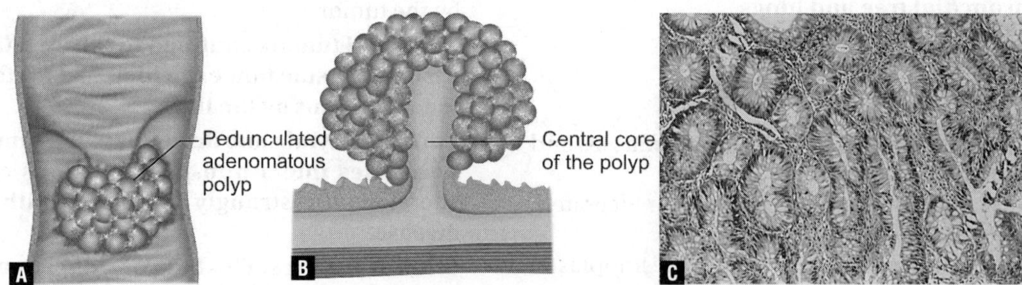

Figs 17.15A to C: Tubular adenoma (A and B diagrammatic). (A) Shows a pedunculated tubular adenomatous polyp; (B) Cut section of tubular adenoma shows a central core; (C) Photomicrograph shows closely packed tubular glands with dysplasia of lining epithelium

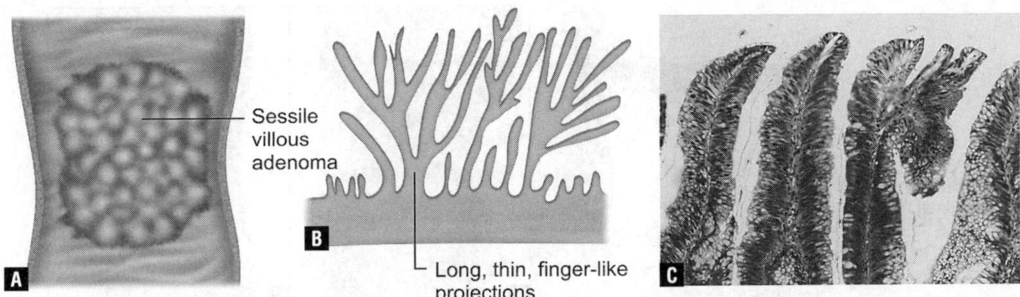

Figs 17.16A to C: Villous adenoma (A and B diagrammatic); (C) Thin, long, finger like projections covered by dysplastic epithelium

COLORECTAL CANCER: ADENOCARCINOMA

Adenocarcinoma of the colon (colorectal carcinoma) is the **most common malignant tumor of the GI tract**.

Etiology

The rate of colorectal cancer has increased significantly, probably as a result of changes in lifestyle and diet.

Dietary Factors

Closely associated with increased colorectal cancer rates.

- **Low intake of dietary fiber**.
- **Dietary high intake of refined carbohydrates and fat**.
- **Other dietary factors: Diets rich in cruciferous vegetables** (e.g. cauliflower, Brussels sprouts, and cabbage) and **vitamin A** may be associated with a **lower incidence of colorectal cancer**. **Deficiencies of vitamins A, C, and E,** which act as antioxidants (free-radical scavengers) may increase the damage caused by oxidants.

Adenoma-carcinoma Sequence

The colonic adenocarcinoma may evolve from the pre-existing adenomas, referred to as adenoma-carcinoma sequence.

Hereditary Non-polyposis Colorectal Cancer

Colon cancers in Hereditary non-polyposis colorectal cancer (HNPCC) patients develop at **younger ages** than sporadic colon cancers and are often found in the **right colon.**

Risk Factors

- **Increasing age**.
- **Family history of colonic cancer** in first degree relative.
- **Prior colorectal cancer:** It increases the risk for a subsequent tumor.
- **Ulcerative colitis and Crohn disease:** They have increased risk of colorectal cancer.
- **Others:** Physical inactivity, obesity (body and abdominal), smoking, alcohol excess (especially beer) and sugar consumption are some of the other risk factors.

Morphology

Gross

Location: Colonic adenocarcinomas can be found in **any location** of the colon.

Types (Fig. 17.17)**:** Grossly, colonic carcinomas can be categorized into four general types:

- **Exophytic polypoid mass in the right-side of colon:** They rarely cause intestinal obstruction.
- **Annular and constricting tumors in the left-side of colon:** These tumors are annular lesions that produce the characteristic **"napkin-ring"** or "**apple core**" **constrictions** and luminal narrowing. It **may be associated with intestinal obstruction** and dilatation with attenuation and flattening of the mucosal folds of colon proximal to the tumor.
- **Diffuse/tubular tumors**.
- **Infiltrative and ulcerating tumors**.

Microscopy (Fig. 17.18)

- Majority of colonic cancers are **adenocarcinomas** and are similar on microscopic examination. Adenocarcinoma may be **well-differentiated, moderately or poorly differentiated**.

Clinical Features

- Tumors in the cecum and other **right-sided colon** cancers usually present with **fatigue and weakness** due to **iron deficiency anemia.** Thus, it is important

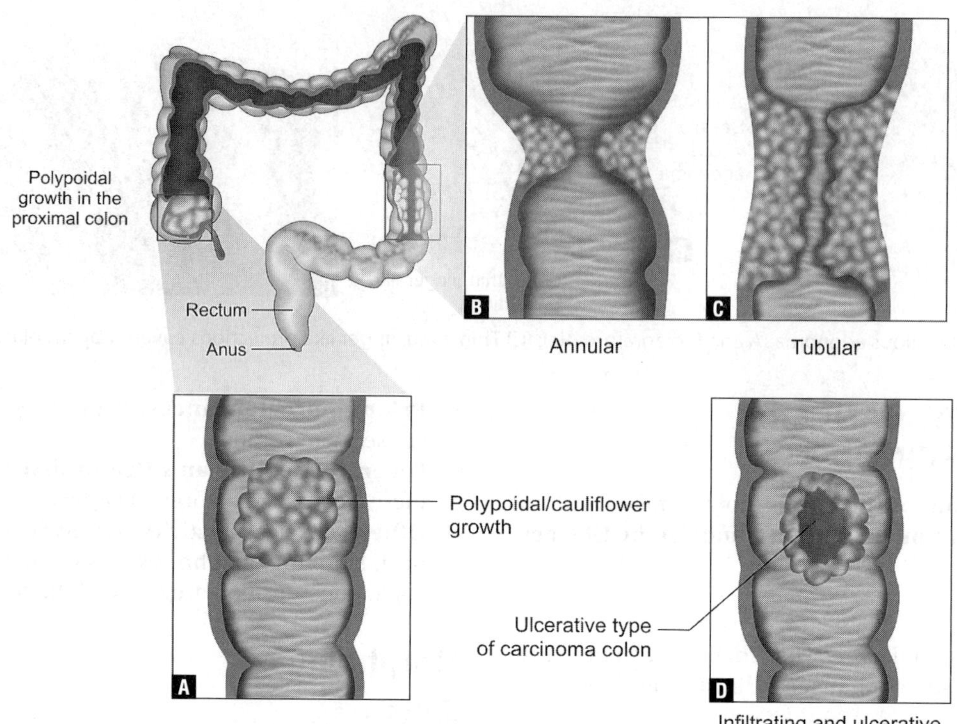

Figs 17.17A to D: The four common macroscopic varieties of carcinoma of the colon. (A) Exophytic/cauliflower/polypoidal; (B) Annular; (C) Tubular; and (D) Infiltrating and ulcerative. Carcinoma of proximal colon are usually polypoidal and exophytic. Carcinoma of distal colon are usually annular

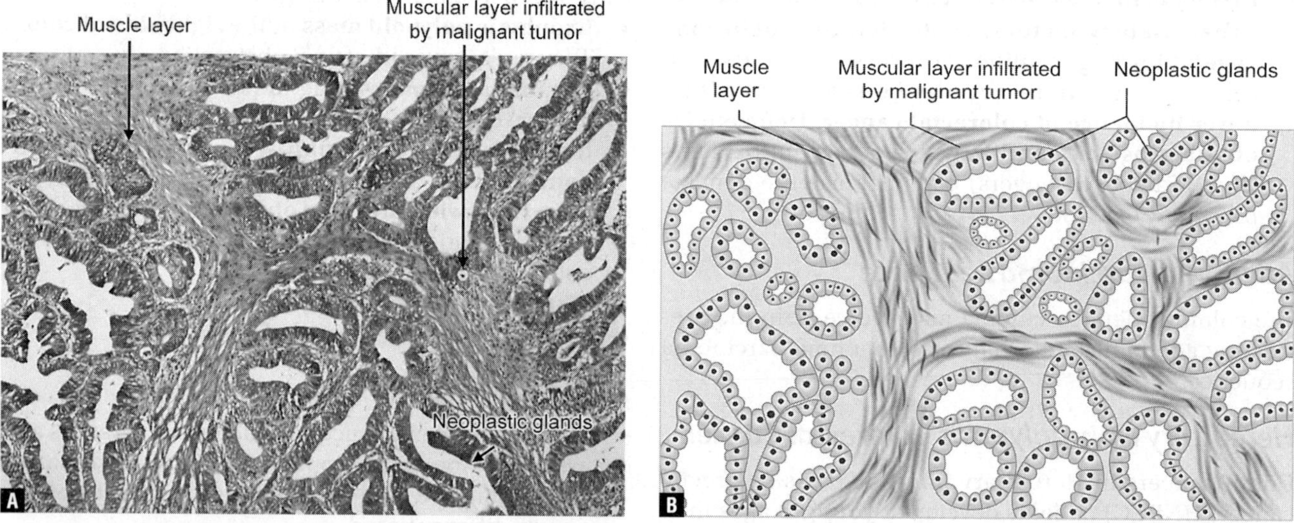

Figs 17.18A and B: Adenocarcinoma of colon composed of tumor cells arranged in glandular pattern. (A) Photomicrograph; (B) Diagrammatic

that **iron deficiency anemia in an older man or postmenopausal woman should be consider as due to GI cancer until otherwise proved**.

- **Left-sided cancers** may produce ***occult bleeding*, altered *bowel habits or pain and* discomfort** in the left lower quadrant.

Methods of Investigation of Colon Cancer

- **Occult blood** loss in the stool by Guaiac test.
- **Tumor markers: Elevated levels of carcinoembryonic antigen (CEA) and CA 19-9**.
- Flexible sigmoidoscopy.

- **Colonoscopy helps in direct visualization of cancer and may be used to take a biopsy:** Investigation of choice.
- **Radiology:**
  - **Double-contrast barium enema:** It is the radiological investigation of choice, when colonoscopy is contraindicated. It characteristically shows **"apple core" appearance**.
  - **Ultrasonography:** Used as a screening investigation for liver metastases.
  - **Spiral CT:** Elderly patients when contrast enemas or colonoscopy are not diagnostic or are contraindicated.

Staging and Prognosis

- **Two most important prognostic factors are depth of invasion and the presence or absence of lymph node metastases.**
- Invasion into the muscularis propria reduces the survival rate which is reduced further in the presence of lymph node metastases.
- Poorly differentiated and mucinous carcinomas are associated with poor prognosis.

Dukes and Kirklin, and Astler-Coller staging were used being presently replaced by **TNM (tumor-nodes-metastasis) classification** and staging system from the American Joint Committee on Cancer.

Spread

- **Direct spread:** The tumor can spread in a transverse, longitudinal, or radial direction.
- **Lymphatic spread:** Tumor may spread through lymphatics into the regional lymph nodes.
- **Blood spread: Venous invasion** may give rise to blood-borne metastases in the **liver** (through portal vein). It may also spread to **lungs and bones**.
- **Transcoelomic spread:** Rarely, it can spread by dislodging tumor cells from the serosa of the bowel or via the subperitoneal lymphatics to other structures within the peritoneal cavity.

ACUTE APPENDICITIS

- The appendix is prone to acute and chronic inflammation.
- Acute appendicitis is an acute inflammatory process involving the appendix.
- Acute appendicitis can occur in any age group but is most common in adolescents and young adults.

Morphology

Gross

- The appendix may be **swollen and erythematous**.
- The **serosa** initially appears dull and gray and later may be **covered by a purulent exudate**
- Perforation secondary to gangrene can follow and form abscess.

Microscopy (Fig. 17.19)

- The early lesions show **mucosal erosions**.
- Later, the inflammation extends into the lamina propria, and collections of neutrophils may also be seen in the lumen of the appendix.
- Diagnosis of acute appendicitis should be made when **muscularis propria shows infiltration by neutrophils**.
- In severe cases, neutrophilic exudate produces fibrinopurulent reaction in the serosa. When focal abscesses develop within the wall, it is termed as **acute suppurative appendicitis**.
- When appendix shows large areas of hemorrhagic ulceration and gangrenous necrosis, it is known as **acute gangrenous appendicitis**. This may rupture leading to suppurative peritonitis.

Clinical Features

Acute appendicitis presents with pain in the periumbilical region, which ultimately localizes to the right lower quadrant. This is followed by nausea, vomiting, low-grade fever, and a mild leukocytosis.

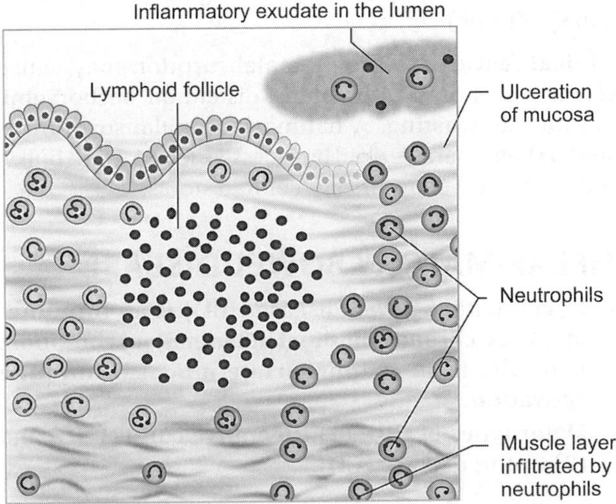

Fig. 17.19: Diagrammatic appearance of acute appendicitis

McBurney's sign: A classic physical finding is deep tenderness located two-thirds of the distance from the umbilicus to the right anterior superior iliac spine (McBurney's point).

Complications: Gangrenous appendicitis, perforation, pyelophlebitis, portal venous thrombosis, liver abscess, and bacteremia.

MALABSORPTION SYNDROME

Definition: Malabsorption is a general term which **most commonly presents as chronic diarrhea** and is **characterized by defective absorption of fats, fat- and water-soluble vitamins, proteins, carbohydrates, electrolytes and minerals, and water.**

Normal absorption: Some nutrients are absorbed in the stomach and colon, but only absorption from the small intestine (chiefly in the proximal portion) is clinically important. Bile salts and vitamin B_{12} are absorbed mainly in the distal small intestine. Normal intestinal absorption occurs in two phase namely: (1) luminal phase and (2) an intestinal phase.

- **Luminal phase:** It occurs in the lumen of small intestine. In this phase, nutrients is altered in such a way that they can be taken up by absorptive cells.
- **Intestinal phase:** This includes processes within the intestinal wall.

Causes of malabsorption: It is caused by many different conditions such as Celiac sprue, tropical sprue, Whipple's disease, damage of small intestinal mucosa (e.g. in tuberculosis, Crohn's disease, lymphoma, radiation injury), pancreatic insufficiency, short or stagnant bowel (blind loop syndrome).

Clinical features: Chronic malabsorption may cause weight loss, anorexia, abdominal distention, borborygmi, and muscle wasting. A hallmark of malabsorption is **steatorrhea**, characterized by excessive fecal fat and bulky, frothy, greasy, yellow or clay-colored stools.

INFLAMMATORY BOWEL DISEASE

- Inflammatory bowel disease (IBD) is an **immune-mediated chronic intestinal inflammatory condition**. It results from **inappropriate mucosal immune activation.**
- **Major types of IBD: (1) Ulcerative colitis (UC)** and **(2) Crohn disease (CD)**.

Epidemiology

- **Age of onset:** Both UC and CD occurs between **15 and 30 years** of age. A second peak is between the ages of **60 and 80 years.**
- **Cigarette smoking:** Risk of UC in smokers is 40% more than that of nonsmokers. Smoking is associated with a two-fold increased risk of CD.
- **Oral contraceptives** use: Increased risk of CD.

Etiology and Pathogenesis

- IBD is an **idiopathic disorder**. The exact trigger for inflammatory bowel disease is not known. Present evidences suggest that IBD represents the outcome of three main interactive factors: **Genetic, environmental and host factors.**

Crohn Disease

Crohn disease (regional enteritis) is a **chronic multifocal relapsing and remitting, progressive inflammatory bowel disease** of unknown cause that **can involve any portion of the gastrointestinal tract**.

Morphology

- Commonly occurs in the **terminal ileum**, but can involve any portion of the gastrointestinal tract.
- Lesions are usually **multiple** and each lesion is **sharply demarcated** from intervening normal bowel giving rise to **characteristic skip lesions.** It **helps in differentiating it from ulcerative colitis.**
- **Mucosal lesions: Aphthous ulcer** is the **earliest lesion. Later** the ulcer become deeper and form linear clefts or **fissures** that may extend deeply **to become fistula tracts or sites of perforation**. The **islands of normal mucosa between the ulcers** show edema and produce a **cobblestone** appearance.
- The **involved region,** shows **fibrotic thickening** and is **rubbery**. The **lumen is narrowed** and strictures are common. It appears **like a hosepipe**. Radiologically, characteristic **string sign** is due to only a trickle of contrast medium passing through the narrowed affected segment.
- **Microscopy:** Two major characteristic features: (1) **Transmural inflammation** (all layers of bowel) (2) **Skip lesions** (inflamed segments separated by normal intestine).

Clinical features: Intermittent attacks of **mild diarrhea, fever** and **abdominal pain.**

Complications: (1) Iron-deficiency anemia, (2) malabsorption, (3) stricture and fistula formation and rarely (4) development of carcinoma.

Ulcerative Colitis

Ulcerative colitis (UC) is a **severe, chronic crypt destructive, ulcerating inflammatory bowel disease** of unknown cause.

Morphology

- Ulcerative colitis is a **diffuse disease limited to colon and rectum**. Usually involves the rectum and extends proximally for a variable distance (continuous lesion) to involve part or the entire colon. It is **limited to the colon and rectum** and inflammation **involves** only the **mucosa and submucosa** of the intestinal wall. **Skip lesions are not seen** in UC.
- Chronic ulcerative colitis shows distortion of crypt architecture, cryptitis chronic inflammatory infiltrate, plasma cell infiltrate at the base of crypts (basal plasmacytosis) and mucosal atrophy.

Clinical features: Presents with **attacks of bloody diarrhea** with mucoid material, **lower abdominal pain** and cramps. It is clinically associated with exacerbations and remissions of bloody diarrhea.

Complications: Toxic megacolon (colonic dilation and toxic megacolon → may lead to perforation), **colorectal cancer, hemorrhage** from intestinal lesions and **electrolyte disturbances**.

PERITONEUM

The peritoneum is the mesothelial lining of the abdominal cavity and its organs/viscera. It consists of two layers namely visceral and parietal peritoneum. The visceral peritoneum invests the gastrointestinal tract from stomach to rectum and encircles the liver. The parietal peritoneum lines the abdominal wall and retroperitoneal space. The cavity between visceral and parietal peritoneum is called peritoneal cavity. The omentum is a double layer of peritoneum that encloses blood vessels and a variable amount of fat.

Peritonitis

Inflammation of the peritoneum is termed as peritonitis. Peritonitis may result from bacterial invasion or chemical irritation.

Bacterial Peritonitis

- Bacterial peritonitis is the peritonitis caused by bacteria.
- **Types:** (1) acute bacterial peritonitis or (2) chronic bacterial peritonitis

Etiology

- **Acute bacterial peritonitis:** It develops when **bacteria present in the gastrointestinal lumen** are released into the abdominal cavity. The most common cause of bacterial peritonitis is perforation of an abdominal viscus (e.g. an inflamed appendix, peptic ulcer or diverticulum of colon). The bacteria released from the gastrointestinal tract into the peritoneal cavity vary according to the site of perforation and the duration of the peritonitis. It includes both aerobic and anaerobic microorganisms such as including *E. coli, Bacteroides* spp., various *Streptococcus* spp., enterococci, and *Clostridium perfringens.*
- **Chronic bacterial peritonitis:** Associated with subacute intestinal obstruction.

Morphology

- Peritoneum shows dense collections of **neutrophils and fibrinopurulent debris** that coat the viscera and abdominal wall.
- Peritoneal cavity initially contains **serous or slightly turbid fluid** which becomes suppurative as infection progresses. Subhepatic and subdiaphragmatic abscesses may be formed.

Spontaneous Bacterial Peritonitis

- **Spontaneous bacterial peritonitis** (SBP) may occur in the absence of an obvious source of contamination. It is a **common and severe complication of ascites.** It is characterized by **spontaneous infection of ascitic fluid in the absence of a recognizable intra-abdominal source of peritonitis.** It is seen mostly in patients with cirrhosis and ascites and less frequently in children with nephrotic syndrome.
- **Causative agents:** Most common organisms are *Escherichia coli, Klebsiella* or enterococci or other gut bacteria. Others include streptococci and enterococci.
- **Route of infection:** The infecting organisms in the gut flora traverse the intestine into mesenteric lymph nodes, leading to bacteremia and seeding of the ascitic fluid by hematogenous spread.

Chemical Peritonitis

It is most often due to:

- **Bile peritonitis:** Leakage of bile usually from a perforated gallbladder.

- In **acute hemorrhagic pancreatitis:** Due to leakage of pancreatic enzymes, which produces severe *peritonitis* with fat necrosis.
- **Hydrochloric acid or hemorrhage** from a perforated peptic ulcer of the stomach or duodenum.
- **Foreign material:** For example, introduced by surgery (e.g. talc and sutures) or by trauma that induces foreign body-type granulomas and fibrous scarring.
- **Endometriosis:** Causes bleeding into the peritoneal cavity.
- **Ruptured dermoid cysts:** It release keratins and produces granulomatous reaction.
- **Leakage of urine**.

Sclerosing Retroperitonitis

Sclerosing retroperitonitis, also termed as idiopathic retroperitoneal fibrosis or Ormond disease. It is characterized by dense fibrosis which may extend to involve the mesentery.

Tuberculous Peritonitis

- Tuberculous peritonitis is infection of peritoneum by *Mycobacterium tuberculosis*.
- **Pathogenesis:** Tuberculosis spreads to involve peritoneum by or more of the following sources:
  - Through hematogenous seeding of peritoneum.
  - Through lymphatics or mesenteric nodes.
  - From genitourinary source.
- **Morphological features:** Peritoneum shows typical tuberculous granuloma.

Peritoneal Dialysis Induced Changes

- Chronic peritoneal dialysis can cause of **bacterial peritonitis**, due to contamination of instruments or dialysate. The clinical course is usually milder than with a perforated viscus. Most common causative organisms include *Staphylococcus* and *Streptococcus* spp.
- Chronic dialysis can also produce **aseptic peritonitis**, probably by chemical in the dialysate.
- May show **narrowing or obliteration of the lumen of blood vessel** in the peritoneal layer. Peritonitis promotes **peritoneal fibrosis** in 50% and 80% of patients within 1 and 2 years.

SELF-ASSESSMENT EXERCISES

I. Essay

1. Discuss the etiology and pathogenesis of peptic ulcer.
2. Discuss the etiology and pathogenesis of gastric carcinoma.

II. Short Notes

1. Peptic ulcer.
2. Pathogenesis of peptic ulcer.
3. Morphology of peptic ulcer.
4. Carcinoma stomach.
5. Pathogenesis of typhoid fever.
6. Amebic ulcer of intestine.
7. Amebiasis.
8. Carcinoid tumor.

CHAPTER 18

Liver, Biliary Tract and Pancreas

CHAPTER OUTLINE

- Normal Structure and Function of Liver
- Jaundice
- Viral Hepatitis
- Alcoholic Liver Disease
- Cirrhosis
- Liver Abscess
- Hemochromatosis
- Tumors of Liver
- Pathology of Gallbladder
- Pathology of Pancreas

NORMAL STRUCTURE AND FUNCTION OF LIVER

Structure

The normal adult liver weighs 1400–1600 g. It is situated in the right upper quadrant of the abdomen immediately below the diaphragm. It consists of two lobes, a larger right lobe and a smaller left lobe (Fig. 18.1). The gallbladder is located inferiorly in a fossa of the right hepatic lobe. The liver has **blood supply from two sources** namely: (1) the **hepatic artery** and (2) the **portal vein**.

Structural unit of liver is hepatic lobule. The classic lobule is hexagonal in shape arranged around the central vein. The **lobule consists of terminal hepatic vein (central vein) in the center with portal triads (or portal tracts) in the periphery** at the angles of the polygon of the lobule (Fig. 18.2). The portal triad consists of (1) bile ducts, (2) hepatic artery and (3) portal vein. The hepatocytes are polygonal having granular cytoplasm and central round nuclei. The space between the hepatocyte is lined by fenestrated endothelial cells and forms the sinusoids. The lining cells also contain Kupffer cells which belong to mononuclear phagocyte system. The space between the endothelial cells and hepatocytes is called **space of Disse** and **contains stellate cells** which store vitamin A and are responsible for fibrosis seen in cirrhosis.

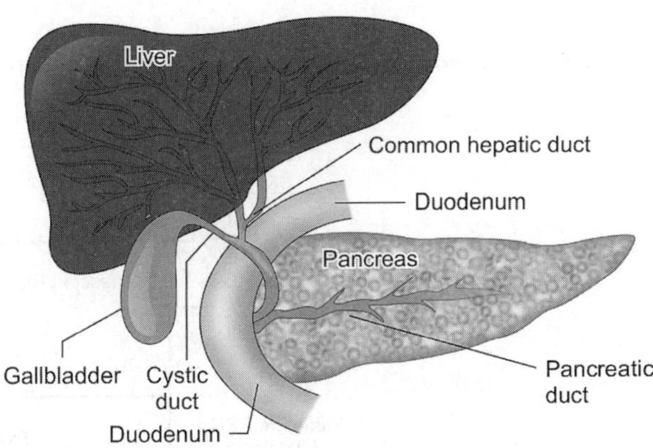

Fig. 18.1: Normal anatomical components of hepatobiliary system

Functions of Liver

- Production and excretion of bile.
- Synthesis of plasma proteins such as albumin, fibrinogen and prothrombin.
- Metabolism of proteins, carbohydrates and lipids.
- Storage of vitamins (A, D and B_{12}) and iron.
- Detoxification of toxic substances such as alcohol and drugs.

JAUNDICE

Definition: Yellow discoloration of skin and mucus membranes (jaundice) and sclera (icterus) due to increased bilirubin in the blood is known as jaundice.

Bilirubin Metabolism (Fig. 18.3)

Bilirubin Production

Source of bilirubin

Bilirubin is derived from the degradation of hemoglobin, mainly from break-down of senescent red blood cells. Hemoglobin is converted into heme and globin. The heme is oxidized to biliverdin, which is reduced to bilirubin by biliverdin reductase.

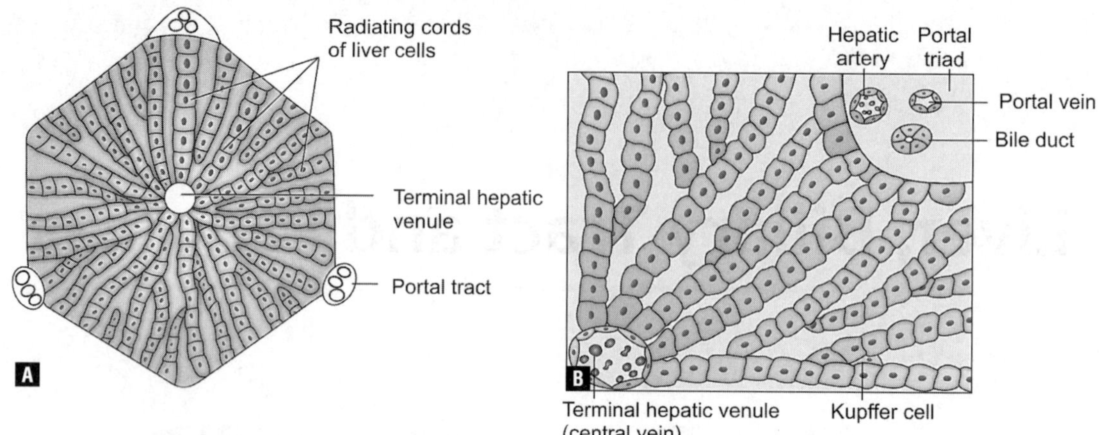

Figs 18.2A and B: (A) Diagrammatic appearance of hepatic lobule; (B) Microscopic appearance of part of the liver lobule

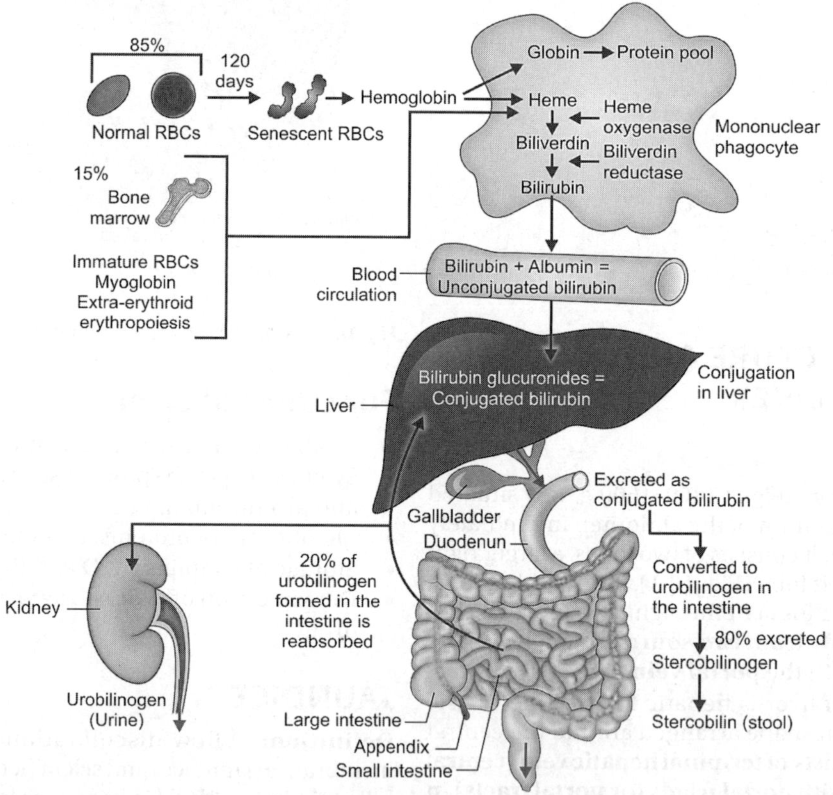

Fig. 18.3: Bilirubin metabolism. Major bilirubin is derived from the break-down of senescent circulating RBCs. The bilirubin binds to serum albumin and delivered to the liver. In the liver, bilirubin forms conjugated water soluble bilirubin and excreted into bile. In the gut bacteria deconjugate the bilirubin and degrade it to colorless urobilinogens. The 80% urobilinogens are excreted in the feces, and about 20% is reabsorbed. The minor fraction of reabsorbed urobilinogen is excreted into urine

Bilirubin Binding

Bilirubin formed is bound to serum albumin for transport to the liver. This bilirubin is known as unconjugated bilirubin and is not soluble in water. Unconjugated bilirubin is toxic to the brain in newborns and in high concentrations causes irreversible brain injury, termed **kernicterus**.

Conjugation

In the **liver**, unconjugated bilirubin is conjugated with glucuronic acid and **forms** water-soluble **conjugated bilirubin**.

Excretion

The conjugated bilirubin is nontoxic and excreted into **bile**. In the small intestine, the conjugated bilirubin is degraded to colorless urobilinogens. Most (80%) of the urobilinogen is excreted in the feces. But a small proportion (approximately 20%) of urobilinogen is reabsorbed in the terminal ileum and colon, returned to the liver and re-excreted into the bile.

Pathophysiology of Jaundice

- Serum bilirubin levels in the normal adult range from 0.3–1.2 mg/dL, and the rate of bilirubin production is equal to the rate of biliary excretion.
- Jaundice occurs when the equilibrium between bilirubin production and clearance is disturbed. Jaundice becomes evident when the serum bilirubin levels rise above 2.0–2.5 mg/dL; levels as high as 30–40 mg/dL can occur with severe disease.
- Jaundice develops due to increase in unconjugated bilirubin and/or conjugated bilirubin. Unconjugated bilirubin is insoluble in water and cannot be excreted in the urine even when its levels in the blood are high. Conjugated bilirubin is water-soluble, nontoxic, and when its level in the blood is increased, it can be excreted in urine. The various causes of jaundice are shown in Box 18.1.

Box 18.1: Causes (types) of jaundice

Predominantly unconjugated hyperbilirubinemia

- Excess production of bilirubin, e.g. hemolytic anemias, ineffective erythropoiesis
- Reduced hepatic uptake of bilirubin, e.g. Gilbert's syndrome
- Impaired bilirubin conjugation in liver, e.g. physiologic jaundice of the newborn, Crigler–Najjar syndrome types I and II, viral or drug-induced hepatitis, cirrhosis

Predominantly conjugated hyperbilirubinemia

- Dubin–Johnson syndrome, Rotor's syndrome, drugs
- Impaired bile flow: Obstruction by gallstones or tumors

Table 18.1: Various classifications of jaundice

1.	Prehepatic	Hepatic	Posthepatic
2.	Hemolytic	Hepatocellular	Obstructive
3.	Medical	Medical	Surgical

Box 18.2: Causes of large bile duct obstruction

- In adults:
  - Gallstones: Most common cause
  - Malignancies of the biliary tree or head of the pancreas
  - Strictures resulting from previous surgical procedures
- In children:
  - Biliary atresia, cystic fibrosis, choledochal cysts

These obstructions **can produce obstructive jaundice**. Prolonged obstruction can result in biliary cirrhosis.

Classification of Jaundice (Table 18.1)

Clinical Features

Bilirubin has affinity for connective tissue and stains it yellow. Clinically, it is better detected in the sclera and skin. Other features depend on the exact cause of jaundice.

Laboratory diagnosis of jaundice: It is by performing **liver function test (LFT).**

Large Bile Duct Obstruction (Box 18.2)

Laboratory Findings

- Raised serum bilirubin
- Raised alkaline phosphatase, especially when associated with obstruction
- Liver function tests show abnormalities depending on the cause
- Urine shows bile salts and pigments.

Neonatal Cholestasis

Prolonged conjugated hyperbilirubinemia in the neonate is termed as neonatal cholestasis. Normally, physiologic jaundice of the new born subsides by two weeks. Hence, infants who have jaundice beyond 14–21 days after birth should be investigated for neonatal cholestasis. Major causes are (1) cholangiopathies, primarily **biliary atresia** and (2) **neonatal hepatitis.**

Neonatal Hepatitis

It is not a specific entity, nor the disorders to be necessarily inflammatory in nature (because term hepatitis means inflammatory condition of hepatocytes). It constitutes a variety of disorders causing conjugated hyperbilirubinemia in the neonate. Neonatal cholestasis may be caused by toxic, metabolic, and infectious liver diseases. Hence, after excluding all the causes, **idiopathic neonatal hepatitis** constitutes only 10 to 15% of cases of neonatal hepatitis.

Clinical presentation: Affected infants have jaundice, dark urine, light or alcocholic stools, and hepatomegaly. Variable degrees of hepatic synthetic dysfunction (e.g. hypoprothrombinemia) may be present.

Morphology: The morphologic features include lobular disarray with focal liver cell apoptosis and necrosis. There is panlobular **giant-cell transformation** of hepatocytes with prominent hepatocellular and canalicular cholestasis.

VIRAL HEPATITIS

Hepatitis is the inflammation of the liver, caused by infectious or toxic agents. The most common cause of hepatitis is viral. Thus, the term hepatitis is commonly used for viral hepatitis.

Definition: Viral hepatitis is an **infection of hepatocytes by virus** which produces necrosis and inflammation in the liver.

Hepatotropic Virus

The term viral hepatitis is usually applied for hepatic infections caused by a group of **five** viruses known as hepatotropic viruses (hepatitis viruses **A, B, C, D and E**) that have a particular affinity for the liver. **All except HBV are RNA viruses**.

Hepatitis A Virus

Hepatitis A virus (HAV) is a non-enveloped, RNA-virus. The hepatitis caused by HAV is known as hepatitis A.

Source of infection

The source of infection is person with acute infection.

Mode of spread

Fecal-oral route by ingestion of contaminated water and foods.

Incubation period

It has a **short incubation period** of 3–6 weeks (with a mean of about 4 weeks).

Hepatitis A tends to be mild or asymptomatic. Affected individuals have nonspecific symptoms such as fatigue and loss of appetite. They often develop jaundice.

Hepatitis B Virus

Hepatitis B virus (HBV) is a DNA virus. The complete virion is called as "**Dane particle**".

Various antigens of HBV

- **HBsAg (hepatitis B surface antigen/Australia antigen):** It is the **first antigen** which appears before the onset of symptoms and declines within 3–6 months. When HBsAg disappears its antibody namely anti-HBs appears. **Anti-HBs is a protective antibody.** Persistence of HBsAg after 6 months indicates development of chronic hepatitis.
- **HBcAg (hepatitis B core antigen):** HBcAg cannot be demonstrated in the blood. But its antibody appears in serum a week or two after the appearance of HBsAg.
- **HBeAg (hepatitis B "e" antigen):** HBeAg appear in serum soon after HBsAg, and signify active viral replication. **Persistence of HBeAg indicates infectivity, and progression to chronic hepatitis.**

Source of infection

Human beings are the only source of HBV infection.

Mode of transmission of HBV

The various routes of HBV infection are shown in Table 18.2.

Incubation period

HBV has a prolonged incubation period (4–26 weeks).

Hepatitis B can produce acute hepatitis, chronic hepatitis and carrier state.

Hepatitis C Virus

Hepatitis C virus (HCV) is enveloped, single-stranded RNA virus. HCV is a major cause of chronic liver disease **(chronic hepatitis or cirrhosis)**.

Mode of spread

Hepatitis C is spread predominantly by the parenteral route.

Incubation period

Ranges from 2–26 weeks, with a mean between 6 and 12 weeks.

Table 18.2: Various routes of infection of HBV

Route of infection of HBV	Causes
Horizontal transmission	Injection in drug addicts, infected unscreened blood products, tattoos/accupuncture needles, sexual (homosexual and heterosexual) contact
Vertical transmission	HbsAg positive mother to fetus

Hepatitis D Virus

Hepatitis D virus (HDV) is **incomplete RNA virus.**

Mode of infection

By parenteral route and sexually.

Incubation period

HDV has a prolonged incubation period (1–4 months).

Hepatitis caused by HDV is known as **Delta hepatitis.** HDV requires HBV for its replication. Delta hepatitis occurs in two clinical patterns:

- **Acute coinfection** occurs when there is **simultaneous infection with HDV and HBV.**
- **Superinfection** occurs when a **chronic carrier of HBV is exposed to new inoculums of HDV.**

Hepatitis E Virus

Hepatitis E virus (HEV) is an unenveloped RNA virus.

Mode of spread

Hepatitis E is an **enterically transmitted, water-borne** infection. It occurs primarily in young to middle-aged adults. **HEV infection is associated with high mortality rate among pregnant women.**

Incubation period

The average incubation period following exposure is **6 weeks.**

In most of the cases, the disease is **self-limiting**; HEV is not associated with chronic liver disease.

Various features of hepatotropic viruses are summarized in Table 18.3.

Clinical Features

The symptoms of acute viral hepatitis are almost same for any of the hepatotropic viruses. It presents with malaise, nausea, poor appetite, vague abdominal pain and jaundice.

Biochemical findings

Increase in serum bilirubin and **aminotransferase levels.**

Serological findings

Appearance of hepatitis viral genome in the liver and serum followed by antibodies to viral antigens.

Microscopic Features of Acute Hepatitis (Fig. 18.4)

- **Ballooning degeneration:** During early stages, **hepatocytes show** diffuse swelling of the cytoplasm known as **"ballooning degeneration".**
- **Necrosis of hepatocytes:** Later, hepatocytes may show necrosis and/or apoptosis.
  - **Dropout necrosis:** Necrosis may appear as focal loss of hepatocytes **(dropout necrosis) surrounded by aggregates of macrophages.**
  - **Councilman bodies:** Apoptosis of hepatocytes results in shrinkage of hepatocytes which become intensely **eosinophilic, with fragmented nuclei.** The remnants of these necrotic hepatocytes appear as **acidophilic or Councilman bodies.**
- **Inflammation:** The **portal tracts** are usually **infiltrated with a mixture of inflammatory cells.**

Chronic Hepatitis

Definition: Chronic hepatitis is defined as symptomatic, biochemical, or serologic evidence of continuing or relapsing **hepatic disease for more than 6 months.**

Causes

- **Viral hepatitis:** HBV, HCV and HDV.
- **Other causes:** Wilson disease, autoimmune hepatitis, drugs (such as methotrexate, isoniazid, alpha methyl dopa) and idiopathic.

Microscopy

The histological features of chronic hepatitis (Fig. 18.5) range from mild to severe.

- **Milder form:** In the mildest forms, inflammation is limited to portal tracts and consists of **lymphocytes, macrophages, and occasional plasma cells.**

Table 18.3: Summary of hepatotropic viruses

Virus	Hepatitis A	Hepatitis B	Hepatitis C	Hepatitis D	Hepatitis E
Type of virus	RNA	DNA	RNA	RNA	RNA
Mode of transmission	Feco-oral (food or water)	Parenteral, sexual contact, perinatal	Parenteral	Parenteral	Feco-oral
Incubation period	3–6 weeks	1–4 months	2–26 weeks	1–4 months	6 weeks
Development of chronic liver disease	Never	About 10%	About 80%	With coinfection 5% and with superinfection ≤70%	Never

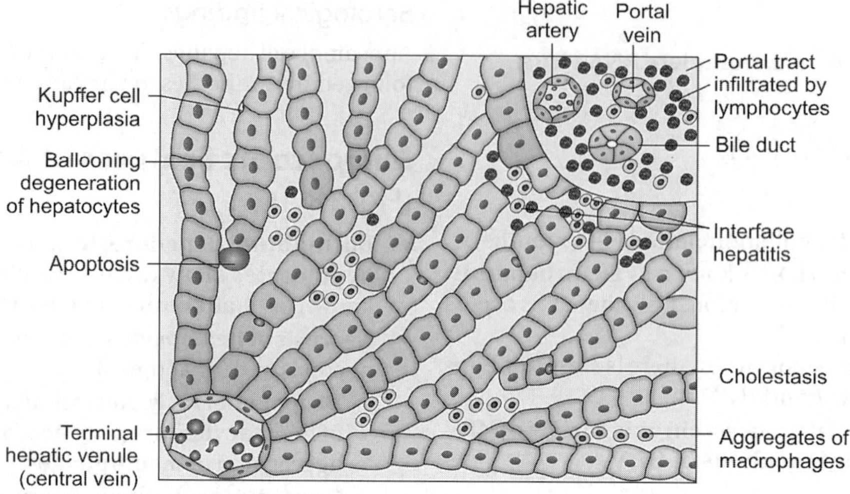

Fig. 18.4: Diagrammatic representation of the microscopic features of acute hepatitis

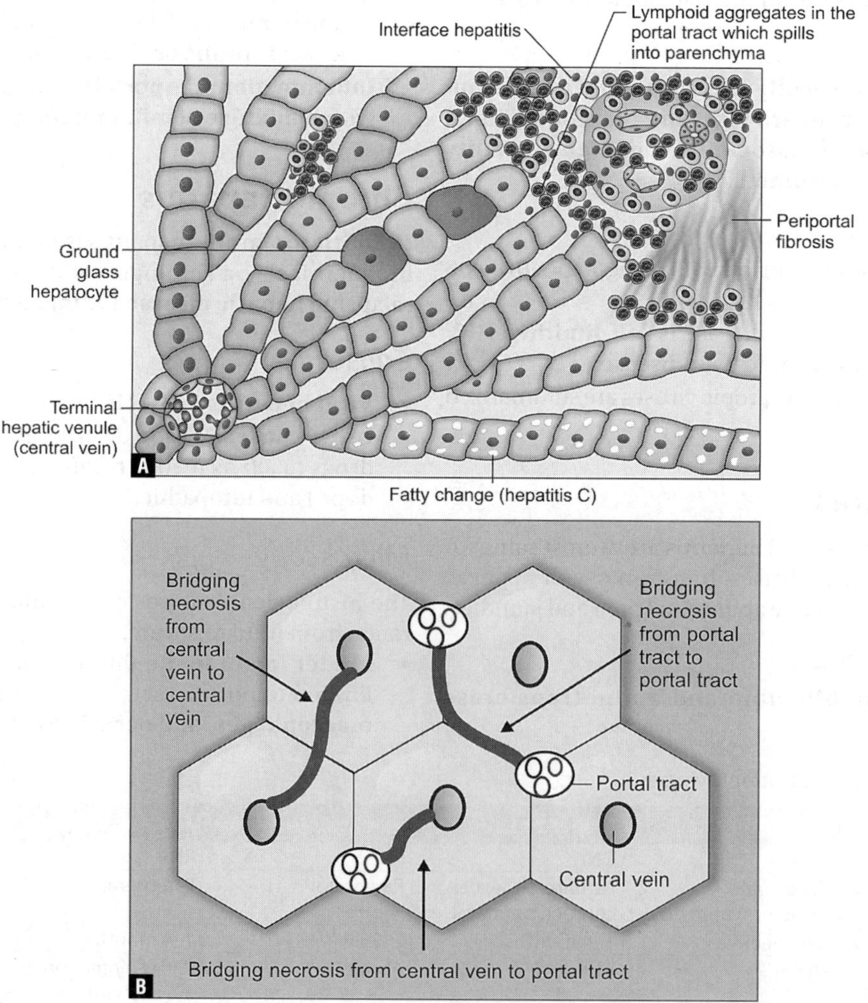

Figs 18.5A and B: (A) Diagrammatic representation of the microscopic features of chronic hepatitis; (B) Types of necrosis seen in chronic hepatitis

- **Severe form:** It may show features of progressive liver damage. These include:
  - **Interface hepatitis:** The inflammatory infiltrate may spill over from portal tract into the adjacent parenchyma, causing apoptosis of periportal hepatocytes. This is known as piecemeal necrosis/interface hepatitis (Fig. 18.5A).
  - **Bridging necrosis:** It is the band of necrosis between portal tracts and portal tracts-to-terminal hepatic (central) veins (Fig. 18.5B).
  - **Features of chronic liver damage:** The characteristic feature of chronic liver damage is the **deposition of fibrous tissue**. Continued loss of hepatocytes and fibrosis results in cirrhosis.

Carrier State

Definition: A "carrier" is an individual who harbors and can transmit an organism. Carrier state is categorized as inactive or active.

- **Inactive carriers (healthy carriers)** carry one of the viruses but have no liver disease.
- **Active carriers** harbor the viruses and have non-progressive liver damage, but are essentially free of symptoms or disability. In HBV carriers, the liver shows **"ground-glass hepatocytes"** due to HBsAg in the cytoplasm (Fig. 18.5A).

In both cases, particularly the latter, these individuals constitute reservoirs for infection.

ALCOHOLIC LIVER DISEASE

- Chronic and excessive alcohol (ethanol) consumption is **one of the major causes** of liver disease.
- Alcoholic liver disease (ALD) constitutes a **spectrum of disorders** directly related to the excessive alcohol use.
- ALD consists of **three major, distinctive, but overlapping lesions**: (1) hepatic steatosis (fatty liver—refer pages 10-1), (2) alcoholic hepatitis, and (3) alcoholic cirrhosis (described later).

Alcoholic Hepatitis

Morphology

- **Gross:** The liver may be **enlarged**; **yellow** due to steatosis and **firm** due to increased fibrosis.
- **Microscopy:** Alcoholic hepatitis has four characteristic features and the lesions are predominantly centrilobular.
  1. Ballooning degeneration of hepatocyte. **Variable degree of steatosis** is also seen in hepatocytes.
  2. **Mallory bodies (Mallory–Denk bodies/Mallory hyaline):** They consist of **tangled skeins of cytokeratin intermediate filaments.** They appear as **dense, eosinophilic ropey cytoplasmic inclusions/clumps**, usually situated in a **perinuclear** location, in the degenerating hepatocytes. Mallory bodies are a **characteristic but not specific** feature of alcoholic liver disease.
  3. **Neutrophilic infiltration: Around ballooned hepatocytes**, particularly those containing Mallory bodies.
  4. **Fibrosis: In pericellular/perisinusoidal region**.

CIRRHOSIS

Definition: Cirrhosis is defined as a **diffuse process** characterized by **fibrosis** and conversion of normal architecture of liver to **structurally abnormal nodules** of hepatocytes.

Classification

Cirrhosis can be the final stage of any chronic liver disease and is classified in two ways.

Morphological Classification

Cirrhosis can be classified according to the average size of the regenerating nodules (Fig. 18.6).

- **Micronodular:** The regenerating nodules measure up to 3 mm in diameter.
- **Macronodular:** The regenerating nodules are greater than 3 mm in diameter.
- **Mixed:** It consists of combination of both types of nodules.

Etiological Classification

The etiological classification is shown in Box 18.3.

Box 18.3: Etiological classification of cirrhosis

Alcohol
Viral hepatitis (HBV and HCV)
Non-alcoholic steatohepatitis (NASH)
Hemochromatosis
Autoimmune liver disease (autoimmune hepatitis and primary biliary cirrhosis)
Recurrent biliary obstruction (e.g. gallstones)
Wilson's disease
'Cryptogenic' (hidden cause) or idiopathic

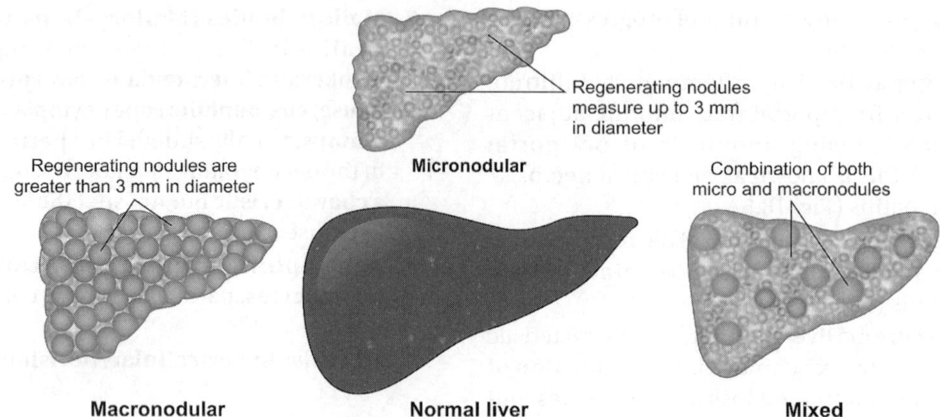

Fig. 18.6: Morphological classification of cirrhosis

Pathogenesis

The important pathogenic processes in cirrhosis are (1) death of hepatocytes, (2) deposition of extracellular matrix (ECM), and (3) vascular reorganization. The death of liver cells and fibrosis stimulate the surviving hepatocytes to form regenerative nodules surrounded by the fibrous septa. This results in a fibrotic, and nodular liver.

Clinical Features

Cirrhosis present with **nonspecific** clinical manifestations: anorexia, weight loss, weakness, and in advanced disease, signs and symptoms of hepatic failure. Increased resistance to portal blood flow may result in **portal hypertension**. Portal hypertension is defined as elevation of the hepatic venous pressure above normal limits. The four major clinical consequences of portal hypertension (Fig 18.7) are: **Ascites, formation of portosystemic venous shunts, congestive splenomegaly, and hepatic encephalopathy**.

Ascites is the accumulation of excess fluid in the peritoneal cavity. It is due to **sinusoidal hypertension, hypoalbuminemia** and **retention of sodium**.

Complications

The complication of cirrhosis results from portal hypertension is the development of portosystemic collaterals.

- **Portosystemic shunts/varices and variceal hemorrhage:** In portal hypertension, shunts between portal system and systemic circulation may cause **esophagogastric varices** (which may cause massive hematemesis) and dilated subcutaneous veins extending from the umbilicus toward the rib margins (**caput medusae**).
- **Splenomegaly:** Long-standing congestion may cause congestive splenomegaly. The spleen may weigh upto 1,000 g.

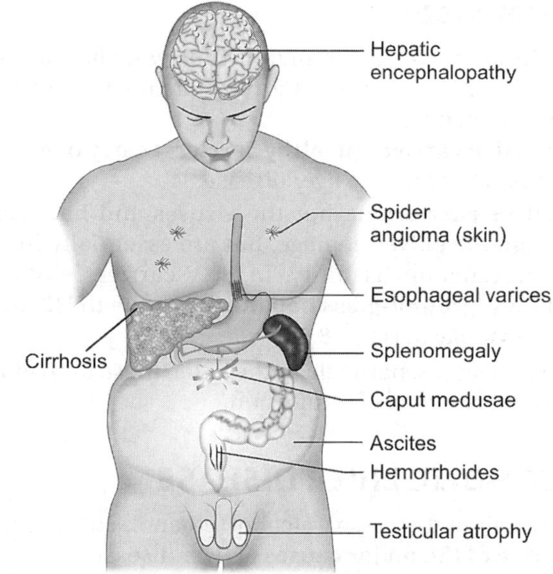

Fig. 18.7: Major clinical consequences of portal hypertension in cirrhosis

- **Endocrine complications:** Chronic liver failure in men leads to feminization, characterized by gynecomastia, testicular atrophy, impotence, and loss of libido.

Alcoholic Cirrhosis

Alcohol is the **most common cause of cirrhosis**. The cirrhosis caused by alcohol is also known as Laennec cirrhosis, portal cirrhosis and nutritional cirrhosis.

Etiology

Chronic and excessive alcohol ingestion is one of the major causes of cirrhosis. Two most important risk factors involved in the development of cirrhosis are the quantity and duration of alcohol intake. About 10–15% of alcoholics develop cirrhosis.

Ethanol metabolism in liver

The liver is the main organ responsible for ethanol (alcohol) metabolism. Ethanol is metabolized to acetaldehyde in the liver. Acetaldehyde is a potentially toxic compound and plays an etiologic role in alcoholic liver disease.

Pathogenesis

Two main mechanisms involved in the pathogenesis of alcoholic cirrhosis are: Destruction of liver cells and development of fibrosis.

Destruction of liver cells

The liver cells may be destroyed by various mechanisms.

- **Oxidative stress/reactive oxygen species:** Metabolism of ethanol in the liver overproduces **reactive oxygen species** and cause destruction of liver cells.
- **Reduced NAD in cytoplasm.**
- **Mitochondrial dysfunction.**
- **Direct hepatotoxicity by ethanol.**
- **Immune and inflammatory mechanisms:** Acetaldehyde, when forms adducts with chemical molecules, may stimulate the host's immune response and cause autoimmune-like destruction of liver cells.
- **Hypoxia:** Chronic alcohol intake increases oxygen demand by the liver resulting in hypoxia to the liver cells.
- **Malnutrition and deficiencies of vitamins:** Alcohol can become a major source of calories in the diet and may lead to malnutrition and deficiencies of vitamins (such as thiamine).

Development of fibrosis

- Hepatic stellate cells (Ito cells or perisinusoidal cells) are located in the space of Disse between hepatocytes and sinusoidal endothelial cells. The fibrosis developing in cirrhosis is due to the **activation of hepatic stellate cells**.
- The **activated stellate cells** proliferate and **secrete extracellular matrix.** They also develop myofibroblast-like contractile property.

Morphology

Gross: Initial stages, the cirrhotic liver is **yellow tan, fatty and enlarged**. Later, it is transformed into a **shrunken brown** organ with **micronodules** which create a **"hobnail"** appearance on the surface of the liver (Fig. 18.8).

Microscopy (Fig. 18.9)

- **Loss of architecture:** Cirrhosis is characterized by loss of the architecture of the **entire liver**.

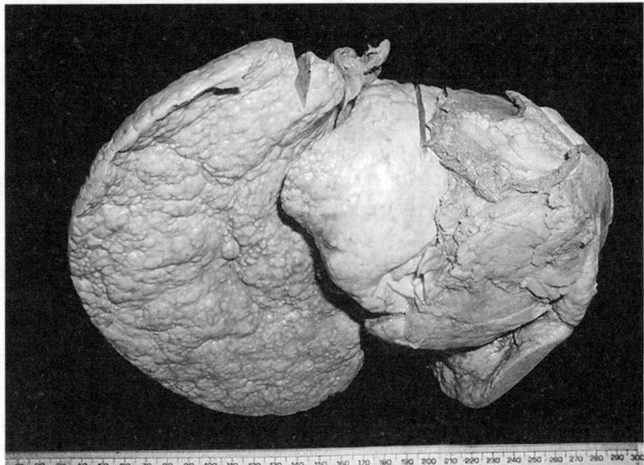

Fig. 18.8: Gross appearance of cirrhosis of liver with numerous nodules throughout the liver

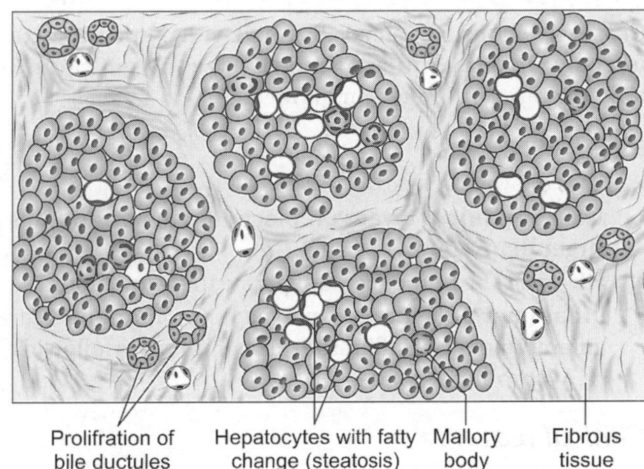

Fig. 18.9: Microscopic appearance of alcoholic cirrhosis composed of regenerating nodules separated by dense fibrous tissue

- **Regenerating nodules/nodular regeneration:** The hepatic parenchyma shows uniform micronodules (less than 3 mm in diameter) which are separated by fibrous tissue. The hepatocytes may show **Mallory bodies.**
- **Fibrosis:** Initially, the fibrous septa are delicate and extend through sinusoids from **central to portal regions as well as from portal tract to portal tract.** Later the fibrous septa may be thick.

Postnecrotic Cirrhosis

Postnecrotic cirrhosis is also known as posthepatitic cirrhosis, macronodular cirrhosis and coarsely nodular cirrhosis.

Liver shows large and irregular nodules of with broad bands of fibrous connective tissue. It is most commonly develops after previous viral hepatitis.

Etiology

- **Viral hepatitis:** Most common viral hepatitis associated with postnecrotic cirrhosis is hepatitis B and C.
- **Drugs and chemical hepatotoxins:** For example, phosphorus, carbon tetrachloride, mushroom poisoning, acetaminophen and α-methyldopa.
- **Others:** Include certain infections (e.g. brucellosis), parasitic infestations (e.g. clonorchiasis), metabolic diseases (e.g. Wilson's disease) and advanced alcoholic liver disease.
- **Idiopathic:** Where the etiology is unknown.

Morphology

Typically, postnecrotic cirrhosis is macronodular type.

Gross: Liver is usually small, distorted with numerous with **irregular macronodules of varying sizes** ranging from 3 mm to a few centimeters in diameter.

Microscopy

- Loss of architecture.
- **Macronodules:** Liver is replaced by macronodules larger than 3 mm.
- **Fibrosis:** The fibrous septa separate the macronodules.
- **Inflammation:** Fibrous septa may show mononuclear inflammatory cell infiltrate especially in cases following HCV chronic hepatitis.

Clinical features

- More common in females than in males.
- Features of cirrhosis similar to alcoholic cirrhosis.
- Splenomegaly and hypersplenism may be observed.
- Postnecrotic cirrhosis following hepatitis B and C virus infection in early life, is more frequently may develop hepatocellular carcinoma later.

Biliary Cirrhosis

Biliary cirrhosis may be secondary or primary biliary cirrhosis.

1. **Secondary biliary cirrhosis:** It develops when there is complete obstruction of the extrahepatic biliary tree (e.g. gallstones, chronic pancreatitis and tumors of biliary tract or pancreas).
2. **Primary biliary cirrhosis:** It is an autoimmune mediated disease due to destruction of the intrahepatic biliary tree.

LIVER ABSCESS

Definition: Localized collection of pus inside the liver parenchyma is known as liver abscess. Liver abscesses are common in developing countries.

Causes

- ***Entameba histolytica:*** Amebic liver abscess is caused by **entameba histolytica** (refer page 209-10).
- **Liver abscess by other protozoa and helminthic organisms:** Secondary infection of hydatid cyst caused by echinococci and less commonly other organisms.
- **Pyogenic abscess:** Such abscesses usually represent a complication of bacterial infection elsewhere.
- **Fungal abscess:** For example, candida.

Mode of Infection

The causative agent may reach the liver by any one of the following routes.

- **Portal vein:** The majority of hepatic abscesses used to result from portal spread of intra-abdominal infections (e.g. appendicitis, diverticulitis, colitis).
- **Artery:** Through hepatic artery, e.g. during septicemia.
- **Ascending infection** in the biliary tract (ascending cholangitis).
- **Direct invasion of the liver from a nearby source** or a penetrating injury.

Morphology

- **Number:** Liver abscesses may be single or (Fig. 18.10) multiple in number. Bacteremic spread through the arterial or portal system usually produces multiple

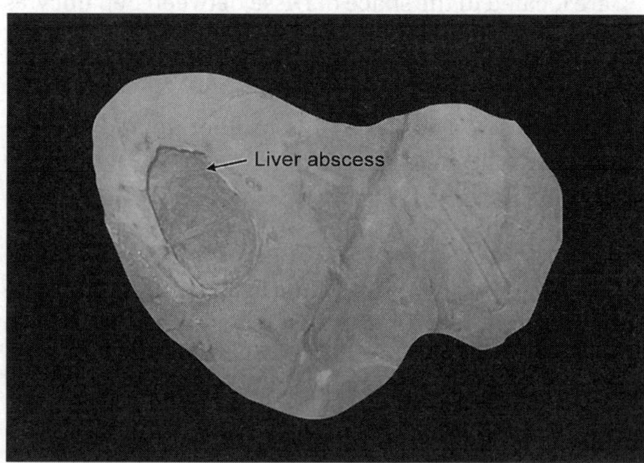

Fig. 18.10: Liver with an abscess in the right lobe

small abscesses. Direct extension and trauma usually cause solitary/single large abscess.

- **Size:** The size of the abscess may range from few millimeters to massive lesions of many centimeters in diameter.

Clinical Features

Liver abscesses are associated with fever, right upper quadrant pain and tender hepatomegaly. Jaundice may develop when there is extrahepatic biliary obstruction.

HEMOCHROMATOSIS

Liver is one of the major organs involved in hemochromatosis. Excessive deposition of iron in the reticuloendothelial cells and hepatocytes may cause cirrhosis of liver.

TUMORS OF LIVER

Malignant tumors occurring in the liver can be primary or metastatic. Most of the primary liver cancers arise from hepatocytes and are termed as **hepatocellular carcinoma** (HCC). Less common carcinomas of bile duct origin are termed as **cholangiocarcinoma**.

Hepatoblastoma

Hepatoblastoma is the most common malignant liver **tumor of childhood**. The tumor is usually fatal within a few years. This tumor has two anatomic types:

- **Epithelial type:** It is composed of small polygonal fetal cells or smaller embryonal cells forming acini, tubules, or papillary structures.
- **Mixed epithelial and mesenchymal type:** It contains foci of mesenchymal differentiation that may consist of primitive mesenchyme, osteoid, cartilage, or striated muscle.

Hepatocellular Carcinoma

Hepatocellular carcinoma (HCC) is a malignant tumor derived from hepatocytes. It is more common in males with a male to female ratio of 2.4: 1.

Etiology and Pathogenesis

It is multifactorial and various risk factors for HCC are shown in Table 18.4.

Table 18.4: Risk factors for hepatocellular carcinoma

Major risk factors	Minor risk factors
• Chronic hepatitis **B** virus infection • Chronic hepatitis **C** virus infection • **C**irrhosis • Dietary exposure to **a**flatoxin B_1	• **H**ereditary hemochromatosis • Oral **c**ontraceptives • **C**igarette smoking
Remember risk factors as	
Major ABCC (A = aflatoxin, B = HBV, C = HCV, C = Cirrhosis)	**Minor HCC (H = hemochromatosis, C = Cigarette, C = contraceptive)**

Morphology

Gross: Hepatocellular carcinoma may appear grossly as **unifocal** (usually large) circumscribed mass, **multifocal**, or **diffusely infiltrative** cancer (Fig. 18.11). They are usually **light brown, yellowish-white** in color. **Areas of necrosis and hemorrhage** are common. They may **cause liver enlargement. HCCs have a strong tendency for invasion of blood vessels.**

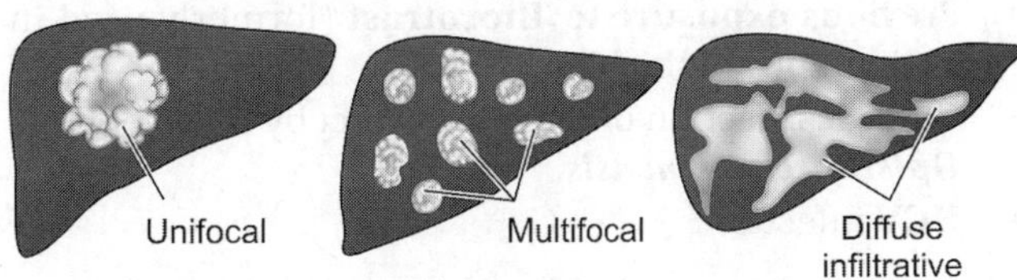

Fig. 18.11: Gross types of hepatocellular carcinoma

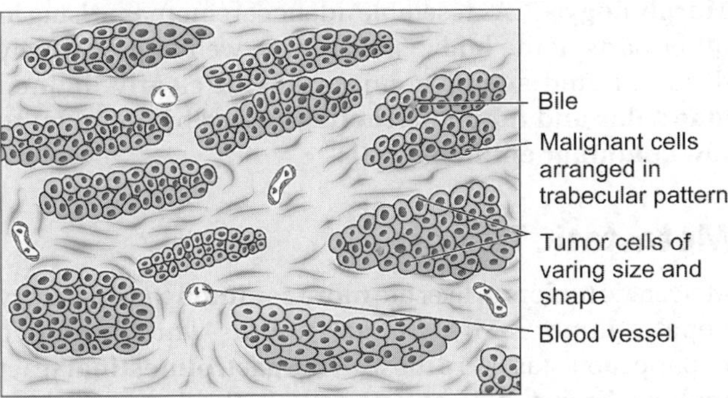

Fig. 18.12: Hepatocellular carcinoma composed of malignant hepatocytes arranged in trabecular pattern

Microscopy: Hepatocellular carcinoma may be graded as **well-differentiated, moderately differentiated and undifferentiated forms**. In well-differentiated tumors, the tumor cells can be identified as hepatocytic in origin. These **malignant cells are arranged in trabecular and acinar** (pseudoglandular) patterns (Fig. 18.12).

Spread

- **Lymphatic spread:** It spreads to the regional lymph nodes (portal lymph nodes).
- **Hematogenous spread:** It may spread into the lungs.

Clinical Features

Most of the patients present with upper abdominal pain, malaise, fatigue and weight loss. Liver is enlarged, irregular or nodular. **Elevated levels of serum α-fetoprotein** are found in 50% of the patients with HCC.

Cholangiocarcinoma

Cholangiocarcinoma (CCA) arises anywhere in the biliary tree.

Risk factors: The risk factors for development of CCA include:

- Previous **exposure to Thorotrast** (formerly used in radiography of the biliary tract).
- Chronic infection of the biliary tract by the liver fluke ***Opisthorchis sinensis***.
- **HCV** infection.

Classification: According to their localization, CCAs are classified into intrahepatic and extrahepatic forms.

Morphology: CCAs resemble adenocarcinomas arising in other parts of the body. Majority are well to moderately differentiated adenocarcinomas with clearly defined **glandular and tubular structures lined by cuboidal to low columnar epithelial cells.**

Metastatic Tumors

Metastatic tumors to liver are **more common than primary** hepatic tumors. The primary tumors which produce hepatic metastases are those of the **gastrointestinal tract (colon), breast, lung and pancreas.** The liver may show only a single nodule or **multiple nodules of metastases** (Fig. 18.13). These tumors are seen on the surface of the liver as **umbilicated masses**, because of central necrosis and hemorrhage. **Microscopically**, the metastatic deposits appear similar to the primary tumor.

Clinical Features

It usually presents with weight loss. Obstruction of the major bile ducts or replacement of most of the liver parenchyma leads to **jaundice.** Laboratory findings may show **increase** in the **serum alkaline phosphatase** level. Most of the patients die within a year of the diagnosis of liver metastases.

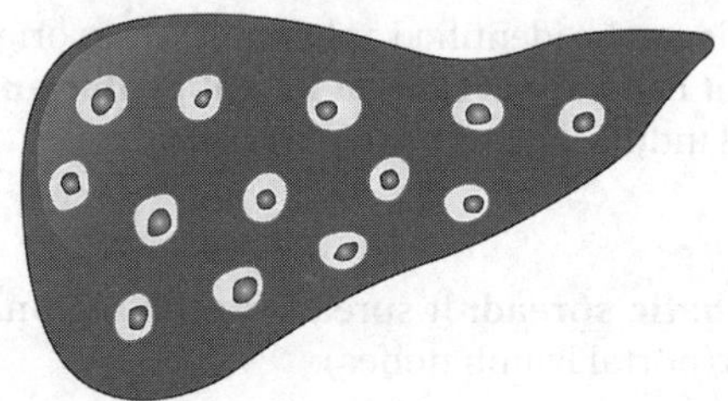

Fig. 18.13: Metastasis to liver showing multiple nodules with umbilication

PATHOLOGY OF GALLBLADDER

Cholecystitis

Inflammation of the gallbladder is known as cholecystitis. It may be acute, chronic, or acute superimposed on chronic. Mostly, it occurs in association with gallstones.

Acute Cholecystitis

Acute cholecystitis is a diffuse inflammation of the gallbladder, usually secondary to obstruction of the gallbladder outlet (passage of exit).

- **Acute calculous cholecystitis:** It develops as a complication of gallstones.
- **Acalculous cholecystitis:** Cholecystitis without gallstones is called **acalculous cholecystitis**. It occurs in severely ill patients and may be due to **ischemia.**

Morphology

Gross: The gallbladder is usually **enlarged** and **tense**. The **serosal surface** may show **exudates or pus**. In calculous cholecystitis, the lumen contains one or more stones (Fig. 18.14).

Microscopy

Microscopically, the wall of the gallbladder shows **edema, hemorrhage** with acute and chronic **inflammation**. The mucosa may show focal ulcerations.

Complications

- **Empyema of the gallbladder** in which gallbladder is filled with pus.
- **Gangrenous cholecystitis** is associated with widespread necrosis of gallbladder.
- **Perforation:** It results in **bile peritonitis, pericholecystic abscess** or creating a **cholecystenteric fistula**.

Clinical features

Acute cholecystitis presents with **right upper quadrant** or epigastric pain, mild fever, anorexia, tachycardia, sweating,

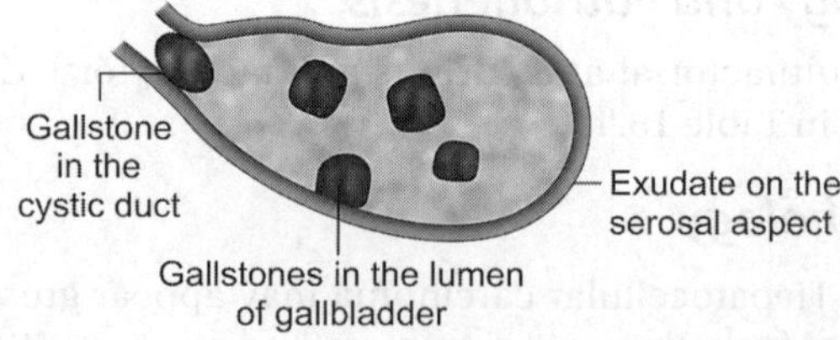

Fig. 18.14: Acute calculous cholecystitis showing enlarged gallbladder containing gallstones and exudate on the serosal surface

nausea and vomiting. Acute calculous cholecystitis usually present with mild symptoms, however it may appear as **acute surgical emergency**. Recurrence is common in patients who recover. Clinical symptoms of **acute acalculous cholecystitis are more insidious.**

Laboratory findings

It may show mild to moderate leukocytosis and mild elevations in serum alkaline phosphatase values.

Chronic Cholecystitis

Chronic cholecystitis is the most common disease of the gallbladder. It is usually associated with gallstones. Chronic cholecystitis may also develop from repeated attacks of acute cholecystitis.

Morphology

Gross (Fig. 18.15): The **size** of the gallbladder may be **decreased** and the **wall** may be **thickened**. The serosa is usually smooth and glistening. The lumen usually contains stones.

Microscopy: The gallbladder wall shows infiltration by **lymphocytes, plasma cells, and macrophages** in the mucosa. The proliferation of the mucosa and fusion of the mucosal folds may give rise to buried crypts of epithelium within the gallbladder wall. These are called **Rokitansky–Aschoff sinuses** (Fig. 18.16).

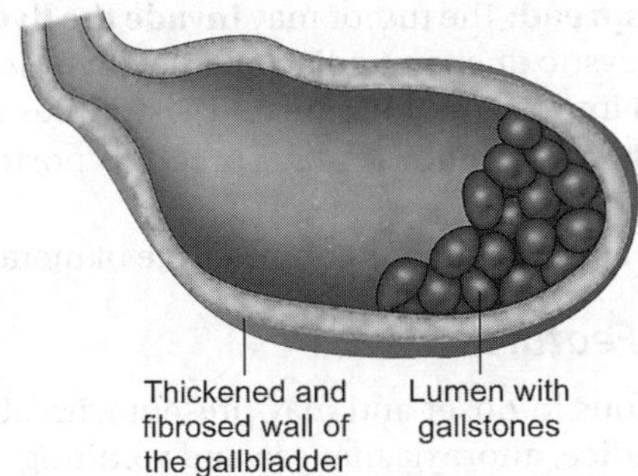

Fig. 18.15: Diagrammatic gross appearance of chronic cholecystis with gallstones

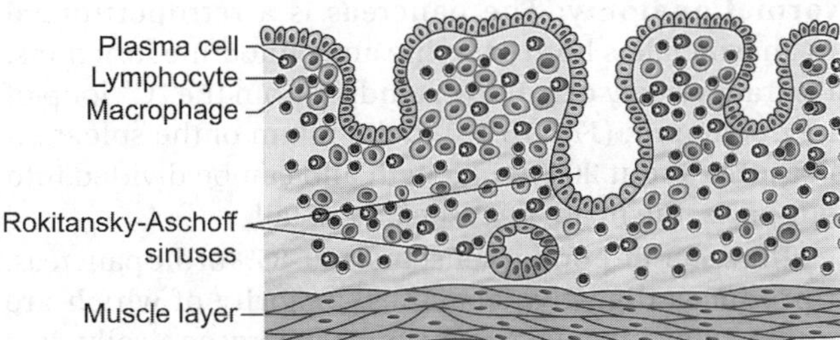

Fig. 18.16: Microscopic appearance of chronic cholecystitis

Clinical features

Chronic cholecystitis presents with recurrent attacks of either steady or colicky epigastric or right upper quadrant pain. Other symptoms include: nausea, vomiting and intolerance for fatty foods.

Complications

These include: bacterial superinfection, gallbladder perforation/rupture with diffuse peritonitis, biliary enteric (cholecystenteric) fistula, gallstone-induced intestinal obstruction and porcelain gallbladder, with increased risk of cancer.

Cholelithiasis (Gallstones)

A stone (pathological concretion) formed from the normal or abnormal constituents of bile in the gallbladder or in a bile duct is called gallstone.

Types

There are two main types of gallstones.

- **Cholesterol stones:** They contain cholesterol and are the most common type of gallstones.
- **Pigment stones:** They are composed of bilirubin calcium salts. Pigment stones are subclassified as **black and brown pigment** stones.

Gallstones were also classified as **pure, mixed and combined**.

Etiology and Risk Factors (Box 18.4)

Pathogenesis of cholesterol stones

It is a multifactorial disease. When the bile gets supersaturated with cholesterol, it forms solid cholesterol monohydrate crystals. Hypomotility of gallbladder and hypersecretion of mucus leads to bile stasis and promotes stone formation.

Box 18.4: Risk factors for gallstones

Cholesterol stones 5Fs: Fat, Fertile, Forty, Female, Familial
• Genetic predisposition such as genetic hyperlipoproteinemias • Increasing age • Female sex hormones: Female sex, oral contraceptives, pregnancy, parity • Environmental factors: Obesity, drugs (e.g. clofibrate) • Familial predisposition • Metabolic abnormalities: Diabetes.
Pigment stones
• Hemolytic anemia • Infection of biliary tract • Gastrointestinal disorders, e.g. Crohn disease, pancreatic insufficiency

Pathogenesis of pigment stones

- **Black pigment stones** form in the gallbladder as a result of **increased production of unconjugated bilirubin** (e.g. hemolytic anemia).
- **Brown pigment stones** develop secondary to stasis and **biliary infections** (predominantly *E. coli*) and with ascending cholangitis.

Morphology

Cholesterol stones: They are usually single. They are **yellow, round** with finely granular external surface and **may grow up to 5 cm.** Cut section shows **glistening**, long, thin **radiating palisading crystals of cholesterol**. Cholesterol stones are **radiolucent.**

Pigment gallstones (Fig. 18.17)

- ***Black pigment stones:*** They occur in patients with cirrhosis and chronic hemolytic states. The black stones are usually **multiple** and less than **1.5 cm in diameter**. They are usually **spiculated and molded.**
- ***Brown pigment stones:*** They tend to be **laminated and soft** and may have a **soap-like or greasy consistency**. They can be **crushed easily**.

Clinical Features

The majority of gallstones (>80%) are silent and patients remain **asymptomatic**. When symptomatic, patients present with **biliary pain**, which is either excruciating and constant or "colicky" (spasmodic).

Complications

- **Cholecystitis:** Both acute and chronic cholecystitis may develop with gallstones.

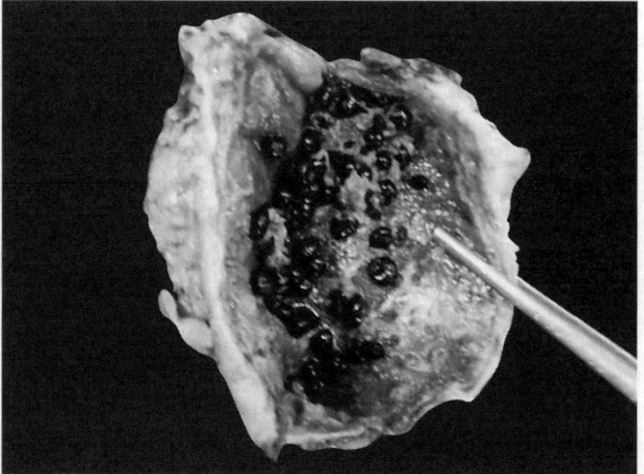

Fig. 18.17: Gallbladder shows multiple black-pigment stones

- **Biliary fistulas:** Formation of fistula between biliary system and bowel or gallbladder and skin.
- **Gallstone ileus or Bouveret's syndrome:** A large stone may erode directly into an adjacent loop of small bowel, causing intestinal obstruction (**gallstone ileus**).
- **Hydrops of the gallbladder (mucocele):** When there is obstruction of the cystic duct, the lumen of gallbladder may be distended with clear mucinous fluid secreted by the gallbladder. This is termed as hydrops of the gallbladder.
- **Increased risk for carcinoma** of the gallbladder.
- **Pancreatitis.**
- **Obstructive jaundice.**

Carcinoma of the Gallbladder

Carcinoma of the gallbladder arises from the mucosa of the gallbladder. It is slightly more common in females in the seventh decade of life. The most important **risk factor is gallstones** (cholelithiasis).

Morphology

Gross: Carcinomas of the gallbladder show two patterns of growth: **Infiltrating** and **exophytic**.

Microscopy: These tumors are **adenocarcinomas** consisting of tumor cells arranged in glandular pattern.

Spread of Tumor

- **Local spread:** The tumor may **invade the liver,** extend to the cystic duct and adjacent bile ducts. It may also spread into the peritoneum and gastrointestinal tract.
- **Lymphatic spread:** It may spread to porto-hepatic lymph nodes.
- **Blood spread:** Lung is common site of metastasis.

Clinical Features

It is insidious in onset and may present with abdominal pain, jaundice, anorexia, nausea and vomiting.

PATHOLOGY OF PANCREAS

Normal anatomy: The pancreas is a retroperitoneal organ which has both exocrine and endocrine functions. It is transversely oriented extending from the "C" loop of the duodenum (Fig. 18.18) to the hilum of the spleen. It measures about 20 cm in length and can be divided into four parts: the head, neck, body and tail.

The exocrine portion constitutes 80–85% of the pancreas. It produces digestive enzymes, majority of which are produced as inactive proenzymes. Microscopically, it is composed of acinar cells.

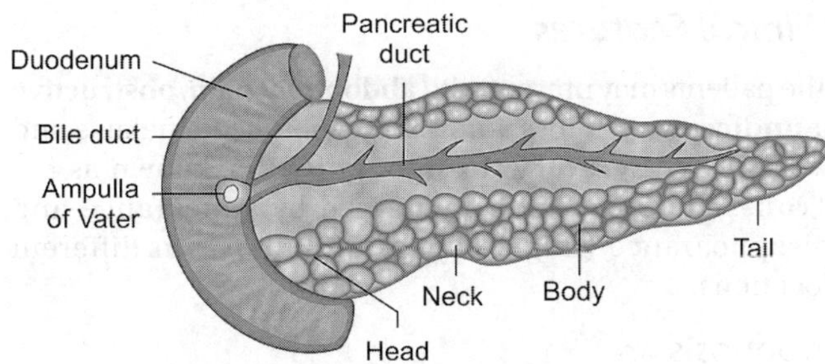

Fig. 18.18: Normal anatomy of pancreas

Box 18.5: Etiologic factors in acute pancreatitis

Metabolic, e.g. alcoholism
Genetic
Mechanical, e.g. gallstones
Vascular, e.g. ischemic injury, shock
Infectious, e.g. mumps

The endocrine portion is composed of the islets of Langerhans. The islet cells secrete hormones such as insulin, glucagon and somatostatin.

Pancreatitis

Pancreatitis is **inflammation of the exocrine pancreas.** It may be acute or chronic.

Acute Pancreatitis

Acute pancreatitis is pancreatic parenchymal injury associated with inflammation. Acute pancreatitis is relatively common.

Etiology

Biliary tract disease and alcoholism account for majority of cases (Box 18.5).

Pathogenesis

The changes of acute pancreatitis are due to **autodigestion of the pancreatic substance by inappropriately activated pancreatic enzymes.** Inappropriate activation of trypsinogen is an important triggering event in acute pancreatitis. The pancreatic enzyme activation may be initiated with **obstruction of the pancreatic duct** (e.g. gallstones). Direct acinar cell injury caused by certain viruses (e.g. mumps), drugs, alcohol and direct trauma to the pancreas, as well as ischemia or shock may also lead to pancreatitis.

Morphology: The pancreas shows edema, acute inflammation, enzymatic fat necrosis (by lipase), destruction of pancreatic parenchyma (by protease), and destruction of blood vessels (by elastase) leading to hemorrhage.

Clinical features

Abdominal pain which is constant and intense is the predominant symptom. This pain is referred to the upper back and occasionally referred to the left shoulder. Anorexia, nausea, and vomiting may accompany the pain.

Laboratory findings

- **Serum amylase:** It is **markedly raised** during the first 24 hours.
- **Serum lipase:** It is **raised** following the raised amylase level.
- **Hypocalcemia:** It is due to precipitation of calcium in necrotic fat cells of fat necrosis.

Radiography

Direct visualization of inflamed pancreas by radiography may be helpful in the diagnosis.

Complications of acute pancreatitis

- Peripheral vascular collapse and **shock** during the first week of illness.
- **Acute respiratory distress syndrome.**
- **Acute renal failure.**
- **Hemolysis.**
- **Disseminated intravascular coagulation.**
- **Diffuse fat necrosis.**
- **Sterile pancreatic abscess.**
- **Pancreatic pseudocyst.**

Chronic Pancreatitis

Definition: Chronic pancreatitis is defined as inflammation of the pancreas with **destruction of exocrine parenchyma**, and in the late stages, the destruction of endocrine parenchyma.

Etiology

The most common cause of chronic pancreatitis is **long-term alcohol abuse**. Other less common causes are: long-standing **obstruction** of the pancreatic duct by pseudocysts, calculi, trauma, neoplasms, or pancreas divisum.

Pathogenesis

The pathogenesis of chronic pancreatitis is not well-known. Repeated attacks of acute pancreatitis may lead to chronic pancreatitis.

Morphology

The **pancreas feel hard**, sometimes with dilated ducts and visible calcified concretions.

Microscopy

Chronic pancreatitis is characterized by:

1. **Parenchymal fibrosis.**

2. **Reduced number and size of acini** with relative **sparing of the islets of Langerhans.**
3. Variable **dilation of the pancreatic ducts.**
4. **Chronic inflammatory infiltrate** around lobules and ducts.

Clinical features

- **Repeated attacks of abdominal pain** or persistent abdominal and back pain.
- **It may remain silent** until pancreatic insufficiency and diabetes mellitus develop. Diabetes mellitus develop when there is destruction of islets of Langerhans.

Complications chronic pancreatitis

- Severe pancreatic exocrine insufficiency and chronic malabsorption.
- Diabetes mellitus.
- Pancreatic pseudocysts.
- Risk of developing pancreatic cancer.

Pancreatic Carcinoma

Pancreatic cancer is one of the visceral cancers occurring between the ages of 60 and 80 years.

Risk factors: These include: Cigarette smoking, consumption of a diet rich in fats, chronic pancreatitis, diabetes mellitus, alcohol consumption and familial clustering.

Morphology

Site: Majority of the pancreatic carcinomas arise in the head, followed by body and tail of the pancreas.

Gross: They are usually hard, stellate, gray-white, and appear as poorly defined masses.

Microscopy: They are **adenocarcinomas** in which tumor cells are arranged in glandular pattern.

Clinical Features

The patients may present with **abdominal pain, obstructive jaundice**, weight loss, anorexia, generalized malaise and weakness. **Migratory thrombophlebitis**, known as the **Trousseau sign**, is characterized by appearance and disappearance (migratory) of thrombosis in different locations.

Prognosis

The course of pancreatic carcinoma is brief and progressive.

Endocrine Tumors of Pancreas

- **Insulinomas:** The tumor cells secrete insulin continuously and produce hypoglycemia. Insulin secretion is not regulated by blood glucose levels. Features of hypoglycemia include sweating, visual changes, nervousness and hunger, which may progress to confusion, lethargy and even seizures or coma. Surgical removal is usually curative.
- **Glucagonomas:** They are associated with a syndrome of (1) mild diabetes; (2) a necrotizing, migratory, erythematous rash; (3) anemia; (4) diarrhea; and (5) deep vein thrombosis.
- **Somatostatinomas:** They produce a syndrome of mild diabetes, gallstones, steatorrhea, hypochlorhydria, anemia and weight loss.
- **Pancreatic gastrinoma:** It is composed of G cells, which secrete gastrin that is a powerful hormone which stimulates gastric acid secretion. Pancreatic gastrinoma produces Zollinger-Ellison syndrome which is characterized by (1) intractable gastric hypersecretion, (2) severe peptic ulceration of the duodenum and jejunum and (3) high blood gastrin levels.

SELF-ASSESSMENT EXERCISES

I. Essay

1. Define and classify cirrhosis. Discuss the pathogenesis and morphology of alcoholic cirrhosis.

II. Short Notes

1. Name five hepatotropic viruses.
2. Morphology of liver in acute viral hepatitis.
3. Chronic hepatitis.
4. Liver abscess.
5. Hepatocellular carcinoma.
6. Causes of obstructive jaundice.
7. Gallstones.
8. Cholecystitis.
9. Acute pancreatitis.
10. Pancreatic carcinoma.
11. Portal hypertension.

CHAPTER 19

Urinary System

CHAPTER OUTLINE

NORMAL ANATOMY

Kidneys are paired, bean-shaped organs in the retroperitoneal space. Each adult kidney weighs about 150 g. They are covered by a thin capsule. Cut section shows, an outer cortex and an inner medulla (Fig. 19.1). The medulla consists of renal pyramids, the apices of which are known as papillae, and is related to calyx. There is a funnel-shaped structure called as renal pelvis that collects and empties into the ureter.

The nephron (Fig. 19.2) is the functional and structural unit of the kidney. Nephron consists of glomerulus, tubule, and the collecting system. The glomerulus (Fig. 19.3) consists of an anastomosing network of capillaries. It has visceral epithelium, basement membrane and the

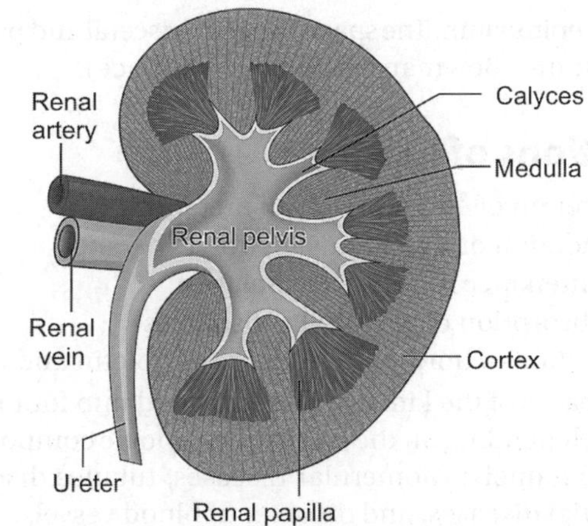

Fig. 19.1: Cut section of renal parenchyma showing different components

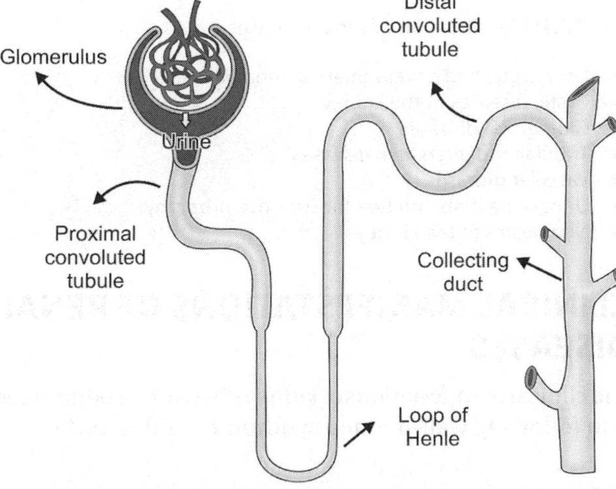

Fig. 19.2: Different components of nephron

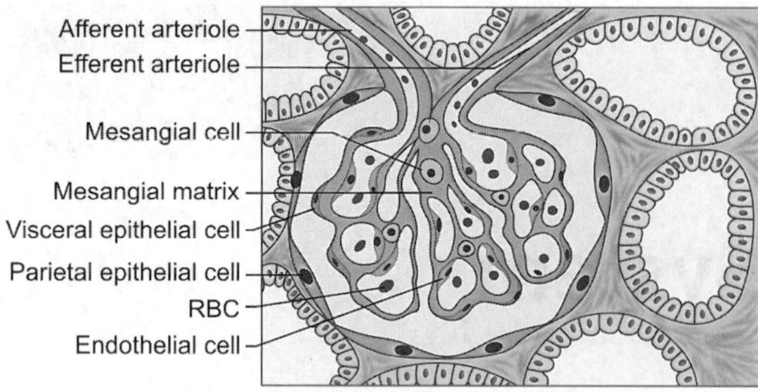

Fig. 19.3: Light microscopic appearance of glomerulus (diagrammatic)

parietal epithelium. The space between visceral and parietal epithelium is Bowman space (urinary space).

Functions of Kidney

- Excretion of end products of metabolism
- Regulation of water and electrolyte balance
- Maintenance of acid-base balance
- Reabsorption of essential substances
- Secretion of hormones like erythropoietin and renin.

Diseases of the kidney can be divided into four major groups depending on the basic morphologic components affected namely: Glomerular diseases, tubules diseases, interstitial diseases, and diseases of blood vessels.

CLASSIFICATION OF RENAL DISEASES (BOX 19.1)

Box 19.1: Classification of renal diseases

- Congenital and developmental anomalies
- Cystic diseases of the kidney
- Glomerular diseases
- Tubular and interstitial diseases
- Vascular diseases
- Urinary tract obstruction (obstructive uropathy)
- Neoplasms of the kidney

CLINICAL MANIFESTATIONS OF RENAL DISEASES

The clinical manifestations of kidney disease can be grouped into following well-defined syndromes (Table 19.1).

CONGENITAL AND DEVELOPMENTAL ANOMALIES

Congenital renal disease may be hereditary or acquired (most commonly) developmental defect during gestation.

Agenesis of the Kidney

Renal agenesis is the **complete absence of renal tissue**. It may be unilateral or bilateral.

- **Bilateral agenesis** is **incompatible with life**, and most infants are stillborn. It is usually associated with other congenital disorders (e.g. limb defects, hypoplastic lungs).
- **Unilateral agenesis** is uncommon, not serious and compatible with normal life if no other abnormalities exist. The contralateral solitary kidney enlarges due to compensatory hypertrophy and can maintain normal renal function. Some patients may develop progressive glomerular sclerosis in the remaining kidney.

Hypoplasia

Hypoplasia is the failure of the kidneys to develop to a normal size. They are smaller, but histologically normal. It may be unilateral or bilateral. It is more commonly unilateral but when bilateral, it results in renal failure in early childhood. True renal hypoplasia is seen in low birth weight infants and it increases the lifetime risk for chronic kidney disease. Hypoplasia must be differentiated from small kidneys due to atrophy (congenital and acquired) or scarring. Hypoplastic kidney shows no scars and has a reduced number of renal lobes and pyramids, usually six or fewer.

Ectopic Kidneys

Renal ectopia is a developmental anomaly in which there is **normal kidney in an abnormal location**. These kidneys are misplaced usually just above the pelvic brim or within the pelvis. One or both kidneys may be affected. They are usually normal or slightly smaller in size. Because of their abnormal location, kinking or tortuosity of the ureters may cause obstruction to urinary flow, which in turn predisposes to bacterial infections.

Horseshoe Kidneys

- Horseshoe kidneys are **common congenital anomaly** in which there is fusion of the upper (10%) or lower poles (90%) of the kidneys.
- It gives a horseshoe appearance to kidneys (Fig. 19.4), which are continuous across the midline anterior to the great vessels.
- It is associated with increased risk for obstruction and renal infection (pyelonephritis) because the ureters are compressed as they cross over the junction between the two kidneys when the kidneys are fused at the lower pole.

Table 19.1: Clinical manifestation of renal diseases

Disease	Manifestations
Glomerular syndromes	
Nephritic syndrome (glomerular disease)	Acute onset of either grossly visible **hematuria** (red blood cells in urine) or microscopic hematuria with dysmorphic red cells and red cell casts on urinalysis, diminished GFR, **mild to moderate proteinuria**, and **hypertension**
Rapidly progressive glomerulonephritis	Nephritic syndrome with rapid decline in GFR (within hours to days)
Nephrotic syndrome (glomerular disease)	Heavy/massive proteinuria (more than 3.5 g/day), hypoalbuminemia, severe edema, hyperlipidemia, and lipiduria (lipid in the urine)
Chronic kidney disease (previously termed chronic renal failure)	Persistently diminished GFR less than 60 mL/minute/1.73 m^2 for at least 3 months, from any cause, and/or persistent albuminuria. It is the end result of all chronic renal parenchymal diseases
Asymptomatic hematuria or proteinuria, or both	Usually due to mild glomerular abnormalities
Others	
Azotemia is biochemical manifestation of kidney injury or extrarenal causes Uremia = azotemia + clinical signs and symptoms + biochemical abnormalities	Raised blood urea nitrogen (BUN) or an elevated serum creatinine due to reduced glomerular filtration rate (GFR) **Renal causes:** Acute or chronic kidney injury **Extrarenal causes:** Prerenal azotemia (e.g. due to hypotension or excessive fluid loss from any cause) or postrenal azotemia (due to obstruction to urine flow distal to the kidney)
Acute kidney injury	**Rapid decline in GFR** (within hours to days), with deranged fluid and electrolyte balance, and **retention** of metabolic waste products normally excreted by the kidney (**urea and creatinine**), **oliguria or anuria** (reduced or no urine flow) in most severe cases. It may be due to glomerular, interstitial, vascular or acute tubular injury
End-stage renal disease (ESRD)	GFR is less than 5% of normal and is the terminal stage of uremia
Renal tubular defects due to diseases that either directly affect tubular structures or cause defects in specific tubular functions	Polyuria (excessive urine formation), nocturia, and electrolyte disorders
Urinary tract obstruction and renal tumors	Features depends on anatomic location and nature of the lesion
Urinary tract infection. It may affect kidney (pyelonephritis) or the bladder (cystitis)	Bacteriuria and pyuria (bacteria and leukocytes in the urine) Infection may be symptomatic or asymptomatic
Nephrolithiasis (renal stones)	Spasms of severe pain (renal colic) and hematuria

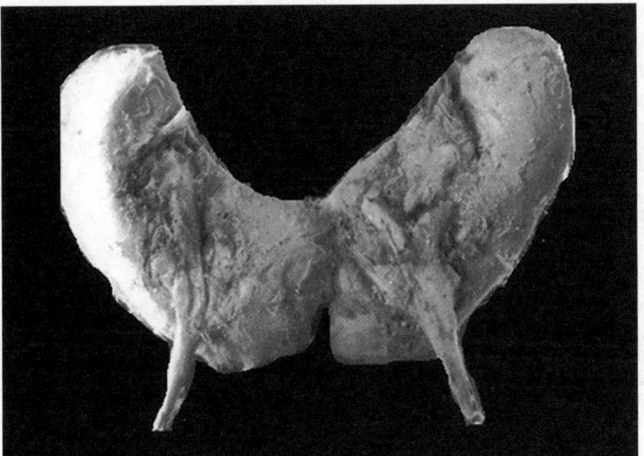

Fig. 19.4: Horseshoe kidney showing fusion at the lower poles

CYSTIC DISEASES OF THE KIDNEY

Definition: Cystic diseases of the kidney represent a **heterogeneous group of hereditary, developmental, and acquired disorders** characterized by the **presence of unilateral or bilateral renal cysts**.

Classification of Renal Cystic Disease (Box 19.2)

Autosomal Dominant (Adult) Polycystic Kidney Disease

Definition: Autosomal-dominant (adult) polycystic kidney disease **(ADPKD)** is a **hereditary disorder** characterized by **multiple cysts in both kidneys**. These cysts expand and cause destruction of kidney parenchyma and leads to renal failure.

Box 19.2: Classification of renal cystic disease

- Polycystic kidney disease
  - Autosomal dominant (adult) polycystic disease
  - Autosomal recessive (childhood) polycystic disease
- Medullary cystic disease
  - Medullary sponge kidney
  - Nephronophthisis
- Multicystic renal dysplasia
- Acquired (dialysis-associated) cystic disease
- Localized (simple) renal cysts

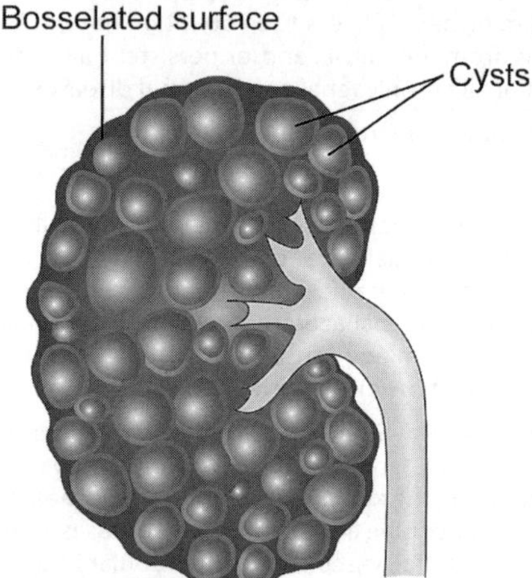

Fig. 19.5: Autosomal-dominant adult polycystic kidney disease (ADPKD) shows markedly enlarged kidney with numerous dilated cysts

Genetics and Pathogenesis

The ADPKD is **genetically heterogeneous disorder** caused by **mutations in *PKD1*** (85% of cases) **and *PKD2* gene** (15%). The exact pathogenesis of ADPKD is unknown.

Morphology

Gross (Fig. 19.5)

- **Bilateral.**
- **Size: Markedly enlarged**; weight is increased and each may reach up to 4 kg.
- **External surface: Bosselated** with **numerous cysts of varying sizes**, measuring up to 3 to 4 cm in diameter, with no intervening parenchyma.

Microscopy

- **Numerous cysts** with functioning nephrons between these cysts.
- **Intervening renal parenchyma:** It may be normal or may show foci of interstitial fibrosis and pyelonephritis.

Clinical Features

- **Majority** of patients remain **asymptomatic until the fourth decade** of life.
- It may present with **flank pain** (heaviness or dragging sensation), **bilateral abdominal masses**, and **renal colic** (due to passage of blood clots in the urine), and **hypertension**. When sufficient quantity of nephrons are destroyed, patient develops **renal failure.**

Extrarenal associated congenital anomalies

1. Large multicystic kidneys, liver cysts
2. Berry aneurysms
3. Mitral valve prolapse.

Autosomal Recessive (Childhood) Polycystic Kidney Disease

Autosomal recessive (childhood) polycystic kidney disease (ARPKD) is **genetically different from adult polycystic kidney disease.**

Etiology

In **majority** of the cases, ARPKD is caused by **mutations of the polycystic kidney hepatic disease gene (*PKHD1*) gene.**

Morphology

Gross

- **Both kidneys** are **markedly enlarged** and have a **smooth external appearance.**
- **Cut section** (Fig. 19.6)**:**

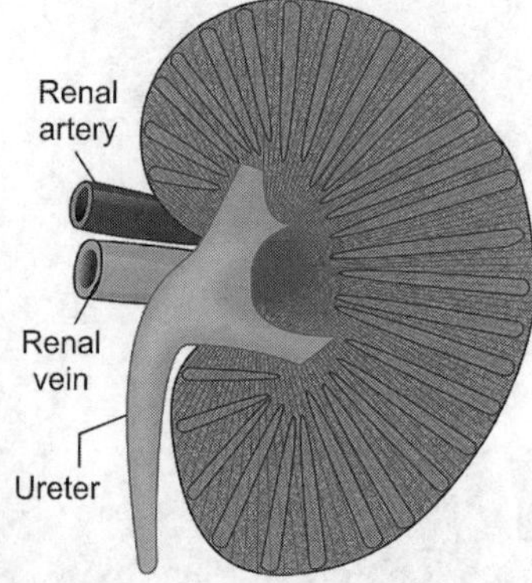

Fig. 19.6: Diagrammatic appearance of cut section of autosomal-recessive childhood PKD, showing smaller cysts and dilated channels at right angles to the cortical surface

- **Medulla and cortex** are completely **replaced by numerous small cysts.**
- The **cysts** tend to be **linear and radiate from the medulla to the outer cortex** (right angles to the cortical surface). It gives a **sponge-like appearance to the kidney**.

Microscopy

- **Shape: Cyst is cylindrical** and appears as dilated tubular structures or, less commonly saccular.
- **Lining: All the cysts are lined** by **cuboidal epithelial cells**, reflecting their **origin from the collecting ducts**.

Features of ARPKD

- All patients also have cysts in the liver.
- Patients who survive infancy (infantile and juvenile forms), may develop **congenital hepatic fibrosis**.

Cystic Diseases of Renal Medulla

Medullary cystic disease of kidney includes: (1) medullary sponge kidney, (2) nephronophthisis and (3) adult onset medullary cystic disease.

Medullary Sponge Kidney

- It is characterized by **multiple cystic dilations of the collecting ducts in the medulla**.
- Medullary sponge kidney occurs in adults. It is usually asymptomatic and is usually discovered radiographically. Renal function is usually normal.
- **Pathogenesis:** Not known.
- **Gross:** The disease is bilateral in 75% of patients. It shows medulla with dilatation of papillary ducts and multiple small cysts (<5 mm in diameter). Unless there is superimposed pyelonephritis, cortical scarring is absent.
- **Microscopy:** The cysts arise from collecting ducts in the renal papillae. These cysts are lined by cuboidal or columnar epithelium or occasionally by transitional epithelium.
- **Complications:** Cysts may predispose to secondary pyelonephritis.

Nephronophthisis and Adult-Onset Medullary Cystic Disease

It is a **group of progressive kidney disorders characterized by variable number of cysts in the medulla, usually concentrated at the corticomedullary junction**. The **cortical tubulointerstitial damage** is **the cause of the eventual renal insufficiency.**

Acquired (Dialysis-Associated) Cystic Disease

- Kidney of patients with end-stage renal disease who have undergone prolonged dialysis may show numerous cortical and medullary renal cysts. The cysts measure 0.1 to 4 cm in diameter, and contain clear fluid.
- Most patients are asymptomatic, but sometimes the cysts bleed producing hematuria.

Simple Cysts

- Simple renal cysts may be single or multiple and usually observed in the cortex. They are translucent and usually measure about 1 to 5 cm in diameter. They are lined by a gray, glistening, smooth membrane, and filled with clear fluid.
- They are common postmortem findings without clinical significance.
- Complications: Occasionally, hemorrhage into the cysts may cause sudden distention and pain. Calcification of the hemorrhage may give produce bizarre radiographic shadows.

GLOMERULAR DISEASES

Diseases of the glomeruli are common. Glomeruli may be injured by a variety of factors and in several systemic diseases (Box 19.3).

Box 19.3: Common glomerular diseases

Primary glomerulonephritis/glomerulopathies
- Acute proliferative glomerulonephritis: Postinfectious, others
- Rapidly progressive (crescentic) glomerulonephritis (RPGN)
- Minimal-change disease (MCD)
- Membranous nephropathy
- Membranoproliferative glomerulonephritis (MPGN)
- Dense deposit disease
- Focal segmental glomerulosclerosis (FSGS)
- IgA nephropathy
- Chronic glomerulonephritis

Systemic diseases with glomerular involvement
- Systemic immunological diseases: For example, systemic lupus erythematosus
- Metabolic diseases: For example, diabetes mellitus
- Vasculitis: Microscopic polyarteritis/polyangiitis, Wegener granulomatosis, Henoch-Schönlein purpura
- Amyloidosis
- Goodpasture syndrome
- Bacterial endocarditis

Hereditary disorders
- Alport syndrome
- Thin basement membrane disease
- Fabry disease

Nephritic Syndrome

It is characterized by **hematuria**, **red cell casts in the urine, azotemia, oliguria** and **hypertension**. Proteinuria and edema are not as severe as in the nephrotic syndrome. One of the main causes of nephritic syndrome is acute proliferative glomerulonephritis.

Acute Proliferative Glomerulonephritis

These are immune complex mediated glomerular diseases. They are characterized histologically by diffuse proliferation of cells in the glomeruli, associated with infiltration by leukocytes. It may be divided into poststreptococcal or non-poststreptococcal type.

Poststreptococcal (postinfectious) glomerulonephritis

Poststreptococcal glomerulonephritis is a common disorder in developing countries.

Etiology and pathogenesis

It follows streptococcal infection usually of the pharynx (pharyngitis). It manifests 1–4 weeks following streptococcal infection. The antibodies produced against streptococci, combine with streptococcal antigens and form antigen-antibody complexes in the circulation. These immune complexes get deposited within glomeruli and initiate inflammation. Thus, it is an immunologically mediated disease.

Microscopy (Fig. 19.7)

- **Hypercellular glomeruli:** The glomeruli are enlarged and hypercellular **with infiltration by leukocytes** (both neutrophils and monocytes).
- **Obliteration of capillary lumen:** Swelling and proliferation of endothelial and mesangial cells along with infiltration by leukocytes lead to obliteration of the glomerular capillary lumina.

Clinical features

Most frequently seen in **children between 6 and 10 years of age**. The child presents with malaise, fever, nausea, oliguria, and hematuria (smoky or cola-colored urine) 1–2 weeks after recovery from a sore throat. Periorbital edema, and mild to moderate hypertension is commonly observed.

Prognosis

It is good in children and more than 95% totally recover.

Nephrotic Syndrome

Definition: It is characterized by **heavy proteinuria** (>3.5 g of protein/24 hours), **hypoalbuminemia, edema, hyperlipidemia and lipiduria**.

Causes

- The most common **systemic causes—diabetes, amyloidosis, systemic lupus erythematosus.**
- **Primary glomerular lesions—minimal-change disease, membranous glomerulopathy and focal segmental glomerulosclerosis.**

Membranous Nephropathy (Membranous glomerulopathy)

Membranous nephropathy is a **common cause of nephrotic syndrome in adults.**

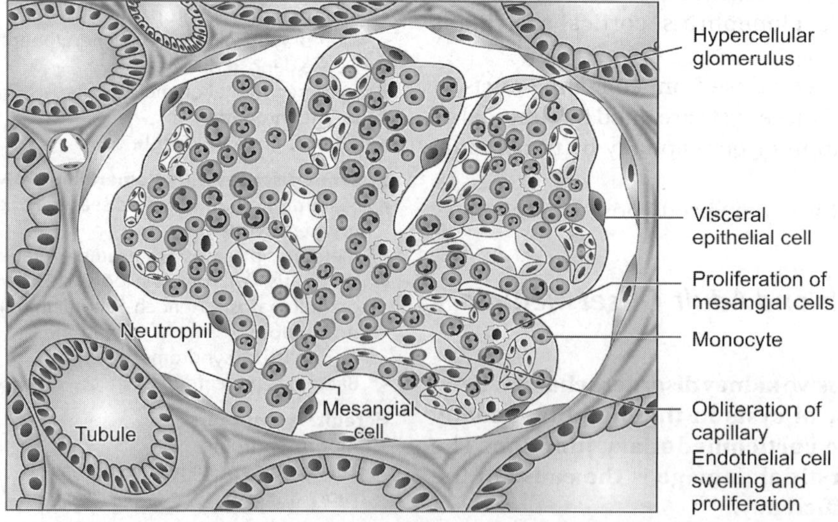

Fig. 19.7: Microscopic features of acute poststreptococcal glomerulonephritis

Etiology and Pathogenesis

It is an **immune complex-mediated disease**. It may develop as a primary disease or secondary to diabetes, malignancy, infections (e.g. hepatitis B virus).

Microscopy

The glomeruli show **uniform, diffuse thickening of the glomerular capillary wall.** There is **neither proliferation nor inflammation**.

Clinical Features

Presents with features of nephrotic syndrome.

Course

Variable but generally indolent.

Minimal-Change Disease (Lipoid Nephrosis/Nil Lesion)

In minimal-change disease (MCD), the glomerular changes are **absent or minimal and glomeruli appear normal under light microscopy**. MCD is the major cause of nephrotic syndrome in children.

Etiology and Pathogenesis

The pathogenesis of MCD is unknown.

Light Microscopy

Glomeruli appear **normal by light microscopy**.

Electron Microscopy

Characteristic feature is **uniform and diffuse effacement** (loss) **of foot processes in the visceral epithelial cells** (podocytes).

Clinical Features

Peak incidence is between 2 and 6 years of age. Classically, it presents as nephrotic syndrome.

Prognosis

Excellent and responds well to corticosteroids.

Membranoproliferative Glomerulonephritis

Membranoproliferative Glomerulonephritis (MPGN) is histologically characterized by thickening of the glomerular basement membrane, proliferation of mainly mesangial cells and leukocyte infiltration.

Etiology and Pathogenesis

It may be primary (idiopathic) or secondary (in association with other systemic disorders). It may be due to activation of both classical and alternative complement pathways.

Light Microscopy

Glomeruli appear **large and hypercellular**, due to proliferation of mesangial and endothelial cells along with infiltration by leukocytes. **Thickening of GBM** is also seen.

Clinical Features

Mainly found in adolescent or young adults. MPGN is responsible for 10–20% of nephrotic syndrome in children and young adults.

Course

Slowly progressive course and about 50% develop chronic renal failure.

Chronic Glomerulonephritis

Chronic glomerulonephritis is an **end-stage of many types of glomerulonephritis** (Table 19.2).

Morphology

Gross (Fig. 19.8)

- **Both kidneys** show **diffusely granular** cortical surfaces and **symmetrical contraction**.
- Cut section: It shows **thinned cortex** and an **increase in peripelvic fat**. The **capsule is difficult to remove** because of adhesions.

Microscopy

- **Glomeruli:** The glomerular changes depend on the stage of the disease:
  - **Early stages:** It may show features of the **primary disease** (e.g. membranous nephropathy or MPGN).
  - **Late stages: Obliteration of glomeruli,** which appear as **acellular eosinophilic masses**.

Table 19.2: Causes of chronic glomerulonephritis

Crescentic glomerulonephritis (RPGN)	Focal segmental glomerulosclerosis (FSGS)
Membranoproliferative glomerulonephritis (MPGN)	IgA nephropathy
Membranous nephropathy	Poststreptococcal glomerulonephritis—rare
Others	

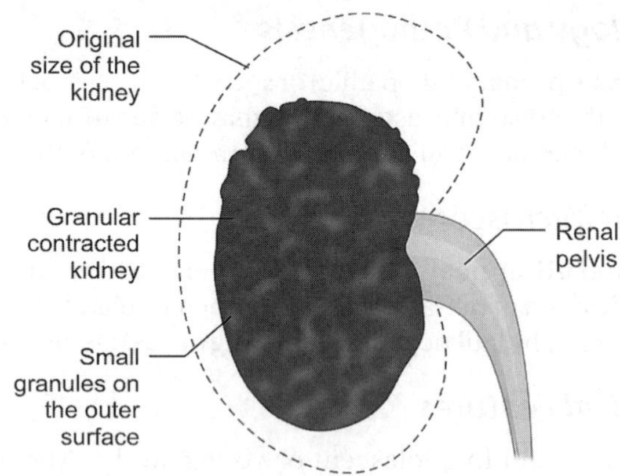

Fig. 19.8: Diagrammatic appearance of chronic glomerulonephritis

- **Tubules:** They show **marked atrophy**.
- **Interstitium:** It **shows fibrosis and mononuclear leukocytic infiltration**.
- **Blood vessels: Hypertension develops** in patients with chronic glomerulonephritis and the **vascular changes of hypertension** such as **arterial and arteriolar sclerosis** may be seen (refer page 113).

Uremic Complications

Patients of chronic renal failure may show complications due to uremia. These include:
- Uremic **pericarditis**
- Uremic **gastroenteritis**
- **Secondary hyperparathyroidism** with nephrocalcinosis and renal osteodystrophy
- **Left ventricular hypertrophy** due to hypertension
- **Diffuse alveolar damage** (uremic pneumonitis).

Clinical Course

Insidious onset: It may **progress to renal insufficiency or uremia** during a span of years. Most patients have **hypertension** and may present with hypertension induce cerebral or cardiovascular diseases.

Nonspecific complaints: These include loss of appetite, anemia, vomiting, or weakness.

It **may be detected during routine medical examination** or during the course of investigation of edema or urinary abnormalities.

TUBULAR AND INTERSTITIAL DISEASES

Most types of tubular injury also involve the interstitium. Hence, diseases affecting tubules and interstitium are discussed together. Two major disease processes are: (1) ischemic or toxic tubular injury, and (2) inflammatory reactions of the tubules and interstitium *(tubulointerstitial nephritis)*.

Acute Tubular Injury/Necrosis (Acute Renal Failure)

- **Definition:** Acute tubular injury (ATI) is a **clinicopathologic entity characterized clinically by acute renal failure** and usually (but not invariably) **accompanied by morphological evidence of tubular injury (necrosis of tubular epithelial cells).**
- Since tubular necrosis is not invariable, the term ATI is preferred than the older term acute tubular necrosis (ATN). ATI is the **most common cause of acute kidney injury (acute renal failure)**. Acute renal failure is characterized by rapid reduction of renal function and with severe oliguria (urine less than 400 mL per day).

Causes of Acute Kidney Injury (Box 19.4)

Pathogenesis

Two important features of AKI (in both ischemic and nephrotoxic) are: (1) Tubule cell injury, and (2) Disturbances in blood flow.

Box 19.4: Causes of acute kidney injury

- **Ischemia:** Due to decreased or interrupted blood flow and is known as *ischemic AKI*.
  - **Reduction of effective circulating blood volume:**
    - Loss of blood: Massive hemorrhage
    - Loss of fluid: Severe burns, dehydration, prolonged diarrhea
    - Septic shock
    - Congestive heart failure
  - **Diffuse involvement of the intrarenal blood vessels:**
    - Microscopic polyangiitis
    - Malignant hypertension
    - Systemic conditions: For example, disseminated intravascular coagulation (DIC)
- **Direct toxic injury to the tubules (nephrotoxic AKI)**
  - Antibiotics (e.g. aminoglycosides, gentamicin, amphotericin B)
  - Poisons such as heavy metals (e.g. mercury, lead, cisplatin)
  - Organic solvents (e.g. carbon tetrachloride, ethylene glycol)
  - Radiation
- **Combinations of ischemic and nephrotoxic AKI**
  - Mismatched blood transfusions
  - Hemolytic crises: For example, sickle cell anemia
  - Skeletal muscle injuries causing myoglobinuria
- **Acute tubulointerstitial nephritis:** Hypersensitivity reaction to drugs
- **Urinary obstruction** (postrenal acute renal failure)
  - Tumors
  - Prostatic hypertrophy

Injury to the tubular epithelial cells

Tubular cells are sensitive to both ischemia and toxins.

- **Ischemia:** Ischemia **may cause reversible injury** (such as swelling, blebbing) or **irreversible injury** (necrosis and apoptosis). **Tubular necrosis** is **focal** and **multiple**, and the **tubular basement membrane** remains **intact**. If the precipitating cause is removed, repair of the necrotic foci and recovery of function can occur.
- **Toxins:** They can cause **direct injury to tubular epithelial cells**.

Consequences of tubular injury

- **Back-leakage of fluid from lumen into the interstitium:** It **occurs in the damaged tubules** → result in **interstitial edema** → causes **increased interstitial pressure**, and **further damage to the tubule**.
- **Luminal obstruction by casts:** Tubular epithelial cells gets detached from injured tubules and form casts leading to obstruction of tubular lumen. **Obstruction results in: (1) increased intratubular pressure**, (2) **decreased GFR,** and (3) **decreased urine outflow**.
- **Interstitial inflammation:** It also causes decreased GFR.

Disturbances in blood flow

Ischemia also causes **vasoconstriction** (intrarenal) and **reduces both glomerular blood flow** and **oxygen supply to tubules.**

Morphology

Ischemic acute kidney injury

Gross

- Both kidneys are **swollen** and show a **pale cortex** and a **congested medulla.**

Microscopy

- **Glomeruli:** Appear normal.
- **Tubules:**
  - **Areas involved:** Tubules show **focal and multiple areas of damage** along the nephron, **with large skip areas** in between. The lesions are **most marked in the proximal tubules** and the **ascending thick limbs of the loop of Henle** in the **outer medulla**.
  - **Tubular epithelial injury**.
- **Interstitium:** It shows edema and accumulations of leukocytes.
- **Blood vessels:** Normal.

Toxic acute kidney injury

Microscopy

- **Areas involved:** Most **common site of toxic injury** is seen in the **proximal convoluted tubules**. The **necrosis** of tubular epithelium is **more-extensive** in toxic ATN than seen in ischemic ATN.

Clinical Course

The clinical course of AKI may be divided into three stages namely: (1) initiation, (2) maintenance, and (3) recovery phases.

Initiation phase

Clinical features depend on the initiating cause of AKI. There is a mild reduction of urine output and increase in BUN.

Maintenance phase

During this phase, there is sustained decrease in urine output in the range of 40 to 400 mL/day (oliguria), salt and water overload, rising BUN level, hyperkalemia, metabolic acidosis, and other features of uremia.

Recovery phase

During this phase, there is a steady increase in urine volume, which may reach up to 3 L/day. There is loss of large amounts of water, sodium and potassium (leading to hypokalemia) in the urine. Once the renal tubular function returns to normal, BUN and creatinine levels also return to normal.

Prognosis: ATN is a **potentially reversible condition** and with modern therapy most patients recover.

Tubulointerstitial Nephritis

Tubulointerstitial nephritis is a **group of kidney diseases characterized by inflammatory injuries of the tubules and interstitium.** These are usually slow in onset and are mainly manifest by azotemia.

Tubulointerstitial nephritis can be acute or chronic. They may be primary as a consequence of progression in diseases that primarily affect the glomerulus or secondary due to a variety of vascular, cystic (polycystic kidney disease), and metabolic (diabetes) renal disorders.

Acute tubulointerstitial nephritis: It is rapid in onset and is characterized microscopically by interstitial edema, leukocyte infiltration of the interstitium and tubules, and tubular injury.

Chronic interstitial nephritis: It is characterized by infiltration by predominantly mononuclear leukocytes, prominent interstitial fibrosis, and widespread tubular atrophy.

Few causes of tubulointerstitial nephritis are listed in Box 19.5.

Box 19.5: Causes of tubulointerstitial nephritis

Infections: For example, acute bacterial pyelonephritis, chronic pyelonephritis
Toxins: For example, drugs, analgesics, heavy metals
Metabolic diseases: For example, urate nephropathy, nephrocalcinosis (hypercalcemic nephropathy)
Physical factors: Chronic urinary tract obstruction
Neoplasms: Multiple myeloma
Immunologic reactions: Transplant rejection
Idiopathic: "Idiopathic" interstitial nephritis

PYELONEPHRITIS AND URINARY TRACT INFECTION

Classification of Urinary Tract Infections

- **Lower urinary tract infections:** These include **cystitis** (bladder) and **urethritis**. Bacterial infection of the lower urinary tract may be completely asymptomatic (asymptomatic bacteriuria). Most of the cases, it remains localized to the bladder. However, lower urinary tract infection always carries the risk of spread to the kidney.
- **Pyelonephritis:** It involves **kidneys and their collecting systems** (pyelonephritis).

Pyelonephritis

Definition: Pyelonephritis is **inflammatory disease** of kidney **affecting the tubules, interstitium, and renal pelvis**.

It is one of the most common diseases of the kidney.

Classification of Pyelonephritis

- **Acute pyelonephritis:** It is caused by bacterial infection and is associated with urinary tract infection.
- **Chronic pyelonephritis:** It is a more complex disorder. However, bacterial infection plays a major role, but other factors (vesicoureteral reflux, obstruction) are also involved in its pathogenesis.

Acute Pyelonephritis

Acute pyelonephritis is an **acute suppurative inflammation** of the kidney affecting the tubules, interstitium, and renal pelvis.

Etiology and Pathogenesis (*Fig. 19.9*)

Causative organisms

Majority (~85%) of urinary tract infection are caused by Gram-negative bacilli, which are normal inhabitants of the intestinal tract (enteric origin).

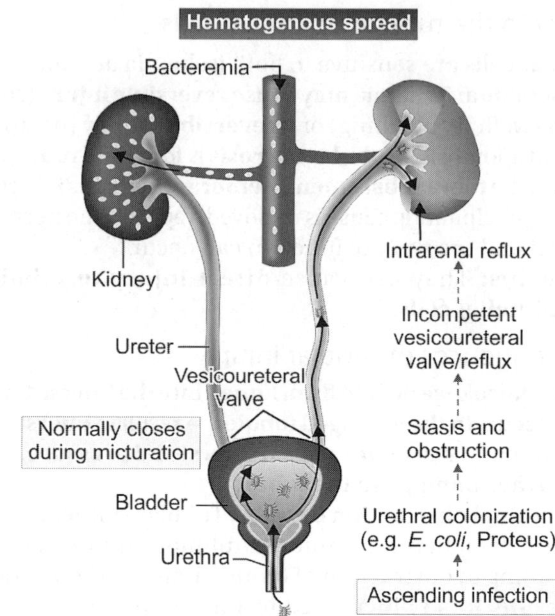

Fig. 19.9: Pathogenesis of acute pyelonephritis. More common mode is ascending infection. Hematogenous infection results from bacteremic spread

- **Most common pathogens:** ***Escherichia coli, Proteus, Klebsiella, and Enterobacter*.**
- **Less common:** *Streptococcus faecalis*, staphylococci, and fungi.
- **In immunocompromized patients:** **Viruses** (polyomavirus, cytomegalovirus, and adenovirus).

Source and route of infection

Bacteria can reach the kidney by **two routes**:

- **Ascending infection:** It is the **most common route** of infection of pyelonephritis. It is a form of endogenous infection, where the source of infecting organisms is the **patient's own fecal flora**. The infection ascends from the lower urinary tract into the renal parenchyma. **Different steps** in the pathogenesis of pyelonephritis are shown in Figure 19.3.
- **Hematogenous route:** It is **less common route of infection**. Because of rich blood supply, bacteria can seed the kidneys during the **course of septicemia or infective endocarditis** through the bloodstream. It occurs with **nonenteric organisms** (e.g. staphylococci), fungi and viruses.

Morphology

Gross

- **Unilateral or bilateral.**
- **Focal abscesses:** It may be seen on the **subcapsular surface** that appear small and **white**. In pyelonephritis

associated with reflux, they are **most common in the lower and upper poles.**
- **Pelvic and calyces:** They may be **hyperemic and covered by purulent exudate.**

Microscopy
- **Interstitium: It shows patchy interstitial neutrophilic infiltration**, which may later become extensive.
- **Tubules: Intratubular aggregates of neutrophils** forms abscess with the destruction of the involved tubules → **tubular necrosis.**
- **Glomeruli:** They appear normal because they are relatively resistant to the infection.

Complications
- **Papillary necrosis:** It is the **necrosis of the tips of the renal papillae.**
  - Seen mainly in **diabetics** and with **urinary tract obstruction.**
- **Pyonephrosis:** It is characterized by accumulation of **pus** (suppurative exudates) **within the renal pelvis, calyces, and ureter** → kidney distended with pus.
- **Perinephric abscess:** It develops when the **suppurative infection breaks the renal capsule** and spread into the perinephric tissue.

Clinical Features
- **Sudden onset of pain at the costovertebral angle, fever and malaise.**
- Dysuria, frequency and urgency.

Urinary Findings
Microscopy
- **Pus cells.**
- **WBC casts.**

Culture and sensitivity: It can **establish the causative organism.**

Course of the disease: Usually, follows a benign course.

Chronic Pyelonephritis and Reflux Nephropathy

Definition: Chronic pyelonephritis is a **chronic inflammation of tubulointerstitial tissue** leading to scarring of calyces, pelvis and renal parenchyma.

Chronic pyelonephritis is an **important cause of end-stage renal disease.**
- **Reflux nephropathy (chronic reflux-associated pyelonephritis)**

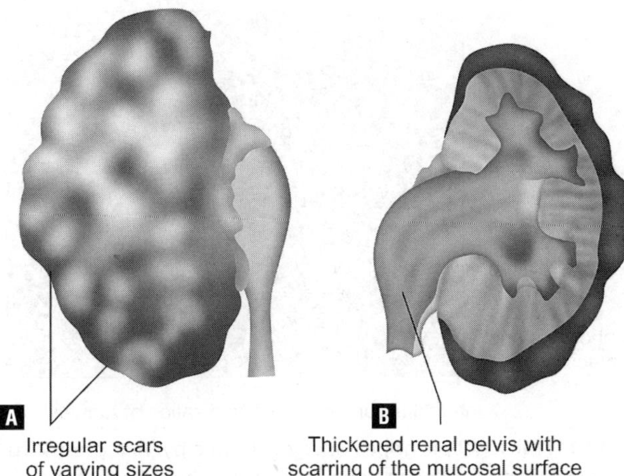

Figs 19.10A and B: Gross appearance of chronic pyelonephritis. (A) Outer aspect; (B) Cut section (diagrammatic)

  - Develops due to **superimposition of a urinary infection on congenital vesicoureteral reflux and intrarenal reflux.**
- **Chronic obstructive pyelonephritis**
  - Develops due to **recurrent infections superimposed on obstructive lesions**, which lead to renal inflammation parenchymal atrophy and scarring.

Morphology
Gross (Fig. 19.10)
- May be **unilateral or bilateral**. When bilateral, the involvement is **asymmetric.**
- **Size:** Kidney is **reduced** in size due to **irregular scars.**
- **Nature of scars:** May affect one or both kidneys.
  - Most are seen in the **upper and lower poles** due to intrarenal reflux.
  - Scars are **coarse, well-defined** and can vary from one to several in number.
- **Calyces and renal pelvis:** It may appear **thickened and irregular** with **scarring of the mucosal surface. Calyces below the scars are dilated, blunted, or deformed. Papillae are flattened.**

Microscopy (Fig. 19.11)

Changes are predominant in the interstitium and tubules.
- **Interstitium:** It shows dense **chronic inflammatory infiltrate** of lymphocytes and macrophages and fibrosis. Few neutrophils may be found with active infection.
- **Tubules:** It may show **atrophy** in some places and hypertrophy or dilation in others.
  - **Thyroidization: Dilated tubules** with flattened epithelium may be **filled with eosinophilic hyaline**

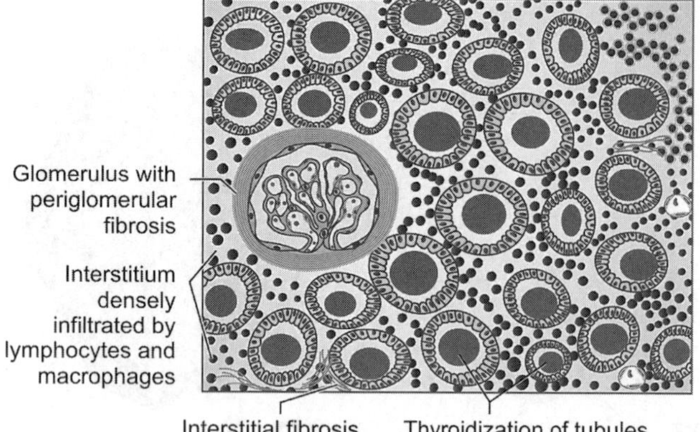

Fig. 19.11: Microscopic appearance of chronic pyelonephritis. Tubules containing hyaline material resembling the colloid of thyroid follicles (thyroidization), interstitium with chronic inflammatory cell infiltrate and periglomerular fibrosis

material and resemble colloid containing thyroid follicles.

- **Glomeruli:** It may appear normal except for **periglomerular fibrosis**.
- **Calyces:** Shows calyceal epithelium surrounded by **fibrosis** and infiltrated by **dense chronic inflammatory infiltrate**.

Clinical Features

Chronic pyelonephritis associated with reflux **may be silent** onset. Usual symptoms are **back-pain, fever, pyuria and bacteriuria**.

TUBERCULOSIS OF THE URINARY TRACT

Tuberculosis of the urinary tract results from hematogenous spread from a distant primary focus of infection that is often impossible to identify.

Types of Lesions in Renal Tuberculosis (Fig. 19.12)

Etiology and Pathology

- Tuberculosis usually involves one kidney. Rarely, tuberculosis may be bilateral as part of the generalized process of military tuberculosis.
- Tuberculous granulomas in the region of renal pyramid may coalesce to form an ulcer and discharge mycobacteria and pus cells into the urine.
- Fibrosis at the necks of the calyces and the renal pelvis may cause tuberculous pyonephrosis.
- Extension of tuberculous pyonephrosis or renal abscess may result in perinephric abscess and the kidney may be progressively replaced by caseous material (putty kidney). This may become calcified (cement kidney).
- Renal tuberculosis is often followed by infection of the ureters and bladder leading to ureteral stricture and contraction of bladder.
- Rarely, cold abscesses may form in the loin. In male, tuberculous epididymo-orchitis may develop even without any lesion in bladder.
- Untreated lesions of renal tuberculosis may enlarge and form tuberculous abscess in the parenchyma.

DIABETIC NEPHROPATHY

Diabetic nephropathy is the term used for **collective lesions that often occur together in the diabetic kidney**. Diabetic nephropathy can develop in both insulin-dependent type 1 diabetes and type 2 diabetes (refer page 309).

Pathogenesis

Diabetic glomerulosclerosis represents a part of the generalized diabetic microangiopathy that involves small vessels throughout the body (refer pages 307-9).

Diabetic Nephropathy—Renal Changes in Diabetes

- The **kidneys** are **main targets** of diabetes.
- **Renal failure** is second only to myocardial infarction as a **cause of death** in diabetes.

Renal lesions in diabetes can be involve any component. Four lesions are encountered namely:

Glomerular Lesions

They are most **important and common renal lesions**. These include (a) Thickening of capillary basement membrane (GBM), (b) diffuse mesangial sclerosis and (c) **nodular glomerulosclerosis (Kimmelstiel-Wilson nodules)**.

Renal Vascular Lesions

- **Hyaline arteriosclerosis** (hyalinosis).
- **Renal atherosclerosis**.

Glomerular and arteriolar lesions together produce **renal ischemia** → leads to atrophy of tubules, interstitial fibrosis, and contraction of kidney.

Pyelonephritis

It is a tubulointerstitial inflammation of the kidneys.

- Both the **acute and chronic pyelonephritis** occurs in nondiabetics as well as in diabetics. It is **more common**

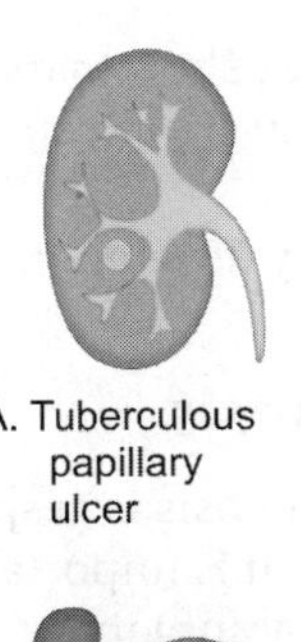

A. Tuberculous papillary ulcer

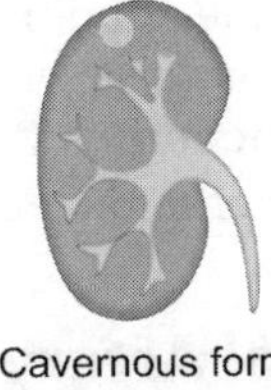

B. Cavernous form it tends to burst like a bombshell

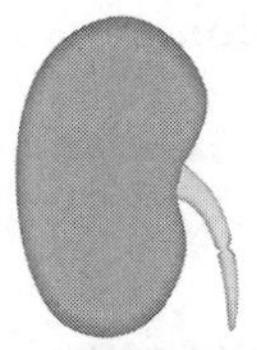

C. Hydronephrosis (rare)

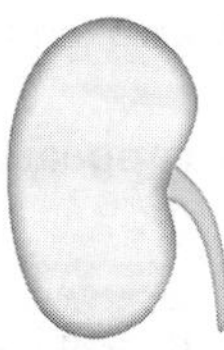

D. Pyonephrosis secondary infection *Escherichia coli*, etc.

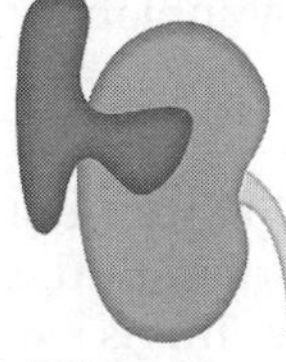

E. Tuberculous perinephric abscess

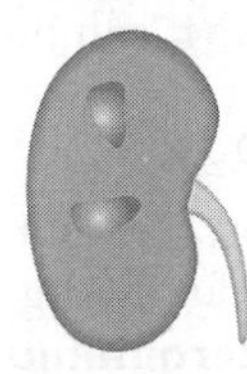

F. Pseudocalculi on X-ray simulate calculi

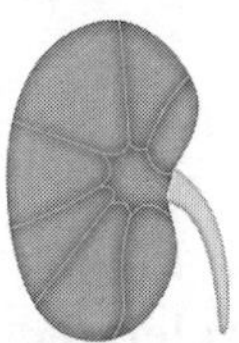

G. Gaseous kidney divided by fibrous septa

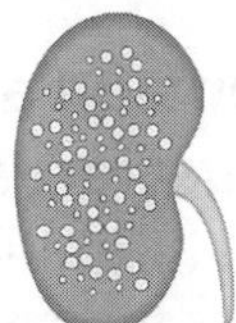

H. Miliary tuberculosis

Figs 19.12 A to H: Various types of lesions in tuberculosis of kidney

and tends to **more severe** in diabetics than in the general population.

- **Necrotizing papillitis** (or papillary necrosis).

Tubular Lesions

The basement membrane of the tubules show thickening. In patients with high blood sugar level, the **epithelial cells of the proximal convoluted tubules show extensive deposits of vacuoles of glycogen**. These are known as **Armanni-Ebstein lesions**.

Amyloidosis

Kidney is the most common and the most serious form of organ involvement in amyloidosis (Renal amyloidosis—refer pages 70-1).

RENAL VASCULAR DISEASES

Almost all kidney diseases secondarily involve the renal blood vessels. Systemic vascular diseases (e.g. vasculitis) also affect renal vessels. Hypertension is closely linked with the kidney, because kidney disease can be both a cause and consequence of increased blood pressure.

Benign Nephrosclerosis

Definition: Benign nephrosclerosis is defined as the **renal pathology associated with sclerosis of renal arterioles and small arteries.**

- Sclerosed vessels with thickened walls → cause narrowing of lumens → result in focal ischemia of renal parenchyma → glomerulosclerosis + chronic tubulointerstitial injury → reduction in functional renal mass.

Causes

Benign nephrosclerosis is associated with:

- Hypertension } increases the incidence and
- Diabetes mellitus } severity of the lesions
- Increasing age and may be seen in the absence of hypertension.

Morphology

Gross

- **Involvement:** Bilateral.
- **Size:** Kidneys are either **normal or smaller** (atrophic).
- **Outer surface:** It shows a **fine, even granularity** resembling grain leather.

Microscopy

- **Blood vessel:** Changes in the kidney depend on the size of the vessel.
  - **Arterioles and small arteries:** They show thickening and hyalinization of the walls causing narrowing of their lumens called as **hyaline arteriolosclerosis.**
  - **Interlobular and arcuate arteries:** They show a characteristic **fibrotic thickening of intima** with **reduplication of the elastic lamina, medial hypertrophy** known as **fibroelastic hyperplasia** → narrow the lumen.
- **Tubules:** They show atrophy.

- **Interstitium:** Fibrosis and chronic inflammatory infiltrate.
- **Glomeruli:** Most of them appear normal.

Clinical Features

Uncomplicated benign nephrosclerosis does not cause renal insufficiency or uremia. There are usually associated with moderate reductions in renal blood flow, but the GFR is either normal or slightly reduced.

Malignant Hypertension and Accelerated Nephrosclerosis

Definition: Malignant nephrosclerosis is defined as **renal disease associated with the malignant or accelerated phase of hypertension**.

- Malignant or accelerated phase of hypertension is relatively uncommon.
- It is often superimposed on pre-existing **essential benign hypertension, secondary forms of hypertension**, or an underlying chronic renal disease, particularly glomerulonephritis or reflux nephropathy.
- **Age and sex:** Pure form usually seen in younger age and more often in men.

Pathogenesis: Exact pathogenesis is not known.

Morphology

Gross

- The size of the kidney depends on the duration and severity of the hypertension.
- **Flea-bitten kidney:** It is characterized by the presence of **small, pinpoint petechial hemorrhages on the cortical surface** due to **rupture of arterioles or glomerular capillaries**.

Microscopy

Histological changes of blood vessels → narrowing of vascular lumens→ ischemic atrophy.

- **Fibrinoid necrosis of arterioles.**
- **Onion-skinning** (hyperplastic arteriolitis).

Clinical Features

- Malignant hypertension is characterized by systolic pressures more than 200 mm Hg and diastolic pressures more than 120 mm Hg, papilledema, retinal hemorrhages, encephalopathy, cardiovascular abnormalities and renal failure.
- Initial symptoms are due to raised intracranial pressure and include headaches, nausea, vomiting and visual impairments.
- Urine examination may show marked proteinuria and hematuria without any significant alteration in renal function.
- Later renal failure may develop.

Renal Artery Stenosis

Unilateral renal artery stenosis is **responsible for about 2 to 5% of hypertension**. It is important to diagnose this because it can be cured by surgery.

Etiology

- Most common (about 70%) cause of renal artery stenosis is narrowing at the origin of the renal artery by an **atheromatous plaque**. This is more commonly found in men, and the incidence increases with advancing age and diabetes mellitus.
- Second most frequent cause of stenosis is **fibromuscular dysplasia** of the renal artery. This is characterized by fibrous or fibromuscular thickening of the wall.

Pathogenesis: Hypertension secondary to renal artery stenosis is due to increased production of renin from the ischemic kidney.

Morphology: Kidney is reduced in size and shows **diffuse ischemic atrophy**.

Clinical course: Resemble those with essential hypertension.

URINARY TRACT OBSTRUCTION (OBSTRUCTIVE UROPATHY)

Urinary tract obstruction is caused by **structural or functional abnormalities** and results in **obstruction to the flow of the urine** (Fig. 19.13).

Consequences:

- Unrelieved obstruction almost always leads to:
  - Renal dysfunction **(obstructive nephropathy)** and permanent renal atrophy.
  - Dilation of the collecting system (hydronephrosis).
- Increased **susceptibility to infection** and to **stone formation**.

Hydronephrosis

Definition: Hydronephrosis is defined as an aseptic **dilation of the renal pelvis and calyces due to obstruction of urinary outflow**. It is associated with **progressive atrophy of the kidney**.

Causes (Fig. 19.13)

It may be classified as structural or functional disorders.

- **Structural disorders:**
  - **Urinary calculi**
  - **Tumors:** Carcinoma of the prostate, bladder tumors, carcinoma of the cervix or uterus
  - **Benign prostatic hypertrophy**
  - **Congenital anomalies:** Urethral strictures, meatal stenosis, bladder neck obstruction
  - **Inflammation:** Prostatitis, urethritis, retroperitoneal fibrosis
  - Pregnancy, uterine prolapse and cystocele.
- **Functional disorders:**
  - Neurogenic bladder (spinal cord damage or diabetic nephropathy).

Pathogenesis

- **Obstruction:** It may be **complete or incomplete.** Obstruction in the urinary tract→ leads to **accumulation of urine proximal to the obstruction.**
- **Dilatation:** Even with complete obstruction, **glomerular filtration** does not stop but **continues for sometime** and → leads to **accumulation of urine** → causes **dilatation of affected calyces and pelvis** due to back pressure. Raised pressure in the renal pelvis → transmitted back through the collecting ducts into the renal parenchyma.
- **Reduced GFR:** If obstruction persists, the functional alterations of tubule results in loss of concentrating function and later **reduces the glomerular filtration rate.**

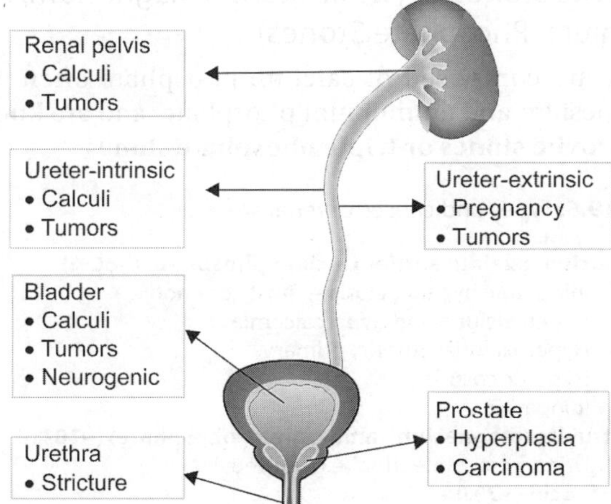

Fig. 19.13: Various common obstructive lesions of the urinary tract

- **Interstitial inflammation:** Obstruction also initiates an **interstitial inflammatory reaction** and interstitial **fibrosis.**

Morphology

Types of obstruction and it consequences

- **Sudden and complete obstruction:** It reduces the glomerular filtration and leads to **mild dilation** of the pelvis and calyces.
- **Subtotal or intermittent obstruction:** It does not suppress glomerular filtration, and **produces progressive dilation.**

Level of obstruction

Depending on the level of urinary obstruction, the dilation may first affect the bladder, or ureter and then the kidney.

Gross

- Depending on the level of obstruction, it may be **unilateral or bilateral** and **may be accompanied by dilatation of ureter (hydroureter).**
- Depending on the degree and the duration of the obstruction, kidney may show **slight to massive enlargement.**
  - **Kidney may be appear** like a **thin-walled, cystic structure** having a diameter of up to 15 to 20 cm.
  - **Renal parenchyma shows destruction due to severe pressure atrophy and thinning of the cortex.** A kidney destroyed by long-standing hydronephrosis appear as a thin-walled, lobulated, fluid-filled sac (Fig. 19.14).

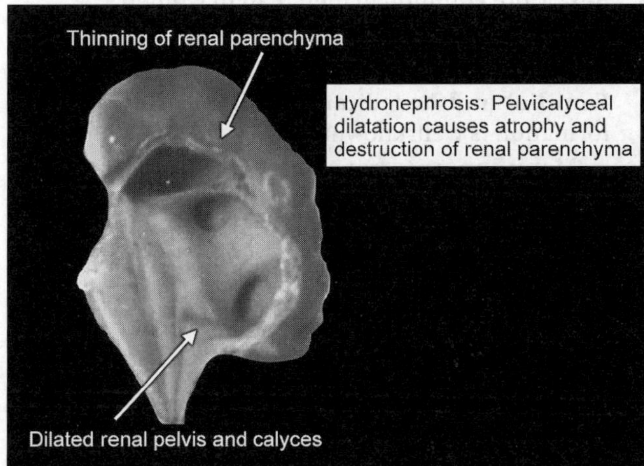

Fig. 19.14: Marked hydronephrosis of the kidney showing marked dilation of the pelvis and calyces and thinning of the renal parenchyma

Microscopy

- **Tubules:** Dilatation and atrophy.
- **Glomeruli:** Partial or complete sclerosis.
- **Interstium:** Marked chronic inflammatory infiltrate and fibrosis.

Clinical Features

- Clinical features **depend on the cause of obstruction**. For example, calculi in the ureters may present with renal colic, and prostatic enlargements may present with bladder symptoms.
- Unilateral complete or partial hydronephrosis may be silent due to maintenance of adequate renal function by the unaffected kidney.
- **Bilateral partial obstruction** may manifest as **polyuria and nocturia** due to inability to concentrate the urine (tubular dysfunction).
- **Complete bilateral obstruction** present with **oliguria or anuria**.
- **Ultrasonography** is a **useful** in the diagnosis of obstructive uropathy.

Urolithiasis (Renal Calculi, Stones)

Stones may be formed anywhere in the urinary tract, but most are found in the renal pelvis and calyces kidney.

- **Terminology**
  - **Nephrolithiasis (renal stones)**—stones within the collecting system of the kidney.
  - **Urolithiasis (urinary calculi/stones)**—stones anywhere in the collecting system of the urinary tract.
- **Age: Peak is between 20 and 30 years**.
- **Sex:** More common in men than in women.

Etiology

- **Familial and hereditary predisposition** to stone formation is well-known.
  - Many inborn errors of metabolism (like gout, cystinuria, and primary hyperoxaluria) are characterized by excessive production and excretion of stone-forming substances.
- **Other factors:**
  - Individual factors
  - Geography
  - **Diet:** Deficiency of vitamin A causes desquamation of epithelium and these cells may form a nidus on which a stone can be deposited.
  - Metabolic alterations
  - **Altered urinary solutes and colloids:** Dehydration increases the concentration of urinary solutes and are liable to precipitate.
  - **Infection:** It favors the formation of calculi. Stone formation are common when urine is infected with urea-splitting streptococci, staphylococci and, especially *Proteus*.
  - **Decreased urinary citrate:** Citrate in urine present as citric acid and is under hormonal control. It tends to keep otherwise relatively insoluble calcium phosphate and citrate in solution. Urinary excretion of citrate is decreased during menstruation.
  - Changes in urinary pH.
  - Urinary stasis: It favors stone formation.

General Features of Renal Stones

- Stones are **unilateral** in **about 80%** of patients.
- **Number:** It may be **single or multiple**.
- **Sites:** Renal **calyces** and **pelvis** and in the **bladder**.
- **Shape:** Stones may have **smooth contours or** may be **irregular, jagged mass of spicules**.

Types and Causes of Renal Stones (Box 19.6)

Calcium stones (Oxalate Calculus/Calcium Oxalate)

Most (80%) renal stones are **composed of calcium complexed with oxalate** (calcium oxalate) or **phosphate** (calcium phosphate) or a mixture of these (calcium oxalate + calcium phosphate). These stones are radiopaque.

- **Morphology: Calcium oxalate** stone: It is irregular in shape **hard** and covered with **sharp projections. Hemorrhage** from the mucosa of the renal pelvis may be produced by its sharp edges and blood may cover the stone **making it to appear black**. It is radiodense.
- **Calcium phosphate** stone: **Soft and pale**.

Struvite stones or (Triple stones/Magnesium, Ammonium, Phosphate Stones)

They are composed of calcium phosphate often with magnesium and ammonium phosphate, and are **known as struvite stones or triple phosphate stones**.

Box 19.6: Types and causes of renal stones

- **Calcium oxalate and/or calcium phosphate (~80%)**
  - Idiopathic hypercalciuria—most common
  - Hypercalciuria and hypercalcemia
  - Hyperoxaluria: Enteric, primary
  - Hyperuricosuria
  - Idiopathic
- **Struvite (magnesium, ammonium, phosphate) (~10%)**
  - Urinary tract infection (e.g. Proteus)
- **Uric acid (~7%)**
  - Associated with hyperuricemia
  - Associated with hyperuricosuria
  - Idiopathic
- **Cystine (~2%)**
- **Others/Unknown (~1%)**

Morphology

- **Yellow-white** and **solitary**.
- **Hard to soft** and **friable.**
- **Largest stones**, because normally large amounts of urea is excreted.
- **Sometimes fill the pelvis and calyces** to **form a cast** of these spaces → referred to as a **staghorn calculus.**
- Even a very large staghorn calculus may be clinically silent for years until it produces hematuria, urinary infection or renal failure.
- Easily seen on radiographic films.

Complications: Intractable urinary tract infection, pain, bleeding, and perinephric abscess.

Uric acid and urate stones

Morphology

- Uric acid stones are **radiolucent;** this is in contrast calcium stones, which are radiopaque.
- **Smooth, hard, and** vary from yellow to reddish-brown. Sometimes have multifaceted appearance.
- Usually **multiple** and are **less than 2 cm** in diameter.
- Show **lamination on cut section**.

Cystine stones

Morphology

- Cystine stones are **small**, **round**, **smooth** and usually **multiple.**
- **Yellow and waxy.**
- They are very hard and radiopaque because of their sulfur content.

Clinical Features of Renal Stones

- Stones may be **asymptomatic** or **may obstruct urinary flow or produce ulceration and bleeding**.
- Small stones **may pass into the ureters**, producing **colic** and ureteral obstruction.
- **Larger stones** cannot enter the ureters and likely to **remain silent** within the renal pelvis. Larger stones may present with **hematuria.**
- Stones also **predispose to superimposed infection** and may also **cause significant renal damage**.

Complications of Renal Stones

- **Hematuria**
- **Hydronephrosis** due to obstruction
- **Pyelonephritis and pyonephrosis**
- **Carcinoma:** Stones can cause squamous metaplasia and later squamous cell carcinoma.

CHRONIC KIDNEY DISEASE

Chronic kidney disease previously termed chronic renal failure or insufficiency.

Chronic kidney disease refers to a **spectrum of long-standing (more than 3 months),** usually progressive processes associated with **irreversible worsening of renal function and decline in glomerular filtration rate (GFR).** CKD spectrum ranges from abnormalities detectable only by laboratory testing to uremia. **Causes of CKD** are listed in Table 19.3.

Clinical Features/Manifestations (Box 19.7)

- Unfortunately, **early stages** of CKD **may be asymptomatic**, despite the progressive loss of kidney function and accumulation of numerous metabolites.
- Usually, there is a rough correlation between serum urea and creatinine levels and symptoms. Symptoms are common when the serum urea level exceeds 40 mmol/L.

Table 19.3: Important causes of chronic kidney disease

Glomerulonephritis* • Proliferative glomerulonephritis • Crescentic glomerulonephritis • Membranoproliferative glomerulonephritis (MPGN)	**Systemic and metabolic diseases** • Diabetes mellitus* • Systemic lupus erythematosus • Polyarteritis nodosa • Amyloidosis
Tubulo-Interstitial • Chronic interstitial nephritis * • Chronic pyelonephritis*	**Obstructive*** • Calculus • Tumors • Prostatic enlargement
Vascular • Essential hypertension (accelerated)*	**Congenital** • Polycystic kidney disease*

* common causes of chronic renal failure

Box 19.7: Major systemic manifestations of chronic kidney disease and uremia

Fluid and electrolytes: Dehydration, edema, hyperkalemia, metabolic acidosis
Calcium phosphate and bone: Hyperphosphatemia, hypocalcemia, renal osteodystrophy secondary hyperparathyroidism
Hematologic: Anemia, bleeding disorder
Cardiopulmonary: Hypertension, congestive heart failure, cardiomyopathy, uremic pericarditis, pulmonary edema
Gastrointestinal: Nausea, vomiting, esophagitis, gastritis, colitis, bleeding
Neuromuscular: Myopathy, peripheral neuropathy, encephalopathy
Cutaneous: Itching, dermatitis, sallow color

Box 19.8: Options of renal replacement therapy

Dialysis • Hemodialysis • Peritoneal dialysis
Ultrafiltration
Hemofiltration
Hemodiafiltration
Continuous renal replacement therapies

RENAL REPLACEMENT THERAPIES

Requirement

Renal replacement therapies (RRT) may be required on a temporary measure in patients with AKI or on a permanent measure for CKD.

Main options of renal replacement therapy (Box 19.8)**:** (1) peritoneal dialysis, (2) intermittent hemodialysis (HD) combined with ultrafiltration, if necessary, (3) intermittent hemofiltration, (4) continuous arteriovenous or venovenous hemofiltration, (5) hemodiafiltration and (6) renal transplantation.

Hemodialysis

Hemodialysis is the most common form of RRT used in end stage renal disease (ESRD) and also in acute kidney injury (AKI).

Basic Principles

- In hemodialysis, blood from the patient is pumped through an array of semipermeable membranes (the dialyser, often called an 'artificial kidney').
- This brings the blood into close contact with dialysate (dialysis fluid) flowing countercurrent to the blood on the other side of membrane.

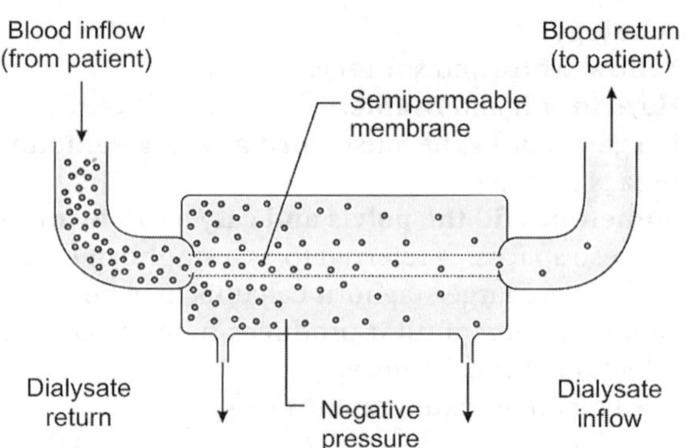

Fig. 19.15: Hemodialysis showing changes across a semipermeable dialysis membrane

- This allows accumulated uremic toxins (e.g. urea and creatinine) and electrolytes (e.g. potassium) to diffuse across a semipermeable membrane (Fig. 19.15) from the blood (where they are in high concentrations), to the dialysis fluid on the other side (where they are in low concentrations). This in turn results in changes in the plasma biochemistry towards that of the dialysate due to the diffusion of molecules down their concentration gradients.

Peritoneal Dialysis

- In peritoneal dialysis, the **peritoneal membrane of the patient acts as a semipermeable membrane.** Through this diffusion of water and solutes takes place and this avoids the need of extracorporeal circulation of blood.
- **Very simple, low-technology** treatment when compared to hemodialysis.

Renal Transplantation

Successful renal transplantation offers the best chance of long-term survival with almost complete rehabilitation in ESRD.

- **Transplantation** is a **procedure for replacement of irreparably damaged tissue or organ to restore their lost function.**
- **Tissue or organ transplanted** is called as **transplant or graft.**
- Individual from which transplant is obtained is known as **donor** and the individual who receives it is called **recipient.**
- **Allograft** is the term used for **a graft from individual of the same species.**

Advantages

- Treatment of choice for most patients with advanced (end-stage) renal failure.

- Method of renal replacement therapy having significant survival advantage when compared to dialysis patients.
- Freedom from dietary and fluid restriction.

Donor is usually a living close relative or a cadaveric donor.

Rejection of Transplants

- A **major barrier for transplantation** is the process known as **rejection**, in which the recipient's immune system recognizes the graft as being foreign and mounts the immunological reactions against it.
- Transplantation **rejection is a complex phenomenon** and it is **mainly due to antigenic differences between a donor and recipient's MHC molecules**.
- Graft survives when MHC antigens of recipient closely matches with the donor.

Classification of Rejection Reaction

Depending on time of occurrence, the rejection reactions are classified as: **(1) hyperacute**, **(2) acute** and **(3) chronic**.

Hyperacute rejection

- **Occurs within minutes or hours after transplantation.**
- It is a special type of rejection, **occurs if the host has preformed anti-donor antibodies in the circulation before transplantation.**
- Results in rapid and irreversible destruction of the graft.

Acute rejection

- Occurs **within days to weeks** after transplantation in the non-immnuosuppressed host
- Types:
  - **Acute cellular rejection.**
  - **Acute humoral rejection (rejection vasculitis).**

Chronic rejection

- Also known as **chronic allograft failure.**
- It is a major cause of graft loss.
- **Occurs months to years after transplantation.**
- Pathogenesis is poorly understood and may be due to both immunological and non-immunological mechanism.

MALIGNANT TUMORS OF THE KIDNEY

Both benign and malignant tumors can occur in the kidney. Most common malignant tumors are renal cell carcinoma and Wilms tumor. WHO classification (abridged) of tumors of the kidney is presented in Box 19.9.

Box 19.9: WHO classification (abridged) of tumors of the kidney

• **Renal cell tumors** – Clear cell renal cell carcinoma – Papillary renal cell carcinoma
• **Nephroblastic tumors** – Nephroblastoma (Wilms tumor)
• **Metanephric tumors** – Metanephric adenoma
• **Mesenchymal tumors**
Others • Metastatic tumors

Renal Cell Carcinoma (Adenocarcinoma of the Kidney, Hypernephroma, Grawitz Tumor)

Renal cell carcinoma (RCC) is a **malignant tumor** of kidney.

- **Cell of origin:** The tumors arise from renal tubular epithelium.
- Because of their **gross yellow color** and the **microscopic resemblance of the tumor cells to clear cells of the adrenal cortex**; these tumors were **originally** thought to arise from embryonic adrenal rests and **were called hypernephroma**.
- **Age:** Usually in the **sixth and seventh decades** of life.
- **Sex: More common in males** with male to female ratio of 2:1.

Etiology

Risk factors

- **Tobacco:** Cigarette and pipe smoking
- Obesity (mainly in women)
- Hypertension
- Unopposed estrogen therapy
- Exposure to asbestos, petroleum products, and heavy metals
- Chronic renal failure and acquired cystic disease
- Tuberous sclerosis.

Types

- **Sporadic: Most (96%) of RCC are sporadic.**
- **Hereditary/inherited/familial:** About **4% of RCC are inherited.**

Clear Cell Carcinoma

- **Most common** type (~70%).
- **Most** (95%) are **sporadic**; but they **can be familial**.
- Usually occur as **solitary** and **unilateral lesions.**

Gross

- **General features of RCC:**
  - **Site:** May arise in **any part** of the kidney. More commonly affects the poles, **mostly upper pole**
- **Cut surface (Fig. 19.16):**
  - Tumor is **solid, bright yellow-gray-white** and shows **areas of hemorrhage, necrosis** and **cystic change,** which give a **variegated appearance**. The **yellow color** is due to **prominent lipid** in the tumor cells.
- **Venous invasion:**
  - **One of the characteristics of RCC** is its **tendency to invade the renal vein**.

Microscopy (Fig 19.17)

- **Growth pattern:** Varies from **solid to trabecular (cord-like) or tubular** (resembling tubules or glands).
- **Tumor cells:** Tumors are **composed of cells with clear or granular cytoplasm** and are **nonpapillary**.
  - The clear cytoplasm is due to **glycogen and lipids.**
  - **Nucleus:** It is **centrally located** and **small,** which falsely mask the malignant nature of this tumor.
- **Stroma: Consists of branching vasculature**.
- **Most tumors** are well-differentiated with **little cellular or nuclear pleomorphism**.

Clinical features

Classical diagnostic triad (seen in only 10% of cases) of renal cell carcinoma are:

- **Costovertebral or flank pain**
- **Palpable abdominal mass**
- **Hematuria (most reliable)**.

Spread

Patients may **develop wide metastasis** before giving rise to any local symptoms or signs.

- **Local spread:** It invades perinephric fat.
- **Lymphatic spread:** It spreads to regional lymph nodes occurs when tumor extends beyond renal capsule.
- **Hematogenous spread:** Most common route. Most common sites are lungs (cannon ball deposits and pulsating secondaries) > bones > liver > adrenal > brain.

Prognosis: Depends on the extent of tumor.

Wilms Tumor (Nephroblastoma)

- Wilms tumor is **most common primary renal tumor of childhood**.
- **Highly malignant primary embroynal tumor**.
- **Age group:** Most common between **2 and 5 years of age**, and more than 95% occur below 10 years of age.

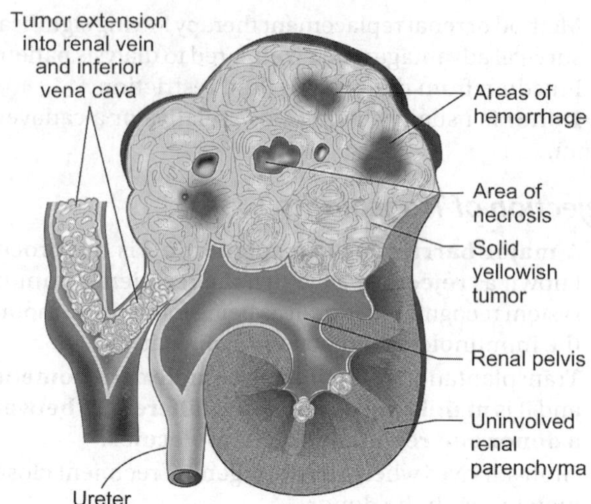

Fig. 19.16: Cut surface of renal cell carcinoma showing a yellowish, spherical, circumscribed, variegated tumor at the upper pole of kidney.

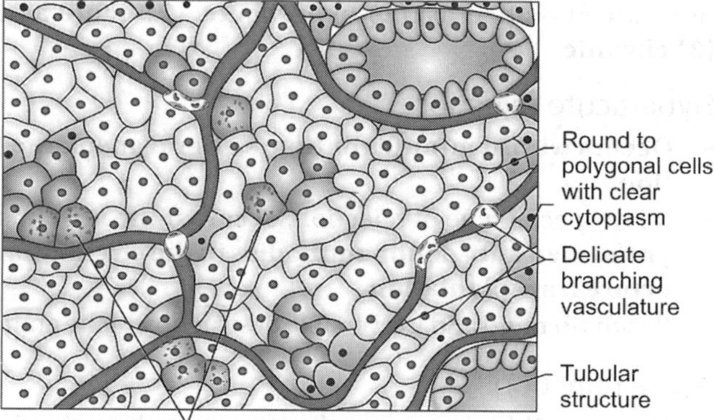

Fig. 19.17: Renal cell carcinoma of clear cell type showing solid groups of clear cells separated by vascular stroma

Morphology

Gross

- Wilms tumor is **usually large, single, round, well-circumscribed** mass.
- **Usually unilateral** but 10% is either bilateral or multicentric.
- **Cut section:**
  - Tumor is **soft, bulging, homogeneous, and tan to gray.**
  - Foci of hemorrhage, cyst formation, and necrosis may be seen.

Microscopy (Fig. 19.18)

- Tumor shows **three major components**, which resemble normal fetal tissue. These cells attempt to recapitulate different stages of nephrogenesis.

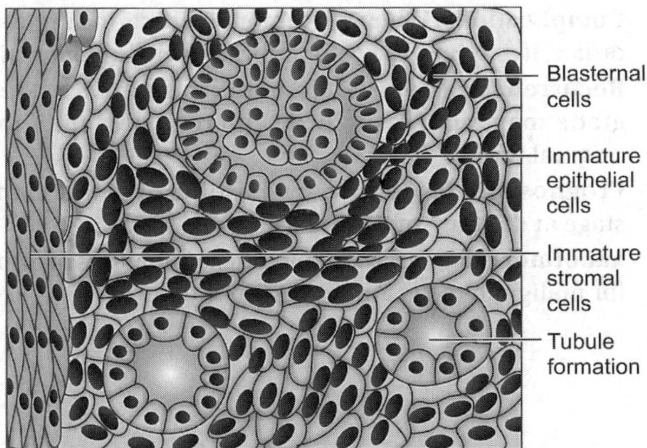

Fig. 19.18: Wilms tumor shows highly cellular areas composed of tightly packed blue cells (undifferentiated blastema) separated by loose stroma containing undifferentiated mesenchymal cells, and immature (primitive) tubules

- The **three types of cells** are:
  - **Blastemal component:** It consists of **small, round to oval blue cells** with **scanty cytoplasm**. These cells are arranged in sheets, nests and trabeculae.
  - **Immature stromal** (mesenchymal) **component:** It consists of **undifferentiated fibroblast-like spindle cells.**
  - **Immature epithelial component: Epithelial cells show differentiation** in the form of **small abortive (embryonic) tubules or immature glomeruli**.

Classically, the tumor shows **triphasic** (all three cell types) combination, although the percentage of each component varies.

Clinical Features

- Most children present with an **abdominal mass**, when large it may extend across the midline and down into the pelvis.
- Others: **Hematuria, pain in the abdomen**, intestinal obstruction, and pulmonary metastases are other patterns of presentation.

Spread

- **Local spread:** It spreads to perirenal soft tissues.
- **Lymphatics:** It spreads to regional lymph nodes.
- **Hematogenous:** Lungs, liver and peritoneum.

UROTHELIAL TUMORS

- **About 95% of bladder tumors are of epithelial origin**. Most of the epithelial tumors of the bladder are composed of urothelial (transitional) cell type and are known as **urothelial or transitional tumors.**
- Urothelial tumors form about 90% of all bladder tumors. These tumors may range from small **benign lesions to aggressive cancers.**
- Many of urothelial tumors are **multifocal** and are most commonly seen in the **bladder**. But they may develop at any site where there is urothelium, from the renal pelvis to the distal urethra.

Box 19.10: Risk factors for urothelial carcinoma

- Cigarette smoking
- Aromatic amines and azo dyes
- *Schistosoma haematobium*
- Analgesics
- Cyclophosphamide
- Radiation

Epidemiology

- **More common in developed** than in developing countries, and in **urban** than in rural dwellers.
- These tumors are usually **not familial**.
- **Sex:** Higher in **males** than in females (male-to-female ratio is 3: 1).
- **Age:** Most between **50–80 years** of age.

Risk factors of urothelial carcinoma (Box 19.10).

Morphology

Site: Most urothelial tumors arise from the **lateral or posterior walls at the bladder base**.

Gross

- **Purely papillary:** These tumors appear as **red, elevated excrescences**. Size varies from small (less than 1 cm in diameter) to large masses (up to 5 cm in diameter). Majority of papillary tumors are low-grade.
- **Nodular.**
- **Flat.**

Microscopy

They range from benign papilloma to highly aggressive anaplastic cancers.

- **Urothelial papilloma.**
- **Papillary urothelial neoplasms of low malignant potential (PUNLMPs)**
- **Low-grade papillary urothelial carcinomas**
- **High-grade papillary urothelial carcinoma**

Metastasis

About 40% of invasive tumors may metastasize.
- Regional lymph nodes
- Hematogenous dissemination to liver, lungs, and bone marrow.

Clinical Course of Bladder Cancer

- **Painless hematuria:** Sometimes, it may be the only clinical feature. Sometimes the hematuria may be associated with frequency, urgency and dysuria.
- **Complications:** When the tumor obstructs the ureteral orifice, it may lead to pyelonephritis or hydronephrosis.
- **Recurrences:** Urothelial tumors, irrespective of their grade may recur, usually at different sites than the original tumor.
- **Prognosis:** It depends on the histologic grade and the stage at the time of diagnosis.
- **Laboratory diagnosis:** Cytologic examinations of urine for malignant cells and biopsy of the tumor.

SELF-ASSESSMENT EXERCISE

I. Short Notes

1. Nephrotic syndrome.
2. Nephritic syndrome.
3. Pyelonephritis.
4. Renal stones.
5. Acute kidney injury.
6. Polycystic kidney disease.
7. Renal transplant.
8. Renal cell carcinoma.

CHAPTER 20

Male Genital System

CHAPTER OUTLINE

- Introduction
- Inflammation of Epididymitis and Orchitis
- Testicular Tumors
- Pathology of Prostate
- Carcinoma of Penis

INTRODUCTION

Male genital system includes: testis, epididymis, spermatic cord, prostate and penis. Testis is composed of structural units called seminiferous tubules separated by interstitium. The seminiferous tubules are lined by germ cells which mature to form spermatozoa. The germ cells are supported by Sertoli cells. The interstitial tissue contains Leydig cells which secrete testosterone. Tunica vaginalis is a mesothelial-lined surface exterior to the testis.

Hydrocele

It is collection or accumulation of serous, clear, translucent fluid in the mesothelially lined scrotal sac between the two layers of the tunica vaginalis. It is a benign condition and causes considerable enlargement of the scrotal sac (Fig 20.1). Hydrocele may be congenital or acquired.

- **Congenital hydrocele:** It is the most common cause of scrotal swelling in infants and is often associated with inguinal hernia.
- **Acquired hydrocele** in adults: It is due to some other disease affecting the scrotum (e.g. infection such as filariasis, tumor or trauma).

Diagnosis: The diagnosis is made by ultrasound or by transluminating the fluid in the cavity.

Complications: Long-standing hydrocele may cause testicular atrophy or compress the epididymis, or the fluid may become infected.

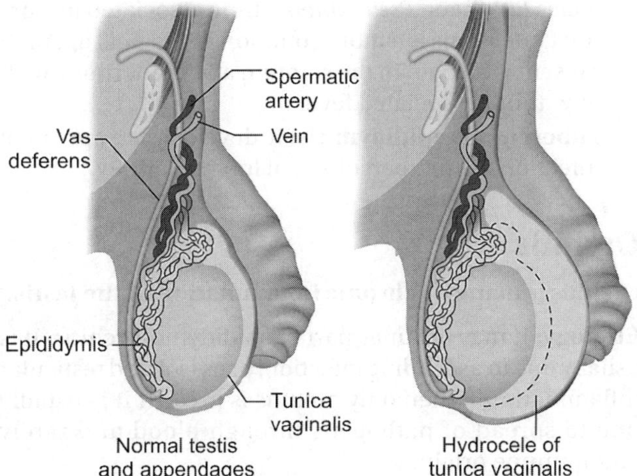

Fig 20.1: Diagrammatic appearance of normal testis with appendages and hydrocele

Hematocele

It is the presence of blood in the tunica vaginalis. It may develop following testicular trauma or torsion, or in individuals with systemic bleeding disorders.

Varicocele

It is characterized by dilated testicular veins in the spermatic cord. It appears as a nodularity on the lateral side of the scrotum.Varicoceles may be asymptomatic but may be cause of male infertility. It can be corrected by surgical repair.

INFLAMMATION OF EPIDIDYMITIS AND ORCHITIS

Inflammations are more common in the epididymis than in the testis. Epididymitis and subsequent orchitis are commonly due to infections in the urinary tract (cystitis, urethritis, prostatitis). The infection reaches the epididymis and the testis through either the vas deferens or the lymphatics of the spermatic cord.

Epididymitis

Epididymitis is **acute or chronic inflammation of the epididymis.** It is **usually caused by bacteria.**

- **Bacterial epididymitis:** The cause of epididymitis varies with the age of the patient. In young males, it is commonly acute and develops as a complication of gonorrhea (caused by *Neisseria gonorrheae)* or a sexually acquired *Chlamydia (C. trachomatis)* infection. In older males *E. coli* and *Pseudomonas* from associated urinary tract infections is a more common etiological agent. It present with pain in the scrotum and tenderness, with or without associated fever.
- **Tuberculous epididymitis:** It develops as a spread of infection from tuberculosis of lung or kidney.

Orchitis

Orchitis is **acute or chronic inflammation of the testis.**

Etiology: It may occur as part of epididymo-orchitis. It is usually due to ascending infection, or as isolated testicular inflammation. When only orchitis is present it is usually due to spread of pathogens through blood and rarely autoimmune origin.

- **Gram-negative bacterial orchitis:** It is the **most common cause** of orchitis usually secondary to urinary tract infection and is typically associated with epididymitis.
- **Syphilitic orchitis:** The testis and epididymis may be affected in both acquired and congenital syphilis. In many cases the epididymis is spared. Morphologically, it has two forms: (1) diffuse interstitial inflammation, with plasma cells, lymphocytes and macrophages; or (2) the production of gummas (refer pages 40-1).
- **Mumps orchitis:** Mumps is a systemic viral disease. It most commonly affects school-aged children. About 20–30% of men who develop mumps develop mumps orchitis. Most often, an acute interstitial orchitis develops about 1 week after the onset of swelling of the parotid glands. It presents with testicular pain and gonadal swelling, most often unilateral. Interstitial inflammation leads to destruction and loss of seminiferous epithelium.
- **Tuberculous orchitis:** Almost invariably tuberculosis begins in the epididymis and then it may spread to the testis. The infection produces the classic morphologic feature of caseating granulomatous inflammation characteristic of tuberculosis elsewhere (refer page 34).
- **Granulomatous (autoimmune) orchitis:** Cause is not known probably may be autoimmune in origin. It is an uncommon disorder of middle-aged men. It presents acutely as painful, moderately tender, testicular enlargement or insidiously as induration sometimes associated with fever. Microscopically, it shows noncaseating granulomas without any organisms or sperm remnants (which may also cause granulomatous reaction). Variable numbers of seminiferous tubules are destroyed by the inflammatory process, which is considered to be a type IV (cell-mediated) hypersensitivity reaction.

TESTICULAR TUMORS

Classification: Testicular neoplasms are divided into two major categories (Box 20.1).

Germ Cell Tumors

Etiology: The exact etiology of testicular tumors is not known. Risk factors are as follows:

- **Environmental factors**.
- **Cryptorchidism:** Undescended testis is the most important risk factor.
- **Testicular dysgenesis syndrome (TDS)**.
- **Genetic/familial predisposition.**
- **Klinefelter syndrome:** It is associated with 50 times greater risk (than normal) for the mediastinal germ cell tumors, but they do not develop testicular tumors.

Seminoma

Seminomas are the **most common type of germ cell tumors**, and constitute about 50% of germ cell tumors. An

Box 20.1: Classification of testicular tumors

I. Germ cell tumors
- **Seminomatous tumors**
  - Seminoma
  - Spermatocytic seminoma
  - Anaplastic seminoma
- **Non-seminomatous tumors**
  - Embryonal carcinoma
  - Yolk sac (endodermal sinus) tumor
  - Choriocarcinoma
- **Teratoma**
  - Mature
  - Immature
  - Teratoma with malignant transformation
- **Mixed germ cell tumors**

II. Sex cord-stromal tumors
- Leydig cell tumor
- Sertoli cell tumor

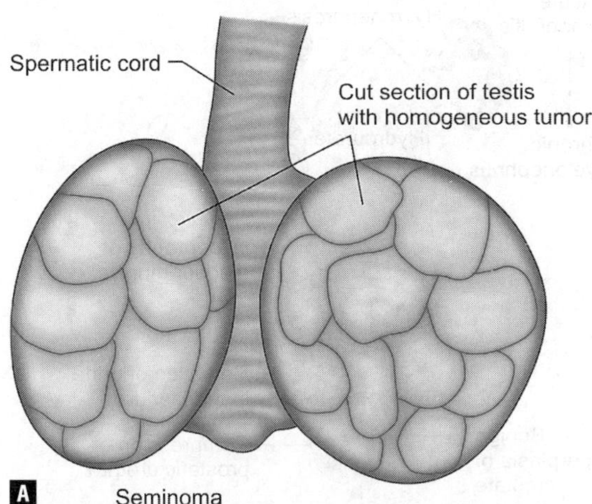

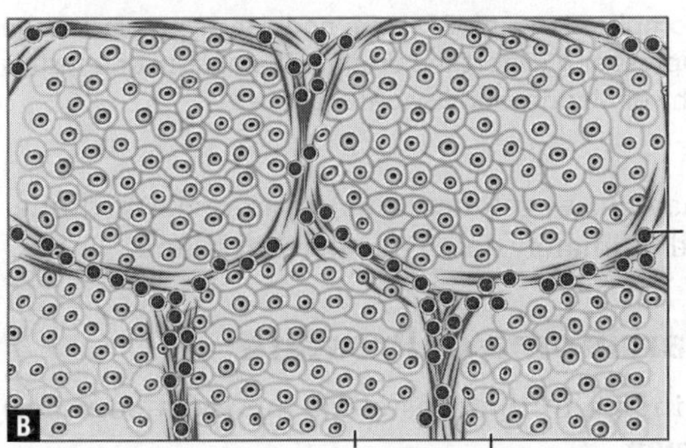

Figs 20.2 A and B: Gross (A) and microscopic (B) appearances of seminoma testis

identical tumor which occurs **in the ovary** is known as **dysgerminoma**.

Age group: The peak incidence is during **third decade (between 30 and 40 years)**.

Morphology (Fig. 20.2)

- **Gross:** Seminomas are **solid, large, firm tumors.** On cut section, the tumor is **homogeneous, gray-white without any hemorrhage or necrosis.**
- **Microscopy:** It is composed of sheets or nests or cords of uniform seminoma cells. These seminoma cells are **large, round to polyhedral with clear (watery) cytoplasm. Nucleus is large, central, and vesicular** with **one or two prominent nucleoli.** The seminoma cells are divided into lobules separated by **delicate fibrous septa.** These septa are infiltrated with moderate amount of **lymphocytes and plasma cells.**

Prognosis: Seminoma are extremely radiosensitive with a very good prognosis.

Clinical Features of Germ Cell Tumors of Testis

Characteristic presentation of germ cell tumor is **painless enlargement of the testis**. Any solid testicular mass should be considered neoplastic unless otherwise proved.

Spread of Testicular Tumors

Testicular tumors have a characteristic mode of spread.

- **Local spread:** It may spread into testis and its surrounding structures.
- **Lymphatic spread:** Initially to retroperitoneal para-aortic nodes and later to mediastinal and supraclavicular nodes.
- **Hematogenous spread:** Lungs, liver, brain, and bones.

Clinical Stages of Testicular Tumors

- **Stage I:** Tumor confined to the testis, epididymis, or spermatic cord.
- **Stage II:** Distant spread confined to retroperitoneal nodes below the diaphragm.
- **Stage III:** Metastases outside the retroperitoneal nodes or above the diaphragm.

PATHOLOGY OF PROSTATE

Prostate is a gland situated close to the male urethra. It consists of two lateral lobes and a median lobe. Microscopically, it consists of glands surrounded by fibromuscular stroma.

Benign Prostatic Hyperplasia or Nodular Hyperplasia

Benign prostatic hyperplasia (BPH) is a very common disorder in men ≥50 years of age. It forms nodules in the **periurethral region** of the prostate. When the nodules become large, they compress and narrow the urethral canal and obstruct the urine outflow.

Etiology and Pathogenesis

It is characterized by hyperplasia of both prostatic stromal cells and epithelial cells. **Androgens** play a role in the pathogenesis of BPH. They increase cellular proliferation and also inhibit cell death.

Morphology

Gross (Fig. 20.3)

Nodular hyperplasia of the prostate **begins in the submucosa of the proximal urethra (transition zone)**.

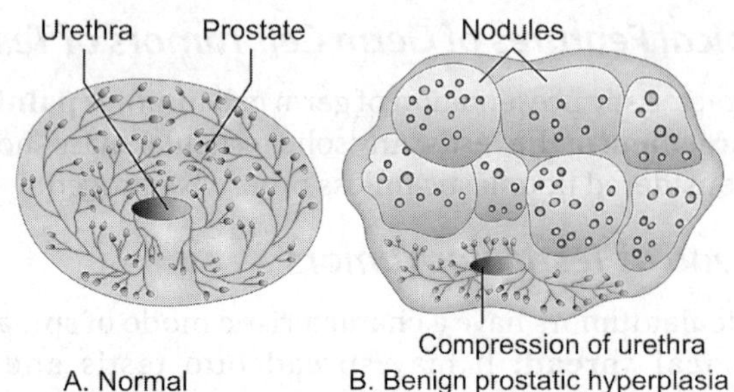

Figs 20.3A and B: (A) Diagrammatic appearances of cross section of normal prostate and (B) nodular hyperplasia of prostate

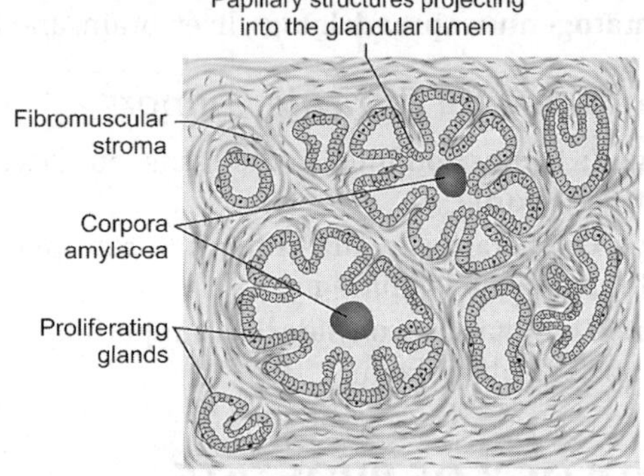

Fig. 20.4: Microscopic appearance of nodular hyperplasia of prostate

It usually involves both the lateral lobes of prostate. Cut section shows multiple circumscribed nodules which vary in color and consistency.

Microscopy (Fig. 20.4)

The characteristic feature of BPH is **nodularity. Epithelial cell proliferation** shows **small to large dilated glands or acini**. These glands are **lined by two layers of cells**, an inner tall columnar and an outer basal layer of cuboidal or flattened epithelium. Corpora amylacea (eosinophilic laminated concretions) are commonly seen within the acini. These **glands are surrounded by smooth muscle cells and fibroblasts.**

Clinical Features

Symptoms of nodular hyperplasia are due to compression of the prostatic urethra and resulting **bladder outlet obstruction, increasing urinary frequency, difficulty in urination and urine retention**.

Complications

Obstruction to urinary outflow leads to hypertrophy and distension of the bladder (Fig. 20.5) accompanied by retention of urine, infection (cystitis, and consequent ascending infection may cause pyelonephritis), hydroureter, hydronephrosis, and ultimately death due to renal failure.

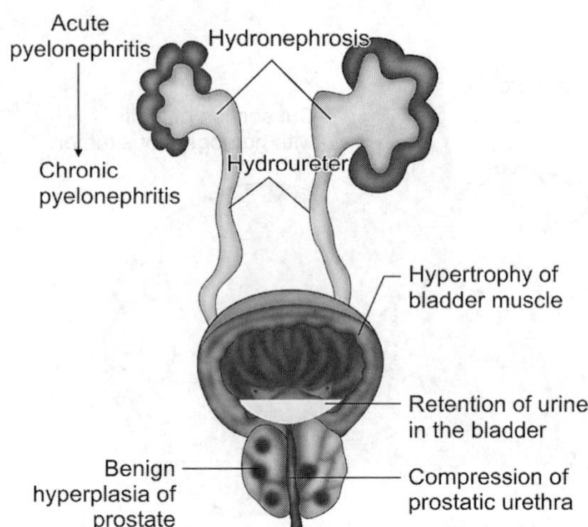

Fig. 20.5: Complications of BPH. In nodular hyperplasia, the nodules compress and distort the urethra. The obstruction results in hypertrophy of bladder and its consequences

Adenocarcinoma of Prostate

Adenocarcinoma of the prostate is the **most common cancer in men**.

Etiology

Several factors are suspected to play a role.

- **Age:** It usually presents in men over age of 50 years.
- **Environmental factors:** They may play a role in the pathogenesis of prostatic cancer.
- **Dietary factors:** Increased consumption of fat increases the risk.
- **Hormones: Androgens** play an important role.
- **Family history:** Strong family history increases risk to two-fold and cancer develops at an earlier age.
- **Hereditary factors.**

Morphology

Gross

Carcinoma of the prostate arises in the **peripheral zone of the gland** (70%), usually in a **posterior location** (Fig. 20.6A). The tumor is **gritty and firm.**

Microscopy

Most of the prostate cancers are **adenocarcinomas** and consist of well-defined glandular patterns (Fig. 20.6B). **Glands are lined by a single uniform layer of cuboidal or low columnar cells**. Perineural tumor invasion is usual.

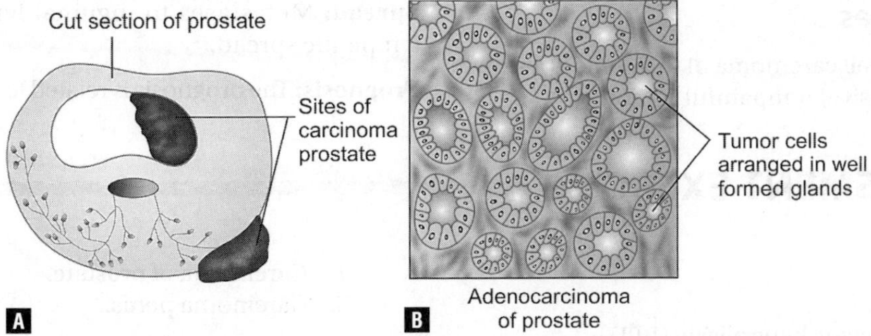

Figs 20.6A and B: Sites (A) and microscopic appearance (B) of carcinoma prostate

Spread

- **Local spread:** Tumor may infiltrate capsule of the prostate and spread into periprostatic tissue, seminal vesicles, and the base of the urinary bladder.
- **Lymphatic spread:** It spreads first to the obturator nodes, later to iliac and to the para-aortic lymph nodes.
- **Hematogenous spread:** Mainly to the bones of the axial skeleton. The bony metastases are **osteoblastic (with formation of bone)** in contrast to other tumors which are osteolytic (destruction of bone). The bones involved, in descending order of frequency, are lumbar spine, proximal femur, pelvis, thoracic spine and ribs.

Grading

Prognosis of prostatic cancer depends on the grade. Prostate cancer is categorized into five grades (grade 1 to grade 5) on the basis of glandular differentiation using **Gleason system**.

Clinical Features

Prostatic carcinoma is **asymptomatic** during early stages when it is localized to the prostate. Advanced prostatic cancer may present with **urinary symptoms**, like dysuria, frequency, or hematuria. **Vertebral metastases** may present as back pain and has fatal outcome. **Transrectal needle biopsy is needed to confirm the diagnosis**.

CARCINOMA OF PENIS

Usual histological type of carcinoma of penis is squamous cell carcinoma.

Etiology

- **Circumcision protects** against carcinoma penis.
- **Smegma** is supposed to contain carcinogenic agents.

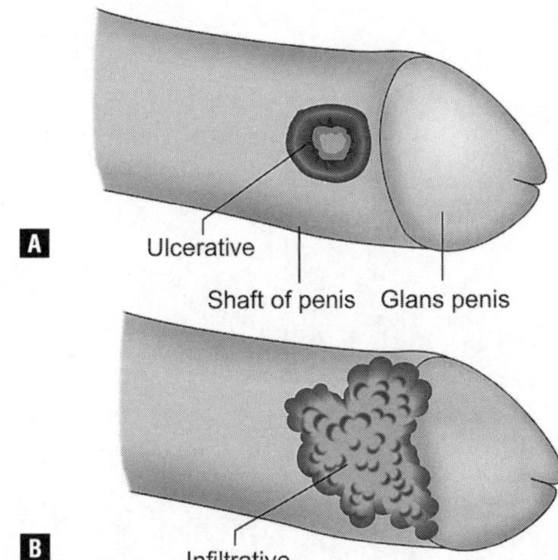

Figs 20.7A and B: Gross appearance of carcinoma penis. (A) Ulcerative type; (B) Cauliflower-like infiltrative mass

- **Human papilloma virus** (HPV) may play a role in carcinoma penis.
- **Cigarette smoking** increases the risk of cancer of the penis.
- **Premalignant lesions of penis:** Bowen's disease, Bowenoid papulosis and erythroplasia of Queyrat.

Age group: Carcinomas are usually found in patients between the ages of **40 and 70 years**.

Morphology

Gross: Squamous cell carcinoma of the penis usually begins on the glans or inner surface of the prepuce. It usually produces a **cauliflower-like fungating mass or an ulcerative lesion** (Figs 20.7A and B).

Microscopy: It shows squamous cell carcinoma with varying degrees of differentiation.

Clinical Features

Invasive squamous cell carcinoma of the penis is a slowly growing, locally invasive, nonpainful tumor.

Spread: Metastases to inguinal lymph nodes through lymphatic spread.

Prognosis: The prognosis is related to the stage of the tumor.

SELF-ASSESSMENT EXERCISE

I. Short Notes

1. Orchitis.
2. Seminoma.
3. Benign prostatic hyperplasia (BPH).
4. Carcinoma of prostate.
5. Carcinoma penis.

CHAPTER 21

Female Genital System

CHAPTER OUTLINE

- Introduction
- Uterine Cervix
- Uterus
- Gestational Trophoblastic Disease
- Ovary

INTRODUCTION

The female genital system consists of vulva, vagina, uterine cervix, uterus, ovaries and fallopian tubes (Fig. 21.1).

UTERINE CERVIX

Normal Anatomy

The lower portion of the uterus is uterine cervix and it communicates with the uterine cavity through internal os and with the vagina through external os. The portion of cervix which is exposed to the vagina is known as **ectocervix** and is lined by stratified squamous epithelium. The inner part is the cervical canal which communicates with endometrial cavity of the uterus and is called **endocervix**. It is lined by mucosa with glandular tissue consisting of endocervical glands. The junction between endocervix and ectocervix is called transitional zone or squamocolumnar junction.

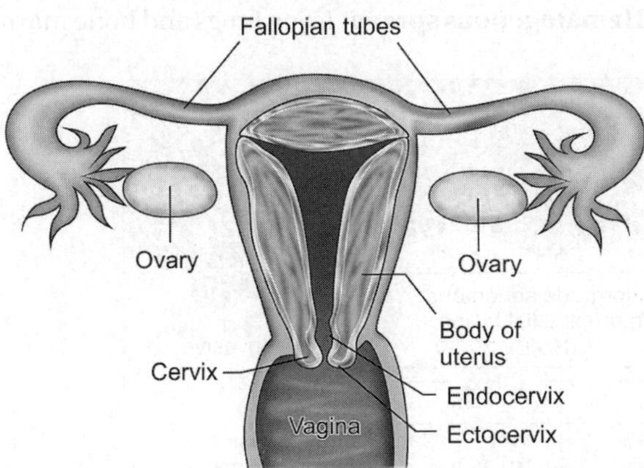

Fig. 21.1: Normal anatomical components of female genital tract

Lesions of Cervix

These include cervicitis (acute and chronic), cervical intraepithelial neoplasms and carcinoma of cervix.

Cervicitis

Inflammation of the cervix is termed as cervicitis and is a common condition of cervix. It may be acute or chronic cervicitis.

Etiology: Normally vaginal pH is below 4.5 which suppresses the growth of other saprophytic and pathogenic organisms. Acute and chronic cervicitis are caused by many organisms, mainly endogenous vaginal aerobes and anaerobes, *Streptococcus, Staphylococcus* and *Enterococcus.* Other specific organisms include *C. trachomatis, mycoplasmas, N. gonorrhoeae* and occasionally herpes simplex (HCV) type 2.

Mode of infection: Either sexually transmitted or may be introduced by foreign bodies, such as residual fragments of tampons and pessaries. If the pH of the vagina becomes alkaline due to bleeding, sexual intercourse, or vaginal douching, antibiotic therapy, it favors the overgrowth of microorganisms.

Morphology

Acute cervicitis: Grossly, the cervix is red, swollen and edematous, with pus "dripping" from the external os. Microscopically, there is dense polymorphonuclear leukocyte infiltration and stromal edema.

Chronic cervicitis: It is more common. The cervix shows chronic inflammatory infiltrate (lymphocytes and plasma cells).

Cervical Intraepithelial Neoplasia

Cervical intraepithelial neoplasia (CIN) is a **precancerous lesion** of cervix. It begins as minimal atypical changes (similar to the malignant cells) in the stratified squamous epithelium and progresses to marked atypical changes and finally as invasive squamous cell carcinoma.

Classification of Cervical Precancers

There are three interchangeably used terminologies for cervical precancer (Fig. 21.2). They are: carcinoma in situ (**CIS**), cervical intraepithelial neoplasia (**CIN**), and squamous intraepithelial lesion (**SIL**).

- **Carcinoma in situ system:** This is the oldest classification in which **mild dysplasia** is at one end of the spectrum and severe **dysplasia/carcinoma in situ** on the other end.
- **Cervical intraepithelial neoplasia** (CIN) **classification:** According to this, mild dysplasia is termed CIN I, moderate dysplasia as CIN II, and severe dysplasia termed as CIN III.
- **Squamous intraepithelial lesion:** The classifications presently being used is **Bethesda system.** According to this, these lesions are divided into low- and high-grade squamous intraepithelial lesions.
  - CIN I is renamed as **low-grade squamous intraepithelial lesion (LSIL)**. It is associated with productive HPV infection.
  - CIN II and CIN III are combined into one category and are known as **high-grade squamous intraepithelial lesion (HSIL)**.

Invasive Carcinoma of Cervix

It is a malignant tumor of cervix.

Precursor lesion: HSIL is an immediate precursor of invasive squamous cell carcinoma.

Age: The peak age is at 45 years.

Etiology and Risk Factors

Human papilloma virus (HPV) infection

HPV is a sexually transmitted DNA virus and plays a role in both CIN and cervical cancer.

Environmental factors

These factors include: cigarette smoking (contains co-carcinogen), **microbial infections** and **hormonal changes**, etc.

Morphology

Gross

Invasive cervical carcinoma may present as either a **fungating (exophytic)** cauliflower-like growth, **ulcerated or infiltrative mass.**

Microscopy

The histological types include:

- **Squamous cell carcinoma:** It is the **most common** (about 80%) histological type of cervical cancer. It is composed of solid nests and groups of malignant squamous cells (either keratinizing or nonkeratinizing) invading the underlying stroma of the cervix. Depending on the cytological features, it can be **divided into 3 subtypes** namely: **keratinizing, nonkeratinizing and small cell carcinoma**
- Other histological types include: adenocarcinoma and rarely adenosquamous.

Spread

- **Local spread:** The tumor may spread into the **surrounding tissues** and organs (urinary bladder and rectum, ureters and vagina).
- **Lymphatic spread:** To paracervical, hypogastric, and external iliac nodes.
- **Hematogenous spread:** Liver, lungs and bone marrow.

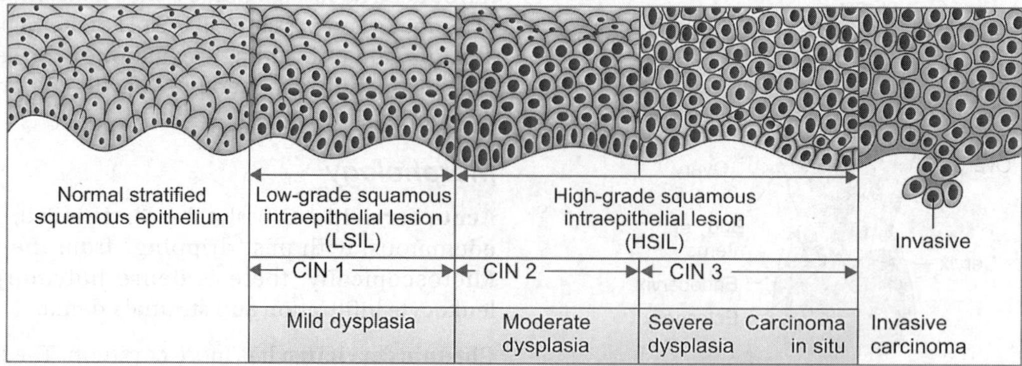

Fig. 21.2: Various stages in the progression of cervical intraepithelial neoplasia

Table 21.1: Staging of cervical cancer

Stage	Extent of cervical cancer
Stage 0	Carcinoma in situ (CIN III, HSIL)
Stage I	Carcinoma confined to the cervix
Stage II	Carcinoma extends beyond the cervix but not to the pelvic wall. Carcinoma involves the vagina but not the lower third
Stage III	Carcinoma has extended to the pelvic wall. The tumor involves the lower third of the vagina
Stage IV	Carcinoma has extended beyond the true pelvis or has involved the mucosa of the bladder or rectum. This stage also includes cancers with metastatic dissemination

Staging of Cervical Cancer (Table 21.1)

Clinical Features

During early stages of cervical cancer, patients most often present with vaginal bleeding after intercourse.

Prognosis

Prognosis for invasive carcinomas depends largely on the stage of the carcinoma.

Cervical Cancer Screening

The cervical cancer screening can be done by:

- **Pap smear examination:** Pap tests are cytological preparations of cells shed from the cervix that are stained with the Papanicolaou method.
- **Schiller test:** In this test, Lugol's iodine (a solution of iodine and potassium iodide) is painted in the suspected area. The region in which there is cancer will not be stained by this solution because cancer cells lack glycogen.
- **Biopsy: Histological diagnosis.**
- **Surgical removal of invasive cancers.**

UTERUS

Normal Components

The body of the uterus consists of lining endometrium and outer wall composed of myometrium.

Endometrium

The endometrium consists of glands separated by stroma. They respond to the hormonal changes that occur during the menstrual cycle or during pregnancy. During the first half of menstrual cycle, the endometrial glands show proliferative changes due to estrogen and is known as **proliferative phase** of the endometrium. In the next half of the menstrual cycle, the glands show secretory activity under the influence of progesterone and is known as **secretory phase.** This is followed by **menstrual phase** during which the endometrium is shed out.

The endometrial stroma is compact during proliferative phase and becomes loose and edematous during secretory phase. During **pregnancy,** there is interruption of menstrual cycle. During this period, the stromal cells become polygonal and show abundant granular cytoplasm and this change is called **decidual reaction.**

After menopause the endometrial glands become small and **atrophic.**

Myometrium

It is composed of smooth muscle bundles which show both hyperplasia and hypertrophy during pregnancy.

Adenomyosis

It is the **presence of endometrial tissue within the myometrium.** The uterus may be enlarged and may show hemorrhagic spots. Microscopically, it shows **endometrial glands and stroma in the myometrium.** It may present as uterine bleeding, polymenorrhea or dysmenorrhea.

Endometriosis

The **presence of endometrial tissue in the extrauterine sites** is known as endometriosis. The sites of endometriosis include: **ovary, fallopian tube, uterine ligaments,** etc.

Leiomyoma

Uterine leiomyomas (commonly called **fibroids**) are **benign smooth muscle neoplasms** and are the most common tumors in females.

Morphology

Gross

Leiomyomas are sharply **circumscribed** (without encapsulation), **round, firm, gray-white** tumors. They **vary in size** from small nodules to massive tumors which fill the pelvis. They may be **single or multiple. Cut section** has a characteristic **whorled pattern** of smooth muscle bundles and has a raw (watered) silk appearance.

Sites (Fig. 21.3)

- **Intramural** (within the myometrium) is the **most common** site.

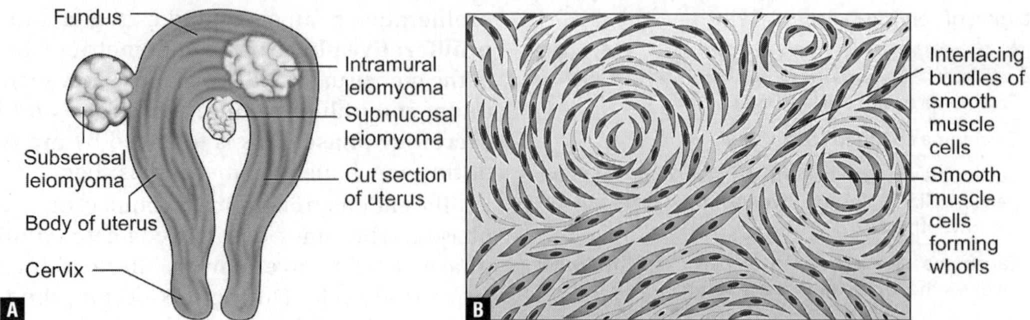

Figs 21.3A and B: Gross (A) and microscopy (B) of uterine leiomyoma

- **Submucosal** (just beneath the endometrium).
- **Subserosal** (beneath the serosa) and may be pedunculated.

Microscopy

- It is composed of **interlacing fascicles/whorled bundles of smooth muscle cells** (Fig. 15.5). The individual muscle cells are uniform in size and shape. They have the characteristic elongated oval nucleus with blunt ends.
- **Secondary changes:** These include:
  - **Hyaline change** (degeneration), mucoid or myxomatous degeneration, calcification, cystic changes and fatty metamorphosis.
  - **Red degeneration:** It shows extensive coagulative necrosis and may be **associated with pregnancy** or the use of contraceptive drugs.

Clinical Features

They are rare before age 20 years, and usually regress after menopause. Leiomyomas of the uterus **may be asymptomatic**. Common symptoms are: **abnormal bleeding, urinary frequency** (compression of the bladder) or **infertility**. Leiomyomas **usually grow slowly,** but occasionally enlarge rapidly during pregnancy.

Carcinoma of the Endometrium

Endometrial carcinoma is the most common pelvic invasive cancer of the female genital tract.

Age group: Carcinoma of the endometrium is uncommon before 40 years of age, and mainly occurs in postmenopausal women with a peak **between 55–65 years**.

Etiopathogenesis: Endometrioid carcinoma is the most common type (more than 80%), and develops from precursor lesions of endometrial hyperplasia. They are associated with the conditions such as **obesity, diabetes, hypertension, infertility and unopposed estrogen stimulation**.

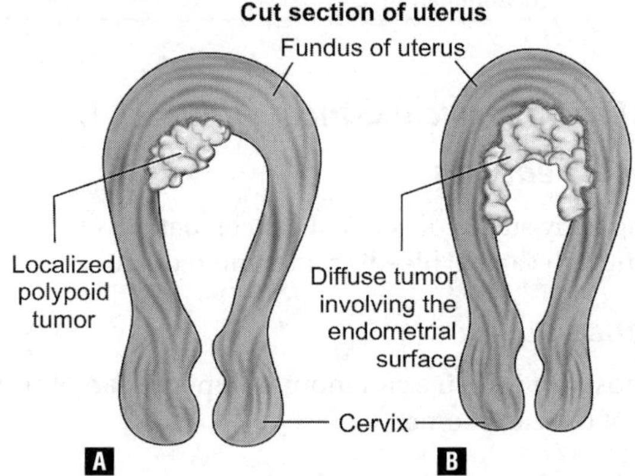

Figs 21.4A and B: Gross types (A and B) of endometrial carcinoma

Morphology

Gross (Fig. 21.4)

Endometrial carcinoma may present either as a **diffuse tumor** involving the endometrial surface or as a **localized polypoid tumor.** Large tumors usually show areas of hemorrhage and necrosis.

Microscopy

Most of the endometrial carcinomas are well-differentiated and characterized by **tumor cells arranged** in **glandular patterns** resembling normal proliferative endometrial glands. The **nuclei** of tumor cells range from **bland to markedly pleomorphic.** Usually, the nuclei show **prominent nucleoli**. Abundant mitotic figures are seen.

Grading

Endometrial carcinomas are graded according to the glandular differentiation as: well-differentiated **(grade 1)**, moderately differentiated **(grade 2)** and poorly differentiated **(grade 3)** adenocarcinoma.

Spread

- **Direct spread:** Direct invasion of myometrium, periuterine structures and the broad ligaments.
- **Lymphatic spread:** To the regional lymph nodes.
- **Hematogenous:** Lungs, liver, bones and other organs, in the late stages.

Clinical Features

They present as **abnormal (postmenopausal) bleeding**.

Prognosis

It depends on the age of the patient and grade of the tumor.

GESTATIONAL TROPHOBLASTIC DISEASE

Gestational trophoblastic disease consists of tumors and tumor-like lesions characterized by **proliferation of placental tissue**. The lesions included are:

- Hydatidiform mole
- Invasive mole
- Choriocarcinoma.

Hydatidiform (Vesicular Mole)

Definition: It is **benign gestational trophoblastic disease** characterized histologically by **cystic swelling of the chorionic villi**, accompanied by variable **trophoblastic proliferation**.

Significance: Hydatidiform mole is associated with an **increased risk of invasive mole or choriocarcinoma**.

Age: It can develop at any age.

Risk factors:

- **Maternal age:** Risk is higher in girls younger than 15 years of age. Risk increases progressively after 40 years.
- **Ethnic background** and **obstetric history:** Both of them influence the risk of developing hydatidiform mole.

Morphology

Gross (Fig. 21.5)

The chorionic villi are delicate and form a friable thin-walled, translucent, cystic mass which resemble **bunches of grapes**.

Microscopy (Fig. 21.5)

Abnormalities involve all or most of the villi. Individual **chorionic villi are edematous and enlarged.** The **central area of the villi is acellular and lack** adequately developed **vessels**. They **show fluid-filled spaces.** There is **diffuse trophoblast proliferation (hyperplasia)** which involves the entire circumference of the villi. Trophoblast consists of syncytiotrophoblast, cytotrophoblast and intermediate trophoblast. **Fetal parts** are **absent.**

Clinical Features

Majority present in the fourth or fifth month of pregnancy with **vaginal bleeding**.

Human chorionic gonadotropin (hCG)

- hCG levels are **high** compared to normal pregnancy.
- Serial hormone determination shows increase in the hCG levels faster than for the pregnancy.
- Monitoring serum concentrations of hCG is necessary to determine the early development of invasive moles or gestational choriocarcinoma.

Majority of moles are treated by thorough curettage.

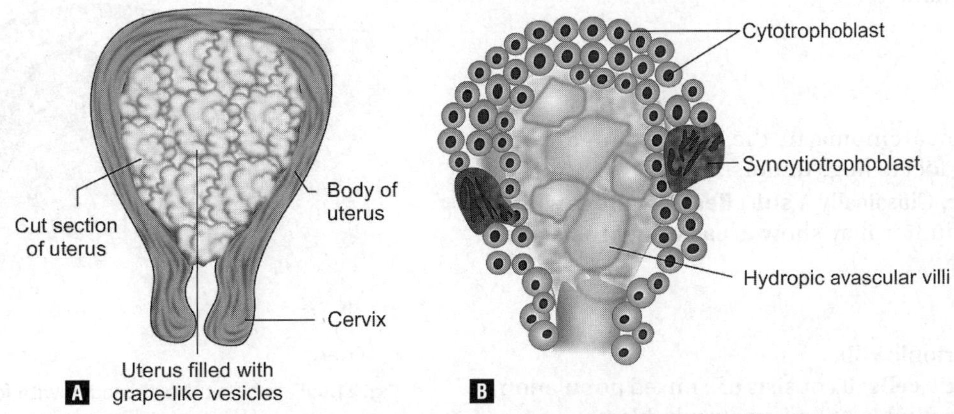

Figs 21.5A and B: Complete hydatidiform mole. (A) Grossly enlarged uterus filled with grape-like vesicles and light microscopic; (B) Appearance showing hydropic avascular chorionic villi lined by trophoblastic cells

Invasive Mole

Definition: It is defined as a **mole that penetrates or even perforates the uterine wall.**

Microscopy: It is characterized by **invasion of the myometrium by hydropic chorionic villi**. There is accompanied proliferation of both cytotrophoblast and syncytiotrophoblast.

Spread

- **Local spread:** The tumor may invade parametrial tissue and blood vessels.
- **Blood spread:** Hydropic villi may embolize to distant sites, such as lungs and brain.

Clinical Features

Presents as **vaginal bleeding** and irregular uterine enlargement.

Laboratory Findings

Persistently elevated serum hCG.

Treatment

Responds well to chemotherapy.

Choriocarcinoma

Definition: Gestational choriocarcinoma is a rapidly **invasive malignant neoplasm of trophoblastic cells** which metastasizes widely. It responds well to chemotherapy.

Incidence: Choriocarcinoma is preceded by:

- Hydatidiform moles
- Previous abortions
- Normal pregnancies
- Ectopic pregnancies.

Morphology

Gross

- **Size:** Choriocarcinoma in the uterus range from microscopic foci to huge tumors.
- **Appearance:** Classically a **soft, fleshy, yellow-white tumor**. The tumor may show **areas of necrosis and hemorrhage**.

Microscopy

Absence of chorionic **villi.**

- **Trophoblastic cells:** It consists of a mixed population of syncytiotrophoblasts and cytotrophoblasts.
- **Abnormal mitosis:** Mitoses are abundant and sometimes abnormal.
- **Invasion:** The tumor invades the underlying myometrium, frequently penetrates blood vessels and lymphatics. It may extend to the uterine serosa and adjacent structures.

Clinical Features

Uterine choriocarcinoma usually manifests as irregular vaginal spotting of a bloody, brown fluid.

Laboratary findings

hCG is elevated more than that found in hydatidiform moles.

Spread

Widespread metastases are characteristic of choriocarcinoma. Frequent sites are **lungs, brain, bone marrow, liver, vagina** and other organs.

Ectopic Pregnancy

Definition: Ectopic pregnancy/gestation is the **implantation of the fetus** in any site **other than a normal intrauterine location**.

Sites of Ectopic Pregnancy

- Within the **fallopian tubes** (Fig. 21.6): It is the most common site (~90%).
- **Other sites:** Ovary, abdominal cavity, and the intrauterine portion of the fallopian tube (cornual pregnancy).

Predisposing Conditions

- Prior pelvic inflammatory disease resulting in fallopian tube scarring

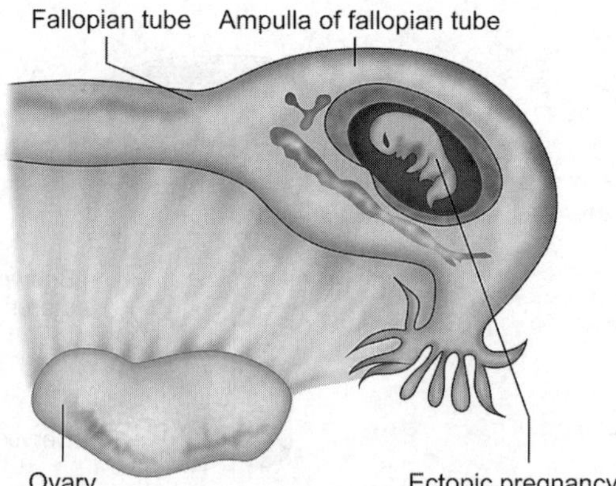

Fig. 21.6: Fallopian tube distended with fetus at the fimbrial end

- Other causes of peritubal scarring and adhesions such as appendicitis, endometriosis, and previous surgery
- Intrauterine contraceptive devices also increase the risk of ectopic pregnancy.

Morphology

Tubal pregnancy is the most common **cause of hematosalpinx** (blood-filled fallopian tube). Microscopic examination, usually shows blood clot admixed with chorionic villi.

Clinical Features

The ectopic pregnancy presents as **severe abdominal pain** due to rupture of the tube leading to pelvic hemorrhage and constitutes a medical emergency. It most commonly develops about 6 weeks after a previous normal menstrual period. The patient may rapidly develop **hemorrhagic shock** with signs of an acute abdomen.

OVARY

Normal Anatomy

Each female has two ovaries, each measuring 3 cm in length and 2 cm in breadth. Cut section of the ovary shows outer cortex and inner medulla. Microscopically, ovaries are covered by celomic epithelium. The cortex consists of numerous follicles. Each follicle consists of an ovum surrounded by stromal cells. The stromal cells are called as granulosa and theca cells. The fully developed follicle is called Graafian follicle. During ovulation, the Graafian follicle ruptures and releases ovum and is transformed into corpus luteum. The medulla of ovary consists of blood vessels, nerves and lymphatics.

Non-Neoplastic and Functional Cysts

These are common lesions seen in ovary.

Follicular and Luteal Cysts

Cystic follicles in the ovary are very common. They arise from an unruptured Graafian follicles or follicle that have ruptured and immediately sealed.

Morphology

They are usually multiple. They range in size up to 2 cm in diameter. The cavity of the cysts is filled by a clear serous fluid. Cysts larger than 2 cm are called as **follicular cysts.**

Microscopy

They are lined by inner granulosa cells and the outer theca cells. The theca cells may be conspicuous because of increased amounts of pale cytoplasm (luteinized).

Granulosa Luteal Cysts (Corpora Lutea)

They are normally present in the ovary. Grossly these cysts are lined by a rim of bright yellow tissue. Microscopically, this yellow tissue consists of luteinized granulosa cells.

Polycystic Ovaries and Stromal Hyperthecosis

Polycystic ovarian disease (PCOD; formerly termed **Stein Leventhal syndrome**) are found in 3–6% of women in the reproductive age.

The ovaries show numerous cystic follicles or follicular cysts and are often associated with oligomenorrhea. Women with PCOD have anovulation, obesity and hirsutism.

Morphology

Gross: The size of the ovaries is usually twice that of normal size. They have a smooth, gray-white outer cortex with numerous subcortical cysts 0.5–1.5 cm in diameter.

Microscopy: Ovary shows thick, superficial cortex beneath which there are numerous follicular cysts associated with hyperplasia of the theca interna (follicular hyperthecosis).

Tumors of Ovary

Incidence: Ovarian cancers constitute the third most common female genital tract cancers. The incidence of ovarian cancer is below only carcinoma of the cervix and the endometrium.

Classification (Box 21.2)

Tumors are broadly classified as **primary** tumor and **secondary** (or metastatic to the ovary). The primary tumors are classified according to the tissue of origin.

Box 21.2: WHO classification of ovarian neoplasms

Primary Tumors

Surface epithelial tumors
- Serous tumors: Benign, borderline tumors and malignant
- Mucinous tumors: Benign, borderline, malignant
- Other tumors: Endometrioid tumors, Brenner tumor, etc.

Germ cell tumors
- Teratoma: Mature, immature and monodermal teratoma and somatic-type tumors arising from dermoid cyst
- Dysgerminoma
- Yolk sac tumor (endodermal sinus tumor)

Sex cord-stromal tumors
- Pure stromal tumors: Fibroma, thecoma, Leydig cell tumor
- Pure sex cord tumors: Adult and juvenile granulosa cell tumor, Sertoli cell tumor

Metastatic Cancer From Nonovarian Primary

Tumors of Surface Epithelium

Surface epithelial tumors are the most important and common primary neoplasms in the ovary.

Origin

These tumors are derived from the surface germinal epithelium which covers the outer aspect of the ovary.

Surface epithelial tumors are classified depending on the type of epithelial differentiation as: Serous, mucinous and endometrioid. Each of these types is further subdivided into benign, borderline and malignant categories. Benign serous and mucinous tumors are cystic whereas malignant serous and mucinous tumors are cystic with solid areas or completely solid.

Serous Tumors

Serous tumors account for about 30% of all ovarian tumors and about over 50% of ovarian epithelial tumors. About 70% are benign or borderline and about 30% are malignant. Serous carcinomas are the most common malignant ovarian tumors and account for about 40% of all cancers of the ovary.

Morphology

- **Benign:** These are usually **large unilocular cysts** and are called as **serous cystadenomas** (Fig. 21.7A). They measure from 15–30 cm in diameter. The **lumen** of the cyst contains clear **serous fluid**. Some of the tumors may show small **papillae** projecting into the cystic cavity. Microscopically, **cysts** are **lined by single layer of tall, columnar** epithelial cells. The **papillae** are also lined by similar epithelium and may show **psammoma bodies** (Fig. 21.7B).
- **Borderline tumors:** These tumors are **predominantly cystic**. Microscopically, the **lining epithelium is multilayered** but there will not be any invasion of the stroma.
- **Malignant serous adenocarcinoma:**
  - It shows a **mixture of solid and cystic areas** with numerous **papillae** may show psammoma bodies. **Areas of necrosis and hemorrhage** are usually found in the solid area of the tumor.
  - Microscopically, these are **adenocarcinomas** and may vary from well-differentiated to poorly differentiated type. **Stromal and capsular invasion** by the tumor cells is seen. The tumor cells in the high-grade carcinomas display marked **nuclear atypia, including pleomorphism, atypical mitotic figures, and multinucleation.**
  - Tumor may get deposited on the peritoneal surfaces and omentum and produce ascites. Umbilical metastasis ("Sister Joseph's nodule"), metastasis to the other ovary and abdominal viscera (bowel, liver, spleen) may also develop.

Mucinous Tumors

Mucinous tumors are less common than serous tumors. They constitute about 30% of all ovarian neoplasms. About 80% of mucinous tumors are benign or borderline, and about 15% are malignant.

Morphology

- **Benign mucinous cystadenoma:** These tumors tend to be **large** and **multiloculated** (Fig. 21.8A). The **cystic spaces contain** sticky semi-solid **mucinous material**. Microscopically, the lining epithelial cells are **uniform tall, columnar**, and nonciliated (Fig. 21.8B). These cells have abundant apical mucin and basally located nuclei.
- **Borderline:** These tumors grossly appear similar to mucinous cystadenoma. Microscopically, there is

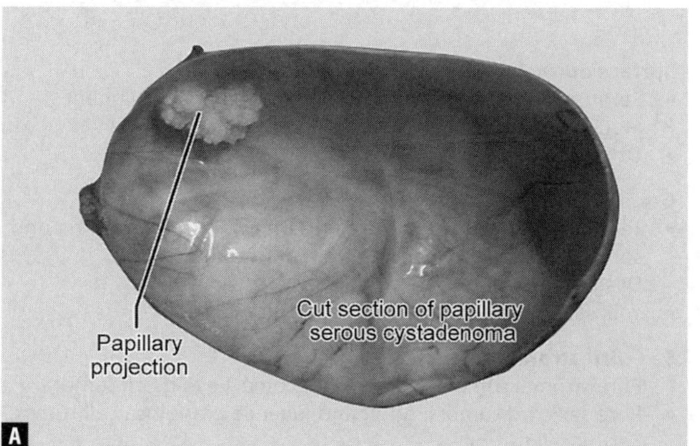

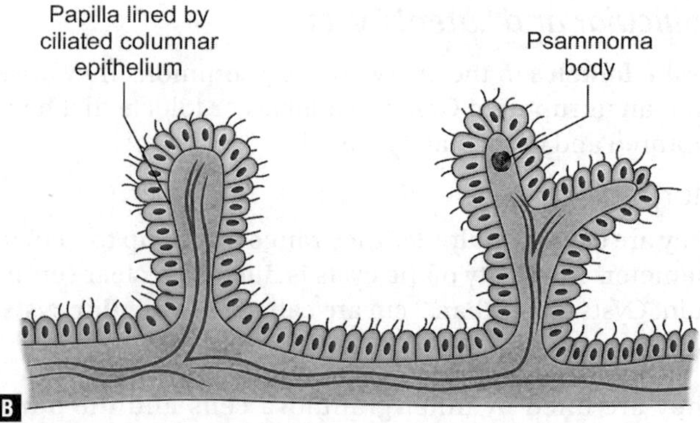

Figs 21.7A and B: Papillary serous cystadenoma of ovary. (A) Cut section with papillary projection; (B) Microscopic features of papillary serous cystadenoma of ovary (Diagrammatic)

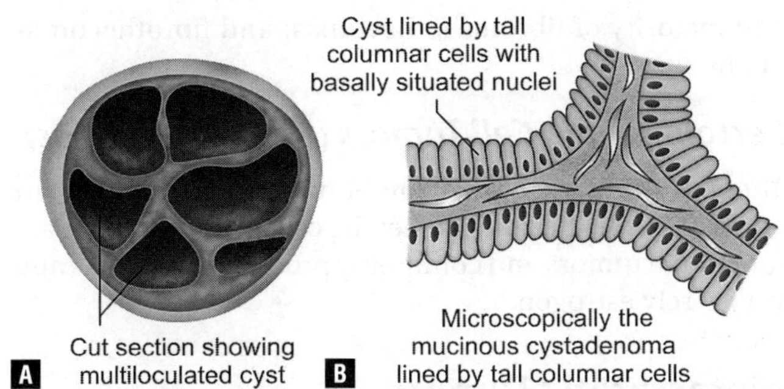

Figs 21.8A and B: (A) Cut section of mucinous cystadenoma of ovary; (B) Microscopy of mucinous cystadenoma of ovary lined by single layer of columnar mucinous cells and basally located nuclei

stratification/multilayering of the epithelium and absence of stromal invasion.

- **Mucinous cystadenocarcinomas:**
  - These tumors appear similar to mucinous cystadenoma but with **solid areas.** These solid areas show **areas of necrosis and hemorrhage**.
  - Microscopically, they range from well to poorly differentiated **adenocarcinomas**. Clear-cut **stromal invasion** is characteristic of carcinoma which is not seen in borderline tumors.
  - **Peritoneal implant** and local invasion into neighboring structures like bowel, abdominal wall, and bladder may be seen. Metastases to distant organs are infrequent.

Endometrioid Tumors

Endometrioid tumors show tubular glands resembling benign or malignant endometrium.

Brenner Tumor

Brenner tumors may be solid or cystic. Microscopically, they show nests of epithelial cells resembling the epithelium of the urinary tract (transitional-type) separated by fibrous stroma, similar to that of the normal ovary. The nuclei of epithelial cells show **nuclear grooves** which resemble coffee-bean.

Germ Cell Tumors

Germ cell tumors constitute about 20% of all ovarian tumors. Most of the germ cell tumor in adults are benign (mature cystic teratoma, dermoid cyst), whereas in children and young adults, they are largely malignant.

Teratomas

Teratoma **contains mature or immature cells or tissues representative of more than one germ cell layer** (at least two) and sometimes tissues derived from all three embryonic layers. The embryonic layers are ectoderm, endoderm and mesoderm. These cells or tissues are arranged in a helter-skelter fashion.

Classification

Teratomas are divided into **three categories**:

- **Mature (benign) teratoma** which consists of all **well-differentiated tissue** components or elements.
- **Immature (malignant) teratomas** consist of less well-differentiated or immature elements.
- **Monodermal or highly specialized**.

Mature (benign) teratomas

Grossly, teratomas may be cystic or solid. Most of the benign ovarian teratomas are cystic and are known as **dermoid cysts** (mature cystic teratoma). Dermoid cysts are usually **unilocular, thick-walled** with a smooth, shiny outer surface. The cyst contains yellow or grey, buttery or cheesy (pultaceous) **sebaceous material** with variable amount of **hair. Tooth structures** and areas of calcification are common (Fig. 21.9A).

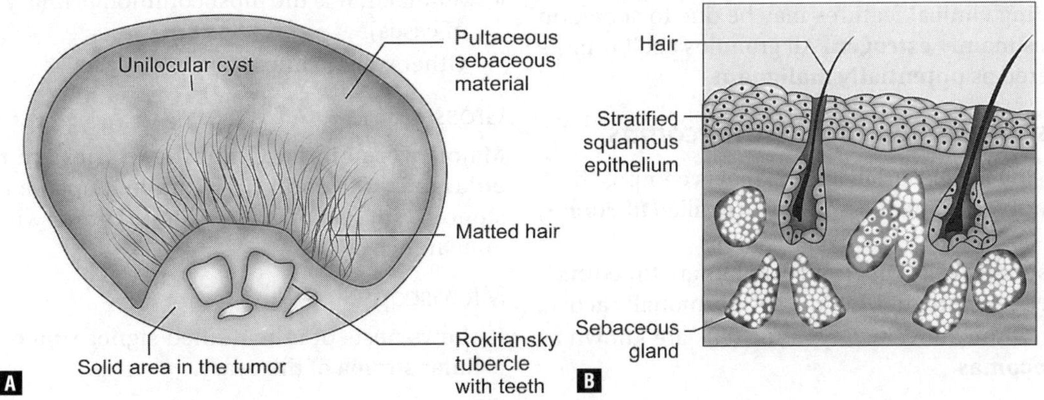

Figs 21.9A and B: Gross (A) and microscopic (B) features of benign cystic teratoma of ovary

Microscopy (Fig. 21.9B)

The cyst wall mainly shows differentiation along ectodermal lines and thus **lining of the cysts consists of skin** (stratified squamous epithelium) **with skin appendages** (sebaceous glands, hair shafts, and other skin adnexal structures). In most of the cases, structures from all three germ layers can be identified, which includes:

- **Ectoderm** (e.g. skin, neural tissue, glia)
- **Mesoderm** (e.g. smooth muscle, cartilage, bone, fat)
- **Endoderm** (e.g. respiratory tract epithelium, gut, thyroid).

Dysgerminoma

Dysgerminoma is the ovarian counterpart of the seminoma of the testis. These are **solid, firm, lobulated and,** encapsulated tumors. On cut section, they are **cream colored. Microscopy** is **similar to seminoma** (Fig. 20.2B).

Sex Cord–Stromal Tumors

Ovarian stroma is derived from the sex cords of the embryonic gonad. So, this group of tumors is known as sex cord-stromal tumors. Some of these cells normally secrete estrogens (granulosa and theca cells) or androgens (Leydig cells). The corresponding tumors may be either feminizing (granulosa–theca cell tumors) or masculinizing (Leydig cell tumors).

Granulosa–Theca Cell Tumors

Granulosa cell tumor of the ovary is associated with estrogen secretion. These neoplasms may be composed almost entirely of granulosa cells or a varying mixture of granulosa and theca cells. **Size varies** from microscopic foci to large, solid, and cystic encapsulated masses. Hormonally active tumors have a **yellow color**, due to intracellular lipids.

Clinical features

The presenting clinical features may be due to secretion of hormones mainly **estrogen**. All granulosa cell tumors are considered as **potentially malignant**.

Fibromas, Thecomas and Fibrothecomas

Tumors arising from ovarian stroma that is composed of:

- Only fibroblasts (spindle-shaped) are called **fibromas**, and are hormonally inactive.
- Plump spindle cells with lipid droplets are **thecomas.** Pure thecomas are rare, but may be hormonally active.
- Mixture of the above two types of cells are known as **fibrothecomas**.

The majority of fibromas, thecomas, and fibrothecomas are benign.

Sertoli–Leydig Cell Tumors (Androblastomas)

These are rare sex cord-stromal tumors in which tumor cells resembles Sertoli and Leydig cells of testis. These are functional tumors and commonly produce androgens and very rarely estrogen.

Metastatatic Tumors

About 3% of ovarian tumors are metastatic carcinomas. Ovary may be the site of metastasis for many primary tumors.

- **From genital tumors:** Most common metastatic tumors of the ovary are derived from tumors of the uterus, fallopian tube, and contralateral ovary.
- **Extragenital tumors:** Most common are from carcinomas of the breast and gastrointestinal tract, biliary tract, and pancreas or hemopoietic malignancies.

Morphology

Gross

Features which point to metastatic carcinoma are **bilateral** ovarian involvement and **multinodularity**. These tumors vary in size from microscopic lesions to large masses.

Krukenberg tumors

A characteristic form of **metastatic ovarian tumor** is known as Krukenberg tumor which was first described by Krukenberg in 1896.

Age

Usually found between 30 and 60 years.

Sources of primary

- Stomach: It is the most common primary site (in 75% of cases).
- Others: Large intestine and breast.

Gross

Majority are **bilateral** and the ovaries are **moderately enlarged** and **retain their shape**. Capsule is intact and smooth. Cut section shows a **solid tumor** with variegated appearance.

Microscopy

It shows nests of mucin filled signet-ring cells within a cellular stroma of the ovary.

SELF-ASSESSMENT EXERCISES

I. Essay

1. Define carcinoma in situ (CIN) and describe in detail the morphological changes.
2. Describe the etiology, pathology and spread of carcinoma of cervix.
3. Classify ovarian tumors. Describe the morphological features of serous tumors of ovary.

II. Short Notes

1. Adenomyosis of uterus.
2. Leiomyoma of uterus/types of leiomyoma.
3. Teratoma of ovary.
4. Hydatidiform mole.

CHAPTER 22

Breast

CHAPTER OUTLINE

- Normal Anatomy
- Mastitis
- Benign Tumors
- Carcinoma of the Breast

NORMAL ANATOMY

Breast is a specialized skin gland. Its primary function is to produce milk for the nutrition of the newborn. Till puberty, both male and female breasts are morphologically similar in appearance. But at puberty, the female breast undergoes hyperplasia under sex hormones. This leads to proliferation of ducts, acini and stroma.

The functional unit of the breast is a lobule. The glandular unit is composed of acini which proliferate during pregnancy and produce milk after delivery.

MASTITIS

Inflammation of the breast parenchyma is called mastitis. It may develop in females during lactation. Mastitis may be acute or chronic. It is usually caused by bacteria which reach breast through either skin or ducts. The inflammation may lead to formation of abscess.

BENIGN TUMORS

Fibroadenoma

- **Most common benign tumor** of the female breast.
- **Age group:** Mostly occur in females between **20 to 30 years.**
- **Origin:** Arise from intralobular stroma.
- **Clinical presentation:** Young women usually present with a **palpable and freely movable mass (mouse in the breast)**.

Morphology

Gross (Fig. 22.1)**:** Fibroadenomas can be single or multiple and unilateral or bilateral.

Spherical nodules and are usually well-circumscribed and freely movable. The tumor can compress the surrounding breast tissue, but is not fixed. This accounts for its mobility on clinical examination → known as 'breast mouse'.

Cut section (Fig. 22.1)**:** It appears as rubbery, glistening, grayish-white nodules that bulge above the surrounding tissue and often contain slit-like spaces.

Size: Varies, usually 1 to 4 cm in diameter.

Microscopy (Fig. 22.2)**:**

- Composed of a **mixture of duct-like structures** and **fibrous connective tissue**.
- **Fibrous connective tissue stroma:**
  - Constitutes most of the tumor
  - Stroma is **delicate, cellular**, often myxoid and resembles normal intralobular stroma.

Classification: According to the microscopic appearance:

- **Pericanalicular** (Fig. 22.2A)**:** In this type, regular round or oval glandular configuration of the glands is

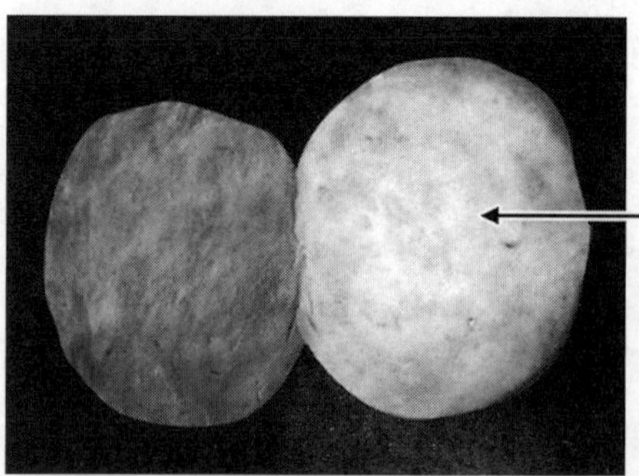

Fig. 22.1: Fibroadenoma of breast showing a well-circumscribe tumor

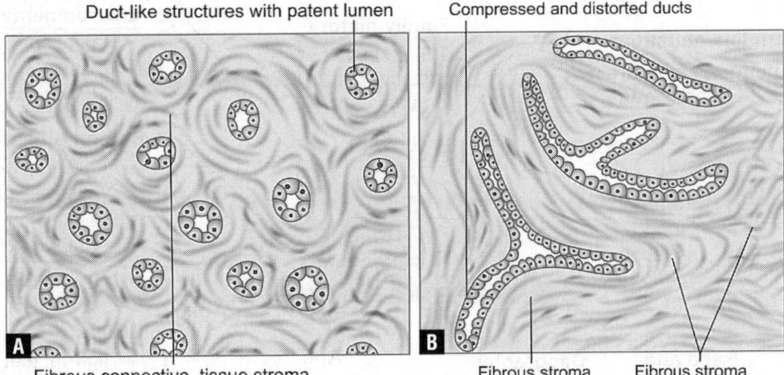

Figs 22.2A and B: Fibroadenoma of breast. (A) Pericanalicular type showing ducts with patent lumen, surrounded by delicate stroma; (B) Intracanalicular type composed of slit-like compressed ducts surrounded by fibrous tissue

maintained. The epithelium forms ducts with patent lumen.

- **Intracanalicular** (Fig. 22.2B)**:** In this type, the proliferated ducts are compressed and distorted by, fibrous tissue reducing them to form curvilinear slits.
- Usually both patterns coexist.

Phyllodes Tumor

Phyllodes tumor is a circumscribed **biphasic neoplasm** that arises from **intralobular stroma** (like fibroadenomas). Majority are detected as palpable masses. Mostly occur **between 30 and 70 years of age**.

Morphology

- Depending on the appearance of the stromal component, phyllodes tumors are divided into (1) low-grade (benign) and (2) high-grade (malignant) phyllodes. **Cut surface** shows characteristic whorled pattern with **curved cleft-like spaces** that **resemble the leaf-buds (phyllodes** is Greek for "leaflike").
- **Gross: Low-grade (benign)** phyllodes tumor is **round, sharply circumscribed. Malignant phyllodes** is usually **poorly circumscribed and locally invasive**.
- **Microscopy: Two key features:** (1) presence of benign epithelial elements and (2) stromal hypercellularity.

Recurrence

- Low-grade tumors may recur locally but rarely metastasize.
- High-grade lesions frequently recur and may also develop hematogenous metastases.

CARCINOMA OF THE BREAST

Carcinoma of the breast is the **most common cancer in women**.

Etiology

Risk Factors (Fig. 22.3)

Most important risk factor is gender and of breast cancer cases occur in only 1% of male.

- **Age:** Breast cancer **develops usually after the age of 25**. Its incidence rises as the age advances **and at 70 to 80 years and then declining slightly thereafter**.
- **Geographic variations:** They are observed and may be related to following:
  - **Type of diet:** Consumption of **coffee (caffeine) may decrease the risk.**
  - **Reproductive patterns:** These include number and timing of pregnancies.
  - **Nursing habits/breastfeeding: Longer the women breastfeed**, the **greater the reduction in risk.**
  - **Obesity: Physical activity (exercise)** may have a **protective role**.
  - **Factors which reduce risk of breast carcinoma: Breastfeeding**, exercise, healthy body weight.
- **Race/ethnicity:** The variation in breast cancer risk genes across ethnic groups is in part responsible for racial or ethnic differences. For example, incidence of ***BRCA1*** and ***BRCA2*** mutations occur at different frequencies in different ethnic groups.
- **Prolonged exposure to estrogens: It increases the risk of breast carcinoma.** It may be seen in the follwoing conditions:
  - **Endogenous hormone exposure** occurs with **long duration of reproductive life:**
    - **Early menarche** (<12 years) and **late menopause** (>55 years).
    - **Late age at first-term pregnancy (>35 years) and nulliparity.**
    - **Postmenopausal obese.**
    - **Carcinoma of the contralateral breast or endometrium.**

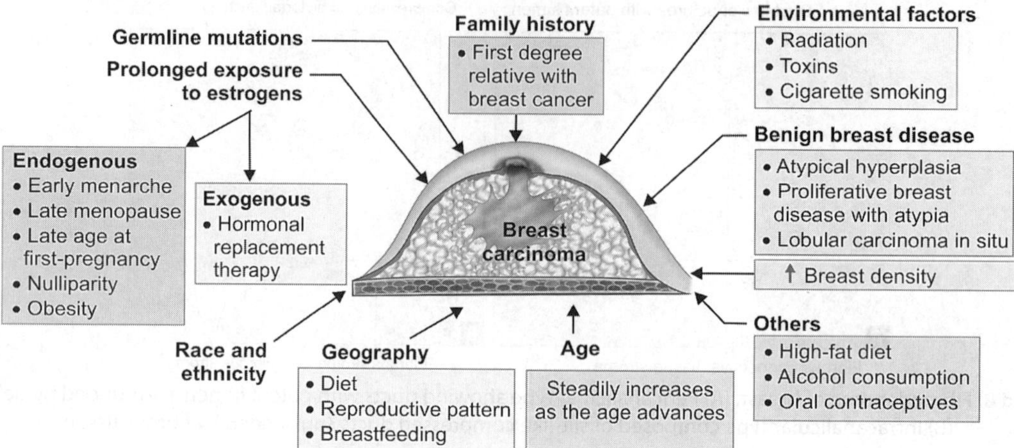

Fig. 22.3: Risk factors involved in the development of breast cancer

- **Exogenous hormone exposure:** It may be due to **postmenopausal hormonal replacement therapy**.
- **Germline mutations.**
- **Family history of first-degree relatives with breast cancer:** First degree relatives include mother, sister or daughter. It is strongly associated with increased risk for breast cancer.
- **Environmental risk factors:**
  - **Radiation exposure:** Radiation to the chest due to cancer therapy, atomic bomb exposure, or nuclear accidents.
  - **Environmental toxins:** For example, organochlorine pesticides, have estrogenic effects.
  - **Cigarette smoking.**
- **Benign breast disease:** Atypical hyperplasia/proliferative breast disease with atypia/lobular carcinoma in situ.
- **High breast density.**

Classification of Breast Carcinoma

More than 95% of breast cancers are adenocarcinomas. They are mainly divided into:

- **In situ carcinomas (carcinoma in situ/CIS):** In carcinoma in situ, malignant cells are limited to ducts and lobules and do not penetrate the basement membrane. These tumors are further divided into **lobular carcinoma in situ and ductal in situ carcinomas.**
- **Invasive carcinomas (infiltrating carcinoma):** These tumors show penetration of the basement membrane and infiltration into the stroma. The malignant cells can invade into the lymphatics and blood vessels and cause metastasis in the regional lymph nodes and distant sites. There are several histological subtypes of invasive carcinoma such as: **invasive ductal carcinoma** (not otherwise specified/no-special-type carcinoma), **medullary carcinoma, mucinous carcinoma, papillary carcinoma, inflammatory carcinoma, invasive lobular carcinoma** and others.

Invasive (Infiltrating) Carcinoma, No Special Type (NST/invasive Ductal Carcinoma)

Invasive carcinomas of no special type constitute the majority of carcinomas (70–80%).

Morphology

Gross (Fig. 22.4)**:** Most of the tumors are **firm to hard** and have an **irregular border**. On cut section, they produce a characteristic grating sound (similar to cutting a water chestnut or unripened pear).

Microscopy (Fig. 22.5)**:** They may range from well-differentiated to poorly differentiated carcinomas. The

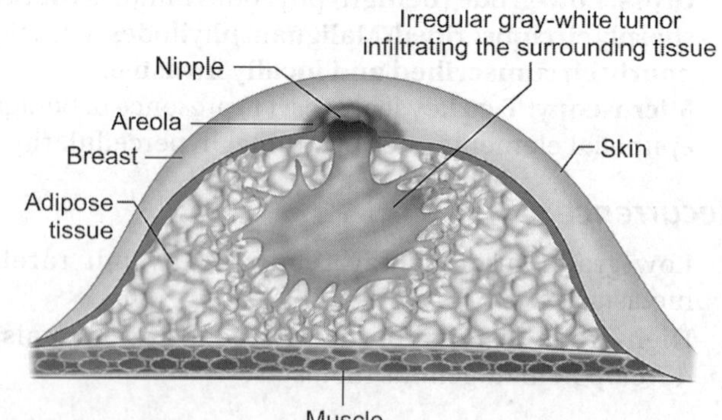

Fig. 22.4: Gross features of infiltrating duct carcinoma. The tumor is irregular in shape and shows infiltration into to nipple causing retraction

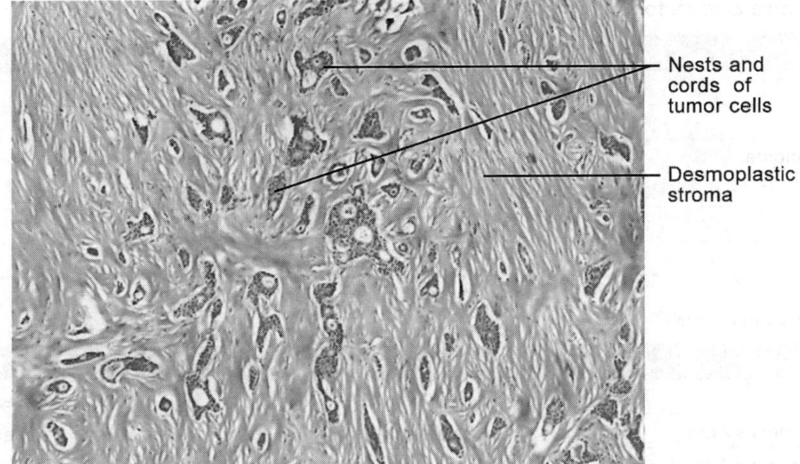

Fig. 22.5: Microscopy of infiltrating duct carcinoma showing nests and cords of tumor cells with desmoplastic stroma extensive fibrous reaction

tumor cells are arranged in nests, cords or as glands. Some tumors may show extensive fibrous reaction in the stroma known as **desmoplasia.**

Invasive Lobular Carcinoma

Lobular carcinomas tend to be bilateral. Microscopically, the infiltrating tumor cells are arranged in single file (Indian file) or in loose clusters or sheets. Tubule formation and desmoplasia are not seen.

Spread

Local spread: It may spread into overlying skin, into the surrounding breast tissue and skeletal muscle.

Lymphatics: Regional lymphnodes, mainly axillary or internal mammary chain.

Blood spread: It may spread to opposite breast, lung, liver, bone, ovaries or brain.

Clinical Features

Invasive carcinoma presents as a **palpable breast lump**. They range in consistency from **firm to hard**. Larger carcinomas may infiltrate the surrounding structures and thus may be fixed to the chest wall or cause **dimpling of the skin**. When the cancer develops in the central portion of the breast, **retraction of the nipple** may develop.

Diagnosis

Following can help in the diagnosis of breast cancer.

- **Clinical examination**
- **Mammography:** It is a radiological method that can detect even smaller lesions before the cancer can be detected by clinical examination.
- **Fine needle aspiration cytology (FNAC):** It is an out-patient procedure by which cells are obtained through aspiration using needle.
- **Intraoperative imprint cytology**
- **Stereotactic biopsy/surgical biopsy**
- **Frozen section**
- **Excision biopsy:** lumpectomy/mastectomy.

Prognostic and Predictive Factors (Table 22.1)

Prognosis is determined by the the biologic features of the carcinoma (molecular or histologic type) and the extent of cancer spread (stage) at the time of diagnosis. **Two important prognostic factors** are **tumor size and lymph node status**.

Staging of Breast Carcinoma (Table 22.2)

Table 22.1: Prognostic and predictive factors of breast cancer

Major factors	Minor factors
Lymph node metastases	Histologic subtype
Tumor size	Histological grade
In situ versus invasive carcinoma	Estrogen and progesterone receptors (ER and PR)
Distant metastases	HER2/neu
Locally advanced disease	Lymphovascular invasion
Inflammatory carcinoma	Proliferative rate

Table 22.2: Staging of breast carcinoma

Stage	T: Primary cancer	N: Lymph nodes (LNs)	M: Distant metastasis
0	DCIS or LCIS	No metastases	Absent
I	Invasive carcinoma ≤2 cm	No metastases	Absent
II	Invasive carcinoma >2 to <5 cm	No metastases/ 1–3 positive LNs	Absent
III	Invasive carcinoma >5 cm	≥4 positive LNs	Absent
IV	Invasive carcinoma of any size	Negative or positive lymph nodes	Present

DCIS, ductal carcinoma in situ; LCIS, lobular carcinoma in situ

SELF-ASSESSMENT EXERCISE

I. Short Notes

1. Fibroadenoma
2. Carcinoma of breast/Infiltrating duct carcinoma

CHAPTER

23

Bones, Joints and Soft Tissue Tumors

CHAPTER OUTLINE

INTRODUCTION

The skeletal system consists of the bones, their associated cartilages, and the joints. Bone is a specialized connective tissue which has structural, protective, metabolic and hematopoietic functions (produces blood cells).

Different Regions in the Bone (Fig. 23.1)

- **Epiphysis:** It is the area of the bone which extends from the base of the articular surface (the site of close approximation of two bones) to the region of the growth plate.
- **Metaphysis:** It is the region which extends from the region of the growth plate to area where the diameter of the bone becomes significantly narrow (becomes funnel-shaped).
- **Diaphysis (shaft):** It is the zone which extends from base of one metaphysis to the base of the opposing metaphysis.

Cells of the Bone Tissue

- **Osteoblasts** produce osteoid and are thus bone forming cells. Osteoid is unmineralized organic bone matrix.

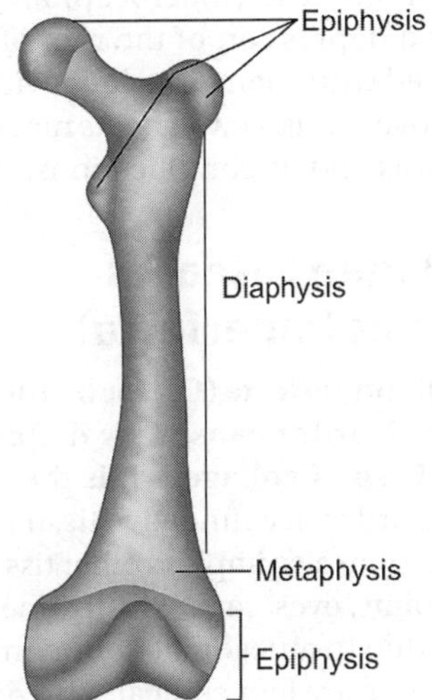

Fig. 23.1: Different regions of bone

- **Osteocytes:** When osteoblast is enveloped by bone matrix it becomes osteocyte. With time osteocytes lose the capacity for matrix synthesis.
- **Osteoclasts:** These are mature multinucleated cells (on an average 6–12 nuclei) that are responsible for bone resorption (removal by absorption).

CONGENITAL DISORDERS

- **Dysostoses:** Abnormalities in a single bone or a localized group of bones are called **dysostoses.** They manifest as absent, supernumerary or abnormally fused bones. The most common congenital disorders include complete absence of a bone or entire digit (aplasia), extra bones or digits (supernumerary digit), and abnormal fusion of bones (e.g. syndactyly, craniosynostosis).
- **Dysplasia:** The term dysplasia with regard to bone implies abnormal (disorganized)growth of bone and/

or cartilage rather than a premalignant lesion as used in the context of neoplasia.
- Genetic factors play role in congenital disorders.

Achondroplasia

- It is the **most common skeletal dysplasia and a major cause of dwarfism.**
- It is transmitted as an autosomal dominant disorder resulting in retarded cartilage growth due to **arrest of growth plate**.
- **Clinical appearance:** These individuals have shortened proximal extremities, a trunk of relatively normal length, and an enlarged head (macrocephaly) with bulging forehead and depression of the root of the nose. It is not associated with changes in longevity, intelligence, or reproductive status. Few patients may develop severe kyphoscoliosis and its complications.

Type 1 Collagen Diseases (Osteogenesis Imperfecta)

- **Osteogenesis imperfecta (OI), or brittle bone disease, is group of disorder caused by deficiencies in the synthesis of type I collagen.** It is the most common inherited disorder of connective tissue.
- It affects bone, but also impacts other tissues rich in type I collagen (joints, eyes, ears, skin, ligaments and teeth).
- It usually is due to autosomal dominant disorder.
- **Subtypes:** There are four clinical subtypes namely type I,II, III and IV.
- **Basic abnormality in OI is too little bone, leading to extreme fragility of skeleton.**

Osteopetrosis

- Osteopetrosis, also known as **marble bone disease** and Albers-Schönberg disease. It refers to a group of rare inherited diseases in which **skeletal mass is increased** as a result of abnormally dense bone.
- There is reduced bone resorption and diffuse symmetric skeletal sclerosis due to impaired formation or function of osteoclasts.
- The term osteopetrosis refers to the stone-like quality of the bones in this disorder. However, the bones are abnormally brittle and easily fracture, like a piece of chalk.
- Osteopetrosis is classified into variants based on both the mode of inheritance and the severity of clinical findings.
- Osteopetrosis was the first genetic disease treated with hematopoietic stem cell transplantation.

INFECTIONS—OSTEOMYELITIS

Definition: Osteomyelitis is defined as **inflammation of the bone and marrow**.

Types of osteomyelitis: Any infectious (bacteria, viruses, parasites, fungi) agent may cause osteomyelitis, but infections by certain pyogenic bacteria and mycobacteria are the most common.
- **Pyogenic**
- **Tuberculous**
- **Others:** Chronic nonspecific osteomyelitis.

Pyogenic Osteomyelitis

Etiology

It is almost always caused by bacteria.
- **Most common** pathogens are ***Staphylococcus*** species (*aureus* in 80–90% of the cases).
- **Other organisms** include: *Escherichia coli, Pseudomonas, Klebsiella, Neisseria gonorrhoeae, Hemophilus influenzae*, and *Salmonella* species.

Portal of entry of organisms: Causative organisms may reach the bone **directly** or through the **bloodstream** (during bacteremia-presence of bacteria in the blood), or **extend from a contiguous site**.

Location of infection: The location of the infection varies with age. **Metaphysis** of long bones (knee, ankle and hip) is the most **common location** of infection in **children**.

Pathogenesis and Morphology (Figs 23.2A to D)

- Normally, in the metaphysis, capillaries form loops, this slows the flow of blood in the metaphyseal region of the bone. During bacteremia (bacteria in the blood), the **infective organism reaches metaphysis of long bone.** The slowing of blood in the metaphysis allows time for bacteria to penetrate blood vessel walls and establish infective foci (the starting point of a disease process) within the marrow in the region of metaphysis.
- Once in the bone, the bacteria grow and induce an **acute inflammatory reaction** with formation of inflammatory **exudates. Exudate increases the pressure,** produces death of **bone (necrosis)** and promotes **formation of pus**. The necrotic bone fragment gets trapped in the exudates. The fragment of **dead necrotic bone** embedded in the pus is known as **sequestrum**.
- The **pus penetrates the periosteum** and **forms an abscess in the surrounding soft-tissue.** The pus may further penetrate the overlying skin to form a **draining sinus**.

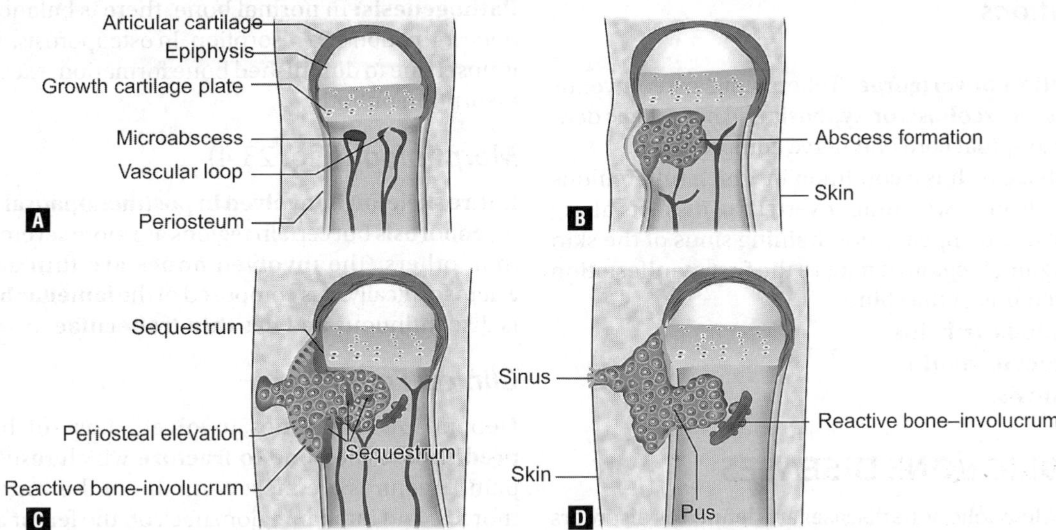

Figs 23.2A to D: Pathogenesis of hematogenous osteomyelitis. (A) A small, septic microabscess is formed at the capillary loop; (B) Abscess expands and stimulates reactive bone formation by the periosteum; (C) Abscess continues to expand through the cortex into the subperiosteal tissue; (D) The extension of this process into the skin produces a draining sinus.

- Reactive new bone gets deposited in the periphery of the inflammatory reaction. This **reactive new bone** formed **is known as involucrum**.

Complications

- **Septicemia:** Organisms may disseminate through the bloodstream and cause septicemia (presence of pathogenic microorganisms in the blood).
- **Acute suppurative arthritis:** Infection may spread into a joint, producing suppurative arthritis.
- **Pathologic fractures.**
- **Squamous cell carcinoma:** It may arise from the epithelialized sinus tract.
- **Secondary amyloidosis** (deposition of proteinaceous substance/amyloid between cells).
- **Chronic osteomyelitis.**

Clinical Features

Presents with **malaise, fever, chills, leukocytosis** (an increase in the number of leukocytes), and **throbbing pain over the affected region.**

Diagnosis

- **Radiography:** Lytic (dissolving) focus of bone destruction surrounded by a zone of sclerosis (hardening or induration).
- **Blood cultures** are positive for the causative microorganisms.
- **Biopsy and bone cultures.**

Tuberculous Osteomyelitis

Tuberculous osteomyelitis is caused by *Mycobacterium tuberculosis.*

Age: Usually seen in **adolescents or young adults** in developing countries.

Source and route of infection: Usually bloodborne infection from a focus of active pulmonary or extrapulmonary disease.

Sites: Spine (thoracic and lumbar vertebrae) is commonly involved and is known as **Pott disease** (Fig. 23.3). Other sites include knees and hips.

Microscopically, it shows tuberculous granuloma (refer Fig. 4.2).

Clinical features: Low-grade fever with evening rise of temperature, pain on movement, localized tenderness and weight loss are common symptoms.

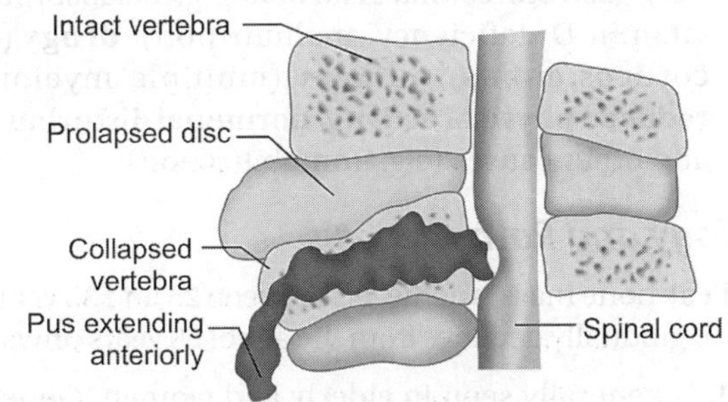

Fig. 23.3: Tuberculosis of spine

Complications

Spine

- **Destruction of vertebrae:** Tuberculous osteomyelitis causes severe **scoliosis or kyphosis** and neurologic deficits due to spinal cord and nerve compression.
- **Psoas abscess:** It is a condition in which tuberculous infection from lower lumbar vertebrae dissects along the pelvis, and appears as a draining sinus of the skin in the inguinal region. It may be the first manifestation of tuberculous of the spine.
- **Tuberculous arthritis**
- **Sinus tract formation**
- **Amyloidosis.**

METABOLIC BONE DISEASES

Definition: Metabolic bone diseases are defined as disorders of metabolism that result in secondary structural effects on the skeleton. These effects include diminished bone mass due to decreased synthesis or increased destruction, reduced bone mineralization or both.

Osteoporosis

Osteoporosis is a disease of bone characterized by **low bone mass** (quantitative reduction) which leads to porosity of bones.

Types

Osteoporosis may be:

- **Localized:** It is usually due to disuse and is seen as a complication of some other disease. For example, local immobilization following fracture due to other causes.
- **Generalized:** Involves the entire skeleton. It may be **primary or secondary**.
  - **Primary** osteoporosis occurs without any known cause. These include senile and postmenopausal.
  - **Secondary** osteoporosis develops due to a large variety of conditions. These include **endocrine disorders** (hyperparathyroidism, hyperthyroidism, etc.), **gastrointestinal disorders** (e.g. malabsorption, vitamin D deficiency, malnutrition), **drugs** (e.g. corticosteroids), **tumors** (multiple myeloma) **reduced physical activity, hormonal disturbances** and other causes (e.g. immobilization).

Etiology and Pathogenesis

Age: Peak bone mass is achieved between 25 and 35 years of age and gradually declines from the age of 50 years onwards.

Sex: It is generally seen in elderly and women. Genetic/ hereditary factors also play an important role.

Pathogenesis: In normal bone, there is balance between bone formation and resorption. In osteoporosis, the balance is upset due to diminished bone formation, excessive bone resorption or both.

Morphology (Fig. 23.4)

Entire skeleton is involved in postmenopausal and senile osteoporosis but certain regions are more severely involved than others. The **involved bones are thin and brittle**. Microscopically, it is composed of the **lamellar bone** which is discontinuous and has **thin trabeculae.**

Clinical Features

Depend on the bones involved. Loss of bone mass **predisposes** the bone **to fracture** which results in bone pain. Fractures are most common in the vertebra in the thoracic and lumbar region, neck of the femur and Colles' fracture (fracture of distal radius).

Complications

- Pulmonary embolism and pneumonia as a complication of fractures of the femoral neck, pelvis or spine.
- When fractures of vertebra are multiple, it may lead to lumbar lordosis and kyphoscoliosis (forward bending).

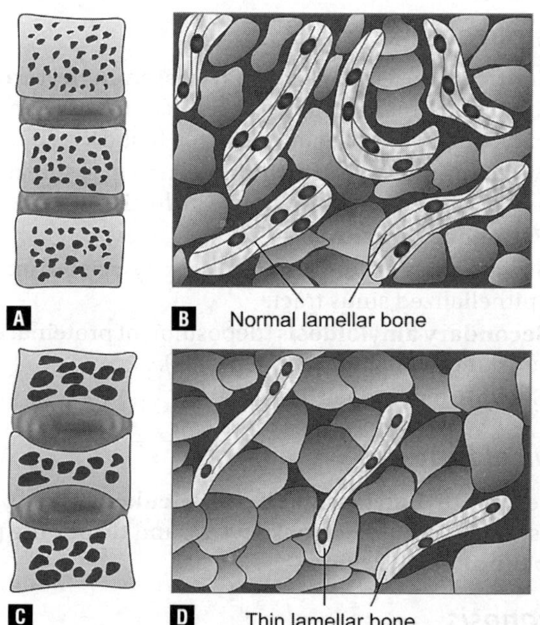

Figs 23.4A to D: (A) Normal gross appearance of bone-vertebral column; (B) Normal microscopic appearance of trabecular bone and fatty marrow. The trabecular bone is lamellar and contains evenly distributed osteocytes; (C) Gross appearance of osteoporosis; (D) Microscopic appearance of osteoporosis composed of the lamellar bone which are discontinuous and have thin trabeculae

Diagnosis

- **Plain X-ray:** Not reliable till 30 - 40% of the bone mass is lost.
- **Dual-energy X-ray absorptiometry** and **quantitative computed tomography.**
- Bone biopsy.

Paget Disease (Osteitis Deformans)

Paget disease of bon is a chronic disorder characterized by increased, but disordered and structurally unsound, bone mass.

Age: Usually begins in late adulthood (average age at diagnosis, 70 years).

Etiology and Pathogenesis

The cause of Paget disease remains uncertain. Probably both genetic and environmental factors contribute. Probably chronic infection of osteoclast precursors by measles or other RNA viruses may play a role.

Morphology

Paget disease may be **monostotic/solitary** (about 15%) and **polyostotic/multiple bones** (85% of case). The axial skeleton or proximal femur is involved in about 80% of cases.

Phases: It has three sequential phases: (1) osteolytic stage, (2) mixed osteoclastic-osteoblastic stage, which evolves ultimately into (3) final burned-out quiescent osteosclerotic stage.

1. **First osteolytic resorptive stage:** In this phase, there are waves of osteoclastic activity with resorption of bone. The osteoclasts are abnormally large and have many more than the normal 10 to 12 nuclei; sometimes 100 nuclei are present.
2. **Mixed osteoclastic-osteoblastic stage:** In this phase there is bone resorption by osteoclasts and formation of new woven or lamellar bone. The cortex in the mixed phase is thickened.
3. **Osteosclerotic (cold or burnt-out) phase: The histological hallmark is a mosaic pattern of lamellar bone observed in this final sclerotic phase**. This is characterized by jigsaw puzzle-like appearance produced by unusually **prominent cement lines**. The findings during the other phases are less specific. The bone is vulnerable to deformation under stress and easily undergoes fracture.

Clinical Course

- Clinical features are extremely variable and depend on the extent and site of the disease.
- Enlargement of the craniofacial skeleton may produce *leontiasis ossea* (lion face) and a cranium is heavy.
- Weight bearing causes anterior bowing of the femurs and tibiae and develops severe **secondary osteoarthritis**.
- **Chalk stick-type fractures** develops in the long bones of the lower extremities. Compression fractures of the spine result in spinal cord injury and the development of kyphosis.
- **Development of tumor and tumor-like conditions develop in pagetic bone**. The benign lesions include giant cell tumor and most malignant include sarcoma (osteosarcoma or fibrosarcoma).

Osteomalacia and rickets (refer Chapter 8 page 87–8).

Primary hyperparathyroidism (refer Chapter 24 page 301).

BONE TUMORS

Classification of Bone Tumors (Table 23.1)

Table 23.1: Classification of primary bone tumors

Histological type	Benign	Malignant
Bone forming	Osteoma	Osteosarcoma
Cartilage forming	Osteochondroma Chondroma	Chondrosarcoma
Hematopoietic		Myeloma Lymphoma
Unknown origin	Giant-cell tumor	Ewing sarcoma
Notochord		Chordoma

Osteochondroma

Osteochondroma (exostosis) is the most common benign cartilage-capped tumor which attaches to the underlying bone by a stalk.

Age group: It occurs in **late adolescence** and early adulthood.

Sex: Men are affected three times more often than women.

Site and location: It arises from the **metaphysis** near the growth plate of **long tubular bones**, especially about the knee.

Morphology (Fig. 23.5): Osteochondromas are **sessile or mushroom-shaped**. The cap is composed of benign hyaline cartilage and underlying lamellar bone.

Clinical features: Slow-growing masses and are detected as an incidental finding.

Osteosarcoma

Osteosarcoma (osteogenic sarcoma) is the most common (20%) primary malignant bone tumor.

Definition: Osteosarcoma is a highly malignant bone tumor **characterized by formation of bone matrix or osteoid** (unmineralized bone) **by** malignant **tumor cells.**

Age group: Osteosarcoma occurs in between **10 and 20** years of age.

Sex: Affects boys more commonly than girls (2:1).

Morphology

Location: It usually arises in the **metaphyseal region** of the long bones of the extremities.

Sites: It usually arises near the knee or shoulder. The common site is:

- Lower femur
- Upper tibia, or fibula
- Proximal humerus.

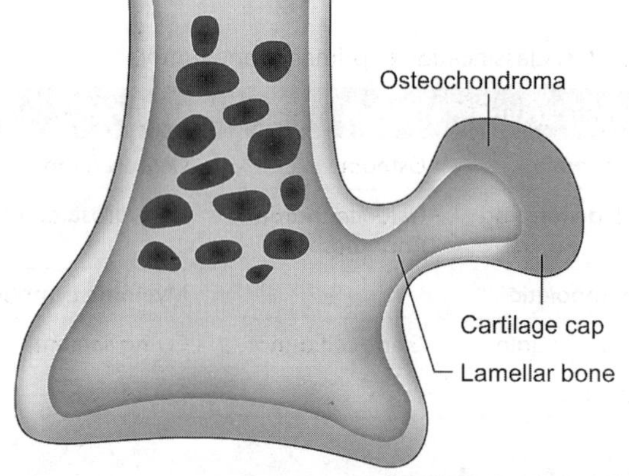

Fig. 23.5: Osteochondroma appears as a mushroom-shaped tumor covered by cartilage

Gross (Fig. 23.6A)**:** Usually, these are **big bulky tumors**. They are **gray-white** in color, **gritty**, shows **areas of hemorrhage and cystic degeneration.** The tumor extends into the adjacent soft tissue giving rise to **mutton leg** appearance.

Microscopy (Fig. 23.6B)**:** It consists of **pleomorphic tumor cells** (cells varying in size and shape) with large hyperchromatic nuclei and often shows mitotic figures. **Bizarre tumor giant cells** are common. **Production of osteoid** (unmineralized/noncalcified) **or bone** (calcified osteoid) **by malignant tumor** cells is the **diagnostic feature** of osteosarcoma.

Clinical Features

Usually presents as painful, progressively enlarging mass around the knee or other involved site. The involved area is swollen and tender, and the function of the adjacent joint becomes reduced.

Radiographic Findings

- It shows a **large destructive mass** which frequently infiltrates the cortex and lifts the periosteum. The space between cortex and elevated periosteum radiologically appears as triangular shadow known as **Codman triangle.**
- When the malignant tumor extends into soft tissues, parallel lines of mineral deposition in the periosteal region gives an appearance of rays of sun. This is called as "**sunburst**" appearance.

Spread

- **Local spread:** It may **invade the adjacent cortex, medullary (marrow) cavity, epiphysis** or into **soft-tissue** and skin.

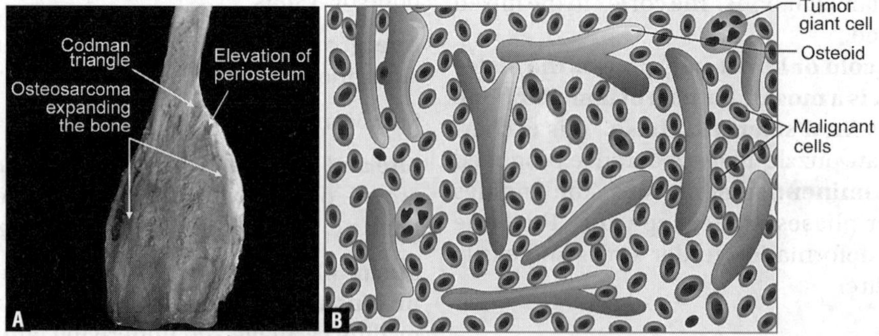

Figs 23.6A and B: (A) Gross appearance of osteosarcoma of the lower part of distal femur showing a tan-white tumor, filling most of the medullary cavity of the metaphysis and proximal diaphysis. The tumor has infiltrated through the cortex, lifted the periosteum and this region on X-ray appears as Codman triangle; (B) Diagrammatic microscopy of osteosarcoma composed of pleomorphic tumor cells separated by osteoid

- **Blood spread:** It may spread to the **lungs**. Less commonly, to other bones (35%), the pleura, brain and the heart.

Giant-Cell Tumor

Giant-cell tumor (osteoclastoma) is a **locally aggressive** and **potentially malignant neoplasm.**

Age: It is usually seen between the ages of **20–40 years.**

Sex: It has a slight predilection for females.

Cell of origin: Primitive stromal cells.

Morphology

Site: Giant-cell tumors arise from **epiphysis.**

Bones involved: Knee area (distal femur and proximal tibia), lower end of the radius, humerus and fibula.

Gross: It appears as a **large circumscribed** tumor. Cut surface is **soft and red-brown** due to **numerous hemorrhagic areas** (Fig. 23.7A). Areas of cystic degeneration and necrosis are common.

Microscopy (Fig. 23.7B): It is composed of **multinucleated osteoclast-type giant cells** (non-neoplastic) uniformly distributed in a **background of mononuclear cells (neoplastic).** Diagnosis of malignancy depends upon the morphology of the mononuclear cells rather than that of the multinucleated giant cells.

Radiological Appearance

The tumor is multiloculated and gives rise to **soap bubble** appearance.

Clinical Features

Giant-cell tumors (GCTs) present as **pain**, usually in the joint adjacent to the tumor and cause arthritis-like symptoms.

Biologic behavior: Majority behave in a benign fashion, but tumors may recur locally.

Spread:

- **Local spread:** It is usually restricted within the involved bone.
- **Metastasis:** Common site is lung.

Ewing Sarcoma/Primitive Neuroectodermal Tumor

Ewing sarcoma is a primary malignant small round-cell tumor of bone and soft tissues.

Age: Mostly seen between **10 and 15 years** of age.

Sex: More frequent in **boys** than girls (2:1), with a predilection for whites.

Origin: Precursor cell of Ewing sarcoma/PNET is a multipotent mesenchymal stem cell.

Morphology

Location and site: They arise in the **medullary cavity** of the **diaphysis** of long bones **(humerus, tibia and femur).**

Gross: It is soft, **grayish white/tan-white,** and frequently shows **areas of hemorrhage and necrosis.**

Microscopy (Fig. 23.8): It consists of **sheets of closely packed, uniform, small and round cells.** Tumor cells have **scant or little cytoplasm. Cytoplasm** appears **clear** because

Articular cartilage
Hemorrhagic and cystic tumor
A

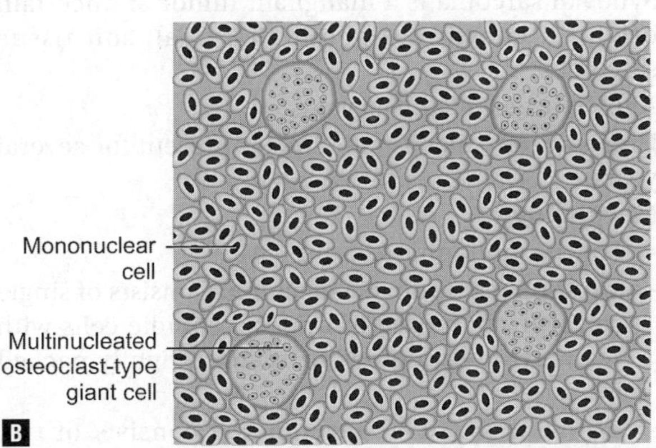

Figs 23.7A and B: Giant-cell tumor of upper part of tibia. (A) Grossly, shows a circumscribed tumor with hemorrhage; Microscopically (B), it is composed of numerous multinucleated giant cells. The background shows mononuclear stromal cells

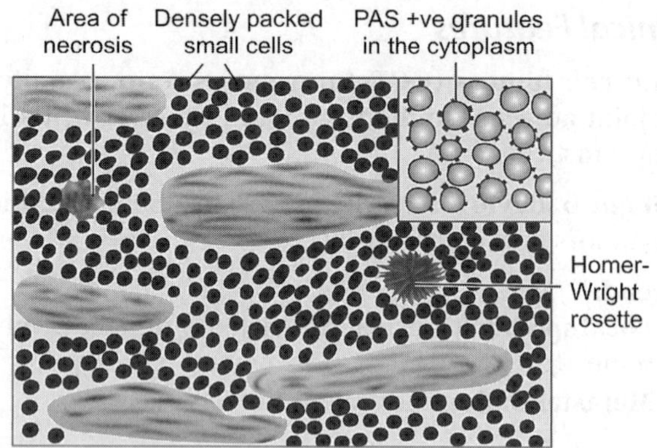

Fig. 23.8: Ewing sarcoma composed of sheets of closely packed uniform small round cells with scanty cytoplasm. The inset shows PAS positive granules in the cytoplasm

it is **rich in glycogen**. The tumor cells may form **Homer-Wright rosettes** in which the tumor cells are arranged in a circle about a central fibrillary space. **Necrosis** may be prominent.

Radiographic Findings

The characteristic layers of periosteal new bone formation produces **onion-skin pattern**.

Clinical features: Presents as **painful enlarging mass** and the affected site is **tender, warm and swollen**.

Spread: Tumor spreads from medullary cavity into cortex, periosteum and surrounding soft tissue. Metastasis may develop to lungs, brain and other bones, mainly skull.

Tumors of Uncertain Origin

Synovial Sarcoma

- Synovial sarcoma is a malignant tumor of uncertain origin. It constitutes about 10% of all soft tissue sarcomas.
- **Age:** Between 20 and 40 years.
- **Presentation:** Deep-seated mass present for several years.
- **Morphology**
  - May be monophasic or biphasic.
  - **Monophasic synovial sarcoma:** Consists of single cell type composed of uniform spindle cells with scant cytoplasm growing in short, tightly packed fascicles.
  - **Biphasic synovial sarcoma:** It consists of two cell types namely the spindle cell component (as in monophasic described above) and gland-like structures composed of cuboidal to columnar epithelioid cells.
- **Treatment:** Treated aggressively with limb sparing surgery and frequently chemotherapy. The 5-year survival varies from 25% to 62% depending on the stage and patient age.

JOINTS

Joints provide movement and mechanical stability to the body. The joints consist of articular cartilage with a joint space (synovial cavity) lined by synovial membrane (Fig 23.9). The articular cartilage provides friction free movement within the joints and acts as a shock absorber. The joints have a wide range of motion. The synovial cavity contains clear and viscous synovial fluid having hyaluronic acid. The fluid acts as a lubricant and supplies nutrition to the articular hyaline cartilage.

Arthritis: Inflammation of the joint is known as arthritis. There are many types of arthritis.

INFECTIOUS ARTHRITIS

- Infectious arthritis is due to direct infection of joints by microorganisms.
- Infectious arthritis is **serious**, because it **can produce joint destruction** leading to permanent deformities.

Suppurative Arthritis

Mode of Infection

- **Blood spread:** Bacterial infections **causing acute suppurative arthritis** usually enter the joints from distant sites by hematogenous route.
- **Direct inoculation or from contiguous spread:** It may occur from a soft tissue abscess or focus of osteomyelitis. In neonates, it can occur due to direct spread from underlying epiphyseal osteomyelitis.

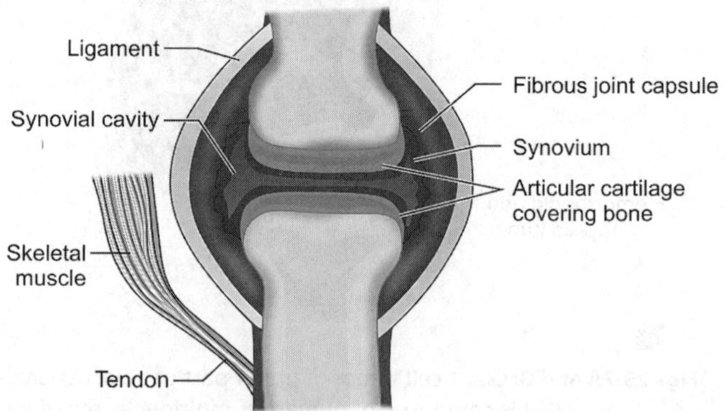

Fig. 23.9: Different parts of the joint

Causative Microorganism

- *H. influenza*: In children younger than 2 years of age.
- *S. aureus:* In older children and adults.
- Gonococcus: During late adolescence and young adulthood.
- *Salmonella:* Patients with sickle cell disease are prone to infection with *Salmonella* at any age.

Clinical Features

- Sudden development of **acute painful and swollen joint** with restriction of joint movement.
- **Systemic features:** These include fever, leukocytosis, and raised ESR common.
- Usually involves single joint. Most commonly affects the knee joint followed by the hip, shoulder, elbow and wrist.
- **Joint aspiration:** It is diagnostic and in the aspirated purulent joint fluid, the causative agent can be identified.

Mycobacterial (Tuberculous) Arthritis

- Mycobacterial **(tuberculous)** arthritis is a chronic progressive monoarticular infection caused by *M. tuberculosis*.
- **Age:** Can occur at any age groups, but common in adults.

Mode of Infection

- **Usually** develops as a **complication of adjoining tuberculous osteomyelitis**.
- Hematogenous dissemination from a visceral (usually pulmonary) site of mycobacterial infection.

Clinical Features

- Onset is insidious with **gradual progressive pain.**
- Systemic symptoms may or may not be present.
- **Joints affected:** Usually affects weight-bearing joints. These include the hips, knees, and ankles in descending order of frequency.
- **Microscopy:** Shows granulomas with central caseous necrosis (refer Fig. 4.2).

Osteoarthritis

Osteoarthritis (degenerative joint disease) is a **noninflammatory, slowly progressive**, most **common joint disease**. It mainly **involves** the **articular cartilage and subchondral** (below the articular cartilage) **bone**. It causes progressive destruction of articular cartilage of weight bearing joints. It develops in genetically susceptible older persons. It leads to narrowing of joint space, subchondral bone thickening, and finally nonfunctioning, painful joint.

Joints Affected

- **Weight bearing joints:** Joints of knee, hips and cervical and lumbar segments of the spine.
- **Non-weight bearing joint:** Proximal and distal interphalangeal joints of the fingers, first carpometacarpal joints, and first tarsometatarsal joints of the feet.

Types

- **Primary osteoarthritis:** Most of the osteoarthritis develop as aging process.
- **Secondary osteoarthritis:** Rarely, osteoarthritis may appear in younger individuals with predisposing condition, like previous injuries to a joint, congenital deformity of a joint(s), and secondary to systemic disease (diabetes, hemochromatosis).

Pathogenesis and Morphological Changes (Figs 23.10A to D)

Osteoarthritis is a multifactorial disease having both **genetic** and **environmental** components. The major environmental factors are **aging** and **biomechanical stress**. This in turn is influenced by obesity, muscle strength, and joint stability. Different changes in the pathogenesis of osteoarthritis are as follows:

- **Chondrocyte injury:** Aging together with genetic and biochemical factors initiate injury to the **chondrocytes of articular cartilage.**
- **Changes in the articular cartilage:** The damaged chondrocytes leads to **cracks on** the surface of the **articular cartilage. Synovial fluid** flows along these cracks and **penetrates deeper into the articular cartilage**. Dead pieces of **articular cartilage fragment** are shed as **loose bodies (joint mice)** in the synovial cavity.
- **Changes in the subchondral bone:** With sloughing of the full thickness of the articular cartilage; the **subchondral bone is exposed** and becomes the new articular surface. The subchondral bone **appears thick, shiny, smooth** giving it the appearance of polished ivory and known as **bone eburnation** (eburnated means ivory like). The eburnated bone allows synovial fluid from the joint surface into the subchondral bone marrow forming **subchondral bone cyst** filled with synovial fluid. The loculated fluid collection increases in size surrounded by reactive bone wall. **Mushroom-shaped** pearly grayish bony outgrowths (spurs) known as **osteophytes** develop at the periphery of the joint surface.

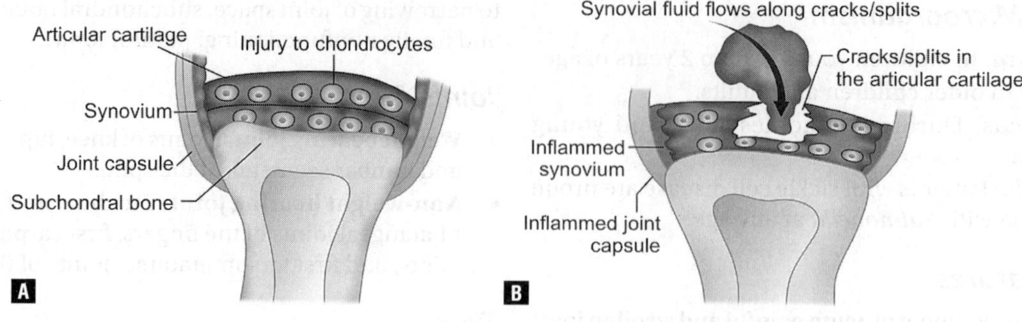

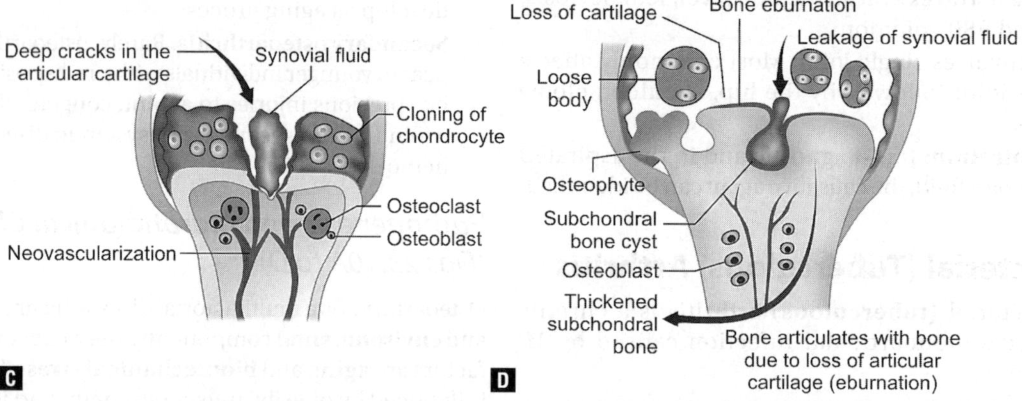

Figs 23.10A to D: Pathogenesis and morphological changes of osteoarthritis

Clinical Features

- Osteoarthritis is an insidious slowly progressive disease, and causes long-term disability.
- Usually, presents with deep, aching pain which worsens with joint movement and is relieved by rest.
- The involved joints may be swollen, tender, and may demonstrate crepitus.
- Osteophytes in spine can cause nerve root compression and neurologic deficits.
- Prominent osteophytes at the distal interphalangeal joints are known as **Heberden nodes,** and seen commonly in women.

Rheumatoid Arthritis

Rheumatoid arthritis (RA) is a **systemic, chronic inflammatory disorder** which **mainly affects the joints** but can affect many other tissues and organs.

Etiology

Cause of rheumatoid arthritis remains unknown. Following three factors play an important role:

- **Genetic factors**
- **Environmental arthritogen agents:** These arthritogenic agents are thought to initiate the disease process. Several microbial agents (e.g. virus, mycobacteria and *Mycoplasma)* have been suggested but not proved.
- **Autoimmunity**.

Morphology

Joints: Rheumatoid arthritis causes most severe changes in the joints. Most commonly affected are **proximal interphalangeal** and **metacarpophalangeal joints**, elbows, knees, ankles and spine.

Synovium:

- **Gross:** The involved synovium shows **edema and thickening**.
- **Microscopy** (Figs 23.11A to E)**:** The characteristic features include:
  - **Synovial hyperplasia** which may form finger-like structures (villi).
  - **Dense inflammatory infiltrate of lymphocytes, plasma cells** and macrophages. Lymphocytes may **aggregate to form lymphoid follicles.**

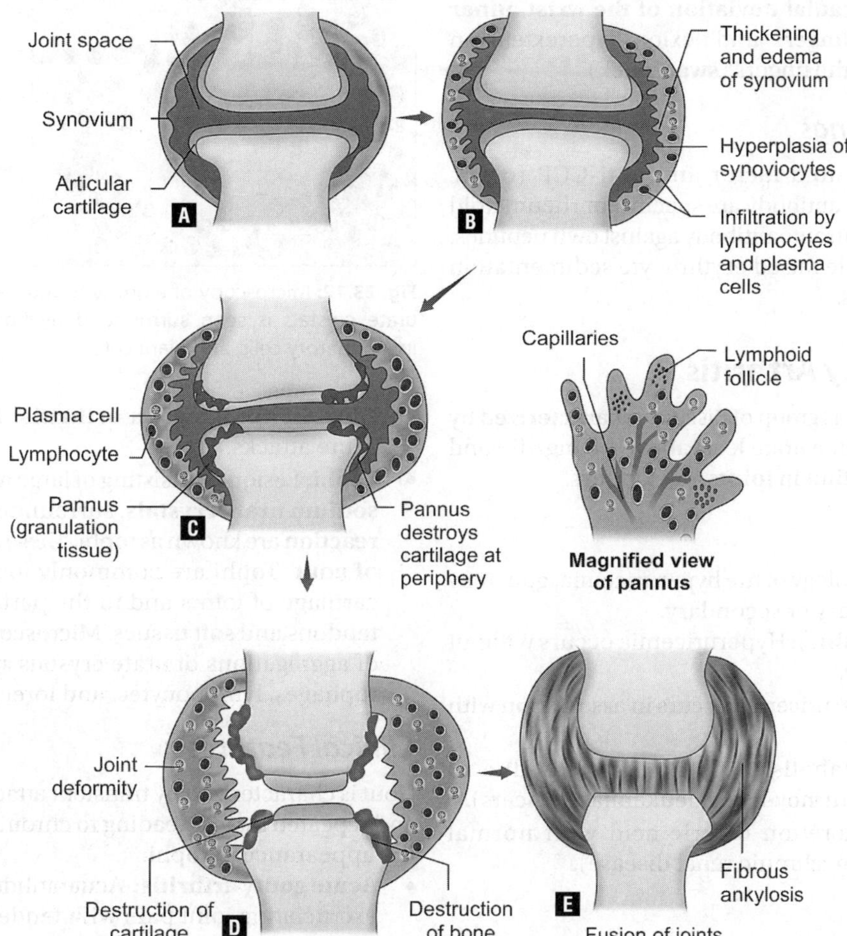

Figs 23.11A to E: Sequence of morphological changes in rheumatoid arthritis. (A) Normal joint; (B) Synovial cells proliferate and synovial tissue is infiltrated by lymphocytes and plasma cells; (C) The synovial hypertrophy and hyperplasia leads to formation of villi. This is accompanied by neovascularization with pannus formation which covers the cartilage. The lymphoid cells form follicles; (D) Proliferating synovium extends into the joint space, destroys cartilage as well as the bone beneath the articular cartilage; (E) The joint is eventually destroyed and becomes fused, a condition termed ankylosis

- **Formation of pannus** which consists of inflammatory cells, granulation tissue, and synovial stroma. **Pannus grows over the articular cartilage** and **destroys** it. After the destruction of cartilage, the pannus bridges the apposing bones to form a **fibrous ankylosis**, which may ossify resulting in **bony ankylosis**.

Other organs/tissues involved

- **Skin: Rheumatoid nodules** are the most common cutaneous lesions.
- **Blood vessels:** Rheumatoid vasculitis.
- **Other tissues:** It may also affect heart, lungs, and muscles.

Clinical Features

- **Age:** RA can occur at any age, but most common between **40 and 70 years.**
- **Sex:** Three to five times more common in **women than men** (3:1).
- Rheumatoid arthritis is usually **slow and insidious in onset**. It presents with malaise, fatigue, and generalized musculoskeletal pain.
- The affected **joints are swollen, warm, painful, and stiff** on arising or following inactivity.
- **Deformities:** Destruction of tendons, ligaments, and joint capsules produces characteristic deformities.

These consist of **radial deviation of the wrist**, **ulnar deviation of the fingers**, and flexion-hyperextension abnormalities of the fingers (**swan neck**).

Laboratory Findings

Presence of rheumatoid factor and anti-CCP (cyclic citrullinated peptide) antibody are specific for rheumatoid arthritis. Anti-CCP is an autoantibody against own peptides. Other findings include raised erythrocyte sedimentation rate and leukocytosis.

Gout and Gouty Arthritis

Gout is a heterogeneous group of diseases **characterized by hyperuricemia** (plasma urate level above 6.8 mg/dL) and **urate crystal deposition in joints** and kidneys.

Classification

Depending on the etiology of the hyperuricemia, gout may be classified as primary or secondary.

- **Primary (idiopathic):** Hyperuricemia occurs without any other disease.
- **Secondary:** Hyperuricemia occurs in association with another illness.
  - Increased catabolism of nucleic acids due to increased cell turnover (e.g. leukemias, cancers).
  - Decreased excretion of uric acid with normal production (e.g. chronic renal disease).

Pathogenesis

- Gout is a **disorder of purine metabolism**. Uric acid is the end product of purine metabolism which is eliminated only in the urine. Human beings do not have uricase, an enzyme which degrades uric acid.
- **Hyperuricemia** is necessary but not sufficient for the development of gout. In gout, the **uric acid crystallizes** in the form of **monosodium urate** (MSU) in joints, on tendon sheaths and in the surrounding tissues. The MSU crystals **trigger inflammatory response** which is characteristic of the acute attack. **Acute arthritis** usually remits in days to weeks. Repeated attacks of acute arthritis lead to **chronic arthritis** and **tophi** formation in the synovial membranes and periarticular tissues.

Morphology (Fig. 23.12)

The morphological changes in gout are:

- **Acute arthritis:** It is characterized by edema, congestion and dense infiltration of synovium by neutrophils.

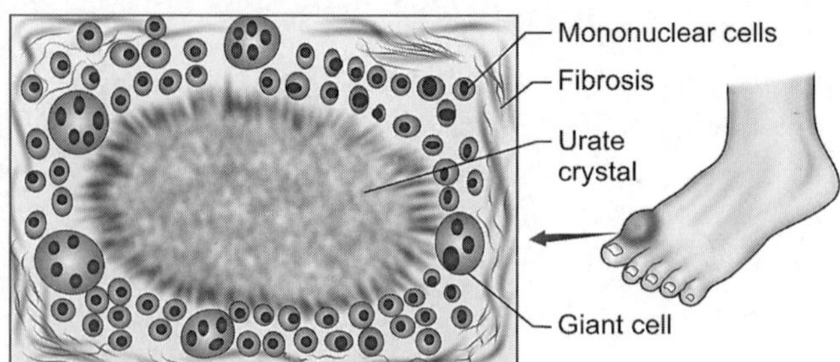

Fig. 23.12: Microscopy of a gouty tophus. Aggregate of dissolved urate crystals is seen surrounded by fibroblasts, mononuclear inflammatory cells, and giant cells

- **Chronic tophaceous arthritis:** It follows repeated acute attacks.
- **Tophi:** Lesions consisting of large **aggregates of monosodium urate crystals**, surrounded by **inflammatory reaction** are known as tophi. These are **pathognomonic of gout**. Tophi are commonly found in the articular cartilage of joints and in the periarticular ligaments, tendons and soft tissues. Microscopically, they consist of aggregations of urate crystals surrounded by macrophages, lymphocytes, and foreign body giant cells.

Clinical Features

Gout is characterized by transient attacks of acute arthritis, and repeated attacks leading to chronic gouty arthritis and the appearance of tophi.

- **Acute gouty arthritis:** Acute arthritis appears as sudden excruciating joint pain with tenderness.
- **Chronic tophaceous gout:** After several years (about 12 years) of acute gouty arthritis, chronic tophaceous gout may develop which may lead to severe crippling disease.
- **Prognosis:** Gout does not reduce the life span, but may cause morbidity.

SOFT TISSUE TUMORS

Soft tissue is the term used for non-epithelial tissue excluding the skeleton, joints, central nervous system, hematopoietic and lymphoid tissues. Sarcomas are malignant tumors of soft tissue.

Liposarcoma

- Liposarcoma is one of the **most common soft tissue sarcomas of adulthood.**
- **Age:** It occurs mainly during 5th to 6th decades of life.
- **Sites:** Deep soft tissues of the proximal extremities and in the retroperitoneum.

Gross

- Liposarcomas appear as nodular masses of 5 cm or more in diameter. Tumors are usually appearing circumscribed but infiltrate into surrounding tissue. Cut section show **gray-white to yellow color** with myxoid and gelatinous appearance.

Microscopy

The cell required for the diagnosis of liposarcoma is **lipoblast**. These cells may be univacuolated or multivacuolated and uninucleated or multinucleated. Liposarcomas are histologically divided into four morphologic subtypes:

1. **Well-differentiated liposarcoma:** Contains adipocytes with scattered atypical spindle cells and lipoblasts.
2. **Myxoid liposarcoma:** Most common histological subtype. Contains abundant basophilic extracellular matrix, arborizing capillaries **(chicken-wire pattern)** and primitive cells at various stages of adipocyte differentiation reminiscent of fetal fat.
3. **Round cell liposarcoma:** It consists of uniform, round to oval cells with central hyperchromatic nuclei. The cytoplasm shows multiple vacuoles.
4. **Pleomorphic liposarcoma:** It is highly undifferentiated/ anaplastic liposarcoma and consists of sheets of anaplastic cells, bizarre nuclei and variable amounts of immature adipocytes (lipoblasts).

Behavior

All histological types of liposarcoma **recur locally** and often repeatedly unless adequately excised. Well-differentiated liposarcoma is relatively indolent; the myxoid/round cell liposarcoma is intermediate in its malignant behavior. The pleomorphic variant usually is aggressive and frequently metastasizes.

Rhabdomyosarcoma

Rhabdomyosarcoma is a **malignant mesenchymal tumor with skeletal muscle differentiation.**

Morphology

Subtypes: Embryonal (60%), alveolar (20%), and pleomorphic (20%).

- **Embryonal rhabdomyosarcoma:** It presents as soft gray infiltrative mass. It consists of **rhabdomyoblasts with cross-striations** may be present. **Sarcoma botryoides** is a variant of embryonal rhabdomyosarcoma that occurs in the walls of hollow, mucosal-lined structures (e.g. nasopharynx, common bile duct, bladder, and vagina).
- **Alveolar rhabdomyosarcoma:** In this, tumor cells are arranged in the alveolar pattern.
- **Pleomorphic rhabdomyosarcoma:** It consists of numerous large, sometimes multinucleated, bizarre eosinophilic tumor cells.

Clinical Features

- Rhabdomyosarcoma (alveolar and embryonal) is the **most common soft tissue sarcoma of childhood and adolescence**. It occurs usually before age 20.
- Pleomorphic rhabdomyosarcoma occurs predominantly in adults. The pediatric type usually arise in the sinuses, head and neck and genitourinary tract (sites that do not normally contain much skeletal muscle.

Rhabdomyosarcomas are **aggressive malignant tumors** usually treated with surgery and chemotherapy, with or without radiation therapy.

Leiomyosarcoma

- Leiomyosarcoma is a **malignant smooth muscle tumor**.
- It occur in adults and common in females than in males.
- **Site:** Most common in the **deep soft tissues of the extremities and retroperitoneum.**
- Leiomyosarcomas **present as painless firm masses**. Retroperitoneal tumors may be large and bulky and cause abdominal symptoms.
- **Microscopy:** They are composed of **eosinophilic spindle cells with blunt-ended, hyperchromatic nuclei arranged in interweaving fascicles**. Immunohistochemically, they are positive for smooth muscle actin and desmin.
- Treatment depends on tumor size, location, and grade.

PEDIATRIC TUMORS

Common malignant neoplasms of infancy and childhood are listed in Table 23.2.

Retinoblastoma

Retinoblastoma is the **most common primary intraocular malignant tumor occurring in children.**

- Cell of origin of retinoblastoma is a neuronal progenitor. About 40% of cases occurs as familial/ hereditary cases in individuals who inherit a germline mutation of one *RB* allele. In the sporadic cases, both RB alleles are lost by somatic mutations.

Table 23.2: Common malignant neoplasms of infancy and childhood

0 to 4 years	5 to 9 years	10 to 14 years
Leukemia **Retinoblastoma** **Neuroblastoma**		Osteogenic sarcoma Thyroid carcinoma Hodgkin disease
Wilms tumor	Ewing sarcoma	
Hepatoblastoma	**Hepatocellular carcinoma**	
Teratomas	Lymphoma	
Soft tissue sarcoma		
Central nervous system tumors		

Morphology

Tumors may contain both undifferentiated and differentiated elements.

- **Undifferentiated elements:** It consists of collections of small, round cells with hyperchromatic nuclei.
- **Well-differentiated tumors:** They show **Flexner-Wintersteiner rosettes.**

Focal zones of dystrophic calcification are characteristic of retinoblastoma.

Spread

Retinoblastoma spread to the brain and bone marrow.

Prognosis

It is adversely affected by extraocular extension and invasion along the optic nerve, and by choroidal invasion.

Other Tumors

These include leukemia (refer pages 148-51), neuroblastoma (refer pages 303-4) Wilms tumor (refer pages 254-5), hepatoblastoma (refer page 229), teratomas, non-Hodgkin and Hodgkin lymphoma (refer pages 167-73), Ewing sarcoma (refer pages 285-6), osteogenic sarcoma (refer pages 284-5), soft tissue sarcoma (refer pages 290-1), and central nervous system tumors (refer pages 329-31)

SELF-ASSESSMENT EXERCISES

I. Essay

1. Write in detail the etiology and pathology of osteomyelitis.

II. Short Notes

1. Pyogenic osteomyelitis.
2. Osteomyelitis.
3. Sequestrum.
4. Osteoarthritis.
5. Osteogenic sarcoma.
6. Callus.
7. Osteoclastoma.
8. Rheumatoid arthritis.
9. Gout.
10. Synovial sarcoma.
11. Liposarcoma.

CHAPTER 24

Endocrine Disorders

CHAPTER OUTLINE

- Pituitary Gland
- Thyroid Gland
- Parathyroid Glands
- Adrenal Glands

PITUITARY GLAND

The pituitary gland is composed of (1) the anterior lobe (adenohypophysis) and (2) the posterior lobe (neurohypophysis).

- The **anterior pituitary** constitutes about 80% of the gland. Anterior pituitary secrets several hormones main being **growth hormone (GH), adrenocorticotropic hormone (ACTH) and thyroid-stimulating hormone (TSH)**.
- The **posterior pituitary** secretes two peptide hormones namely **oxytocin and antidiuretic hormone (ADH),** also called vasopressin**)**.

Clinical Manifestations of Pituitary Disease

It is due to either excess or deficiency of pituitary hormones, or to mass effects.

- **Hyperpituitarism:** The causes of hyperpituitarism include pituitary adenoma, hyperplasia and carcinomas of the anterior pituitary, etc.
- **Hypopituitarism:** The causes of hypopituitarism include ischemic injury, surgery or radiation, inflammatory reactions involving the pituitary gland or hypothalamus.
- **Local mass effects:** These include abnormalities of the sella turcica, including sellar expansion, bony erosion, disruption of the diaphragma sella and visual field abnormalities, etc.

Posterior Pituitary Syndromes

- **Diabetes insipidus: ADH deficiency** causes diabetes insipidus. It is characterized by excessive urination (polyuria) due to an inability of the kidney to resorb water properly from the urine.
  - **Causes of diabetes insipidus:** For example, head trauma, tumors, inflammatory disorders of the hypothalamus and pituitary, and surgical complications.
- **Syndrome of inappropriate ADH (SIADH) secretion:** ADH excess causes resorption of excessive amounts of free water, resulting in hyponatremia. The most frequent causes is the secretion of ectopic ADH by malignant neoplasms (particularly small-cell carcinoma of the lung).

THYROID GLAND

Thyroiditis

Thyroiditis is a group of disorders characterized by **inflammation of the thyroid gland** (Box 24.1).

Hashimoto Thyroiditis

- Hashimoto (**chronic lymphocytic**) thyroiditis is an **autoimmune disease** that leads to gradual failure of thyroid function.
- **Age:** Peak between **45 and 65 years** of age.
- **Sex: More common in women** than in men. Female to male ratio 10: 1–20: 1.

Box 24.1: Various types of thyroiditis

Various types of thyroiditis
• Infectious thyroiditis – Bacterial including mycobacterial – Fungal
• Hashimoto (chronic lymphocytic) thyroiditis
• Granulomatous (subacute/ de Quervain) thyroiditis
• Reidel's thyroiditis

Etiology

Genetic factor/susceptibility: Autoimmune disease, such as Hashimoto and Graves disease are associated with polymorphisms in genes associated with immune regulation.

Pathogenesis

Hashimoto thyroiditis is **autoimmune disease** characterized by the presence of circulating **autoantibodies against thyroglobulin and thyroid peroxidase**.

Morphology

Gross

- **Diffuse and symmetric** enlargement of thyroid gland.
- Gland is **firm and nodular**.
- **Cut surface** is **pale, gray-tan** and shows **accentuation of normal lobulation**.

Microscopy (Fig. 24.1)

- **Inflammation:**
  - **Dense mononuclear inflammatory infiltrate** consisting of small lymphocytes and plasma cells in the thyroid parenchyma.
  - **Lymphoid follicles** with well-developed **germinal centers**.
- **Epithelial changes:**
  - **Atrophy of thyroid follicles:** They appear smaller than normal follicles.
  - **Hürthle cell metaplasia: It** is a **metaplastic response** of the follicular epithelium **to injury. Hürthle cells (Askanazy/oxyphil cells or oncocytes)** have abundant **eosinophilic, granular cytoplasm** and line some of the follicles.
- **Fibrosis:** The **interstitial connective tissue** is **increased (fibrosis)** and may cause atrophy of thyroid follicles. In contrast to Reidel thyroiditis, the **fibrosis does not extend beyond the capsule** of the gland.

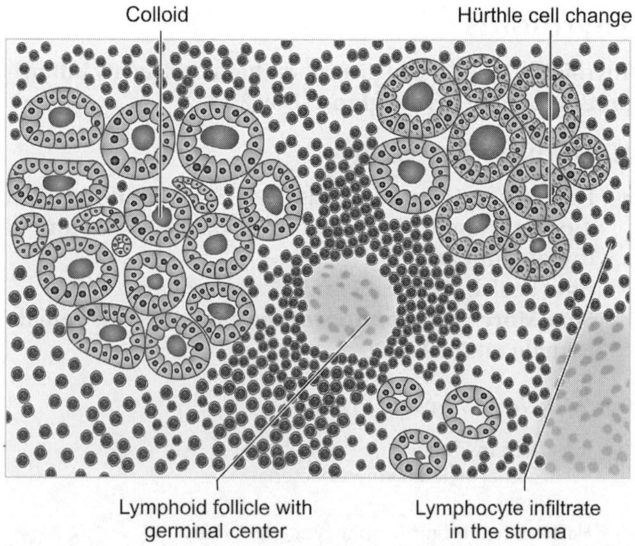

Fig. 24.1: Diagrammatic. Microscopy of Hashimoto thyroiditis shows parenchyma densely infiltrated by lymphocytes with germinal centers. Some of the thyroid follicles lined by deeply eosinophilic Hürthle cells

Fine-needle aspiration cytology (FNAC): It is shows Hürthle cells with a heterogeneous population of lymphocytes.

Clinical course

- **Painless enlargement of the thyroid** in middle-aged woman.
- **Hypothyroidism** gradually develops.
- Early stages may produce transient thyrotoxicosis due to destruction of thyroid follicles, with secondary release of thyroid hormones (Hashitoxicosis).

Subacute (Granulomatous) Thyroiditis

- Subacute (de Quervain) thyroiditis is **less common** than Hashimoto disease.
- **Age:** Common between **40 and 50 years** of age.
- **Sex: Affects women** more often than men (4:1).

Etiology and pathogenesis

Subacute thyroiditis is thought to be **initiated by a viral infection**.

- Pathogenesis is not known.

Morphology

Gross

- **Unilateral or bilateral enlargement** of the thyroid gland.
- **Cut section:** The involved regions are **firm and yellow-white**.

Microscopy

1. **Damaged thyroid follicles** with escape of colloid.
2. **Inflammation:** Consists of aggregates of **lymphocytes, activated macrophages, and plasma cells.**
3. **Granulomatous reaction**.
4. **Fibrosis:** It develops at late stages.

Clinical course

- **Painful** enlargement of the thyroid.
- **Early phase: Hyperthyroidism** with high serum T_4 and T_3 levels and low serum TSH levels.
- **Recovery within 6–8 weeks** and thyroid function returns to normal.

Riedel Thyroiditis

- Less common form of thyroiditis.
- **Etiology:** It is **unknown**, but the presence of circulating antithyroid antibodies in most patients **suggests** an **autoimmune** etiology.

Gross: Thyroid is stony hard and fixed which **clinically simulates a thyroid carcinoma.**

Microscopy: Shows **extensive fibrosis** involving the **thyroid and contiguous neck structures.**

Thyrotoxicosis

Definition: Thyrotoxicosis is a **systemic syndrome** (with hypermetabolic state) caused by exposure to **excessive levels of thyroid hormone** (free T_3 and T_4).

Causes of Thyrotoxicosis (Box 24.2)

Clinical Manifestations of Hyperthyroidism

- Clinical manifestations are due to the **hypermetabolic state** produced because of excess of thyroid hormone and to **overactivity of the sympathetic nervous system** (i.e. an increase in the β-adrenergic "tone"). Excessive thyroid hormone results in an **increase in the basal metabolic rate.**
- **Skin: Soft, warm and moist. Heat intolerance** and **sweating.**
- **Cardiac manifestations: Increased cardiac output, tachycardia, palpitations, arrhythmias** and **cardiomegaly.**
- **Neuromuscular system: Fine tremor, hyperactivity, nervousness, anxiety, emotional liability,** inability to concentrate, and insomnia.
- **Ocular changes: Lid retraction** causes a staring appearance. However, **Graves' disease is associated with proptosis** that comprises Graves' ophthalmopathy.

Box 24.2: Causes of thyrotoxicosis

Associated with Hyperthyroidism
Primary hyperthyroidism • Graves' disease (diffuse toxic hyperplasia) • Toxic multinodular goiter • Toxic adenoma
Secondary hyperthyroidism • TSH-secreting pituitary adenoma (rare)
Not Associated with Hyperthyroidism
• Granulomatous (de Quervain) thyroiditis • Struma ovarii (ovarian teratoma with ectopic thyroid)

- **Gastrointestinal system: Increased stool frequency,** often with diarrhea.
- **Skeletal system: Osteopenia** and a small increase in fracture rate.
- **Thyroid storm:** It is the **sudden onset of severe hyperthyroidism.** It occurs **most commonly in Graves' disease** and **probably due to sudden elevation in catecholamine levels.**

Diagnosis of Hyperthyroidism

- **Clinical findings.**
- **Laboratory** findings:
  - **Serum TSH concentration:** It is the **most useful single screening test** for hyperthyroidism, because it is **decreased even at subclinical stage.**
  - **Free T_4:** It is **increased.**
  - Measurement of **radioactive iodine uptake** by the thyroid gland to determine the cause.

Graves' Disease

Graves' disease (also known as Basedow disease) is the **most common cause of hyperthyroidism.**

Triad of Clinical Findings

1. **Hyperthyroidism:** It is due to diffuse hyperplasia of the thyroid.
2. **Infiltrative ophthalmopathy** → results in exophthalmos.
3. Localized, infiltrative **dermopathy** (pretibial myxedema) in few patients.

Age: Peak between **20 and 40 years** of age.

Sex: Females are affected 10 times **more frequently** than males.

Etiology

Graves' disease (hyperthyroidism) **and Hashimoto thyroiditis** (hypothyroidism) are considered as **two extremes of autoimmune thyroid disorders.**

- Graves' disease has a **strong genetic component.**

Pathogenesis

Graves' disease is an **autoimmune disease** characterized by the **presence of multiple autoantibodies most importantly against** the **TSH receptor.**

Autoantibodies in Graves' disease

1. **Thyroid-stimulating immunoglobulin:** It is an immunoglobulin (Ig) G antibody, which binds to the TSH receptor on the plasma membrane of thyrocytes.

2. **Thyroid growth-stimulating immunoglobulin:** It is also directed **against the TSH receptor.**
   - **Action:** Causes **proliferation of thyroid follicular epithelium and diffuse hyperplasia** of the thyroid gland.
3. **TSH-binding inhibitor immunoglobulin (anti-TSH receptor antibody):** It **prevents normal binding of TSH to its receptor** on thyroid epithelial cells.

Infiltrative ophthalmopathy

Autoimmunity is responsible for infiltrative ophthalmopathy.

Morphology

Gross

- Thyroid gland is **symmetrically enlarged** due to **diffuse hypertrophy and hyperplasia** of thyroid follicular epithelial cells.
- **Cut section:** The parenchyma appears **soft and meaty resembling normal muscle**.

Microscopy (Fig. 24.2)

- Thyroid follicles:
  - **Crowding of epithelial cells:** Epithelial cells lining the thyroid follicles are **tall and more crowded** than normal gland.
  - **Small papillae without fibrovascular cores**
- **Colloid:** It is **pale with scalloped margins.**
- **Lymphocyte infiltration in the interstitium:** Along **with mature plasma cells.** These lymphoid aggregates commonly show **germinal centers**.

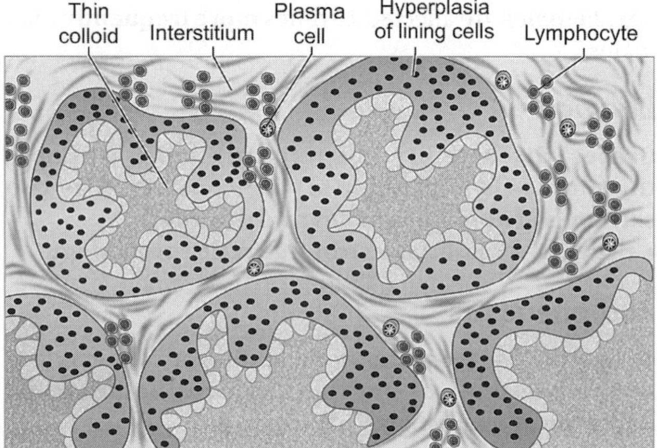

Fig. 24.2: Graves' disease. Microscopic view (diagrammatic) showing follicles lined by tall, columnar epithelium that are crowded and project into the lumens of the follicles. The follicle contains pale colloid with scalloped appearance of the edges. Stroma shows lymphocytes and plasma cells

Clinical Features

- **Thyrotoxicosis:** Its degree varies.
- **Unique features:**
  - **Diffuse hyperplasia of the thyroid:** It is seen in all cases and causes enlargement of thyroid.
  - **Ophthalmopathy.**
  - **Infiltrative dermopathy** or **pretibial myxedema**.

Laboratory Findings in Graves' Disease

- **Elevated free T_4 and T_3 levels.**
- **Decreased TSH levels.**
- **Radioactive iodine uptake is increased**, and **radioiodine scans show a diffuse uptake of iodine**.

Myxedema

Definition: Myxedema is the term applied to hypothyroidism developing in the older child or adult.

Clinical manifestations: Vary with the age of onset of the deficiency.

- Slowing of physical and mental activity.
- Generalized fatigue, apathy and mental sluggishness.
- Slowing of speech and intellectual functions.
- Cold intolerant and usually overweight.
- Constipation and decreased sweating.
- Skin is cool and pale because of decreased blood flow.
- Shortness of breath and decreased exercise capacity probably due to reduced cardiac output.

Laboratory Finding

- **Most sensitive screening test is measurement of the serum TSH level.** The TSH level is increased in primary hypothyroidism and it is not increased in persons with hypothyroidism due to primary hypothalamic or pituitary disease.
- T4 levels are decreased in hypothyroidism due to any cause.

Diffuse and Multinodular Goiters

Definition: Goiter is defined as **enlargement of thyroid without hyperthyroidism.**

- It is the **most common manifestation of thyroid disease.**
- Two morphological forms of goiter are: (1) diffuse nontoxic goiter and (2) multinodular goiter.

Diffuse Nontoxic (Simple) Goiter

- Diffuse nontoxic (simple) goiter is characterized by the **diffuse enlargement of the thyroid gland without any nodularity.**

- Microscopically, it consists of large thyroid follicles distended with colloid and is also known as **colloid goiter**.

Etiology

Types: (1) endemic and (2) sporadic.

Endemic goiter: This term is used **when goiters are present** in **more than 10% of the population in a given region.** The causes are:

- **Deficiency of iodine:** This may be due to **low iodine** in the soil, water, and food.
- **Goitrogens:** These are **substances ingestion of which interferes with thyroid hormone synthesis**. Goitrogenic substances include vegetables which belong to:
  - **Brassicaceae (Cruciferae) family:** For example, cabbage, cauliflower, Brussels sprouts, and turnips.
  - **Cassava root:** It contains a thiocyanate that inhibits iodide transport within the thyroid. Consumption of this may worsen the concurrent iodine deficiency.

Sporadic goiter

- **Less frequent** than endemic goiter.
- **Age:** Puberty or in young adult life.
- **Sex: Female preponderance.**
- **Causes:** In most cases of sporadic goiter, the cause is not known.

Morphology

Diffuse nontoxic goiter has **two phases:**

- **Hyperplastic phase:**
  - **Gross:** Thyroid is **moderately, diffusely, and symmetrically enlarged**. The gland rarely exceeds 100 to 150 grams.
  - **Microscopy: Hyperplasia of lining epithelium** of thyroid follicles. Which may pile up to form **pseudopapillae** (Sanderson's Polster) and project into the follicular lumen.
- **Phase of colloid involution:**
  - Subsequently, if the dietary content of iodine increases or if the demand for thyroid hormone decreases, the stimulated hyperplastic phase goes into phase of colloid involution.
  - **Gross:** Thyroid is **enlarged** and the **cut surface** is usually **brown, glassy, and translucent.**
  - **Microscopy:**
    - **Flattened follicular epithelial lining**.
    - **Abundant colloid** causes enlargement of follicle **(colloid goiter)**.

Clinical course

- **Majority** with simple goiters are **clinically euthyroid**.
- **Mass effects** from the enlarged thyroid gland.
- In children, dyshormonogenetic goiter due to congenital biosynthetic defect may produce cretinism.

Laboratory findings

- Serum T_3 and T_4 levels are normal.
- **Serum TSH is usually elevated** or at the upper range of normal.

Multinodular Goiter

- In long-standing simple goiters (diffuse and symmetric enlargement), **recurrent episodes of hyperplasia and involution** combine to produce a more **irregular enlargement of the thyroid** known as multinodular goiters.
- Since, multinodular goiters are derived from simple goiter, they occur in both **sporadic and endemic** forms.

Morphology

Gross

- **Multiple nodules:** Thyroid is **asymmetrically enlarged**, and **nodular** due to **multiple nodules of varying sizes**.
- **Cut section:**
  - Shows **numerous irregular nodules containing variable amounts of colloid**.
  - **Older lesions** may show areas of **hemorrhage, fibrosis, calcification**, and **cystic change**.

Microscopy (Fig. 24.3)

- Multiple **nodules of varying size and shape**.
  - **Colloid cysts:** They may be formed **fusion (or rupture)** of large **colloid-containing follicles**.
- **Stroma**
  - **Fibrosis and dystrophic calcification are common**.
  - **Areas of hemorrhage** and **chronic inflammation** are common.

Clinical course

- **Usually asymptomatic** and present as a **mass in the neck**.
- **Large** multinodular goiter may cause **compression of surrounding structures** and may cause:
  - **Airway obstruction** due to compression of trachea.
  - **Dysphagia** by compressing the esophagus.
- **Functional status: Most patients are euthyroid** and T_4, T_3, and TSH are normal.
- Fine-needle aspiration biopsy is helpful for diagnosis.

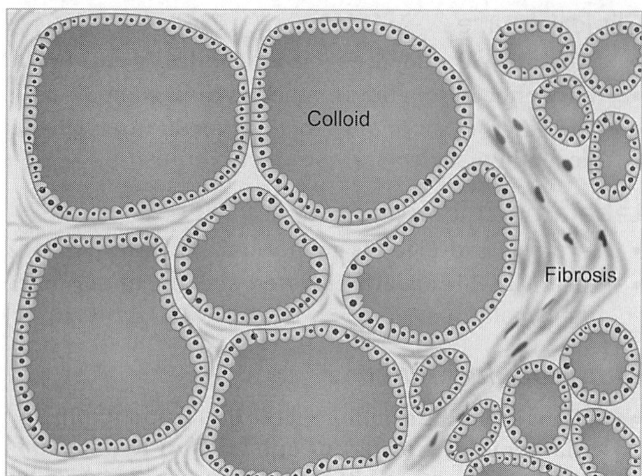

Fig. 24.3: Photomicrograph and diagrammatic. Microscopy of a multinodular goiter composed of thyroid follicles of varying sizes distended with variable amount of colloid

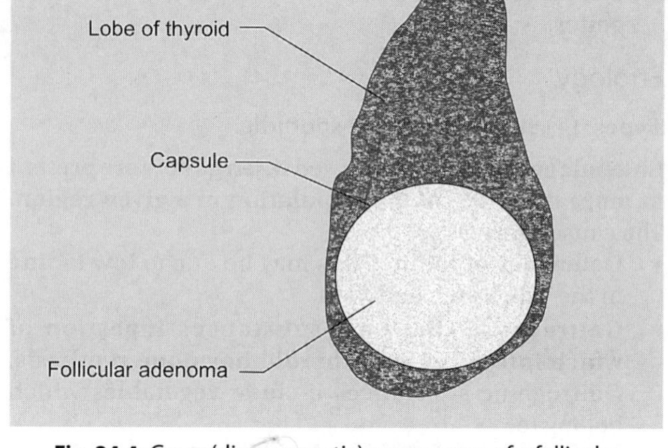

Fig. 24.4: Gross (diagrammatic) appearance of a follicular adenoma

Neoplasms of the Thyroid

Tumors of the thyroid are usually benign.

Follicular Adenomas

Adenomas of the thyroid consist of follicular epithelium.

Morphology

Gross (Fig. 24.4)

- Follicular adenoma is a **solitary** (single)**, spherical, solid** and **encapsulated** tumor.
- **Size:** It ranges from **1 to 3 cm in diameter**.
- **Cut surface:**
  - Tumor is **soft and paler** than the surrounding gland.
  - **Well-demarcated** and surrounded by a **thin intact,** well-formed **fibrous capsule.**
  - **Color** may range from **gray-white to red-brown.**
- **Secondary changes:** They are common and include **hemorrhage, fibrosis, calcification,** and **cystic change.**

Microscopy (Fig. 24.5)

Patterns: Follicular adenomas may show **many histologic patterns,** which **do not have of any significance.** The tumor cells are arranged in follicles, which may **resemble normal thyroid tissue or mimic different stages in the embryonic development of the gland.**

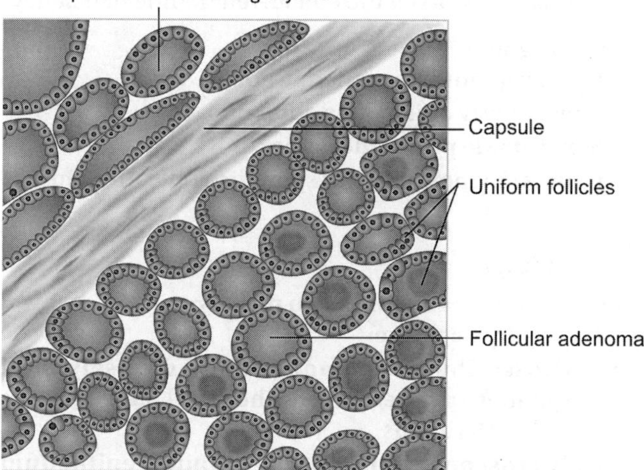

Fig. 24.5: Diagrammatic: Microscopic appearance of part of follicular adenoma of the thyroid showing well-differentiated, uniform thyroid follicles, well-formed capsule and compressed adjacent thyroid follicles

Clinical features

- Mostly present as a **unilateral painless mass.**
- Larger tumors may produce local symptoms.

Investigations

- **Radionuclide scanning:**
  - **Nonfunctioning adenomas:** They **take up less radioactive iodine** than does normal thyroid parenchyma. The nonfunctioning adenomas usually **appear as cold nodules.**
  - **Functioning follicular adenoma** (toxic adenomas): They appear as **hot nodules. Malignancy is rare** in hot nodules.
- **Ultrasonography.**
- **Fine-needle aspiration biopsy.**
- **Histological examination** of surgically resected specimen should be evaluated for capsular integrity, and definitive diagnosis of adenomas.

Prognosis: Excellent and adenomas do not recur or metastasize.

Carcinomas

- Carcinomas of the thyroid are **relatively uncommon**.
- **Sex:**
  - **Early and middle adult** years: **Female** predominance.
  - **Childhood and late adult life:** Males and females **equally** affected.
- **Nature: Majority** of thyroid carcinomas are **well-differentiated**.

Major Subtypes

- Papillary carcinoma (more than 85%).
- Follicular carcinoma (5–15%).
- Anaplastic (undifferentiated) carcinoma (less than 5%).
- Medullary carcinoma (5%).

Pathogenesis of Thyroid Carcinomas

Origin

- **Follicular cell-derived malignancies:** These include three major types of thyroid cancers namely (1) **follicular**, (2) **papillary** and (3) **anaplastic carcinoma**.
- **Non-follicular cancer:** One type namely **medullary carcinomas** do not arise from the follicular epithelium.

Two factors play major role in thyroid carcinoma: (A) genetic factors and (B) environmental factors.

A. Genetic factors: Different genetic changes are involved in the pathogenesis of the four major histologic variants of thyroid cancer.

B. Environmental factors:

1. **Ionizing radiation:** It is the major risk factor mainly during the first 2 decades of life.
2. **Deficiency of dietary iodine** and associate goiter may be associated with a higher frequency of follicular carcinomas.

Papillary Carcinoma

- The **most common** and constitutes ~ 85% of primary **thyroid cancer**.
- **Age:** It **can occur at any age**, but **mostly** found between the ages of **25 and 50**.
- Associated with **previous exposure** to **ionizing radiation**.
- Genetic factors play a role.

Morphology

Gross

- Papillary carcinomas may be **solitary or multifocal** lesions.

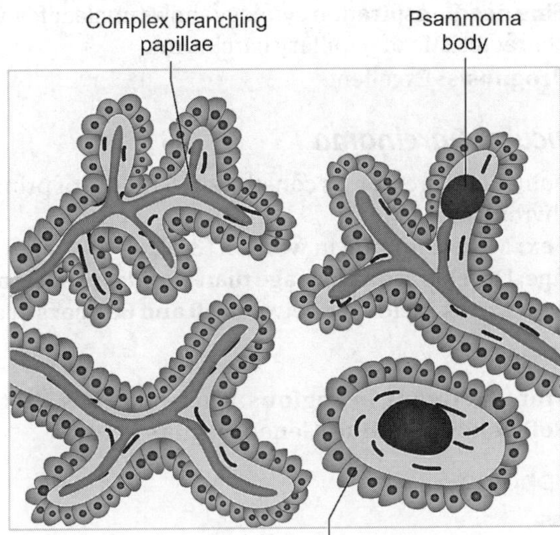

Fig. 24.6: Diagrammatic; Papillary carcinoma of the thyroid shows well-formed, branching papillae lined by cells with characteristic empty-appearing ("Orphan Annie eye") nuclei. Inset in A: upper right shows Orphan Annie eye nuclei and nuclear groove and right lower shows psammoma body

- **Gray white, firm to hard tumor**, which may show areas of fibrosis and calcification.
- **Cut surface** may show **papillary foci**.

Microscopy (Fig. 24.6)

- **Complex branching papillae:** They have a dense central fibrovascular stalk/core. Papillae are covered by **uniform cuboidal to columnar** epithelial **cells**.
- **Nuclear features:** These are **important for diagnosis** of papillary carcinoma, **even in the absence of papillary architecture**.
  - **Ground glass** or **Orphan Annie eye nuclei:** They contain **finely dispersed chromatin**, which gives an **optically clear** or **empty** appearance.
  - **Intranuclear inclusions and intranuclear grooves**.
- **Psammoma bodies** (calcospherites): These are **concentrically calcified structures usually** present **within the papillary core**. They are virtually **diagnostic** of papillary carcinoma, and almost **never found in follicular and medullary carcinomas.**
- **Lymphatic spread: Lymphatic invasion** and **spread** to regional cervical lymph nodes are **common**, but **vascular invasion and blood spread are uncommon**.

Clinical course

Most papillary carcinomas present as **asymptomatic thyroid nodules**, sometimes the presenting symptom may be a mass in a cervical lymph node (due to metastasis).

- **Fine needle aspiration** cytology shows nuclear features characteristic of papillary carcinoma.
- **Prognosis:** Excellent.

Follicular Carcinoma

- Follicular carcinomas constitute ~ 5 to 15% of primary thyroid cancers.
- **Sex:** More common in **women** (3:1).
- **Age:** Develop at **an older age than papillary carcinoma** with a peak incidence between **40 and 60 years** of age.

Etiology

- More **frequent in regions** where there is **dietary deficiency of iodine**. Genetic factors.

Morphology

Gross

- Follicular carcinomas are **single nodules** which may be **either well-circumscribed or infiltrate** into the surrounding thyroid parenchyma.
- Cut section of tumor appears **gray to pink** in color.

Microscopy

- **Follicular pattern of tumor cells:**
  - Tumor consists of **uniform cuboidal to columnar** follicular epithelial **cells.**
  - Tumor cells may form **small follicles containing colloid or** may be arranged in **nests or sheets** without forming follicles.
- **Increased mitotic activity**.
- **Invasion: Depending on the pattern of invasion,** follicular carcinoma can be **subdivided into two** variants.
  - **Minimally invasive follicular carcinomas.**
  - **Widely invasive follicular carcinomas.**
- **Metastasis:**
  - **Lymphatic spread** is **uncommon.**
  - **Hematogenous spread is common to bone, lungs and liver.**

Clinical course: Follicular carcinomas present as **slowly enlarging painless nodules.**

Anaplastic (Undifferentiated) Carcinoma

- Anaplastic carcinomas are **undifferentiated tumors** of follicular epithelium.
- Constitute less than 5% of thyroid tumors.
- **Age: Elderly** with a mean age of 65 years.
- Genetic factors play a role.

Morphology

Gross: Diffusely infiltrative tumor.

Microscopy: Composed of highly anaplastic cells, which includes:

- **Spindle** cells with a sarcomatous appearance.
- Large, pleomorphic **giant** cells.
- **Mixed** spindle and giant cells.

Spread

- **Local spread** Into thyroid capsule and adjacent neck structures.
- **Hematogenous spread** to lungs.

Clinical course

- Usually present as a **rapidly growing bulky neck mass.**
- Symptoms due to **compression and invasion of the neck structures** may cause dyspnea, dysphagia, hoarseness, and cough.

Prognosis: Aggressive tumor with poor prognosis.

Medullary Carcinoma

- Medullary carcinomas of the thyroid are **neuroendocrine tumors derived from** the **parafollicular cells** or **C cells** of the thyroid.
- Similar to normal C cells, they **secrete calcitonin,** measurement of which is **useful in the diagnosis and postoperative follow-up.**
- It constitutes ~ 5% of thyroid neoplasms.
- Genetic factors play a role.

Types

- **Sporadic:** Constitutes about 70% of tumor with a peak incidence in the **40s and 50s**.
- **Familial.**

Morphology

Gross

- **Number of tumor nodules.**
  - **Solitary nodule** in **sporadic** medullary thyroid carcinomas.
  - **Multicentric and bilateral common in familial cases.**
- Tumor is **firm, pale gray, and infiltrative**.
- **Larger lesions** may show areas of **necrosis and hemorrhage**.

Microscopy (Fig. 24.7)

- Tumor cells:
  - **Polygonal to spindle-shaped** cells. **Small, more anaplastic cells** may be found **in some** tumors.
  - Cells are arranged as **nests, trabeculae** and even form follicles.

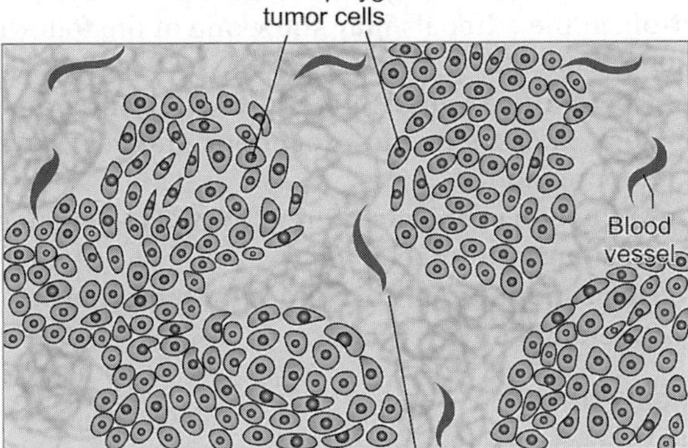

Fig. 24.7: Diagrammatic; Medullary carcinoma of thyroid shows nests and trabeculae of round, spindle to polygonal cells separated by abundant homogeneous, extracellular, pink deposits of amyloid

- Acellular **amyloid** deposits **in the stroma**: It is found in most of the cases. These are **derived from altered calcitonin polypeptides**.

Immunohistochemistry: Calcitonin can be demonstrated within the cytoplasm of the tumor cells and in the stromal amyloid by immunohistochemical methods.

Clinical course

- **Sporadic cases:**
  - Present as a **mass in the neck**.
  - **Tumor markers:** They are useful, mainly for presurgical assessment of tumor load and in calcitonin-negative tumors. These include:
    - Calcitonin.
    - Carcinoembryonic antigen (CEA).
- **Familial cases:** Present with **symptoms localized to the thyroid** or as a component of familial syndromes along with neoplasms in other organs (e.g. adrenal or parathyroid glands).

PARATHYROID GLANDS

There are four parathyroid glands situated on the posterior part of thyroid. They consists of two cell types: Chief cells and oxyphil cells. They secrete *parathyroid hormone (PTH)*. **The function of the parathyroid glands is to regulate calcium homeostasis.**

Hyperparathyroidism

Hyperparathyroidism is caused by raised levels of parathyroid hormone and is classified into primary, secondary, and least commonly, tertiary types.

- **Primary hyperparathyroidism:** Is due to an autonomous overproduction of parathyroid hormone (PTH). It is usually result from an adenoma or hyperplasia of parathyroid tissue.
- **Secondary hyperparathyroidism:** Is characterized by compensatory hypersecretion of PTH in response to prolonged hypocalcemia, most commonly from chronic renal failure.
- **Tertiary hyperparathyroidism:** Is due to persistent hypersecretion of PTH even after the cause of prolonged hypocalcemia is corrected (e.g. after renal transplant).

Symptoms of Hyperparathyroidism

It is due to combined effects of increased PTH secretion and hypercalcemia.

- *Bone disease* and bone pain secondary to fractures of bones weakened by osteoporosis.
- *Nephrolithiasis* (renal stones).
- Gastrointestinal disturbances: For example, constipation, nausea, peptic ulcers, pancreatitis, and gallstones.
- Central nervous system: Depression, lethargy, and eventually seizures.
- Neuromuscular abnormalities: Weakness and fatigue.
- Cardiac manifestations: Aortic or mitral valve calcifications (or both).

Hypoparathyroidism

Hypoparathyroidism is less common than hyperparathyroidism. Acquired hypoparathyroidism is always due to an unknowingly removal of parathyroid during thyroid surgery.

Clinical Features

- The major clinical manifestations are due to hypocalcemia.
- **Tetany:** It is the hallmark of hypocalcemia and is characterized by *neuromuscular irritability*, resulting from decreased serum calcium levels. The symptoms range from circumoral numbness or paresthesias (tingling) of the distal extremities and carpopedal spasm, to life-threatening laryngospasm and generalized seizures.

ADRENAL GLANDS

Introduction

- The adrenal glands are paired endocrine organs.
- They consist of outer cortex and inner medulla. They differ in structure and function.

- **Adrenal cortex synthesizes three different types of steroids.**
  - Glucocorticoids (principally cortisol).
  - Mineralocorticoids: Most important is aldosterone.
  - Sex steroids (estrogens and androgens).
- **Adrenal medulla** secretes **catecholamines,** mainly epinephrine.
- **Diseases of the adrenal cortex:** They can be divided into.
  - Those associated with **hyperfunction**.
  - Those associated with **hypofunction**.

Adrenocortical Hyperfunction (Hyperadrenalism)

Syndromes of adrenal hyperfunction are caused by overproduction of the three major hormones of the adrenal cortex.

- **Cushing syndrome:** Due to an excess of cortisol.
- **Hyperaldosteronism:** Due to excessive aldosterone.
- **Adrenogenital or virilizing syndromes:** Due to an excess of androgens.

Hypercortisolism (Cushing Syndrome)

Pathogenesis

Cushing syndrome is produced by conditions that produce raised glucocorticoid levels.

Causes:

- **Exogenous causes:** Majority of cases are the result of the administration of exogenous glucocorticoids ("iatrogenic" Cushing syndrome).
- **Endogenous causes:**
  - ACTH dependent: ACTH-secreting pituitary adenomas is responsible for about 70% of cases of endogenous hypercortisolism. Other cause is small-cell carcinoma of the lung which may secrete ectopic ACTH.
  - ACTH independent: Primary adrenal neoplasms (e.g. adrenal adenoma and carcinoma) are the most common causes. Other cause is cortical hyperplasia.

Morphology

- Main lesions of Cushing syndrome are observed in the pituitary and adrenal glands.
- **Pituitary:** Most common changes are due to high levels of endogenous or exogenous glucocorticoids and are called as **Crooke hyaline change.** This is characterized homogeneous and pale appearance of the cytoplasm of ACTH-producing cells in the anterior pituitary.
- **Adrenals:** Depending on the cause of the hypercortisolism the adrenals may show one of the following abnormalities.
  - **Cortical atrophy:** Bilateral **cortical atrophy** is seen in cases due to exogenous glucocorticoids, suppression.
  - **Diffuse hyperplasia:** Found in ACTH-dependent Cushing syndrome.
  - **Macronodular or micronodular hyperplasia.**
  - **Adenoma or carcinoma.**

Clinical course

Cushing syndrome develops slowly.

Early stage: May present with **hypertension and weight gain**.

Later:

- More characteristic features characterized by **truncal obesity, moon facies**, and accumulation of fat in the posterior neck and back (**buffalo hump**).
- **Decreased muscle mass and proximal limb weakness**.
- **Hyperglycemia, glucosuria and polydipsia** (secondary diabetes).
- **Skin is thin, fragile, and easily bruised**; and cutaneous striae are particularly common in the abdominal area.
- Bone resorption results in **osteoporosis** and associated with increased susceptibility to fractures.
- Increased risk for a variety of infections.
- Others include several mental disturbances, hirsutism and menstrual abnormalities.

Primary Hyperaldosteronism

Hyperaldosteronism is the generic term for a group of closely related conditions characterized by chronic excess aldosterone secretion.

Causes:

- **Primary hyperaldosteronism:** Due to autonomous overproduction of aldosterone. **Raised blood pressure is the most common manifestation of primary hyperaldosteronism.**
- **Secondary hyperaldosteronism:** It is characterized by increased levels of plasma rennin and is due to an extra-adrenal cause (e.g. renal artery stenosis congestive heart failure, cirrhosis, nephrotic syndrome).

Adrenogenital Syndromes

Adrenal cortex can secrete excess androgens due to either of the following:

- Adrenocortical neoplasms (usually *virilizing* carcinomas).

- Congenital adrenal hyperplasia (CAH): It consists of a group of autosomal recessive disorders characterized by defects in steroid biosynthesis, usually cortisol. Reduced secretion of cortisol causes a compensatory increase in ACTH secretion, which in turn stimulates androgen production.
- Androgens have virilizing effects. These effects include masculinization in females (ambiguous genitalia, oligomenorrhea, hirsutism), precocious puberty in males.

Adrenocortical Insufficiency (Hypoadrenalism)

Causes: Adrenocortical insufficiency, or hypofunction may be caused due to:

- **Primary adrenocortical insufficiency:** Due to primary adrenal disease (primary hypoadrenalism). It can be:
  - Primary *acute* adrenocortical insufficiency (acute adrenal crisis): Waterhouse-Friderichsen syndrome or,
  - Primary *chronic* adrenocortical insufficiency: Addison disease.
- **Secondary adrenocortical insufficiency:** Decreased stimulation of the adrenals due to a deficiency of ACTH (secondary hypoadrenalism).
  - Chronic adrenal insufficiency may be secondary to autoimmune adrenalitis.
  - Other causes: (1) tuberculosis and infections due to opportunistic pathogens associated with the human immunodeficiency virus and (2) tumors metastatic to the adrenals.

Clinical feature: These include: fatigue, weakness, and gastrointestinal disturbances.

Adrenocortical Neoplasms

- These include: adenomas and carcinomas.
- Most cortical neoplasms are sporadic.
- They may be functional (producing steroid hormones) or non-functional. Functional adenomas commonly associated with hyperaldosteronism and Cushing syndrome, whereas a carcinoma is associated with virilization.

Adrenocortical Adenomas

Majority are clinically silent.

Gross: Well-circumscribed, nodule up to 2.5 cm in diameter that expands the adrenal gland. Cut surface usually yellow to yellow brown due to lipid content.

Microscopy: Cells appear similar to those of the normal adrenal cortex.

Adrenocortical Carcinomas

Rare neoplasms and can occur at any age.

More likely to be functional than adenomas and are often produce virilism or features of hyperadrenalism.

Gross: Large, invasive and may be more than 20 cm in diameter. On cut surface, they appear variegated, poorly demarcated lesions with areas of necrosis, hemorrhage, and cystic change.

Microscopy: Composed of well-differentiated cells, resembling cortical adenomas, or bizarre, monstrous giant cells.

Neuroblastic Tumors

Neuroblastic tumors are group of tumors of the sympathetic ganglia and adrenal medulla that are derived from primordial neural crest cells.

Neuroblastoma

- Most **important neuroblastic tumor**.
- **Age: Most common extracranial childhood solid tumor**. It is the most frequently diagnosed during infancy.
- **Sporadic and familial types:** Mostly occur sporadically, but 1–2% is familial.

Morphology

Gross

- **Site:** About 40% of neuroblastomas occur in the **adrenal medulla**.
  - **Other sites:** It may develop along the sympathetic chain.
    - **Paravertebral region of the abdomen** (25%).
    - **Posterior mediastinum** (15%).
    - Pelvis, the neck, and brain (**cerebral neuroblastomas**).
- **Size: Vary** from minute nodules (as in situ lesions) to large tumors weighing 1 kg.
- **Nature: Majority** are **silent** and **regress spontaneously**.
- May be **sharply demarcated** by a fibrous pseudocapsule **or infiltrate** the surrounding structures (kidneys, renal vein, and vena cava, and aorta).
- **Cut section: Soft, and gray-tan. Large tumors** may show areas of **necrosis, cystic change** and **hemorrhage**.

Microscopy (Fig. 24.8)

- **Tumor cells:** They are arranged in solid sheets. The tumor cells appear as:

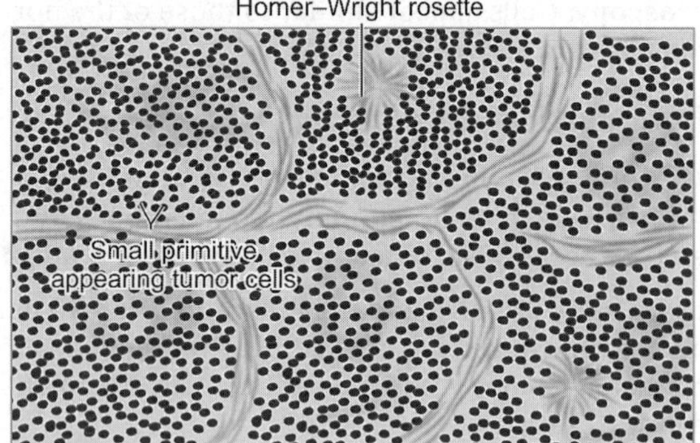

Fig. 24.8: Diagrammatic; Neuroblastoma consists of small primitive appearing cells with scant cytoplasm embedded in a finely fibrillar matrix.

- **Small, primitive cells containing dark nuclei.**
- **Scant cytoplasm with poorly-defined cell borders.**

- **Background:** Shows a faintly **eosinophilic fibrillary material** (**neuropil**), which represents the neuritic processes of the primitive neuroblasts.
- **Homer-Wright pseudorosettes:** It consist of tumor cells concentrically arranged about a central space filled with neuropil may be seen.

Spread of tumor

- Local infiltration.
- Lymph node spread.
- Bloodspread: Liver, lungs, bone marrow, and bones.

Clinical course

- **Children below 2 years of age:** Usually present as **large abdominal masses, fever, and weight loss**.
- **Older children:** Symptoms develop due to metastases such as bone pain, respiratory symptoms, or gastrointestinal complaints.

Laboratory finding

- **Majority** (~90%) of neuroblastomas, **secrete catecholamines** (similar to pheochromocytomas) producing raised blood levels of catecholamines (hypertension is less frequent).
- **Raised urine levels** of the **metabolites vanillylmandelic acid** (VMA) and **homovanillic acid** (HVA).

Course: It is extremely variable.

Pheochromocytoma

- Pheochromocytomas are **neoplasms composed of chromaffin cells.**
- The **tumor cells synthesize and release catecholamines** and some may produce peptide hormones.
- These tumors are the rare cause of surgically correctable **hypertension**.

Rule of 10s

- About 10% of pheochromocytomas are **extra-adrenal**.
  - They occur in organs of Zuckerkandl and the carotid body.
  - Extra-adrenal pheochromocytomas are called as **paragangliomas.**
- About 10% of sporadic adrenal pheochromocytomas are **bilateral**. In pheochromocytomas associated with familial syndromes up to 50% may be bilateral.
- 10% of adrenal pheochromocytomas **metastasize** and are **malignant**. Malignancy is more common in extra-adrenal paragangliomas and tumors developing due to germline mutations.
- 10% of adrenal pheochromocytomas are **not associated with hypertension**.

Morphology

Gross

- **Size: Varies** and may range from small, circumscribed lesions to large hemorrhagic masses.
- **Cut surface:**
  - Small have **yellow tan.**
  - Large show areas of **hemorrhage, necrosis, and cystic changes and typically efface the adrenal gland.**
- **Chromaffin reaction:** When the **fresh tumor tissue is incubated in potassium dichromate solution**; the **tumor turns dark brown in color** due to oxidation of stored catecholamines. This is termed positive **chromaffin reaction**.

Microscopy

- **Zellballen pattern:** Tumor consists of **polygonal to spindle-shaped chromaffin cells or chief cells**, clustered with the sustentacular cells **into small nests or alveoli (Zellballen)** separated by a **rich vascular network**.
- **Cytoplasm:** It has a **fine granular appearance due to** the presence of granules containing **catecholamines**. It is best **demonstrated with silver stains.**
- **Nuclei:** They are **round to oval**, with a stippled **"salt and pepper"** chromatin that is characteristic of neuroendocrine tumors.

Spread

- **Definitive diagnosis of malignancy in pheochromocytomas is made only when there they develop metastases.**

- The tumor may metastasize to regional lymph nodes as well as more distant sites, including liver, lung, and bone.

Clinical course

Hypertension in 90% of patients.

The elevations of blood pressure are induced by the sudden release of catecholamines. This may precipitate congestive heart failure, pulmonary edema, myocardial infarction, ventricular fibrillation, and cerebrovascular accidents.

Complications

Cardiac complications are called **catecholamine cardiomyopathy**, or catecholamine-induced myocardial instability and ventricular arrhythmias.

Laboratory diagnosis

Demonstration of **increased urinary excretion of free catecholamines and their metabolites**, such as vanillylmandelic acid and metanephrines.

SELF-ASSESSMENT EXERCISE

I. Short Notes

1. Hashimoto thyroiditis.
2. Multinodular goiter.
3. Thyrotoxicosis.
4. Myxedema.
5. Papillary carcinoma of thyroid.
6. Medullary carcinoma of thyroid.

CHAPTER 25

Diabetes Mellitus

CHAPTER OUTLINE

INTRODUCTION

Diabetes mellitus is a **group of metabolic disorders having features of hyperglycemia**.

The prevalence of diabetes is increasing sharply in the developing countries because of more sedentary lifestyles. India and China have the largest prevalence of diabetics.

Diagnosis (Table 25.1)

Normally, the **blood glucose levels** are maintained in a very narrow range of **70 to 120 mg/dL**.

- **Euglycemic:** Individuals are considered to be euglycemic, when.
  - **Fasting glucose** level is **less than 100 mg/dL**, or
  - Glucose level **less than 140 mg/dL** following an oral glucose tolerance test (OGTT).
- **Prediabetes:** It is defined as condition in which there is **impaired glucose tolerance**, but elevated **blood sugar does not reach the criterion accepted for an outright diagnosis of diabetes**. The criteria for diagnosis are:
  - **Fasting glucose** level is **greater than 100 mg/dL but less than 126 mg/dL**.
  - Glucose tolerance test (GTT) values **greater than 140 mg/dL but less than 200 mg/dL**.

  Risks in prediabetes: (1) **Progression to frank diabetes** over time and (2) **cardiovascular disease**.
- **Diabetes:** Any **one of three criteria** can be used for the **diagnosis of diabetes**:
  1. A **random glucose** level **greater than 200 mg/dL, with classical signs and symptoms**.

Table 25.1: Levels of blood glucose in normal, prediabetes and diabetes

	Euglycemic	Prediabetes	Diabetes
Fasting glucose level	Less than **100** mg/dL.	Greater than **100** mg/dL but less than **126** mg/dL	Greater than **126** mg/dL on more than one occasion
OGTT	Less than **140** mg/dL.	Greater than **140** mg/dL but less than **200** mg/dL	Greater than **200** mg/dL

Abbreviation: OGTT, oral glucose tolerance test.

  2. A **fasting** glucose level **greater than 126 mg/dL on more than one occasion.**
  3. **An abnormal oral glucose tolerance test** (OGTT), in which the **glucose level is greater than 200 mg/dL, 2 hours after a standard carbohydrate load.**

Classification

Diabetes is classified according to etiopathogenesis into different groups (Box 25.1) but **majority of cases fall into one of two** broad classes namely: **Type 1 and type 2.**

TYPE 1 DIABETES (T1D)

- Accounts for ~ **5–10%** of all cases.
- **Age:** Most common in **childhood** (**younger than 20 years** of age). Since, it can develop at any age, the term "juvenile diabetes" should be avoided.

Cause

- **Autoimmune disease** characterized by:
  - **Pancreatic β-cell destruction.**
  - **Absolute deficiency of insulin.**
- **Idiopathic:** It is a rare form in which there is no evidence for autoimmunity.

Box 25.1: Classification of diabetes mellitus

1. **Type 1 diabetes:** (1) Immune-mediated or (2) idiopathic
2. **Type 2 diabetes**
3. **Other specific types of diabetes** – **Genetic defects of β-cell function:** Maturity-onset diabetes of the young (MODY), neonatal diabetes – **Genetic defects in insulin action** – **Exocrine pancreatic defects:** Chronic pancreatitis, hemochromatosis – **Endocrinopathies:** Acromegaly, Cushing syndrome, hyperthyroidism, pheochromocytoma – **Infections:** Cytomegalovirus, coxsackie B virus – **Drugs:** Glucocorticoids, thyroid hormone – **Genetic syndromes associated with diabetes:** Down syndrome, Klinefelter syndrome, Turner syndrome
4. **Gestational diabetes mellitus**

Pathogenesis of Type 1 Diabetes Mellitus

Involves interplay of both genetic susceptibility and environmental factors.

- **Genetic susceptibility:** Incidence of type 1 diabetes is greater in twins of affected individuals than in the general population, and greater in monozygotic than in dizygotic twins.
- **Environmental factors: Viral infections:** They **may trigger islet cell destruction** and associations have been found between type 1 diabetes and infection with ***mumps, rubella, coxsackie B, or cytomegalovirus***. Viral infection induces autoimmunity.

Mechanisms of β-Cell Destruction

The autoimmune damage starts many years before the disease becomes clinically evident. **Hyperglycemia and ketosis occur after more than 90% of the β cells have been destroyed**.

TYPE 2 DIABETES (T2D)

- Accounts for ~ **90–95% of diabetic patients**.
- **Majority** of patients are **overweight**.
- Though known as "adult-onset," it is now found in children and adolescents also.

Pathogenesis of Type 2 Diabetes Mellitus (Fig. 25.1)

Type 2 diabetes is a **multifactorial disease**.

- **Environmental factors** play a role and includes:
  - **Sedentary lifestyle**.
  - **Dietary habits and associated obesity**.
- **Genetic factors:**
  - Type 2 diabetes has a **concordance rate of 35–60% in monozygotic twins compared with 17–30% in dizygotic twins.**
  - **Lifetime risk** for type 2 diabetes in an offspring is more than double **if both parents** are **affected**.
  - **Diabetogenic genes** have been found.
  - There is **no evidence of an autoimmune basis**.

Metabolic Defects in Type 2 Diabetes

Two important metabolic defects are:

Insulin resistance

Definition: Insulin resistance is **the decrease/failure of target (peripheral) tissues to insulin action. Main factors** in the development of insulin resistance is **obesity**.

- **Consequences of insulin resistance:**
  - **Decreased uptake of glucose in muscle**.
  - **Reduced glycolysis** and **fatty acid oxidation** in the liver.
  - **Inability to suppress hepatic gluconeogenesis**.

β-cell dysfunction

In type 2 diabetes, β-cell dysfunction manifests as **inadequate insulin secretion by the pancreatic β-cells (relative insulin deficiency)** in association with insulin resistance and hyperglycemia. β-cell dysfunction is multifactorial in origin.

PATHOGENESIS OF THE COMPLICATIONS OF DIABETES

Pathogenesis is multifactorial and includes:

- Hyperglycemia (glucotoxicity) is the main mediator.
- Insulin resistance (described already).
- Obesity.

Hyperglycemia

- **Control of blood sugar level** (glycemic control) **can reduce the long-term complications** of diabetes.
- **Glycemic control is assessed by** estimation of **glycosylated hemoglobins (HbA_{1C})**. HbA_{1C} is formed by addition of glucose to hemoglobin in red cells. HbA_{1C} should be maintained below 7% in diabetic patients and its **measurement is helpful in knowing the glycemic control over the lifespan of a red cell** (120 days).

Organ Damage by Hyperglycemia

- The chronic hyperglycemia and the metabolic disorders cause secondary **damage in multiple organ** systems.

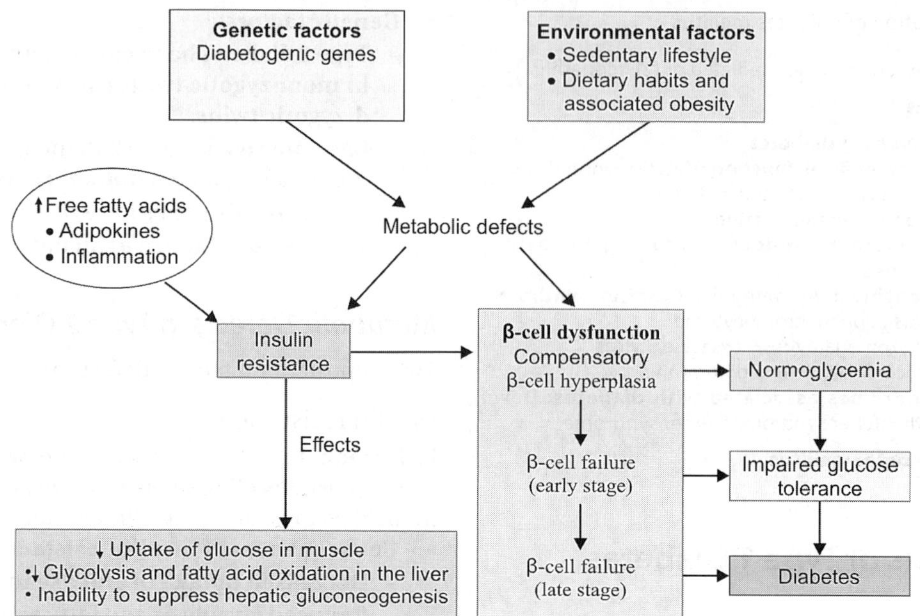

Fig. 25.1: Pathogenesis of type 2 diabetes. Insulin resistance associated with obesity is induced by free fatty acids, adipokines, and chronic inflammation in adipose tissue. Insulin resistance causes β cells of pancreas to undergo compensatory hyperplasia and the resulting hypersecretion of insulin maintains normoglycemia. However, at some point, β-cell compensation is followed by β-cell failure, and diabetes develops

- Common organs damaged are **kidneys** (end-stage renal disease), **eyes** (adult-onset blindness), **nerves,** and **blood vessels** (gangrene of lower extremity).

Effects Hyperglycemia

Harmful effects of persistent hyperglycemia on peripheral tissues can be brought out by **three distinct metabolic pathways.**

Formation of advanced glycation end products (AGEs)

In diabetics, glucose binds to proteins nonenzymatically and **is termed nonenzymatic glycosylation**.

Activation of protein kinase C (PKC)

In patients with hyperglycemia, **intracellular hyperglycemia stimulates synthesis of diacyl glycerol (DAG) from glycolytic intermediates**. DAG **activates intracellular protein kinase C**.

Disturbances in polyol pathways

- **Some tissues** (e.g. nerves, lenses, kidneys, blood vessels) **do not require insulin for glucose transport**.
- **Persistent hyperglycemia increases** the **intracellular glucose in these tissues. The excess intracellular glucose is metabolized by the enzyme aldose reductase to sorbitol (polyol)** and finally to fructose.
- This **reaction uses NADPH** (the reduced form of nicotinamide dinucleotide phosphate) as a cofactor. Reduced NADPH predisposes to increased susceptibility of cells to oxidative stress.

Morphology

Pancreas

Lesions of pancreas are **not diagnostic** and are more common with type 1 than with type 2 diabetes. The morphological changes include:

- **Reduced number and size of islets:** It is seen in type 1 diabetes which is mild in type 2 diabetes.
- **Infiltration of islets (insulitis):** Mainly in type 1 diabetes.
- **Amyloid deposition within islets:** It is observed in and around capillaries and between cells in type 2 diabetes. In advanced stages, the islets may be virtually obliterated and may show fibrosis.

Blood vessels

- **Hyaline arteriolosclerosis:** It is characterized by **amorphous, hyaline thickening of the wall of the arterioles,** which may **narrow the lumen** of the vessel (refer Fig. 11.5).
- **Diabetic microangiopathy:** It is characterized by **diffuse thickening of basement membranes,** which is **mostly**

seen in the capillaries of the skin, skeletal muscle, retina, renal glomeruli, and renal medulla.

- The microangiopathy results in diabetic nephropathy, retinopathy, and some forms of neuropathy.

Diabetic Nephropathy—Renal Changes in Diabetes

Diabetic nephropathy is the term used for **collective lesions that often occur together in the diabetic kidney**. Diabetic nephropathy can develop in both insulin-dependent type 1 diabetes and type 2 diabetes (refer pages 246–7).

- The **kidneys** are **main targets** of diabetes.
- **Renal failure** is second only to myocardial infarction as a **cause of death** in diabetes.

Renal lesions in diabetes can involve any component. Four lesions are encountered namely:

Glomerular lesions

They are most **important and common renal lesions**. These include:

- **Diffuse widespread thickening glomerular capillary basement membrane.**
- **Diffuse mesangial sclerosis.**
- **Nodular glomerulosclerosis:** It is also called as **Kimmelstiel-Wilson disease** and **are pathognomonic**. Glomerular lesion consists of **ovoid or spherical**, often laminated, **nodules of mesangial matrix situated in the periphery of the glomerulus**. The nodules are **PAS-positive.**
- **Insudative lesions:**
  - **Fibrin caps.**
  - **Capsular drops.**

Renal vascular lesions

- **Hyaline arteriosclerosis** (hyalinosis)**:** It involves **both the afferent and the efferent arteriole** at the hilum of glomeruli. **Arteriolosclerosis efferent arteriole is rare in non-diabetics.**
- **Renal atherosclerosis:** It involves arteries and arterioles and are similar to those found in other parts of the body.

Glomerular and arteriolar lesions together produce **renal ischemia** and leads to atrophy of tubules, interstitial fibrosis, and contraction of kidney.

Pyelonephritis

It is a tubulointerstitial inflammation of the kidneys.

- Both the **acute and chronic pyelonephritis** occurs in non-diabetics as well as in diabetics. It is **more common** and tends to **more severe** in diabetics than in the general population.
- **Necrotizing papillitis** (or papillary necrosis)**:** It is one **special pattern of acute pyelonephritis** and is much more frequent in diabetics compared to non-diabetics. **Hyaline arteriolosclerosis** narrows blood vessels and **reduces the blood supply** to the renal medulla. This produces ischemia and causes **necrosis of the tips of papillae** (papillary necrosis).

Tubular lesions

The basement membrane of the tubules show thickening. In patients with high blood sugar level, the **epithelial cells of the proximal convoluted tubules show extensive deposits of vacuoles of glycogen**. These are known as Armanni–Ebstein lesions.

Clinical Features of Diabetes (Fig. 25.2)

Type 1 Diabetes Mellitus

- **Age:** Type 1 diabetes can occur at any age.
- **Classical triad of diabetes:** It consists of **polyuria, polydipsia, polyphagia**, and **in severe cases ketoacidosis**, are due to metabolic derangements.
- **Insulin requirement:** In the **initial 1 or 2 years**, the exogenous insulin required may be **minimal** because of endogenous insulin secretion and **later**, its requirement suddenly **increases.**

Consequences of insulin deficiency

Insulin is an anabolic hormone and its deficiency results in a catabolic state, which affects glucose metabolism, fat and protein metabolism.

1. **Carbohydrate metabolism:**
   - **Diminished transport of glucose** into **muscle cells** and **adipose tissue.**
   - **Reduction of stored glycogen in liver and muscle** due to **glycogenolysis.** This **further aggravates the hyperglycemia.**
   - When **hyperglycemia exceeds the renal threshold** level, it causes **glycosuria** and leads to osmotic diuresis. The resulting **increased quantity of urine known as polyuria,** with **loss of water and electrolytes.**
   - Water loss through urine + hyperosmolarity (due to hyperglycemia)—causes **depletion of intracellular water.** This **stimulates** the osmoreceptors of the **thirst centers** of the brain and results in increased thirst known as **polydipsia.**
2. **Protein and fat metabolism:**
   - Insulin deficiency causes **catabolism of proteins and fats** and produces a **negative energy balance.** This leads to **increased appetite (polyphagia).**
   - In spite of increased appetite, catabolic effects insulin results in paradoxical **loss of weight and muscle weakness.**

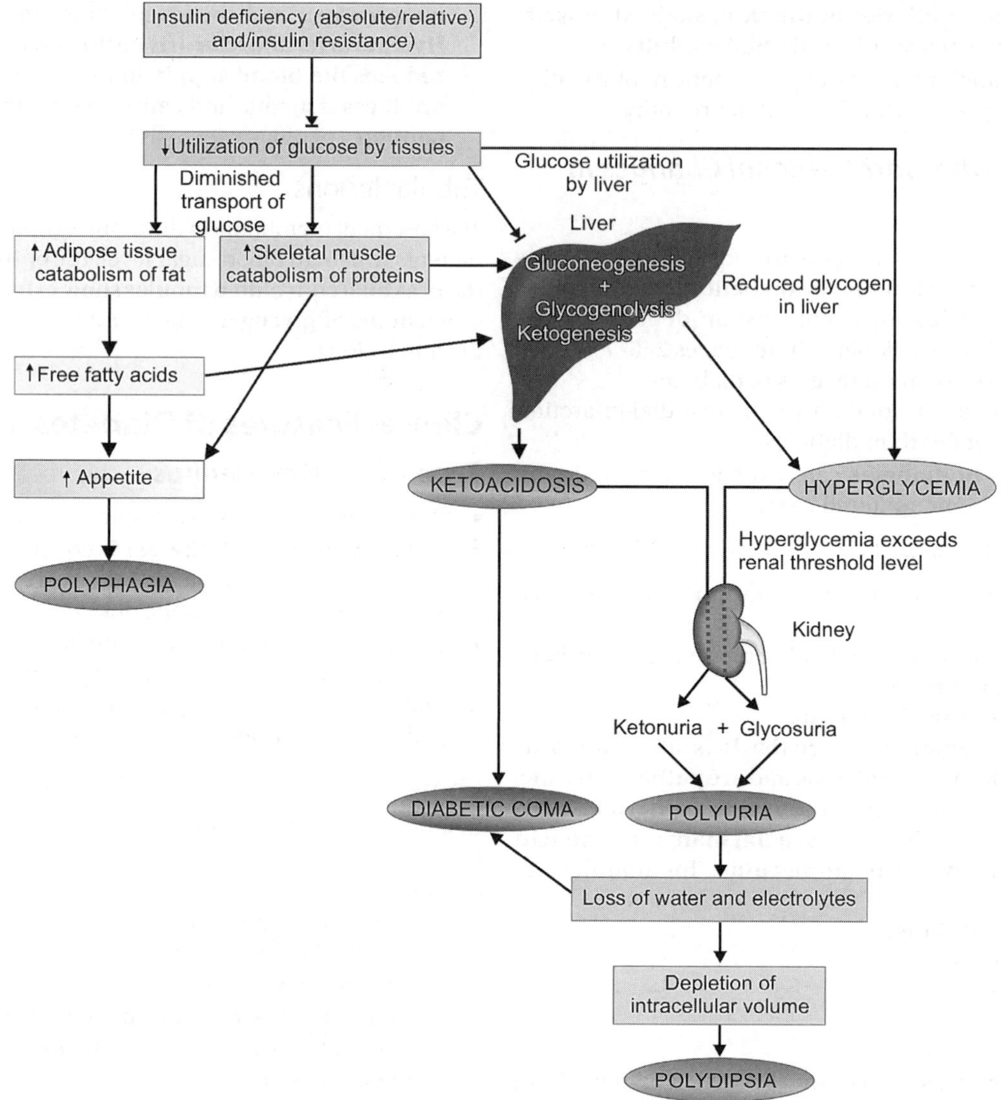

Fig. 25.2: Sequence of metabolic derangements underlying the symptoms and signs of uncontrolled hyperglycemia in diabetes mellitus

3. **Diabetic ketoacidosis:**
   - It is a serious complication of diabetes mellitus.
   - More **common and marked in type 1 diabetes**, but may also occur in type 2 diabetes.
     - **Diuresis and dehydration**.
     - **Activation of the ketogenic machinery** results in ketonemia and ketonuria.

Type 2 Diabetes Mellitus

- **Age:** Usually occurs in older **above the age of 40 years** and frequently in **obese individuals**. Due to increase in obesity and sedentary lifestyle, it is now detected also in children and adolescents.
- **Presentation: Polyuria, polydipsia, unexplained weakness or weight loss. Ketoacidosis is infrequent** and presentation is usually mild.
- In **asymptomatic individuals**, the **diagnosis is made after routine blood or urine testing**.

Complications (Fig. 25.3)

- Complications are similar in both type 1 and type 2 diabetes.
- **Long-term complications of diabetes** usually develop about 15–20 years after the onset of hyperglycemia. They are responsible for the majority of the morbidity and mortality.

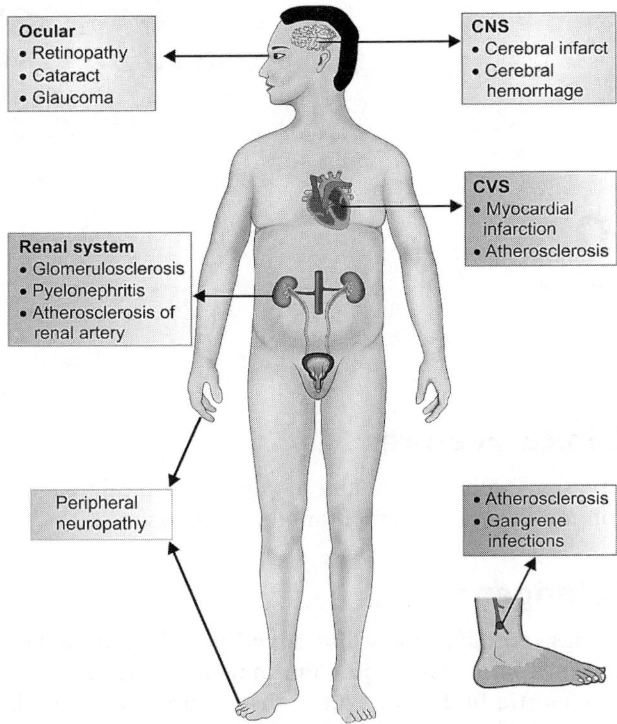

Fig. 25.3: Complications of diabetes

Diabetic Macrovascular Disease

The lesions of large- and medium-sized muscular arteries are the **most common causes of mortality** in long-standing diabetes. These include:

- **Atherosclerosis:** Diabetes is one of the major modifiable risk factor for atherosclerosis and other cardiovascular morbidities. The **atherosclerosis is more severe and occurs at earlier age**.
- **Myocardial infarction:** It is due to atherosclerosis of the coronary arteries and is the **most common cause of death in diabetics.** Diabetics have greater risk of coronary artery disease and cardiovascular complications than non-diabetics.
- **Gangrene of the lower extremities:** It results from advanced vascular disease and is more common in diabetics.
- **Renal vascular insufficiency**.
- **Cerebrovascular accidents** (stroke).

Microvascular Disease (Microangiopathy)

It involves small vessels and is characterized by capillary dysfunction in target organs and is mainly observed in kidneys (nephropathy), retina (diabetic retinopathy) and peripheral nerves (neuropathy).

- **Diabetic nephropathy:** About **30–40% of all diabetics** develop nephropathy (refer page 309) and is **leading cause of end-stage renal disease**.
- **Diabetic retinopathy** (refer page 339)**:** It develops in **~60–80% of diabetics, about 15–20 years after diagnosis**. The basic lesion of retinopathy is **neovascularization caused by hypoxia-induced overexpression of VEGF in the retina**. Diabetics have **increased risk for glaucoma** and **cataract formation**.
- **Diabetic neuropathy:** It may involve the **central and peripheral nervous systems** (refer page 319).

Diabetic Dyslipidemia

It is a condition in which there are **increased blood levels of triglycerides and LDL and decreased levels of the high-density lipoprotein** (protective).

Increased susceptibility to infections

Infections of the skin, tuberculosis, pneumonia, and pyelonephritis are common in diabetes.

Laboratory Diagnosis of Diabetes Mellitus

1. Urine examination for sugar, ketone bodies and protein.
2. Blood glucose level.
3. Glucose tolerance test.
4. Glycated hemoglobin (HbA1c) to measure of glycemic control.

SELF-ASSESSMENT EXERCISE

I. Short Notes

1. Type 1 diabetes mellitus.
2. Type 2 diabetes mellitus.
3. List the complications of diabetes mellitus.

CHAPTER

26

Skin

CHAPTER OUTLINE

- Acute Eczematous Dermatitis
- Psoriasis
- Malignant Tumors of Skin

ACUTE ECZEMATOUS DERMATITIS

The word eczema is derived from Greek, meaning "to boil over" which describes its gross appearance. Acute eczematous dermatitis is one of the most common skin disorders.

Types

Based on initiating factors it can be subdivided into: (1) allergic contact dermatitis, (2) atopic dermatitis, (3) drug-related eczematous dermatitis, (4) photoeczematous dermatitis, and (5) primary irritant dermatitis.

Etiology

- Dermatitis due to external application of an antigen (e.g. poison ivy) or
- Dermatitis due to an internal circulating antigen (derived from ingested food or a drug).

Pathogenesis: Eczematous dermatitis is due to type IV hypersensitivity.

Eczematous dermatitis are characterized by red, papulovesicular, oozing, and crusted lesions.

PSORIASIS

Psoriasis is a chronic, frequently familial **inflammatory dermatosis that appears to have an autoimmune basis**.

Individuals of all ages may develop the disease shows a peak in late adolescence. About 15% of the patients with psoriasis have associated arthritis.

Clinical Features

It presents with chronic, large, erythematous, scaly plaques, commonly on extensor cutaneous surfaces.

Pathogenesis

Psoriasis is multifactorial disease with genetic, immunologic and environmental factors contributing to its development.

- **Genetic factors:** Several observations support the genetic basis of psoriasis.
- **Immunologic factors:** T-lymphocytes play a crucial in the pathogenesis of psoriatic lesions.
- **Environmental factors:** Environmental stimuli such as physical injury, infection, certain drugs and photosensitivity may produce psoriatic lesions in apparently normal skin.

Morphology

- Psoriasis most commonly involves the skin of the elbows, knees, scalp, lumbosacral areas, intergluteal cleft, and glans penis. The typical lesion consists of a well-demarcated, **pink to salmon-colored plaque covered by loosely adherent silver-white scale**.
- **Nail changes occur in about 30% of cases of patients.**

Microscopic Features

- **The stratum granulosum of epidermis is thinned or absent, and extensive overlying parakeratotic** (persistence of nuclei in cells of the stratum corneum, which occurs with increased epidermal turnover) **scale is seen.**
- **Psoriasiform hyperplasia of epidermis:** The nucleated layers of the epidermis is thickened several fold in the rete pegs and appear as sections of cones.
- **Thinning of the portion of the epidermal** cell layer over the tips of dermal papillae (suprapapillary plates) and dilated, tortuous blood vessels within these papillae.

MALIGNANT TUMORS OF SKIN

Squamous Cell Carcinoma

- **Second most common tumor** arising **on sun-exposed sites**.
- **Sex:** More **common in men** than in women.
- **Clinical presentation:** Appear as sharply defined, red, scaling plaques.
- **Sites:** Skin, oral cavity, larynx, penis, cervix, esophagus, lung and sites wherever there is squamous epithelium.

Etiology and Pathogenesis

Risk factors

- **Exposure to UV light:** It **may produce DNA damage** and is the **most important cause** of squamous cell carcinoma of skin. The risk is proportional to the degree of lifetime sun exposure.
- **Chronic immunosuppression:** It may be due to **chemotherapy or organ transplantation** and may contribute to carcinogenesis.
- **Other risk factors:**
  - **Industrial carcinogens: Tars and oils.**
  - **Chronic non-healing ulcers:** For example, chronic osteomyelitis.
  - **Old burn scars (e.g. Marjolin's ulcers).**
  - **Ingestion of arsenicals.**
  - **Ionizing radiation.**
  - **Tobacco and betel nut chewing in the oral cavity.**

Genetics of squamous cell carcinoma

- **Mutations in tumor suppressor *p53* gene**
- **Mutations in DNA repair genes:**
  - **Xeroderma pigmentosum** is a disorder characterized by **inherited mutations in DNA repair genes,** and these **patients are susceptible to squamous cell carcinoma.**
- **Other genes:** Dysregulated RAS signaling may also be responsible.

Morphology

Gross: Invasive lesions are more advanced lesions, which appear as **nodular growth and may ulcerate**. The ulcer is **surrounded by a wide, elevated, indurated border**.

Microscopy: Tumor consists of **irregular masses of epidermal cells** that **proliferate downward into the dermis**. They show variable degrees of differentiation, ranging from well to poorly differentiated.

- **Well-differentiated squamous cell carcinoma** (Figs 26.1A and B): They are composed of **polygonal squamous tumor cells arranged in orderly lobules** and **produce large amounts of keratin**. Some of this keratin form **epithelial or squamous pearls** and are characteristically seen in well-differentiated tumors.
- **Moderately differentiated squamous cell carcinoma:** They consist of **anaplastic squamous cells, which show single-cell keratinization** (dyskeratosis).
- **Poorly differentiated squamous cell carcinoma:** They consist of **highly anaplastic cells.**

Basal Cell Carcinoma

- Basal cell carcinoma is the most common, **slow-growing invasive cancer** that **rarely metastasizes.**
- **Sites:** Occur at **sun-exposed sites** and in fair skinned people. Usual site is **above a line drawn from angle of mouth to the pinna of the ear.**

Etiology and Pathogenesis

The incidence of basal cell carcinoma is also **more in patients with immunosuppression** and **inherited defects in DNA repair** such as **xeroderma pigmentosum**.

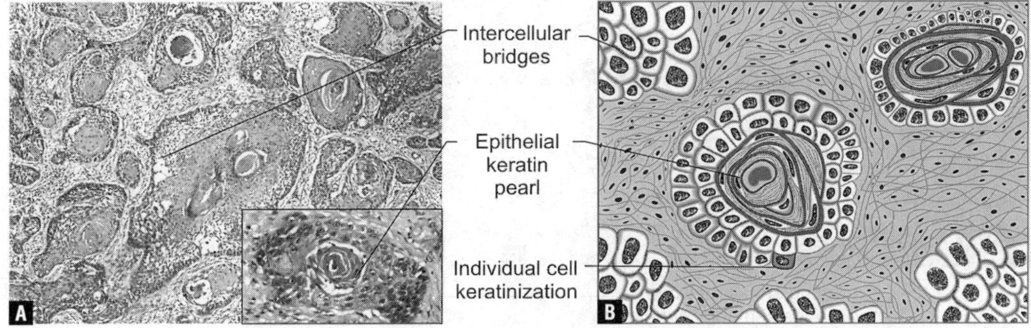

Figs 26.1A and B: (A) Photomicrograph and (B) Diagrammatic; Well-differentiated squamous cell carcinoma composed of polygonal squamous tumor cells arranged in orderly lobules and produce large amounts of keratin. Some of this keratin form epithelial or squamous pearls (inset of A)

Genetics of basal cell carcinoma

- **Mutation in tumor suppressor gene:**
  - **Mutation in *PTCH*: *PTCH* acts as tumor suppressor gene.**
  - ***p53* mutations.**
- **Defect in DNA repair genes: Xeroderma pigmentosum** is a disorder of DNA repair, associated with increased incidence of basal cell carcinoma.

Clinical Presentation

- Appear as **pearly papules** often containing prominent, dilated subepidermal blood vessels.
- Advanced tumors **may ulcerate, and locally invade and erode the underlying bone or facial sinuses like a rodent** and are known as **rodent ulcers**.

Morphology

Gross

- **Appearance varies** and may be **nodular, ulcerative, superficial or erythematous.**
- **Nodulo-ulcerative** basal cell carcinoma is the **most common type** and present as a nodule that increases slowly in size and undergoes central ulceration. A **typical lesion** consists of a **slowly enlarging ulcer surrounded by a pearly, rolled border**. This represents the so-called rodent ulcer (**erodes the underlying structures similar to a rodent**).

Microscopy (Figs 26.2A and B)

- **Tumor cells:** They **resemble the normal basal cell layer** of the epidermis. The tumor cells are **deeply basophilic epithelial cells.**
- **Arrangement:** Tumors cells are arranged in **nests** and are attached to the epidermis and protrude into the subjacent papillary dermis.
- **Peripheral palisading:** At the periphery of each nest, the **columnar cells are arranged radially with their long axes in parallel alignment** known as peripheral **palisading.**
- **Clefting artifact between tumor islands and adjacent stroma.**

Melanoma

Melanoma is a **relatively common** neoplasm.

- **Site:**
  - **Skin:** It is the most common site and may develop in the trunk, leg, face, sole, palm and nail beds.
  - **Other sites:** Oral and anogenital mucosal surfaces, esophagus, leptomeninges, eye, and the substantia nigra.
- **Cell of origin:** Melanocytes.

Etiology and Pathogenesis

Predisposing factors

Sun exposure:

- **Melanomas most commonly develop on sun-exposed surfaces**, particularly the upper back in men and the back and legs in women.
- **Lightly pigmented individuals** are at **greater risk** than darkly pigmented individuals.

Inherited genes: About 10 to 15% of melanomas are familial.

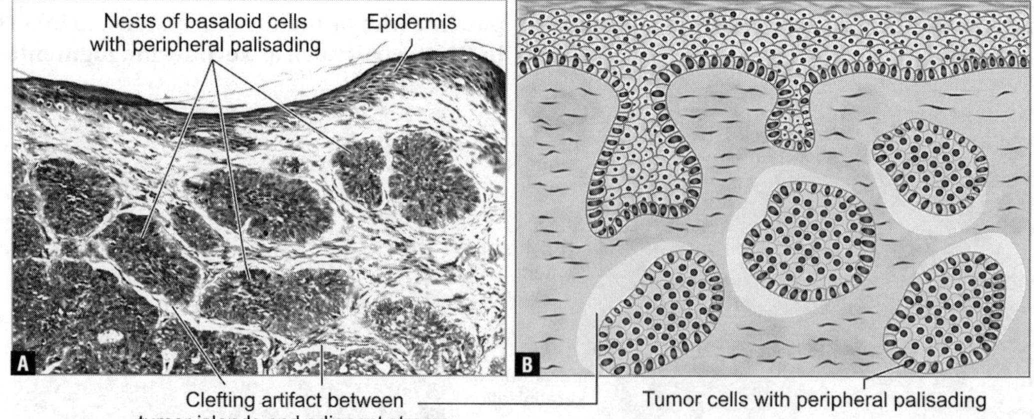

Figs 26.2A and B: Basal cell carcinoma. Composed of nests of uniformly atypical basaloid cells within the dermis, that are often separated from the adjacent stroma by thin clefts. (A) Photomicrograph; (B) Diagrammatic

Morphology (Figs 26.3A to C)

Growth phases

- **Radial growth phase:** During this phase, the **melanoma spread horizontally** within the **epidermis and superficial dermis.** It represents the **initial stage** where the tumor cells **lack the capacity to metastasize.**
- **Vertical growth phase: After a variable and unpredictable period,** melanoma from the radial phase develops a **vertical growth phase. Risk of metastasis** correlates with the **depth of invasion**, which is the distance from the superficial epidermal granular cell layer to the deepest intradermal tumor cells. This measurement is known as the **Breslow thickness.**

Microscopy (Figs 26.4A and B)

- **Tumor cells:** They have **similar appearance in both the radial and vertical phases** of growth.
  - **Size:** Tumor cells are usually **larger than normal melanocytes.**
  - **Nuclei:** They are **large with irregular contours, clumping of chromatin at the periphery** of the nuclear membrane, and **prominent red (eosinophilic) nucleoli. Mitotic figures** are often seen.
- **Pattern of growth:** Tumor cells are arranged in **solid masses, sheets, islands**, etc. Tumor invades upper epidermis as well as deeper dermis.
- **Melanin pigment:** It is **seen in melanoma.** The melanoma, **which does not show the pigment,** is known as **amelanotic melanoma**. Melanin is present **in the cytoplasm as uniform brown fine granules.**

Clinical Features

- Melanoma of the skin is **usually asymptomatic**, but may present with itching or pain at the site of lesion.
- **Changes in pigmented lesions:** These are the **most important clinical signs** of melanoma and include:

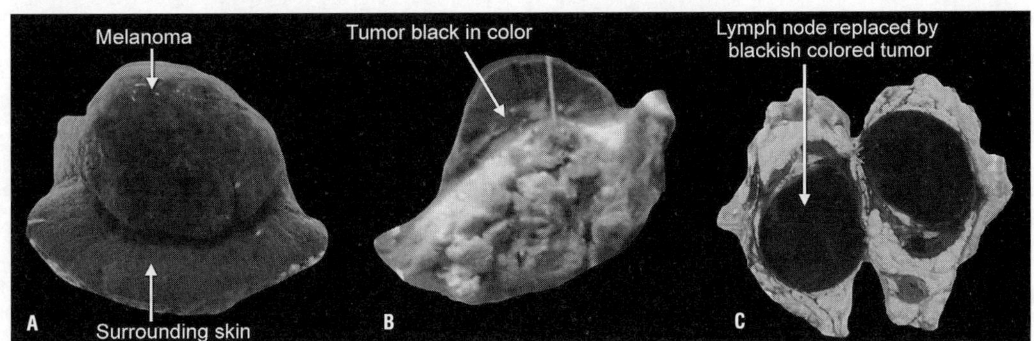

Figs 26.3A to C: Gross features of malignant melanoma. (A) Nodular growth projecting from the skin; (B) Cut section of the same shows blackish pigmentation in the tumor; (C) Lymph node with extensive metastasis from malignant melanoma (black color)

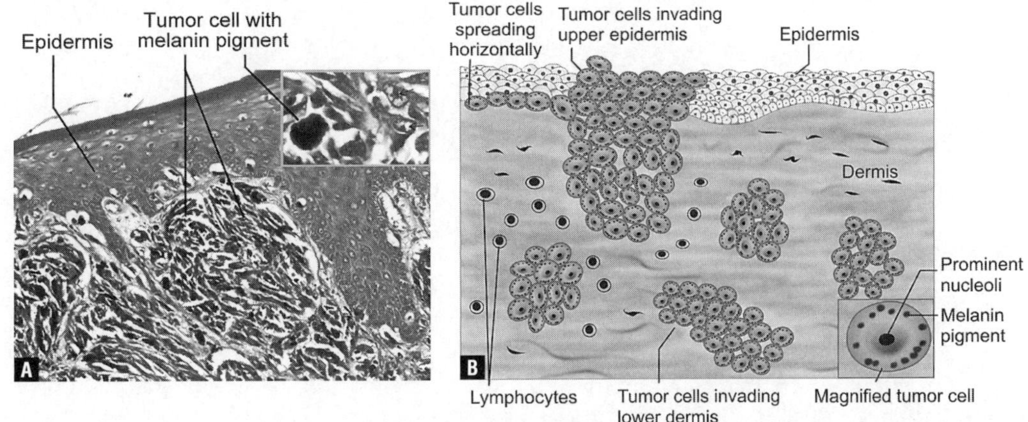

Figs 26.4A and B: (A) Photomicrograph of malignant melanoma showing nests of tumor cells in the upper dermis containing melanin pigment. Inset shows tumor cell with melanin pigment; (B) Diagrammatic microscopic appearance of malignant melanoma showing nests of tumor cells infiltrating epidermis (radial growth phase) and dermis (vertical growth phase)

- **Color:** Unlike benign nevi, **melanomas show variations in color**, ranging from shades of black, brown, red, dark blue, and gray.
- **Size:** Majority are **larger than 10 mm** in diameter at the time of diagnosis. But, if a pigmented lesion is greater than 6 mm a diameter, any change in appearance, and new onset of itching or pain should raise the suspicion of malignancy.
- **Shape:** The borders of melanomas are **irregular and often notched**, whereas they are smooth, round, and uniform in melanocytic nevi.

SELF-ASSESSMENT EXERCISE

I. Short Notes

1. Squamous cell carcinoma.
2. Basal cell carcinoma (rodent ulcer) of skin.
3. Malignant melanoma.

CHAPTER 27

Peripheral Nerves and Skeletal Muscles

CHAPTER OUTLINE

NEUROMUSCULAR DISEASES

- Neuromuscular diseases are a complex group of disorders.
- May be inherited and acquired.
- Typically present with weakness, muscle pain, or sensory deficits.

Classification

- Neuromuscular disorders may be classified as those preferential affect.
  - Peripheral nerves.
  - Neuromuscular junction.
  - Skeletal muscles.

DISEASES OF PERIPHERAL NERVES

- Main components of peripheral nerves are axons and myelin sheaths made by Schwann cells.
- Injuries to either of these components produce peripheral neuropathy.

General Types of Peripheral Nerve Injury

Axonal Neuropathies

In this large group of peripheral neuropathies (Fig. 27.1), **axons are the primary target of the damage.** Degeneration (necrosis) of the axon can occur in many neuropathies. The degeneraion may be limited to distal axons or involve both (proximal and distal) axons and neuronal cell bodies.

Morphology

- The axon degeneration may be initially limited to the distal ends (**dying-back neuropathy or distal axonopathy**) of nerves. Portions of axons that are distal to the point of injury/transection get disconnected from the central neuron and degenerate.

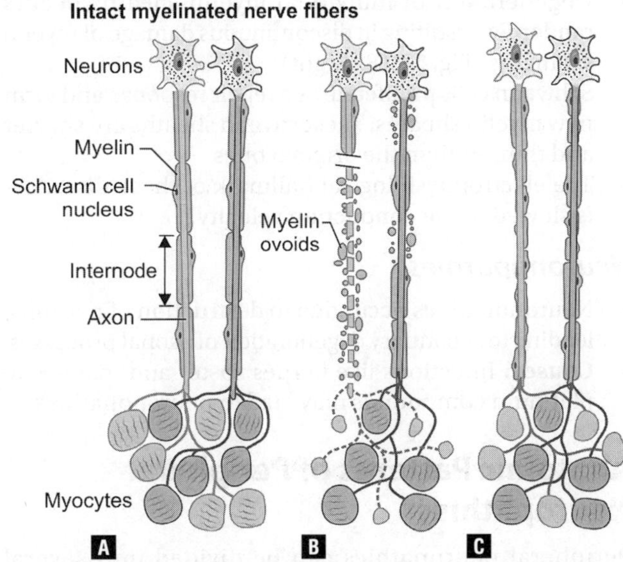

Figs 27.1A to C: Patterns of peripheral nerve damage. (A) Normal motor units; (B) Left axon shows acute axonal injury. It results in degeneration of the distal axon and its associated myelin sheath, with atrophy of denervated myofibers. Right axon shows acute demyelinating disease. It produces random segmental degeneration of individual myelin internodes and spares the axons; (C) Left axon shows regeneration of axons after injury. It allows reinnervation of myofibers. Right axon shows remission of demyelinating disease with remyelination

- Within a day of injury, there is fragmentation of distal axons with separation of the associated myelin sheaths (Fig. 27.1 B-Left) and disintegration into spherical structures (*myelin ovoids*). Macrophages are recruited and remove debris of axon and myelin. The striated muscle shows denervation atrophy.
- Regeneration begins at the site of injury/transection and new sprouts of axon develop from the proximal axon and grow toward their distal target (Fig. 27.1C-Left). Schwann cells and their associated basement membranes guide these sprouting axons. The Schwann cells produce new myelin sheaths around these regenerating axons.
- The repair process is successful only if the two transected ends remain closely approximated.
- With time, damage tends to exceed repair, resulting in progressive loss of axons. The electrophysiological hallmark of axonal neuropathies is a reduction in signal strength.

Demyelinating Neuropathies

Schwann cells with their myelin sheaths are the primary targets of damage in demyelinating neuropathies. The **axons are relatively preserved.**

- Degeneration of individual myelin sheaths occurs randomly, resulting in discontinuous damage of myelin segments (Fig. 27.1B- Right).
- Schwann cells proliferate as a repair response and form new myelin sheaths. These myelin sheaths are shorter and thinner than the original ones.
- The electrophysiological hallmark of these disorders is slowed nerve conduction velocity.

Neuronopathies

- Neuronopathies occur due to destruction of neurons, leading to secondary degeneration of axonal processes.
- **Causes:** Infections like herpes zoster and toxins like platinum compounds may lead to neuronopathies.

Anatomic Patterns of Peripheral Neuropathies

Peripheral neuropathies can be divided into several groups according to the anatomic patterns/distribution of involvement and the associated neurological deficits.

- **Mononeuropathies:** They involve a single nerve and a deficit is restricted to the distribution of the nerve. Causes include: trauma, entrapment, and infections.
- **Polyneuropathies:** They involve multiple nerves, usually in a symmetric fashion. They result in a characteristic "stocking and glove" distribution of sensory deficits.
- **Mononeuritis multiplex:** In this damage occurs in several nerves in a haphazard fashion. Vasculitis is a common cause.
- **Polyradiculoneuropathies:** These show disease affecting nerve roots as well as peripheral nerves. These lead to diffuse symmetric symptoms in proximal and distal parts of the body.

Specific Peripheral Neuropathies

A peripheral neuropathy is a **process that affects the function of one or more peripheral nerves**. It occur in **all age groups** and may be **hereditary or acquired**. Different types of diseases can damage peripheral nerves. These include inflammatory diseases, infections, metabolic changes, toxic injury, trauma, etc.

Inflammatory Neuropathies

Guillain-Barré syndrome (acute inflammatory demyelinating polyneuropathy)

It is a **demyelinating peripheral neuropathy**. It may lead to life-threatening respiratory paralysis.

- **Pathogenesis:**
  - Guillain-Barré syndrome is probably an acute-onset immune-mediated demyelinating neuropathy.
  - Majority of patients have preceding acute, influenza-like illness. Infections preceding Guillain-Barré syndrome may be due to *Campylobacter jejuni*, Cytomegalovirus, Epstein-Barr virus, and *Mycoplasma pneumoniae*, or prior vaccination.
- **Microscopy:**
  - It shows inflammation and demyelination of spinal nerve roots and peripheral nerves (radiculoneuropathy).
    - Inflammation of peripheral nerves accompanied by lymphocytes, macrophages, and a few plasma cells.
    - Segmental demyelination affecting peripheral nerves: Most prominent lesion.
    - Damage to axons when the disease is severe.
    - Inflammation and demyelination can be widespread in the peripheral nervous system but are usually most prominent close to the nerve roots.
- **Clinical features:**
  - Weakness beginning in the distal limbs that rapidly advances to affect proximal muscle function ("ascending paralysis").
  - Loss of deep tendon reflexes (areflexia).
  - Sensory involvement: Loss of pain sensation.

- Nerve conduction velocities: Slowed because of multifocal destruction of myelin segments in many axons within a nerve.
- Cerebrospinal fluid (CSF): Protein levels are raised. Little or no CSF pleocytosis.

Chronic inflammatory demyelinating poly (radiculo) neuropathy

- Most common chronic acquired inflammatory peripheral neuropathy.
- Characterized by symmetrical mixed sensorimotor polyneuropathy that persists for 2 months or more.

Neuropathy associated with systemic autoimmune diseases

- Systemic autoimmune diseases such as rheumatoid arthritis, Sjögren syndrome, or systemic lupus erythematosus (SLE) may be associated with peripheral neuropathies.
- Characterized by distal sensory or sensorimotor polyneuropathies.

Neuropathy associated with vasculitis

- **Vasculitis is a noninfectious inflammation of blood vessels.**
- **Vasculitis can involve and damage peripheral nerves.**
- Vasculitis often presents as mononeuritis multiplex.
- Peripheral nerves involvement typically reveals patchy axonal degeneration and loss.

Infectious Neuropathies

Many infectious diseases affect peripheral nerves. Examples, leprosy, diphtheria, and varicella-zoster.

Metabolic, Hormonal, and Nutritional Neuropathies

These include diabetic neuropathy, uremic neuropathy, neuropathy associated with thyroid dysfunction, Vitamin B_{12} (cyanocobalamin) deficiency, deficiencies of vitamin B_1 (thiamine), vitamin B_6 (pyridoxine), folate, vitamin E, copper, and zinc.

Diabetic peripheral neuropathy

- Diabetes is the most common cause of peripheral neuropathy.
- Both type 1 and type 2 diabetes mellitus patients are affected.
- **Manifestations:**
  - **Ascending distal symmetric sensorimotor neuropathy:** It is the most common type and is characterized by sensory symptoms, like numbness, loss of pain sensation, difficulty with balance, and paresthesias.
  - **Dysfunction of the autonomic nervous system:** It always develops in association with a distal sensorimotor neuropathy. It produces various manifestations such as postural hypotension, incomplete emptying of the bladder (resulting in recurrent urinary tract infections), and sexual dysfunction.

Toxic Neuropathies

Peripheral neuropathies may develop after exposure to industrial or environmental chemicals, biologic toxins, or therapeutic drugs. Important causes include alcohol, heavy metals (lead, mercury, arsenic, and thallium), and organic solvents. Various therapeutic drugs can cause toxic neuropathies, but the most important are chemotherapeutic agents.

Neuropathies Associated with Malignancy

Neuropathies associated with malignancy may develop due to local effects (direct infiltration or compression of peripheral nerves by tumor), complications of therapy (chemotherapy, radiation, poor nutrition and infection), paraneoplastic effects, or tumor-derived immunoglobulins (B-cell lymphomas secreting monoclonal immunoglobulins).

Neuropathies Caused by Physical Forces

Peripheral nerves are commonly injured by trauma or compression/entrapment. Any trauma can damage peripheral nerves. Compression neuropathy (entrapment neuropathy) may develop when a peripheral nerve is chronically subjected to increased pressure, often within an anatomical compartment.

- **Carpal tunnel syndrome:** It is the most common entrapment neuropathy that develops due to compression of the median nerve at the level of the wrist. It is more common in females than males and frequently bilateral. It may be found in association with many disorders (e.g. edema, pregnancy, inflammatory arthritis). Symptoms are restricted to distribution of the median nerve and consist of numbness and paresthesias of the tips of the thumb and first two digits.

Inherited Peripheral Neuropathies

- These are a group of genetically diverse disorders with overlapping clinical phenotypes.
- They often present in adulthood.
- They may be present with sensory, motor, or autonomic dysfunction, alone or in combination.

- Major types include: (1) hereditary motor and sensory neuropathies [Charcot-Marie-Tooth (CMT) disease], (2) hereditary motor neuropathies, (3) hereditary sensory neuropathies, with or without autonomic neuropathy, and (4) other inherited neuropathy.

DISEASES OF THE NEUROMUSCULAR JUNCTION

- **Neuromuscular junction:** It is a complex specialized structure situated at the junction of motor nerve axons and skeletal muscle. It serves to control muscle contraction.
- **Diseases of the neuromuscular junction:** They **present with painless weakness.** Myasthenia gravis (literally, *grave weakness*) due to autoantibodies against neuromuscular junction proteins is the most common cause.

Antibody-Mediated Diseases of the Neuromuscular Junction

Myasthenia Gravis

- Myasthenia gravis literally means **grave weakness**.
- Myasthenia gravis is an **autoimmune disease** associated **autoantibodies directed against acetylcholine receptors** in majority of patients.
- Bimodal age distribution.
- **Pathogenesis:**
  - **Autoantibodies against postsynaptic acetylcholine receptors:** Observed in about 85% of patients receptors.
  - **Antibodies against** the sarcolemmal protein **muscle-specific receptor tyrosine kinase:** Found in about 15% of patients.
- **Clinical features:**
  - Patients with anti-acetylcholine receptor antibodies:
    - Usually present with fluctuating weakness that worsens with exertion.
    - Diplopia and ptosis due to involvement of extraocular.
  - Patients with antibodies against muscle-specific receptor tyrosine kinase: Show more focal muscle involvement (neck, shoulder, facial, respiratory, and bulbar muscles).
  - **Diagnosis:** It is made on the basis of clinical history, physical findings, demonstration of autoantibodies, and electrophysiological studies.

Lambert-Eaton Myasthenic Syndrome

- It is an **autoimmune disorder**.
- **Mechanism:** Caused by **antibodies** that **block acetylcholine release by inhibiting a presynaptic calcium channel.**
- **Causes:** In 50% there is an underlying malignancy (e.g. neuroendocrine carcinoma of the lung). In patients without malignancies have other autoimmune diseases (e.g. vitiligo or thyroid disease).
- **Clinical features:** Weakness of extremities.

Congenital Myasthenic Syndromes

- Genetic defects in neuromuscular junction proteins give rise to congenital myasthenic syndromes.
- These are rare disorders most commonly due to autosomal recessive mode of inheritance and characterized by varying degrees of muscle weakness.
- Mutations have been identified in genes encoding different presynaptic, synaptic, or postsynaptic proteins.
- Mainly present in the perinatal period with poor muscle tone, external eye muscle weakness, and breathing difficulties.

Disorders Caused by Toxins

- *Botulism* is caused by a neurotoxin (known as *Botox*) produced by the anaerobic Gram-positive organism *Clostridium botulinum*. Botox blocks the release of acetylcholine from presynaptic neurons.

DISEASES OF SKELETAL MUSCLE

Skeletal Muscle Atrophy

Atrophy of skeletal muscle is a common feature of many disorders. These include loss of innervation, disuse, cachexia, old age, and primary myopathies. Loss of muscle mass is found in severe atrophy.

Neurogenic and Myopathic Changes in Skeletal Muscle

Altered skeletal muscle function may be to primary muscle process in which there is a direct damage to myofibers (myopathic injury) or due disruption muscle innervation (neurogenic injury). Myopathic processes are characterized by marked by degeneration and regeneration of myofibers.

Inflammatory Myopathies

The three main types of inflammatory myopathies are:

1. **Dermatomyositis:** It is a systemic autoimmune disease in which **muscle injury is due to damage of small blood**

vessels. It presents with proximal muscle weakness and skin changes. It occurs in children and adults. In adults frequently as a manifestation of paraneoplastic disorder. Immune damage to small blood vessels and perifascicular atrophy of skeletal muscle are common features.
2. **Polymyositis:** It is an adult onset myopathy caused by T-cells.
3. **Inclusion body myositis:** It is a chronic progressive disease of older patients (above 50 years of age) associated with rimmed vacuoles. Most patients present with slowly progressive muscle weakness. It is most severe in the quadriceps and the distal upper extremity muscles.

Toxic Myopathies

Toxic myopathies may be produced by prescription or recreational **drugs**, or by few hormonal imbalances. Myopathy is the most common complication of **statins** (widely used cholesterol-lowering drugs). Other drugs include **chloroquine** and **hydroxychloroquine**. **ICU myopathy** or myosin deficient myopathy is a neuromuscular disorder seen in patients in an intensive care unit especially with corticosteroid therapy. **Thyrotoxic myopathy** may precede other signs of hyperthyroidism. **Alcohol** can also cause myopathy.

Inherited Diseases of Skeletal Muscle

Inherited diseases of skeletal muscle are due to inherited **mutations and are responsible for a diverse disorders characterized by defects in skeletal muscle**. In some of these disorders, skeletal muscle is the main target, but in others multiple organs are involved. They can be studied under two broad subheadings.

Congenital Myopathies

They usually present during infancy with muscle defects that tend to be static or even improve over time. They are associated with distinct structural changes in the muscle.

Muscular Dystrophies

Muscular dystrophies consist of several **inherited disorders of skeletal muscle** that have in common **progressive muscle damage** and typically comes to attention between **childhood and adulthood** (after infancy).

X-linked muscular dystrophy with dystrophin mutation/Duchenne and Becker muscular dystrophy

- Most common muscular dystrophies are **X-linked** and are due to **mutations that disrupt the function** of a large structural protein called dystrophin. These diseases are also called as dystrophinopathies.
- **Duchenne muscular dystrophy is the most common early onset form.**
- **Becker muscular dystrophy is a second relatively common** dystrophinopathy that usually manifest later and of milder phenotype. Others are rare.
- **Pathogenesis:** Duchenne and Becker muscular dystrophy are due to mutations in the dystrophin gene on the X chromosome. **Dystrophin provide mechanical stability to the myofiber and its cell membrane during muscle contraction.** Defects in dystrophin trigger events that result in myofiber degeneration.
- **Morphology:** Morphological changes in Duchenne and Becker muscular dystrophy are similar, but differ in degree.
  - Muscle biopsies damage characterized by segmental myofiber degeneration and regeneration associated with atrophic myofibers.
  - No inflammation.
  - As the disease progresses, muscle is replaced by collagen and fat cells ("fatty replacement" or "fatty infiltration"). The remaining myofibers show prominent variation in size, from small atrophic fibers to large hypertrophied fibers.
- **Clinical features:**
  - Boys with Duchenne muscular dystrophy appear normal at birth.
  - Milestones are normal but walking is often delayed.
  - Muscle weakness begins in the pelvic girdle muscles and then extends to the shoulder girdle.
  - Enlargement of the muscles of the lower leg (pseudohypertrophy) associated with weakness.
  - Other features: Joint contractures, scoliosis, worsening respiratory reserve, and sleep hypoventilation. Dystrophin is also expressed in the heart (causes cardiomyopathy and arrhythmias) and the central nervous system (cognitive impairment), hence both are affected.
  - Mean age of death for Duchenne muscular dystrophy is 25–30 years of age where as Becker muscular dystrophy is more slowly progressive with a near normal life expectancy.
- **Diagnosis:** Made based on the history, physical examination, and laboratory studies. Serum creatine kinase is markedly raised during the first decade and then falls as the disease progresses with loss of muscle mass.

Myotonic dystrophy

It is an **autosomal dominant multisystem disorder**.

- **Skeletal muscle weakness is associated with cataracts, endocrinopathy, and cardiomyopathy**. Myotonia is characterized by a sustained involuntary contraction of muscles and is a key feature of the disease. The disease is caused by expansions of CTG triplet repeats in the myotonic dystrophy protein kinase (*DMPK*) gene.

Emery–Dreifuss muscular dystrophy (EMD)

It is **due to mutations in genes that codes nuclear lamina proteins** (emerin and lamin).

Clinical features: Triad of (1) slowly progressive humeroperoneal weakness, (2) cardiomyopathy and (3) early contractures of the Achilles tendon, spine, and elbows.

Fascioscapulohumeral dystrophy

It is characterized by prominent weakness of facial muscles and muscles of the shoulder girdle. It is an autosomal dominant disease.

Limb-girdle muscular dystrophy

These are heterogeneous group autosomal dominant and autosomal recessive disorders. In all forms **muscle weakness preferentially involves proximal muscle groups.**

Diseases of Lipid or Glycogen Metabolism

Many inborn errors of lipid or glycogen metabolism can affect skeletal muscle.

Mitochondrial Myopathies

These are complex systemic disorders which can involve many organ systems, including skeletal muscle.

Spinal Muscular Atrophy and the Differential Diagnosis of a Hypotonic Infant

It is a neuropathic disorder characterized by loss of motor neurons leading muscle weakness and atrophy.

Ion Channel Myopathies (Channelopathies)

These are a group of inherited diseases due to mutations affecting the function of ion channel proteins.

SELF-ASSESSMENT EXERCISE

I. Short Notes

1. Neuropathy.
2. Guillain-Barré syndrome.
3. Diseases of the neuromuscular junction.
4. Myasthenia gravis.
5. Muscular dystrophies.

CHAPTER

28

Central Nervous System

CHAPTER OUTLINE

- Introduction
- Infections
- Cerebrovascular Diseases
- Intracranial Hemorrhage
- Paraplegia
- Hemiplegia
- Demyelinating Diseases
- Neurodegenerative Diseases
- Central Nervous System Tumors

INTRODUCTION

The central nervous system (CNS) consists of brain and spinal cord. Brain is within the cranial cavity in the bony skull and spinal cord is within the vertebral cavity of the bony vertebra. The brain consists of cerebrum, cerebellum, pons and medulla oblongata. Histologically, it consists of neurons and neuroglia. The neurons are specialized cells involved in conduction of impulses. The neuroglial cells include: astrocytes, oligodendrocytes and ependymal cells. These glial cells provide support and nutrition to the neurons. The brain is covered by dura, pia and arachnoid mater. The latter two (pia and arachnoid) constitute leptomeninges.

INFECTIONS

The central nervous system infections can be divided depending upon the location of the infection as:

- **Meningitis:** Inflammation of the meninges.
- **Encephalitis:** Inflammation of the parenchyma of the brain.
- **Meningoencephalitis:** Inflammation of both brain parenchyma and meninges.

Many organisms infect the CNS and include viruses, bacteria and parasites. The infection may be **acute or chronic**.

Routes of infection: Infectious microbes may enter the central nervous system by following routes:

- **Hematogenous:** It is the most common route of entry of infectious agents.
  - **Septicemia and septic embolism** usually through the arterial circulation.
  - **Retrograde spread** can occur through veins of the face.
- **Direct implantation:** Usually follows trauma or is associated with congenital malformations (e.g. meningomyelocele).
- **Local extension:** It may be from adjacent structures like air sinuses, an infected tooth, cranial or spinal osteomyelitis.
- **Transport along the peripheral nervous system:** This route is mainly used by certain viruses, such as rabies and herpes zoster.

Consequences: Bacteria generally cause meningitis. Bacteria can also invade brain and result in brain abscess or enter the subdural space to induce subdural empyema.

Meningitis

Meninges have three layers and from inside out are pia, arachnoid and dura matter.

Meningitis is the term used usually for **inflammation of the meninges.** It is mainly applied to **inflammation within subarachnoid space between pia and arachnoid mater** (and is known as leptomeningitis).

Causes

Meningitis is a dangerous infection caused by a variety of microorganisms.

Table 28.1: Causative agents for different types of meningitis

Infectious meningitis	Causative agent
• **Acute** – Pyogenic (bacterial/ purulent) – Aseptic (usually viral)	*Escherichia coli*, group B *Streptococcus, Haemophilus influenzae*, meningococcus *(Neisseria meningitidis).* Enterovirus, HIV, mumps virus, Epstein-Barr virus and herpes simplex virus
• **Chronic** – Tuberculous – Syphilitic – Cryptococcal	*Mycobacterium tuberculosis* *Treponema pallidum* *Cryptococcus*

- **Infectious meningitis:** It is the most common cause of meningitis. It is classified depending on the characteristics of inflammatory exudate and the clinical features, as **acute and chronic** (Table 28.1).
- **Chemical meningitis:** Due to a nonbacterial irritant introduced into the subarachnoid space.

Pyogenic/Bacterial Meningitis

Clinical features: Common symptoms of meningitis are: headache, vomiting, fever and convulsions (especially in children). Classic signs of meningitis are:
- **Cervical rigidity**/Neck stiffness.
- **Kernig sign:** Knee pain with hip flexion.
- **Brudzinski sign:** Knee/hip flexion when the neck is flexed.

Laboratory tests: Clinical features and classical signs suggest meningitis. Examination of the cerebrospinal fluid (CSF) by lumbar puncture is essential in each case.

Cerebrospinal Fluid Findings

- **Appearance:** Normally CSF is clear. In acute meningitis, it becomes **cloudy or frankly purulent**.
- **Pressure: Increased** (>180 mm of water).
- **Cells:** Presence of **neutrophils** in the CSF is the most definitive feature of meningitis. Neutrophils may be as many as 90,000/μL.
- **Protein concentration: Increased** (>50 mg/dL).
- **Glucose: Markedly reduced** (<40 mg/dL).
- **Smear:** Bacteria may be seen on a smear **(Gram-stain)** or can be cultured.

Complications of Bacterial Meningitis

- Obstructive hydrocephalus.
- Thrombophlebitis of leptomeningeal veins.
- Chronic adhesive arachnoiditis.
- Cerebral abscess.
- Subdural empyema.
- Epilepsy.
- **Waterhouse-Friderichsen syndrome:** It results from meningitis-associated septicemia with hemorrhagic infarction of the adrenal glands and cutaneous petechiae.

Acute Aseptic (Viral) Meningitis

Aseptic meningitis is a term referring to the absence of recognizable organisms in a patient with symptoms of acute meningitis.

Age: Common in children and young adults.

Clinical features: It presents with fever and headache.

Cerebrospinal Fluid Findings

- Appearance: Clear.
- Protein: Moderately increased(>40 mg/dL).
- Glucose: Always normal.
- Microscopy: 10 to 100 **lymphocytes**/μL.

Prognosis

Usually self-limiting.

Cerebrospinal fluid findings in various types of meningitis are summarized in Table 28.2.

Chronic Meningitis

Types: The important types are:
- **Bacterial:** Tuberculosis is caused by *M. tuberculosis* and syphilitic is caused by *T. pallidum*.
- **Fungal:** Cryptococcal.

Tuberculous Meningitis

It is defined as the infection of the meninges by tubercle bacilli. *Mycobacterium tuberculosis* human type is the most common (causative agent).

Mode of infection

- **Hematogenous route:** Tuberculous infection from other sites (most commonly from lungs) may spread through blood. Meningitis develops as a result of **miliary spread**.
- **Direct spread** from adjacent site such as vertebral body.

Morphology

Gross:
- Subarachnoid space contains a greenish, gelatinous or fibrinous exudate, most prominent at the base of the brain and surrounding cranial nerves.
- Leptomeninges may show white granules of tubercles.

Table 28.2: Cerebrospinal fluid findings in meningitis

	Normal	Acute pyogenic	Acute viral	Tuberculous
Physical examination	Clear and colorless	Turbid and forms coagulum	Clear	Clear and colorless, forms cobweb on standing due to coagulation of fibrinogen
CSF pressure	60–150 mm of H_2O	Raised above 180 mm of H_2O	Raised above 250 mm of H_2O	Raised above 300 mm of H_2O
Total protein	20–40 mg/dL	50–200 mg/dL	>40 mg/dL	50–150 mg/dL
Glucose	45–80 mg/dL	0–20 mg/dL	Normal	20–50 mg/dL
Chlorides	720–750 mg/dL	600–700 mg/dL	Normal	450–600 mg/dL
Cells				
Polymorphs	Usually absent	1500–2000/µL	Absent	0–5 cells/µL
Lymphocytes	0–5 cells/µL	5–50 cells/µL	10–100//µL	500–700 cells/µL
Gram-stain/ZN stain	–	Bacteria +	–	AFB +

Microscopy:

- **Granulomas** consisting of epithelioid cells, Langhans giant cells surrounded by lymphocytes. They may show central area of caseous necrosis (refer Fig. 4.2).

AFB stain may show acid-fast bacilli.

Clinical features

Includes headache, malaise, mental confusion, and vomiting. On examination, there will be neck rigidity.

Cerebrospinal fluid findings

- **Physical examination:** Clear and colorless, forms **cobweb on standing** due to coagulation of fibrinogen.
- **CSF pressure: Raised** above 300 mm of H_2O.
- **Protein: Raised** ranges from 50-150 mg/dL.
- **Glucose:** Moderately **reduced** or normal (20-50 mg/dL).
- **Chloride: Decreased** (450-600 mg/dL).
- **Cells:** Moderate CSF pleocytosis (500-700 cells/µL), mainly **lymphocytes**.

Complications

- **Hydrocephalus**.
- **Nerve root damage**.
- **Tuberculous encephalitis**.

Encephalitis

Encephalitis is an **acute inflammation of brain parenchyma**. Encephalitis with meningitis is known as meningoencephalitis.

Cause

- **Virus:** The most common cause is viral encephalitis. The common viruses are rabies, herpes simplex, polio virus and measles virus.
- **Bacterial and other agents:** It can be caused by a bacteria (such as bacterial meningitis, spreading directly to the brain), or may be a complication of syphilis. Certain parasitic and protozoal infestations, such as toxoplasmosis, malaria, or primary amoebic meningoencephalitis, can also cause encephalitis in people with compromised immune systems.

Clinical Features

Adult patients with encephalitis present with acute onset of fever, headache, confusion, and sometimes seizures. Younger children or infants may present with irritability, poor appetite and fever.

- Cerebrospinal fluid usually shows **increased protein and white blood cells with normal glucose**.

CEREBROVASCULAR DISEASES

Cerebrovascular disease is the term for **group of diseases of the blood vessels of the brain**. It includes stroke (ischemic and hemorrhagic stroke) and cerebrovascular anomalies.

Factors determining the extent of brain damage: Brain needs constant blood supply for supplying glucose and oxygen. Diseases of blood vessels of the brain may impair blood supply and oxygenation of brain.

Effects of cerebrovascular diseases: It may lead to ischemia, infarction or hemorrhage.

Stroke (Cerebrovascular Accident)

Definition: Stroke is the term for a group of diseases that begin suddenly and cause neurologic damage due to focal ischemia or hemorrhage. It is a common medical emergency.

Clinical classification of stroke: Depending on the duration and evolution of symptoms stroke can be classified into three types.

- **Transient ischemic attack (TIA):** It is a stroke in which CNS disturbances last for less than 24 hours.
- **Progressing stroke (evolving stroke):** In this type of stroke, the focal neurological deficit worsens after the patient first presents.
- **Completed stroke:** This is characterized by persistence of focal deficit which does not progress.

Causes of Stroke

Depending on the cause, stroke may be divided into ischemic or hemorrhagic.

Hemorrhagic stroke

Approximately 15% of strokes are of hemorrhagic type. It is due to bleeding either into brain tissue (intraparenchymal/ intracerebral hemorrhage) or into the spaces surrounding the brain (i.e. subarachnoid or intraventricular spaces). About two-thirds of hemorrhagic strokes are due to subarachnoid hemorrhages, whereas about a third due to intracerebral hemorrhages. Hemorrhage may be the result of rupture of CNS blood vessels (due to hypertension) or ruptured aneurysm and arteriovenous malformations (AVMs).

Ischemic stroke

About 85% of strokes are of ischemic type. Cerebral **arterial occlusion** may cause **reduced blood supply** and ischemia of the specific area supplied by that artery. If ischemia continues **infarction** develops at that area.

Causes of Cerebral Infarction

Cerebral artery occlusion due to thrombus and embolus are responsible for 65% of all strokes.

- **Thrombosis**.
  - **Atherosclerosis:** Atherosclerosis predisposes to thrombosis and may occlude the lumen of the blood vessel. Cerebral infarction is mostly due to thrombosis in the major extracranial arteries (carotid artery and aortic arch), middle cerebral artery and basilar artery.
- **Embolism:** The most common type of emboli is thromboemboli. The origin of emboli may be:
  - **Heart:** The most common source of emboli is from thrombi in the heart chambers. Important predisposing factors for thrombi in the heart are myocardial infarct, valvular disease, and atrial fibrillation.
  - **Arteries:** Thromboemboli may arise from thrombus developed on atheromatous plaques within the carotid arteries.
  - **Other sources of emboli**.
    - Paradoxical emboli (e.g. in children with cardiac anomalies).
    - Other emboli like tumor, fat, or air.
- **Generalized arterial disease: Vasculitides** may lead to narrowing of lumen and cerebral infarcts. Vasculitis may be due to infections (e.g. syphilis and tuberculosis) or non-infectious (e.g. polyarteritis nodosa).

Morphology

Classification of infarcts: Infarcts are subdivided into two broad groups depending on the presence of hemorrhage.

- **Hemorrhagic (red) infarction:** It is characterized by multiple, petechial hemorrhages and is seen with embolic events.
- **Nonhemorrhagic (pale, bland, anemic) infarcts:** They are usually associated with thrombosis.

Gross:

- Initially, the infarcted area appears **pale, soft, and swollen**, with loss of boundary between normal and infarcted area.

  Later, the involved area of brain undergoes **liquefactive necrosis** and becomes **gelatinous and friable**. The boundary between normal and infarcted area becomes more prominent.

Microscopy of infarct:

- **Liquefactive necrosis** develops at the infarcted area with progressive infiltration by neutrophils.
- Later, neutrophils are replaced by macrophages, which remove all the necrotic tissue.
- **Hemorrhagic infarction**, in addition, shows blood extravasation and resorption.

Clinical features

Defects associated with infarction depend on the region of the brain involved rather than the cause. Neurologic symptoms referable to the area of injury usually develop rapidly, over minutes, and may continue to evolve over hours.

INTRACRANIAL HEMORRHAGE

It may be divided into **intracerebral** and **subarachnoid** type.

Intracerebral (Intraparenchymal) Hemorrhage (Fig. 28.1)

This is characterized by **hemorrhages within the brain parenchyma**. Majority are caused by rupture of a small intraparenchymal vessel. The major cause of **rupture of**

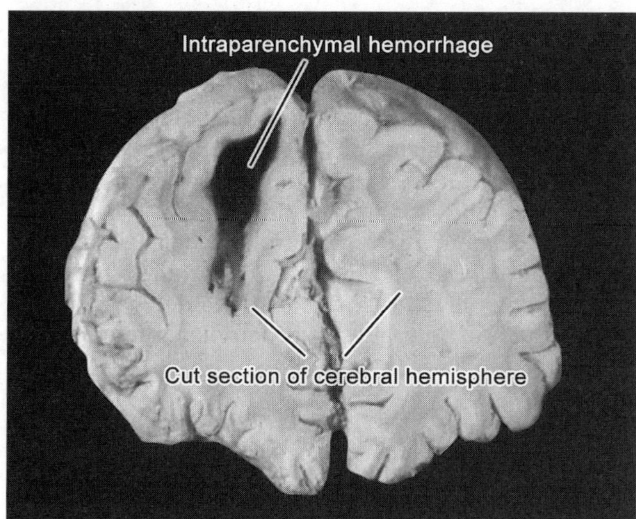

Fig. 28.1: Intraparenchymal hemorrhage appears as dark colored area on the left cerebral hemisphere

vessel is **hypertension**. They are usually spontaneous and occur in middle to late adult life (peak during 60 years of age).

Subarachnoid Hemorrhage

Subarachnoid **hemorrhage** refers to any bleeding **into the subarachnoid space**.

Causes

Subarachnoid hemorrhage may be due to:
- Rupture of a saccular (berry) aneurysm.
- Trauma.
- Extension of a hypertensive intracerebral hemorrhage into the ventricular system.
- Hematologic disorders.
- Vascular malformation.
- Neoplasms.

Clinical features

Subarachnoid hemorrhage is associated with sudden, severe headache followed by loss of consciousness.

PARAPLEGIA

Definition: Paraplegia is impairment in motor or sensory functions of the lower extremities. This results in complete paralysis of the lower half of the body including both legs.

Causes

- Trauma to spinal cord with damage.
- Non-traumatic and congenital factors:
  - Spinal tumors.
  - Scoliosis: It is an abnormal sideward curving of the bones of the spinal cord.
  - Congenital: Spina bifida is a birth defect in which parts of spinal bones do not come together properly that affects the neural elements of the spinal canal.

Areas involved: The area of the spinal canal that is affected in paraplegia is either the thoracic, lumbar, or sacral region.

Clinical features: Depending on the level and extent of spinal damage, paraplegic patients have varying degrees of loss of sensation in the affected limbs. Many patients with paraplegia are dependent on wheelchairs and other supportive measures. They also have various degrees of urinary and fecal incontinence.

Complications: The most common complications includes pressure sores (decubitus ulcers), thrombosis, and pneumonia.

In **quadriplegia both arms and both legs** are affected by paralysis. If only **one limb is affected**, it is termed as **monoplegia**.

HEMIPLEGIA

Definition: Hemiplegia is total paralysis of the arm, leg, and trunk on the one (same) side of the body.

Areas involved: If the damage is on the right side of the brain, the hemiplegia will be on the left side of the body and vice versa.

Causes: The common causes of hemiplegia are:
- In elderly individuals, **strokes** are the most common cause of hemiplegia.
- Other causes include spinal cord injury, brain infections (e.g. viral) and tumors.

Clinical Features

- Hemiplegia patients usually show a characteristic gait (Fig. 28.2).
  - The leg on the affected side is extended and internally rotated. It is swung in a wide, lateral arc rather than lifted in order to move it forward.
  - The upper limb on the same side is also adducted at the shoulder, flexed at the elbow. It is pronated (rotation of the hand so that the palm faces down or back) at the wrist with the thumb tucked into the palm and the fingers curled around it.
- Difficulty in balance while standing or walking.
- Having difficulty with motor activities like holding, grasping or pinching.

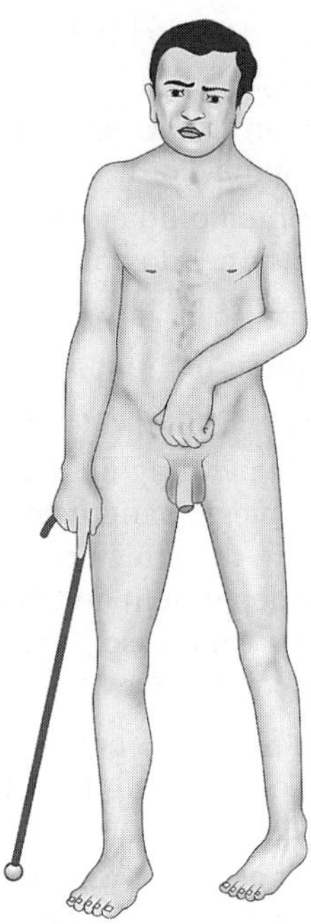

Fig. 28.2: Gait of patient with hemiplegia (left-sided)

- Increasing stiffness of muscles and muscle spasms.
- Difficulty in speech.
- Difficulty swallowing food.

Prognosis: Hemiplegia is not a progressive disorder, except in progressive lesions like a growing brain tumor. Once developed usually the symptoms do not worsen.

Complications: Muscle and joint stiffness, loss of aerobic fitness, muscle spasms, bed sores, pressure ulcers and thrombosis.

DEMYELINATING DISEASES

- Demyelinating diseases of the CNS are **acquired disorders** characterized by preferential **damage to myelin** with relative sparing of axons.
- Damage to myelin produces defect in the transmission of electrical impulses along axons.
- **Causes:**
  - **Immune-mediated destruction of myelin:** For example, **multiple sclerosis**, and infections.
  - **Inherited:** Disorders that affect synthesis or turnover of myelin components (e.g. leukodystrophies).

One of the demyelinating disease is multiple sclerosis.

Multiple Sclerosis

- **Multiple sclerosis (MS) is an autoimmune demyelinating disorder**.
- It is **characterized by distinct episodes of neurologic deficits**.
- Most common demyelinating disorder.
- Clinically manifest at any age. Females are affected twice as often males.
- **Clinical course**: Characterized by **relapses and remission** of variable duration (weeks to months to years) accompanied by neurologic defects, followed by gradual, partial recovery of neurologic function. The frequency of relapses tends to decrease during the course of time, but steady neurologic deterioration occurs.

Pathogenesis

- **Autoimmune disease due to immune response against components of the myelin sheath**.
- Involves both genetic and environmental factors.

Morphology

- Multiple sclerosis is a **disease of white matter of the brain and spinal cord.** The lesions are firmer than the surrounding white matter **(sclerosis)** and appear as well-circumscribed, glassy, gray-tan, irregularly shaped **plaques**. The area of demyelination often has sharply defined borders. The size of lesions varies.
- **Microscopy:**
  - **Active plaque shows myelin breakdown** associated with abundant macrophages containing lipid-rich, PAS-positive debris. Lymphocytes and monocytes are also present. Within a plaque there is relative preservation of axons.

Inactive plaques: As lesions become quiescent, the inflammatory cells slowly disappear. **No myelin is seen within inactive plaques**.

Clinical Features

- Lesions of MS can develop anywhere in the CNS and may show **wide range of clinical manifestations**.
- More common manifestations include **unilateral impairment of vision** due to involvement of the optic nerve (optic neuritis, retrobulbar neuritis), ataxia, nystagmus, and internuclear ophthalmoplegia.
- Spinal cord involvement produces **motor and sensory impairment** of trunk and limbs, spasticity, and difficulties with the voluntary control of bladder function.

NEURODEGENERATIVE DISEASES

- Neurodegenerative diseases are a group of disorders characterized by the **progressive loss of neurons**.

- Morphologic **hallmark** of these diseases is **the accumulation of protein aggregates.** The protein aggregates are resistant to degradation, localize within neurons, and elicit a stress response from the cell. They are often directly toxic to neurons.
- Microscopically, the protein aggregates **appear as** inclusions, which are the **diagnostic hallmark of the disease**.

Two examples of neurodegenerative diseases are Alzheimer disease (AD) and Parkinson disease.

Alzheimer Disease

- Alzheimer disease is the **most common cause of dementia in older adults.**
- Characterized by **progressive increase in the incidence with increasing age**.
- It may be **sporadic or familial** (5–10%).

Clinical manifestations: Insidious impairment of higher cognitive functions. As the disease progresses, deficits in memory, judgment, personality and language develops.

Pathogenesis

- The fundamental abnormality in AD is the **accumulation of two proteins (Aβ and tau) in the brain,** probably as **a result of excessive production and defective removal**.
- **Two pathologic hallmarks**:
  1. **Plaques** are deposits of aggregated Aβ peptides in the neuropil.
  2. **Tangles** are aggregates of the microtubule binding protein tau. This develops intracellularly and appears extracellularly after neuronal death.

Both plaques and tangles are responsible for the neural dysfunction.

Morphology

- **Gross:** Brain shows **cortical atrophy** characterized by widening of the cerebral sulci accompanied by compensatory ventricular enlargement.
- **Microscopy**:
  - **Neuritic (senile) plaques** are focal, spherical collections of dilated, tortuous, neuritic processes (dystrophic neurites).
  - **Neurofibrillary tangles** are bundles of filaments in the cytoplasm of the neurons that displace or encircle the nucleus.
  - Progressive, severe, neuronal loss accompanied by **reactive gliosis** in the region of plaques and tangles.

Clinical Features

- **Initial phase:** Forgetfulness and memory disturbances.
- **With progression:** The progression of AD is slow but relentless and manifests as language deficits, loss of mathematical skills, and loss of learned motor skills.
- **Final stages:** Patient becomes incontinent, mute, and unable to walk.

Parkinson Disease

- Parkinson disease (PD) is a **neurodegenerative disease** characterized by a **prominent hypokinetic movement disorder.**
- It is caused by **loss of dopaminergic neurons from the substantia nigra.**

Clinical Syndrome of Parkinsonism

- It is characterized by **diminished facial expression** (masked facies), **stooped posture, festinating gait** (progressively shortened, accelerated steps), **slowing of voluntary movement**, rigidity, and a **"pill-rolling" tremor**.
- Clinical syndrome of Parkinsonism is **found in many conditions that have in common damage to the nigrostriatal dopaminergic system.**

Presumptive diagnosis of PD: It is based on the central triad of parkinsonism: (1) tremor, (2) rigidity, and (3) bradykinesia—in the absence of a toxic or other known underlying etiology.

- Parkinson disease may be sporadic (majority) but in few genetic causes have been identified.

Morphology

- Characteristic finding is **pallor of the substantia nigra**.
- **Lewy bodies:** They may be found in some of the neurons. These are single or multiple cytoplasmic, eosinophilic, round to elongated inclusions.

CENTRAL NERVOUS SYSTEM TUMORS

Most common tumors of central nervous system are listed in Box 28.1.

Box 28.1: Common CNS tumors

- Gliomas
  - Astrocytoma
  - Oligodendroglioma
  - Ependymoma
- Poorly differentiated neoplasms
  - Medulloblastoma
- Tumors of meninges
  - Meningioma
- Metastatic tumors

Gliomas

Gliomas are the most common group of primary brain tumors. These tumors are derived from the glial tissue and include: astrocytomas, oligodendrogliomas and ependymomas.

Astrocytoma

It is a glioma **derived from astrocytes**. They form about 80% of primary brain tumors in adults.

- **Site:** Usually found in the cerebral hemispheres. Other sites include cerebellum, brain stem, and spinal cord.
- **Age:** Usually in the fourth to sixth decades.

Classification

Astrocytomas can be further categorized according to their histologic differentiation/grades, increasing anaplasia and clinical outcome into:

- **Diffuse astrocytoma (grade II)**.
- **Anaplastic astrocytoma (grade III)**.
- **Glioblastoma (grade IV)**.

Morphology

- **Diffuse astrocytoma** (grade II)
  - **Gross:** It is a **poorly demarcated** tumor which **infiltrates** into the **surrounding** normal **brain tissue. Cut surface** is **gray** in color and **firm.**
  - **Microscopy** (Fig. 28.3A): It is characterized by **glial tumor cells (astrocytes)** with variable degree of nuclear pleomorphism. The **background** is **fibrillary**.
- **Anaplastic astrocytomas** (grade III)
  - **Microscopy:** It shows **increased cellularity**, cellular and nuclear **pleomorphism, anaplasia**, presence of mitotic figures and rapid growth of the tumor.
- **Glioblastoma** (grade IV)
  - **Gross:** It shows **variable consistency and color.**

Microscopy (Fig. 28.3B)

It shows features **similar to anaplastic astrocytoma**. In addition, it also shows **serpentine (snake like) pattern of necrosis** surrounded by the palisading tumor cells which is known as **pseudopalisading** (garlanding) and **endothelial cell proliferation.**

Clinical features

The most common presenting signs and symptoms are seizures, headaches. The focal neurologic deficits are related to the anatomic site of involvement and growth rate of the tumor.

Prognosis

- Well-differentiated diffuse astrocytomas may remain static or progress only slowly over a number of years.
- Glioblastoma has a very poor prognosis.

Oligodendroglioma (WHO grade II)

It is one of the gliomas and constitutes 5–15% of gliomas.

Age

Most common during fourth and fifth decades.

Morphology

Gross: It is **well-circumscribed, gelatinous,** gray tumor. It is common in the white matter of the cerebral hemispheres.

Microscopy: The tumor consists of sheets of **small, round, and regular cells** with spherical nuclei. Nuclei are surrounded by a **clear halo** of cytoplasm giving rise to **fried egg appearance** to the cell. **Calcification** (calcospherites) is common.

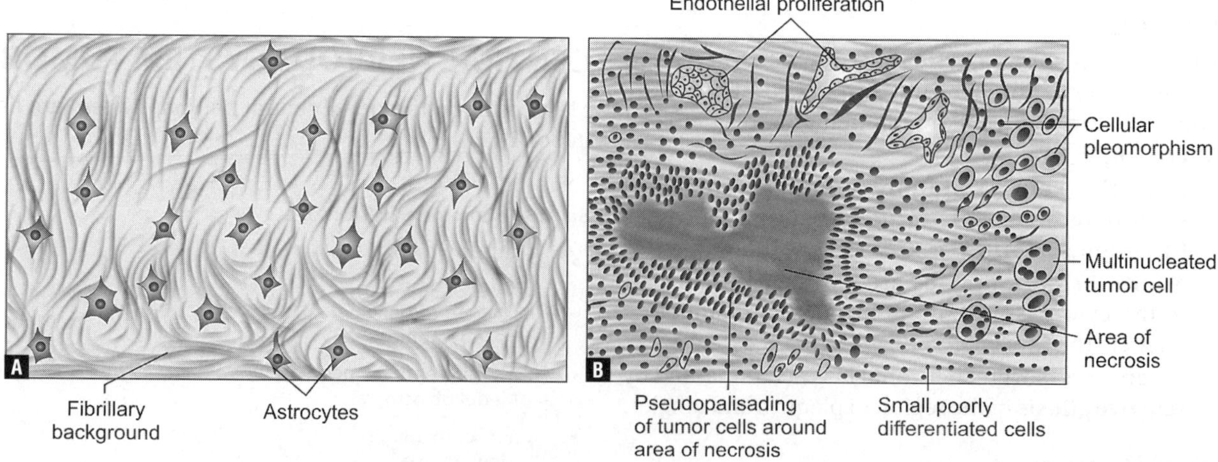

Figs 28.3A and B: Microscopic appearance (diagrammatic) of astrocytoma (A) and glioblastoma (B)

Poorly differentiated Neoplasms

Medulloblastoma

It is a highly malignant poorly differentiated neoplasm.

Age

Occurs predominantly in children; majority towards the end of the first decade.

Morphology

- **Gross:** It arises exclusively in the **cerebellum** as **well-circumscribed, gray and friable** tumor.
- **Microscopy (Fig. 28.4):** It is an extremely **cellular tumor** and consists of sheets of **small, anaplastic cells** with **scant cytoplasm and hyperchromatic nuclei**. **Homer-Wright rosettes** (pseudorosettes) may be seen.

Clinical features

Presents with cerebellar dysfunction and hydrocephalus.

Prognosis

Dissemination through the CSF is common and prognosis is poor.

Tumors of Meninges–Meningiomas

Meningiomas are **benign** intracranial tumors that arise from the meningothelial cells of the arachnoid.

Incidence: They account for about 20% of all primary intracranial neoplasms.

Age: Peak incidence is seen in fourth to fifth decades.

Sex: Female predominance (female-to-male ratio is 3:2).

Morphology

Site: It can occur at any intracranial site both on external surfaces of the brain as well as within the ventricular system.

Gross: Majority are **well-circumscribed**, rounded masses of variable size. They are usually attached to the dura with a well-defined broad base. They compress the underlying brain but do not infiltrate it, so that it can be easily separated.

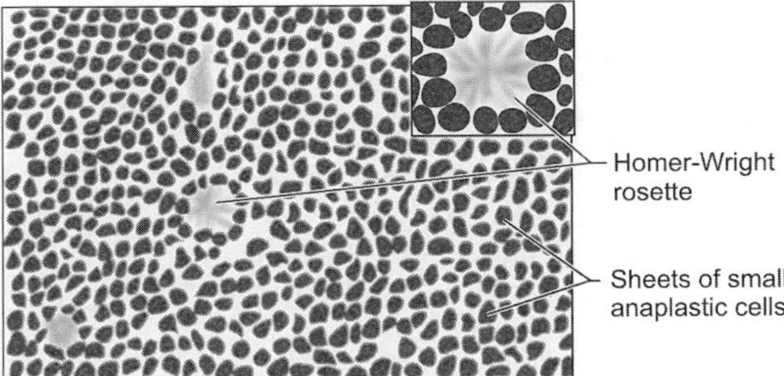

Fig. 28.4: Medulloblastoma (diagrammatic) composed sheets of small anaplastic cells and Homer-Wright rosette (inset)

Microscopy: The characteristic features of meningiomas are a **whorled pattern** of arrangement of meningothelial cells and the presence of **psammoma bodies** (laminated, spherical calcospherites).

- **Histological types:** Many histological types are seen, which do not have prognostic significance. **Syncytial (meningothelial)** type of tumor shows whorled clusters of polygonal cells without visible cell membranes (syncytial). The tumor cells have centrally placed oval nuclei. Other histological types are: **Fibroblastic, transitional/mixed, psammomatous, secretory, angioblastic,** etc.

Grade

Most of the meningiomas are considered as WHO grade I.

Metastatic Tumors

Metastatic tumors are the most common intracranial neoplasms.

Primary site: Mostly from carcinomas and the five most common primary sites are lung, breast, skin (melanoma), kidney and gastrointestinal tract.

Route of spread: Metastatic tumors reach the intracranial compartment through the bloodstream, generally in patients with advanced cancer.

Morphology

- **Gross** (Fig. 28.5): Brain metastases form **multiple, sharply demarcated masses**. They are usually seen at the **junction of gray matter and white matter**.

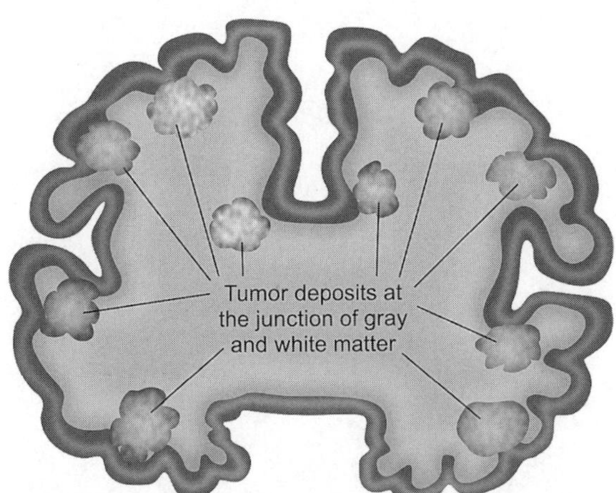

Fig. 28.5: Cross section of cerebral hemispheres showing multiple metastatic tumor deposits at the junction of gray and white matter

SELF-ASSESSMENT EXERCISE

I. Short Notes

1. Pyogenic meningitis.
2. Tuberculous meningitis.
3. Multiple sclerosis.
4. Alzheimer disease.
5. Parkinson disease.
6. Glioma.
7. Meningioma.

CHAPTER 29

Eye

CHAPTER OUTLINE

- Normal Structure
- Eyelids
- Orbit
- Conjunctiva
- Sclera
- Cornea
- Anterior Segment
- Uvea
- Retina and Vitreous
- Optic Nerve

NORMAL STRUCTURE

Different Parts of Eye-ball (Fig. 29.1)

The **globe of the eye** consists of three layers: the cornea-sclera, choroid-iris, and retina.

- **Cornea-sclera:** Cornea is transparent structure continuation of the conjunctiva over the cornea present in the anterior part of the eyeball. Sclera forms the outermost layer of eyeball.
- **Choroid:** Is the vascular membrane in contact with the sclera. The choroid is thickened anteriorly and forms ciliary body, ciliary processes and contains ciliary muscle.
- **Iris:** Is the continuation of the choroid which extends in front of the lens. It is structurally similar to the choroid but contains pigment cells.
- **Uveal tract:** Consists of three parts—the choroid and ciliary body posteriorly, and the iris anteriorly.
- **Retina:** Is part of the central nervous system and is composed of a number of layers of cells and their synapses. The **central fovea** is a specially differentiated region in the retina posteriorly. **Macula lutea or yellow spot** surrounds the central fovea. At the optic disc, the fibers of the nerve fiber layer of the retina pass into the optic nerve.

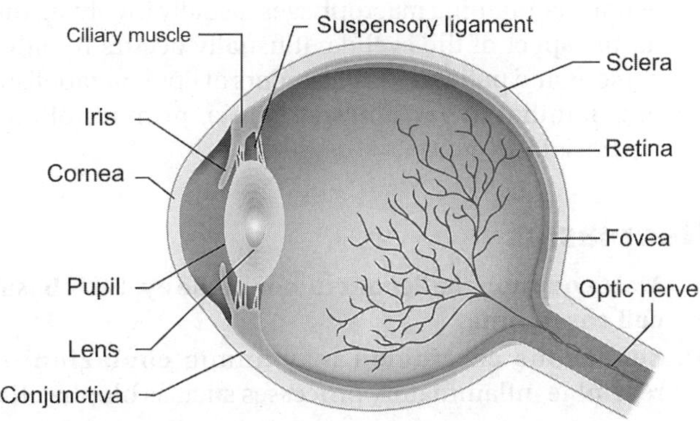

Fig. 29.1: Longitudinal section of eyeball (diagrammatic)

- **Lens:** Is biconvex mass.
- **Anterior chamber:** Is the space filled with the aqueous humor.
- **Posterior chamber:** Containing aqueous humor is the triangular space between the back of the iris, the anterior surface of the lens and the ciliary body.
- **Vitreous chamber:** Is the large space behind the lens containing gelatinous material, the vitreous humor.
- The intraocular pressure is normally 15–20 mm Hg.
- **Eyelids:** Are covered externally by the skin and internally by conjunctiva.
- **Lacrimal glands** are situated at the outer upper angle of the orbit.

EYELIDS

The eyelid is covered by skin on external aspect and mucosa (the conjunctiva) on the internal surface apposed to the eye. It covers and protects the eye. The important conditions affecting the eyelids include:

- **Blepharitis:** It is inflammation of the eyelids. It may be acute or chronic.
- **Hordeolum (or stye):** It is an acute, inflammatory, focal lesion of the eyelid. Acute inflammation involving the Meibomian glands is called as **hordeolum internum**, whereas acute folliculitis of the glands of Zeis is termed **hordeolum externum**.
- **Chalazion:** It is a granulomatous inflammation centered around the Meibomian glands or the glands of Zeis. It is due to granulomatous response against extruded lipid secretions and usually produces a painless swelling in the eyelid.
- **Xanthelasma (lipogranuloma):** It is a yellow plaque of lipid-containing macrophages, usually involving the nasal aspect of the eyelids. It usually occurs in older persons and patients with disorders of lipid metabolism (e.g. familial hypercholesterolemia, primary biliary cirrhosis).

Neoplasms

- **Most common malignant tumor of the eyelid is basal cell carcinoma.**
- **Sebaceous carcinoma** may mimic **chalazion** or resemble inflammatory processes such as blepharitis.

ORBIT

The orbit is a compartment that is closed medially, laterally, and posteriorly.

Physical and Chemical Injuries

Causes

- **Chemicals:** The eye may be injured by a variety of household and industrial caustic chemicals. The damage produced depends on the nature of the chemical.
- **Physical:** Blunt trauma may cause fracture of the bones in the floor of the orbit **(blowout fracture)**. The involvement of inferior rectus muscle in this fracture may cause sinking of the eye to sink into the orbit **(enophthalmos)**.
- **Foreign materials:** A foreign material may damage the eye during entry or because of secondary infection after the introduction of microorganisms. Some foreign bodies may produce acute inflammatory or granulomatous reaction. Others (e.g. those containing iron) may cause retinal degeneration and discoloration of ocular tissues **(siderosis bulbi)**.

Consequences

- **Trauma to eyelid:** may cause ecchymosis of the highly vascular eyelids (black eye).
- **Trauma to cornea:** Superficial disruptions of the corneal epithelium may occur following traumatic abrasions, prolonged wearing of a contact lens, foreign bodies on the eye and exposure to ultraviolet light.
- **Other complications:** For example, cataracts, retinal detachment and glaucoma.

Exophthalmos or Proptosis

Definition: Proptosis is an abnormal forward protrusion/ displacement of the eyeball. The **proptosis** refers to a unilateral protrusion of the eye, whereas it is termed as **exophthalmos** when it is bilateral.

Causes

Proptosis develops from lesions or pathologic changes in tissue that occupy space in the orbit. Most common cause is thyroid disease, orbital dermoid cysts and hemangiomas. Others include: inflammatory lesions, lymphomas, developmental anomalies, neoplasms and lesions of the paranasal sinuses and intracranial cavity.

- **Exophthalmos of hyperthyroidism** (Graves' disease): It usually occurs in early adult life. Females are more commonly affected than males (female-to-male ratio, 4:1).
- **Inflammatory pseudotumor: It is a chronic idiopathic inflammatory condition** associated with a variable degree of fibrosis.

Consequences

The proptotic eye might not be covered completely by the eyelids. Hence, the tear film might not be distributed evenly across the cornea. Chronic corneal exposure to air may predispose to corneal ulceration and infection.

Neoplasms

Most common primary neoplasms of the orbit are vascular in origin: The capillary hemangioma, cavernous hemangioma and the lymphangioma.

CONJUNCTIVA

Conjunctival hemorrhage: It may follow blunt trauma, anoxia or severe coughing.

Conjunctivitis

Inflammation of the conjunctiva may be infectious (viral or bacterial) **or allergic.**

Causes

- Microorganisms present on the surface of the eye may cause conjunctivitis, keratitis (corneal inflammation) or a corneal ulcer.
- **Hematogenous:** The conjunctiva may also become infected by hematogenous spread from a focus of infection elsewhere.
- **Iatrogenic eye infections:** For example, with adenovirus may follow ophthalmic manipulations, (e.g. corneal grafts, intraocular implantation of lens prostheses or use of infected eye drops or diagnostic instruments).

Clinical Features

Conjunctivitis is extremely common eye disease is characterized by hyperemic conjunctival blood vessels (pink eye).The inflammatory exudate accumulates in the conjunctival sac causing the eyelids to stick together in the morning. The conjunctival discharge may be purulent, fibrinous, serous or hemorrhagic.

Conjunctival Scarring

Most of bacterial or viral conjunctivitis cause redness and itching and **heal without sequelae**. Trachoma is a chronic, contagious conjunctivitis caused by *Chlamydia* **trachomatis. Trachoma may produce significant conjunctival scarring. This infection is the most common cause of blindness in the world.** Conjunctival scarring may develop following damage by alkalis or as a sequele to ocular cicatricial **pemphigoid**. The conjunctival scarring may occur iatrogenically through reaction to drugs or as a consequence of surgery.

Ophthalmia Neonatorum

Ophthalmia neonatorum is a **severe, acute conjunctivitis** with a copious purulent discharge, **occurring in the newborn, caused by** *Neisseria gonorrheae.* It can cause of blindness due to corneal ulceration, perforation, scarring and panophthalmitis. Infants acquire the infection usually when passing through the birth canal of an infected mother. Other causative organisms for ophthalmia neonatorum include other pyogenic bacteria and *C. trachomatis.*

Pinguecula and Pterygium

Both **pinguecula** and **pterygium** occur as submucosal elevations located in the sun-exposed regions of the conjunctiva (i.e. in the fissure between both the upper and lower eyelids—the interpalpebral fissure). They are caused due to actinic damage.

- **Pterygium:** It arises in the conjunctiva astride the limbus. It is formed by a submucosal growth of fibrovascular connective tissue that migrates onto the cornea. Pterygium does not cross the pupillary axis. It **grows horizontally onto the cornea in the shape of an insect wing (hence the name)**. Except for inducing mild astigmatism, it does not affect the vision. Most of pterygia are benign. But it is necessary to examine the excised tissue for histopathologic examination because, on occasion it may be the precursor of actinic induced neoplasms (e.g. squamous cell carcinoma and melanoma).
- **Pinguecula:** Similar to pterygium, it appears astride the limbus and appears as a small, yellowish submucosal elevation/lump usually located nasal to the corneoscleral limbus.

Neoplasms

- **Conjunctival nevi:** They are common and are seen in the fornix or over the palpebral conjunctiva.
- **Malignant neoplasm:** These include squamous neoplasms and melanocytic neoplasms.

SCLERA

The sclera consists of collagen and contains few blood vessels and fibroblasts.

Causes of blue appearance of sclera

- Following episodes of scleritis (inflammation of sclera).
- Sclera may be thinned in eyes with high intraocular pressure and the resulting lesion, known as a **staphyloma.**
- In osteogenesis imperfecta.
- In a heavily pigmented congenital nevus of the underlying uvea, a condition known as **congenital melanosis oculi.**

CORNEA

The cornea is anteriorly covered by epithelium that rests on a basement membrane. The Bowman layer, situated below the epithelial basement membrane is acellular and acts a barrier against the penetration of malignant cells from the epithelium into the underlying stroma.

The corneal stroma does not contain blood vessels and lymphatics. This feature is responsible for the transparency of the cornea and high rate of success of corneal transplantation.

Corneal vascularization may develop due to chronic corneal edema, inflammation, and scarring.

Keratitis and Ulcers

Inflammation of cornea is termed keratitis.

Causes

Various pathogens can cause corneal ulceration. These include **bacterial, fungal, viral (especially herpes simplex and herpes zoster), and protozoal *(Acanthamoeba)*.**

Corneal Degenerations and Dystrophies

Corneal disorders can be **divided into degenerations and dystrophies**.

Corneal degenerations may be either unilateral or bilateral and are usually nonfamilial (e.g. band keratopathy).

- **Band keratopathies:** Mainly two types.
  - **Calcific band keratopathy:** It is characterized by deposition of calcium in the Bowman layer. It may develop as a complication of chronic uveitis.
  - **Actinic band keratopathy:** It develops in individuals exposed chronically to high levels of ultraviolet light. It is characterized by sever solar elastosis in the superficial layers of corneal collagen in the sun-exposed inter-palpebral fissure.

Corneal dystrophies are usually bilateral and are hereditary.

ANTERIOR SEGMENT

Anterior chamber is bounded anteriorly by the cornea, laterally by the trabecular meshwork, and posteriorly by the iris. The lens is a closed epithelial system. The basement membrane of the lens epithelium (known as the lens capsule) totally envelops the lens. As the age increases, the size of the lens increases.

Cataract

Cataract is defined as opacity in the lens that may be congenital or acquired.

Causes: Cataracts are a major cause of visual impairment and blindness throughout the world. It may develop in various conditions.

- Systemic diseases: For example, galactosemia, diabetes mellitus, Wilson disease, and atopic dermatitis.
- Drugs: For example, corticosteroids.
- Others: Radiation, trauma, and many intraocular disorders.
- Age-related cataract is due to opacification of the lens nucleus (nuclear sclerosis).
- Physical agents: For example, heat, ultraviolet light, trauma, intraocular surgery and ultrasound.

Pathology

- During the development of cataracts, clefts appear between the lens fibers, and degenerated lens material accumulates in these spaces (morgagnian corpuscles, incipient cataract). Degenerated lens imbibe water and swell. The swollen lens may obstruct the pupil and cause glaucoma (phacomorphic glaucoma).
- In a **mature cataract**, the entire lens degenerates, and the debris escapes into the aqueous humor through the lens capsule. This reduces the volume of the lens (hypermature or morgagnian cataract).

Anterior Segment and Glaucoma

Definition: Glaucoma refers to a **collection of diseases characterized by distinctive changes in the visual field and in the cup of the optic nerve (optic neuropathy).**

Most of the glaucomas are associated with raised intraocular pressure **(ocular hypertension)**. However, some patients with normal intraocular pressure may develop characteristic optic nerve and visual field changes (normal or low-tension glaucoma).

Pathogenesis

Normally, the aqueous humor is produced by the ciliary body enters the posterior chamber. It passes from the posterior chamber through the pupil into the anterior chamber (between the iris and the cornea). From the anterior chamber most of the aqueous humor is drained into veins by way of the trabecular meshwork and the canal of Schlemm. A delicate balance between production and drainage of the aqueous humor maintains intraocular pressure within its physiologic range of 10–20 mm Hg. In certain pathologic states, the drainage of aqueous humor from the eye is impaired, and intraocular pressure increases. Temporary or permanent impairment of vision is produced from pressure-induced degenerative changes in the retina and optic nerve head and from edema and opacification of the cornea.

Classification of Glaucoma

Congenital glaucoma (infantile glaucoma, buphthalmos)

Congenital glaucoma is caused due obstruction to aqueous drainage by developmental anomalies. They are more common in boys (65%), and transmitted as an X-linked recessive mode of inheritance. It may be accompanied by a variety of other ocular malformations.

Adult-onset primary glaucoma

- In **open-angle (primary open-angle) glaucoma** the anterior chamber angle is open and appears normal. The aqueous humor has complete physical access to the trabecular meshwork. The intraocular pressure is raised due to the increased resistance to aqueous outflow in the open angle.
- In **angle-closure (primary closed-angle) glaucoma** the anterior chamber is shallower than normal, and the angle is abnormally narrow. The peripheral zone of the iris adheres to the trabecular meshwork and physically impedes the egress of aqueous humor from the eye.

Secondary glaucoma

Causes: For example, pseudoexfoliation glaucoma, neovascular glaucoma.

Endophthalmitis and Panophthalmitis

When there is intraocular inflammation, the vessels in the ciliary body and iris become leaky, allow cells and exudate to accumulate in the anterior chamber of the eye. The inflammatory cells may adhere to the corneal endothelium. These can be visualized with a slit lamp as visible **keratic precipitates**.

Complications: The presence of exudate in the anterior chamber can lead to adhesions between the iris and the trabecular meshwork or cornea **(anterior synechiae)** or between the iris and anterior surface of the lens **(posterior synechiae)**. Anterior synechiae can raise the intraocular pressure and may lead to optic nerve damage. The formation of synechiae can be prevented by inducing pupillary dilation in individuals with intraocular inflammation.

Endophthalmitis is the term used for inflammation within the vitreous humor. Endophthalmitis is classified as **exogenous** (external environmental agent gaining access to the interior of the eye through a wound) or **endogenous** (delivered to the eye hematogenously).

Panophthalmitis is the term applied to inflammation within the eye that involves the retina, choroid, and sclera and extends into the orbit.

UVEA

Uvea consists of iris, the choroid and ciliary body. The choroid is the most richly vascularized sites in the body.

Uveitis

Uveitis is the term used for any type of inflammation in one or more of the tissues that compose the uvea. Inflammation of the uvea **(uveitis)** also encompasses inflammation of the iris **(iritis)**, the ciliary body **(cyclitis)** and the iris plus the ciliary body **(iridocyclitis)**. Clinically, the term **uveitis** is restricted to chronic diseases that may be either components of a systemic process or localized to the eye. Uveitis may involve the anterior segment (e.g. in **juvenile rheumatoid arthritis**) or may affect both the anterior and posterior segments.

Causes: Uveitis is usually accompanied by retinal pathology. Uveitis may be caused by infectious agents (e.g. *Pneumocystis carinii*), may be idiopathic (e.g. sarcoidosis), or may be autoimmune in origin (sympathetic ophthalmia). Numerous infectious processes can affect the choroid or the retina. Inflammation in one compartment is typically associated with inflammation in the other. Retinal *toxoplasmosis* is usually accompanied by uveitis and even scleritis. Individuals with AIDS may develop cytomegalovirus retinitis and uveal infection such as *Pneumocystis* or mycobacterial choroiditis.

Examples are described later.

Granulomatous Uveitis

It is a common complication of sarcoidosis.

- In the anterior segment it gives rise to an exudate that evolves into "mutton-fat" keratic precipitates.
- In the posterior segment, sarcoid may involve the choroid and retina. The sarcoid granulomas may be seen in the choroid. Retina shows perivascular inflammation which on ophthalmoscopic examination produces "candle wax drippings."

Diagnostic biopsy: Conjunctival biopsy may show granulomatous inflammation and confirm the diagnosis of ocular sarcoid.

Sympathetic Ophthalmia

It is a noninfectious uveitis limited to the eye. It is characterized by bilateral granulomatous inflammation that affects all components of the uvea (panuveitis).

Etiopathogenesis: May complicate a penetrating injury of the eye. It is a delayed hypersensitivity reaction or autoimmune disorder that affects not only the injured eye but also the contralateral, noninjured (sympathizing) eye. It may develop from 2 weeks to many years after injury.

Pathology: It is characterized by diffuse granulomatous inflammation of the uvea (choroid, ciliary body, and iris).

Treatment: Sympathetic ophthalmia is treated by the systemic immunosuppressive agents.

Neoplasms

- **Most common intraocular malignancy of adults is metastasis to the uvea (typically to the choroid).** Metastases to the eye are associated with short survival, and treatment is usually by palliative radiotherapy.
- **Uveal melanoma is the most common primary** intraocular malignancy of adults.

RETINA AND VITREOUS

The retina responds to injury by means of gliosis. Retina has no lymphatics.

Retinal Hemorrhage

Appearance

- Hemorrhages in the nerve fiber layer of the retina are oriented horizontally. They appear as streaks or "flames" on fundoscopy.
- Hemorrhages in the external retinal layers are oriented perpendicular to the retinal surface. These hemorrhages appear as round/dots (the tips of cylinders).

Cause: It may occur in both local and systemic diseases. Important causes of retinal hemorrhages are hypertension, diabetes mellitus, central retinal vein occlusion, bleeding diatheses and trauma.

Retinal Detachment

Retinal detachment is **separation of the neurosensory retina from the retinal pigment epithelium (RPE).**

During fetal development, the space between the neurosensory retina and the retinal pigment epithelium (RPE) is obliterated when these two layers become apposed. However, the neurosensory retina may get separated from the retinal pigment epithelium when fluid (liquid vitreous, hemorrhage or exudate) accumulates within the potential space between these two structures. Such a separation is a common cause of visual impairment and blindness. Laser therapy and surgical management has improved the prognosis for patients with retinal detached.

Etiology

Retinal detachment **follows intraocular hemorrhage** (e.g. after trauma) and develop as a **complication of cataract extractions** and many **other ocular operations.**

Predisposing factors: Include retinal defects (due to trauma or certain retinal degenerations), vitreous traction, diminished pressure on the retina (e.g. after vitreous loss) and weakening of the fixation of the retina.

Consequences: Normally, the photoreceptors and retinal pigment epithelium function as a unit. After retinal detachment, oxygen and nutrients that normally reach the outer retina from the choroid must diffuse across a greater distance. This leads to the degeneration of photoreceptors.

Pathology

Retinal detachment **is broadly classified by etiology based on the presence or absence of a break in the retina into two** varieties.

- **Rhegmatogenous retinal detachment:** This type of retinal detachment is associated with a full thickness retinal defect. Retinal tears may develop after the vitreous collapses with degenerative changes in the vitreous body or peripheral retina. Liquefied vitreous humor then seeps through the tear and gains to the potential space between the neurosensory retina and the RPE.
- **Non-rhegmatogenous retinal detachment (retinal detachment without retinal break):** It may develop as a complication of retinal vascular disorders associated with significant exudation. It may also occur in any condition that damages the RPE and permits fluid to leak from the choroidal circulation under the retina.

Retinal Vascular Disease

Hypertension

Normally, the thin walls of retinal arterioles allow direct visualization of the circulating blood by ophthalmoscopy. Increased blood pressure commonly affects the retina, and produces changes which can be seen with the ophthalmoscope. The changes in hypertension includes: (1) arteriolar narrowing, (2) hemorrhages in the retinal nerve fiber layer (flame-shaped hemorrhages), and (3)exudates, including some that radiate from the center of the macula (macular star), (4) fluffy white bodies in the superficial retina (cotton-wool spots) and (5) microaneurysms (Fig 29.2).

- In **retinal arteriolosclerosis** (characterized by the thickening of the arteriolar wall) the vessels may

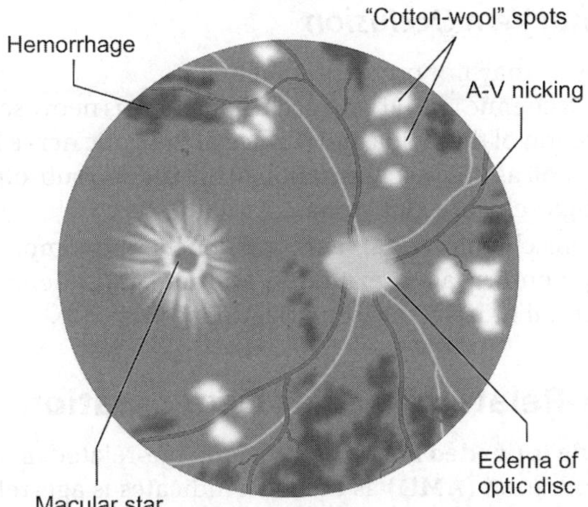

Fig. 29.2: Various features of hypertensive retinopathy

appear narrowed, and the color of the blood column may change from bright red to copper and to silver (depending on the degree of vascular wall thickness). Since retinal arterioles and veins share a common adventitial sheath, in severe retinal arteriolosclerosis the arteriole may compress the vein at points where both vessels cross. Venous stasis distal to arteriolar-venous crossing may occlude the retinal vein branches.

- In **malignant hypertension** vessels in the retina and choroid may be damaged. Damage to choroidal vessels **may produce focal infarcts in the choroid** which is clinically observed as *Elschnig spots*. Damage to the choriocapillaris may damage the overlying RPE and allow the exudate to accumulate in the potential space between the neurosensory retina and the RPE. This may result in **retinal detachment. Exudate** resulting from damaged retinal arterioles usually accumulates in the outer plexiform layer of the retina. The ophthalmoscopic finding of a **macular star** (a spoke like arrangement of exudate in the macula) in malignant hypertension is due to accumulation of exudate in the outer plexiform layer of the macula. Occlusion of retinal arterioles may produce infarcts of the nerve fiber layer of the retina. Accumulation of mitochondria at the swollen ends of damaged axons of nerve fibers produces **cytoid bodies.** Collections of cytoid bodies in the infarcted area are seen ophthalmoscopically as "cotton-wool spots".

Diabetes Mellitus

The eye is commonly affected in diabetes mellitus. Thickening of the basement membrane of the epithelium of the pars plicata of the ciliary body is a reliable histologic marker of diabetes mellitus in the eye and is similar to changes in the glomerular mesangium.

Morphology

One of the most important morphologic features of diabetes mellitus is **diffuse thickening of basement membranes**. The thickening is most evident in the capillaries of the skin, skeletal muscle, retina, renal glomeruli, and renal medulla. Though there is increase in the thickness of basement membranes, **diabetic capillaries are more leaky than normal to plasma proteins.** The **disease of small vessels (capillaries) is termed microangiopathy**. The retinal vasculopathy of diabetes mellitus may be classified as (1) **nonproliferative** and (2) **proliferative diabetic retinopathy**.

- **Nonproliferative diabetic retinopathy:** It consists of a spectrum of changes resulting from structural and functional abnormalities of retinal vessels. The **basement membrane of retinal blood vessels is thickened. Microaneurysms** are an important manifestation of diabetic microangiopathy. They are usually smaller than the resolution of direct ophthalmoscopes, and these microaneurysms observed under ophthalmoscope may in fact be retinal microhemorrhages. The retinal microcirculation in diabetics may be leakier, and produce **macular edema**, which is a common cause of visual loss in diabetic patients. The vascular changes may also produce **exudates** that accumulate in the outer plexiform layer. Degeneration of pericytes and some loss of endothelial cells are found.
- **Proliferative diabetic retinopathy:** After many years, diabetic non-proliferative retinopathy may become proliferative. Proliferative diabetic retinopathy is defined by the **appearance of new vessels** called as **retinal neovascularization**. It is a prominent feature of diabetic retinopathy in which new vessels sprout on the surface of either the optic nerve head ("neovascularization of the disc) or the surface of the retina (neovascularization elsewhere). The term "retinal neovascularization" is used when the newly formed vessels breach the internal limiting membrane of the retina. The newly formed friable vessels **bleed easily**, and **produce vitreal hemorrhages** which can obscure vision. Diabetic retinopathy, glaucoma and age-related maculopathy are the leading causes of irreversible blindness.

Retinopathy of Prematurity (Retrolental Fibroplasia)

Normally, the temporal (lateral) aspect of the retinal periphery is incompletely vascularized whereas the medial aspect is vascularized. This is a developmental disorder occurring in premature or low-birth-weight infants who have been given oxygen-therapy at birth. The basic defect is developmental prematurity of the retinal blood vessels which are extremely sensitive to high dose of oxygen-therapy. They develop constriction of immature retinal vessels in the temporal aspect resulting in ischemia of retinal tissue distal to this constriction. Retinal ischemia may lead to retinal angiogenesis. Contraction of the resulting peripheral retinal neovascular membrane may "drag" the temporal aspect of the retina toward the peripheral zone. This displaces the macula (situated temporal to the optic nerve) laterally. Neovascular membrane contraction may produce sufficient force to cause retinal detachment.

Sickle Retinopathy, Retinal Vasculitis, Radiation Retinopathy

Retinopathy affecting patients with sickle cell anemia is divided into two types that roughly parallel those used for diabetic retinopathy: nonproliferative (intraretinal angiopathic changes) and proliferative (retinal neovascularization). The final common pathway in both types is vascular occlusion. Low oxygen tension within the blood vessels in the retinal periphery results in sickling of red cells and microvascular occlusions.

Retinal Artery and Vein Occlusions

Retinal Artery Occlusion

The central retinal artery or its branches may be occluded by disorders of the vessels in general. For example, the central retinal artery lumen may be narrowed by atherosclerosis and may predispose to thrombosis. Emboli to the central retinal artery can originate from thrombi in the heart or from ulcerated atheromatous plaques in the carotid arteries. Fragments of atherosclerotic plaques can occlude the retinal circulation.

Consequences

- Total occlusion of the central retinal artery can produce a **diffuse infarct** of the retina.
- Complete occlusion of a branch of retinal artery can produce a segmental infarct of the retina.
- When the blood supply to retina is suddenly blocked (acute occlusion), the retina swells acutely and becomes optically opaque. Following an, the retina appears relatively opaque by ophthalmoscopy.
- The central retinal artery occlusion produces **cherry-red spot**. However, it can also be seen in rare storage diseases such as **Tay-Sachs** and **Niemann-Pick** diseases.

Retinal Vein Occlusion

It may or may not produce ischemia.

- In ischemic retinal vein occlusion, there is neovascularization of the retina and surface of the optic nerve head as well as neovascularization of the iris and subsequent angle-closure glaucoma.
- Nonischemic retinal vein occlusion may be complicated by hemorrhages, exudates, and macular edema and retinal or iris neovascularization is very rare.

Age-Related Macular Degeneration

Macula is needed for central vision. Age-related macular degeneration **(AMD)** as the term indicates is age-related degeneration of the macula. Advancing age is a risk factor and its incidence in individuals 75 years of age and older is 8%.

Types: There are two forms of AMD namely dry and wet. They are **distinguished by the presence of neoangiogeneis in the wet form and its absence in the dry form.**

- **Atrophic or "dry" AMD:** It is characterized ophthalmoscopically by diffuse or discrete deposits in the Bruch membrane (drusen) and geographic atrophy of the RPE. Loss of vision is severe in these individuals and there is no neoangiogenesis.
- **Neovascular or "wet" AMD:** It is characterized by **choroidal neovascularization**, defined by the presence of angiogenic vessels which penetrate through the Bruch membrane beneath the retinal pigment epithelium (RPE).

Etiology: Age-related maculopathy is a multifactorial disease in which environmental and genetic factors contribute. Risk factors include advancing age, smoking, carotid/cardiovascular disease and elevated serum cholesterol levels.

Other Retinal Degenerations

Retinitis Pigmentosa

Retinitis pigmentosa (pigmentary retinopathy) is an inherited condition due to mutations in genes that affect rods and cones, or RPE. It can cause **varying degrees of visual impairment including, in some cases, total blindness.** The term "retinitis" is a misnomer since inflammation of the retina is not a feature of this disease.

Etiology: Retinitis pigmentosa may develop due to mutations in over 60 genes that regulate the functions of either the photoreceptor cells or the RPE. They may be inherited as X-linked recessive, autosomal recessive, or autosomal dominant.

Pathology: In retinitis pigmentosa, there is destruction of rods (lead to early night blindness), and subsequently cones (may affect the central visual acuity).by apoptosis. It is followed by migration of retinal pigment epithelial cells into the sensory retina (thus accounting for the "pigmentosa" in the disease name). Melanin accumulates mainly around small branching retinal blood vessels like spicules of bone. The retinal blood vessels then gradually undergo constriction, and the optic nerve head undergo atrophy and produces characteristic waxy pallor of the optic disc.

Retinitis

A variety of pathogens can produce infectious retinitis. Hematogenous spread of pathogens to the retina usually produces multiple retinal abscesses. Cytomegalovirus retinitis is an important cause of visual morbidity in immunocompromised individuals (e.g. AIDS).

Retinal Neoplasms

Retinoblastoma (*refer page 291 chapter 23*)

Retinal Lymphoma

Primary retinal lymphoma is an aggressive tumor. It occurs in older individuals and may clinically mimic uveitis. Microscopically, most are diffuse large B-cell lymphomas. They spread to the brain commonly through the optic nerve.

OPTIC NERVE

Anterior Ischemic Optic Neuropathy

Anterior ischemic optic neuropathy (AION) includes a spectrum of injuries to the optic nerve that ranges from ischemia to infarction. Transient partial obstruction of blood flow to the optic nerve can produce episodes of transient loss of vision, whereas total obstruction in blood flow can lead to an optic nerve infarct which may be segmental or total. Zones of relative ischemia may surround segmental infarcts of the optic nerve. Optic nerve function in this relatively ischemic region without infarct may recover whereas the optic nerve in the infarcted area does not regenerate and visual loss from infarction is permanent.

Papilledema

Papilledema is the **bilateral edema of the head of the optic nerve**.

Cause: It may develop as **consequence of compression of the nerve. Raised cerebrospinal fluid pressure surrounding the optic nerve results in bilateral edema of the optic discs.** It is usually bilateral and is commonly termed *papilledema*. Usually, acute papilledema due to increased intracranial pressure does not cause loss of vision.

Primary neoplasm of the optic nerve when swelling of the nerve head produces unilateral disc edema.

Ophthalmoscopically, the optic nerve head is swollen and hyperemic.

Glaucomatous Optic Nerve Damage

Majority of patients with glaucoma have raised intraocular pressure. However, **few patients develop the visual field and optic nerve changes typical of glaucoma with normal intraocular pressure *(normal-tension glaucoma)*.** Conversely, some patients with raised elevated intraocular pressure may never develop visual field changes or optic nerve cupping.

Morphology

- Diffuse loss of ganglion cells.
- Thinning of the retinal nerve fiber layer.
- Optic nerve cupping and atrophy in advanced stage.

Other Optic Neuropathies

Optic neuropathy may be primary/**inherited or may be secondary**. Causes of secondary optic neuropathies include nutritional deficiencies or toxins (e.g. methanol).

Optic Neuritis

Many unrelated conditions were grouped under the term of optic neuritis. Commonly, the term optic neuritis is used to describe a loss of vision secondary to demyelinization of the optic nerve. One of the important causes of optic neuritis is multiple sclerosis and optic neuritis may be the first manifestation of this disease.

The End-Stage Eye: Phthisis Bulbi

Phthisis bulbi is term used for a **nonspecific, end-stage eye** that is **internally** disorganized and **small (atrophic)**. Congenitally small eyes (hypoplastic or **microphthalmic** eyes) are usually not disorganized internally.

Causes: Many conditions can give rise phthisis bulbi. These include **trauma, intraocular inflammation, and chronic retinal detachment**.

Morphology: Eyes afflicted with phthisis bulbi are enucleated (removed). Phthisical eyes show the following changes:

- Presence of exudate or blood between the ciliary body and sclera and the choroid and sclera **(ciliochoroidal effusion)**.
- Presence of a membrane extending across the eye from one aspect of the ciliary body to the other *(cyclitic membrane)*. The choroid and ciliary body are separated from the sclera. The cornea is flattened, shrunken and opaque.
- Intraocular contents are disorganized by diffuse scarring and with retinal detachment.
- Optic nerve atrophy.
- Presence of intraocular bone, which is probably due to osseous metaplasia of the RPE. This causes extreme hardening of the eyes.
- Sclera is thickened sclera (especially posteriorly) and shows wrinkling and indentation owing to loss of intraocular pressure.
- If present, the lens is displaced and often calcified.

SELF-ASSESSMENT EXERCISE

I. Short Notes

1. Cataract.
2. Glaucoma.
3. Sympathetic ophthalmia.
4. Retinal changes in hypertension.
5. Retinal changes in diabetes.
6. Age-related macular degeneration (AMD).
7. Retinitis pigmentosa.
8. Papilledema.
9. Phthisis bulbi.

SECTION

3

Clinical Pathology

CHAPTER

30

Anticoagulants and Hemoglobin Estimation

CHAPTER OUTLINE

- ➢ Anticoagulants
- ➢ Collection of Blood
- ➢ Hemoglobin Estimation

ANTICOAGULANTS

Blood coagulates when withdrawn from the vessel and anticoagulants are used to prevent blood from clotting. Commonly used anticoagulants are:

Calcium Chelating Agents

These anticoagulants act by binding to calcium present in the blood. Since, calcium is essential for many of the steps in the clotting mechanism, chelation (removal) of calcium prevents clotting.

Ethylenediaminetetraacetic Acid (EDTA)

- **Advantages:** EDTA **preserves the morphology** of the blood cells up to 3 hours and cell counts up to 12 hours after collection of the blood.
- **Disadvantages:** It is **not suitable for coagulation studies.**
- **Uses:** It is the **anticoagulant of choice** for all cell counts and peripheral smear.

Oxalate

Potassium oxalate shrinks RBCs and **ammonium oxalate** causes swelling of RBCs. They are not recommended for hematological investigations.

Double oxalate: To balance the shrinking effect of potassium oxalate and the swelling effect of ammonium oxalate, the two are combined in a mixture in the ratio of two parts of potassium oxalate to three parts of ammonium oxalate Nowadays, they are not used.

Sodium Citrate

Since, it is used as a liquid which results in dilution of cellular elements, it is not suitable for cell counts, and hemoglobin (Hb) estimation.

Uses

- **Coagulation studies**
- **ESR by Westergren method**
- **Blood bank:** Citrate phosphate dextrose adenine (CPDA) used as anticoagulant.

Sodium Fluoride

Sodium fluoride acts an antiglycolytic agent which inhibits the use of glucose by blood cells. It is used for estimation of **blood sugar**.

Heparin

Heparin is used when almost instantaneous (immediate) anticoagulation is required.

Disadvantages

- Expensive.
- Causes clumping of platelets and leukocytes, so it is not used for automated cell counters.
- Imparts bluish discoloration to the background of peripheral blood smears.
- Prevents coagulation for only a limited period of time and its effect slowly disappears.

Uses

- Osmotic fragility test done for diagnosis of hereditary spherocytosis.
- Red cell enzyme studies like G6PD deficiency.
- Electrolyte estimation.
- Arterial blood gas analysis.

COLLECTION OF BLOOD

The blood for the tests is collected in specific container or vacuum tubes which have a colored top (Fig. 30.1). It is essential to use appropriate vacuum tubes with proper ratio of anticoagulant.

Type of Blood Sample

Certain blood chemistry tests require fasting blood sample. For the fasting blood sample, the patient should fast overnight for 8–10 hours. Intake of water is allowed during fasting. The blood sample required may be whole blood, serum or plasma.

Whole Blood

Uses

- For complete hemogram (hemoglobin, ESR, platelet count, reticulocyte count, and peripheral smear evaluation).
- Osmotic fragility test, estimation of HbF (fetal hemoglobin) Hb electrophoresis, Coombs test, etc.

Serum

Serum is obtained by allowing the blood to clot in a tube or in a vial (without adding any anticoagulant).

Uses

- Estimation of bilirubin, creatinine, uric acid, proteins, albumin, globulin, etc.
- Serum enzyme levels like alkaline phosphatase, acid phosphatase, aspartate (AST/SGOT) and alanine aminotransferase (ALT/SGPT).

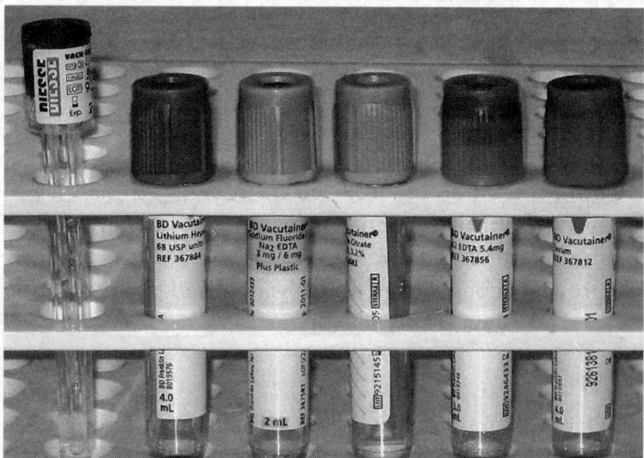

Fig. 30.1: Different types of vacuum tubes and their anticoagulants mentioned in brackets. Black (citrate), green (heparin), gray (fluoride), light blue (sodium citrate), purple (EDTA) and red (without anticoagulant)

- Serum electrophoresis of proteins, lipoproteins and immunoglobulins.

Plasma

Plasma is obtained by centrifugation of the anticoagulated blood (e.g. citrated blood collected for coagulation studies). Red blood cells form the sediment and the supernatant is the plasma.

Uses

- Coagulation studies: Prothrombin time (PT), activated partial thromboplastin time (APTT), thrombin time.
- Assay of various coagulation factors like factor VIII, IX.
- Assay of FDP and D-dimer as in disseminated intravascular coagulation.
- Confirmation of hemoglobinemia where plasma is colored red (e.g. PNH).
- For biochemical investigations like blood glucose.

Methods of Blood Collection

Blood may be collected as follows:

Venous Blood

- It is usually collected from the antecubital vein either by a disposable syringe or vacuum tubes.
- Clean the skin of the antecubital area of the arm with an alcohol swab and allow it to dry.
- Apply a tourniquet about 2 inches above the selected venous puncture site.

By syringe

- Insert the needle of the syringe into the vein.
- Collect the required amount of blood in the syringe.
- Discharge the blood from the syringe into appropriate vial.
- Pour one drop each on 2–3 glass slides and prepare peripheral blood smears.

By vacuum tubes

These are nowadays used in most of the laboratories instead of syringes. The different types of vacuum tubes are shown in Figure 30.1.

Capillary Blood

Capillary blood may be collected either from the finger or heel.

Finger prick method: Using sterile disposable lancet/needle, prick on the lateral side of the tip of the finger (middle or ring) so that blood starts flowing. The free flowing blood is collected in the hemoglobinometer pipette for hemoglobin estimation, total WBC count, platelet count, etc. Peripheral smears are also prepared by placing a drop of blood on one end of the glass slide.

Heel prick method: This method is usually employed for collecting blood from infants.

HEMOGLOBIN ESTIMATION

Hemoglobin is a molecule composed of iron containing pigment called heme and protein globin. One of the important features of anemia is the reduction in the hemoglobin (Hb).

Methods of Hemoglobin Estimation

There are several methods for Hb estimation utilizing different principles. The commonly used methods include colorimetric method namely Sahli's and cyanmethemoglobin method and automated analyzer.

- **Colorimetric methods:** Sahli's method, cyanmethemoglobin method.
- **Physical method:** Specific gravity method.
- **Chemical method:** Iron content of hemoglobin.
- **Gasometric method:** Oxygen combining capacity of hemoglobin.
- **Automated analyzer (Cell counter).**

Colorimetric Methods

Sahli's Method or Acid Hematin Method (Fig. 30.2).

This is the most popular visual colorimetric method.

Principle

When blood is added to N/10 HCl, **hemoglobin is converted into brown colored acid hematin.** The intensity of brown color depends on the amount of hemoglobin.

Technique

- Take N/10 HCl with a dropper into the hemoglobinometer tube upto the lowest mark.
- Draw blood up to 20 cu mm (0.02 mL) mark of Hb (hemoglobin) pipette.
- Blood in the Hb pipette is blown into the hemoglobinometer tube.
- Wait for 10 minutes for the acid to act on the RBCs which causes lysis of RBCs liberating hemoglobin. The acid converts Hb to acid hematin.
- With the help of a glass rod, mix the acid hematin. Place the hemoglobinometer tube into the comparator.

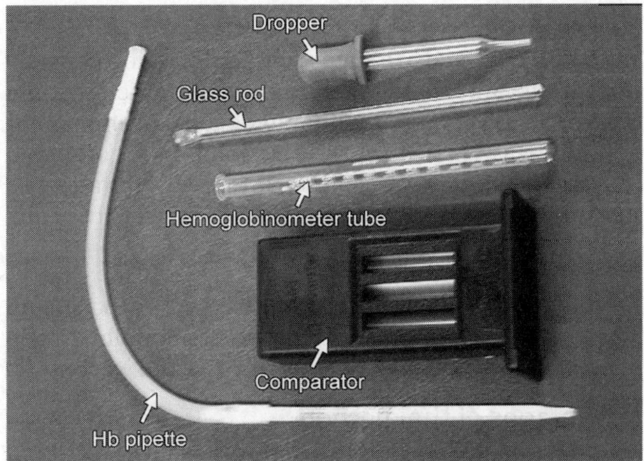

Fig. 30.2: Sahli's hemoglobinometer consisting of Hb pipettes, comparator, hemoglobinometer tube, glass rod and dropper

- Match the color of the solution in the tube with that of the comparator by holding against the natural light or fluorescent tube light.
- Take the tube out of comparator and remove the glass rod. Take the reading from the lower meniscus.
- Hemoglobin is recorded as g/dL (or g%).

Sources of error

- **Technical errors:** Improper venipuncture (puncture of a vein to obtain a specimen of blood) technique and improper mixing of blood sample may give rise to falsely low or high hemoglobin value.
- **Visual errors:** Comparison of colors is very subjective and can vary from person to person. Hence, the results may not be accurate.

Disadvantages of the method

- It is **not an accurate method** and hydrochloric acid **does not convert all hemoglobins** (like carboxyhemoglobin, methemoglobin and sulphemoglobin) into acid hematin. Thus, Hb value obtained may be slightly lower than the actual Hb.

Advantages of the method

Simple, easy and cheap method.

Normal range of hemoglobin: Males 13–17 g/dL, females 12–15 g/dL, newborns 14–19 g/dL.

Cyanmethemoglobin (Hemiglobincyanide) Method

Cyanmethemoglobin is the **most accurate** and preferred method for estimation of hemoglobin concentration. It is the standard method used in most of the laboratories.

Principle

The blood is diluted in a stable standard solution of potassium ferricyanide and potassium cyanide. Hemoglobin is converted to stable cyanmethemoglobin hemiglobincyanide (HiCN). The color of this solution is compared against a standard HiCN solution of known Hb value in a spectrophotometer or photoelectric colorimeter at 540 nm.

Reagent

The diluent is **Drabkin solution** which consists of potassium ferrocyanide, potassium cyanide, potassium dihydrogen phosphate, non-ionic detergent and distilled water.

Advantages of the method

Hb value obtained is **accurate** since almost all forms of hemoglobin (hemoglobin, oxyhemoglobin, methemoglobin, carboxyhemoglobin, but not sulphemoglobin) are converted into cyanmethemoglobin. **No visual error** during matching the color.

Disadvantages of the method

Turbidity interferes with the reading, and the Drabkin's diluent is poisonous and explosive.

Automated Analyzer (Cell Counter)

These instruments measure not only hemoglobin but also various parameters like cell counts, [(Packed cell volume (PCV)] and absolute values [Mean corpuscular volume (MCV), Mean corpuscular hemoglobin (MCH) and Mean corpuscular hemoglobin concentration (MCHC)].

SELF-ASSESSMENT EXERCISE

I. **Short Note**
   1. Anticoagulants.
   2. Hemoglobin estimation.
   3. Methods of collection of blood.

CHAPTER

31

Blood Cell Counts

CHAPTER OUTLINE

INTRODUCTION

Red blood cells, white blood cells and platelets are the formed elements of blood. Their counts are altered in various diseases.

Hemogram (Complete blood counts): It includes hemoglobin, RBC count, total leukocyte count, platelet count, differential leukocyte count, PCV, ESR and peripheral smear examination.

Hemocytometer: The hemocytometer (Fig. 31.1) is an instrument used for counting blood cells. It consists of **RBC pipette, WBC pipette and improved Neubauer counting chamber** (Figs 31.1 and 31.2).

RED BLOOD CELL COUNT

Red blood cell count (RBC) count can be measured by manual method using an improved Neubauer counting chamber or by automated analyzer.

Manual Method

RBC pipette (Thoma red cell pipette): It consists of a graduated capillary tube divided into 10 parts marked 0.5 at the fifth mark and 1.0 at the tenth mark. The capillary tube opens into a mixing bulb containing a

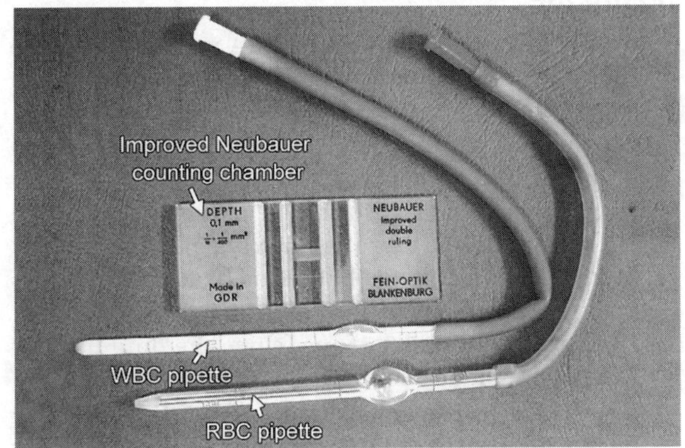

Fig. 31.1: Hemocytometer consisting of improved Neubauer counting chamber (in the center), WBC pipette and RBC pipette

red glass bead which facilitates mixing of the blood and the diluent. There is another short capillary tube above the bulb marked 101. Each pipette is provided with an aspirating tube. In the red cell pipette, blood is drawn up to the 0.5 mark and diluent up to the 101 mark. The resulting dilution is 1:200.

Uses of the RBC pipette: It is used for manual **RBC count, platelet count** and for WBC count when total leukocyte count is very high.

While loading the counting chamber, discard the first 2–3 drops since it contains only diluting fluid.

Principle: The blood is diluted with an isotonic solution and the RBCs in diluted fluid are counted in a hemocytometer under a microscope in the RBC counting area.

RBC diluting fluids: There are two types of RBC diluting fluids.

- **Hayem's RBC diluting fluids** (Table 31.1).
- **Dacie's RBC diluting fluids** (Table 31.1).

Table 31.1: Composition of RBC diluting fluids

Constituents	Quantity	Action
Hayem's fluid		
• Mercuric chloride • Sodium chloride • Sodium sulfate • Distilled water	0.5 g 1.0 g 5.0 g 200 mL	Prevents growth of bacteria Provides iso-osmolarity
Dacie's fluid (formal-citrate solution)		
• Sodium citrate dihydrate • Formalin • Distilled water	5.0 g 1 mL 100 mL	Anticoagulant Fixation of cells, retards bacterial and fungal growth

Technique

- Gently mix the blood in the EDTA vial and draw the **blood up to 0.5 mark** of RBC pipette. Wipe off the excess blood from sides of the tip of the pipette.
- Dip the tip of the pipette in the **RBC diluting fluid** and draw the fluid **up to mark 101**.
- Holding the pipette horizontally in its long axis, rotate it slowly to ensure **thorough mixing of blood and diluent.** This is facilitated by the red bead in the bulb.
- Place the cover slip on the ruled area of the chamber. **Discard the first 2–3 drops** (since the fluid has not mixed with blood) of RBC fluid from the pipette.
- **Charge the improved Neubauer counting chamber** by placing the tip of the pipette just under the cover slip and allow the fluid to flow by capillary action till the counting chamber is just filled.
- Wait for 2–5 minutes for the cells to settle in the chamber.
- **Count RBCs** using high power objective in the **5 black small squares** in the central big square (Fig. 31.2) and total them together. RBC count = counted cells × 10,000 cells per cu mm (mm^3) of blood.

Table 31.2: Normal range for WBC count

	Range
Adult male	4.4–6.0 millions/cu mm
Adult female	3.8–5.0 millions/cu mm
At birth	6.0–7.0 millions/cu mm

Sources of error: Improper blood collection, improper mixing of blood sample and improper charging of improved Neubauer chamber may result in inaccurate values.

Automated Analyzer

- **Advantages:** (1) Easy rapid and time-saving method, (2) large number of blood samples is counted rapidly and (3) high level of precision.
- **Disadvantages:** (1) equipment is expensive (2) calibration error, (3) nucleated RBCs and platelet clumps are counted as leukocytes.

Normal range for RBC count is shown in Table 31.2.

Causes of increased RBC count: Polycythemia (polycythemia vera and secondary polycythemias).

Causes of decreased RBC count: Anemias and hemodilution.

TOTAL WBC COUNT

Total leukocytes/WBC count (TLC) in the blood can be measured either by manual method using an improved Neubauer counting chamber or by automated analyzer.

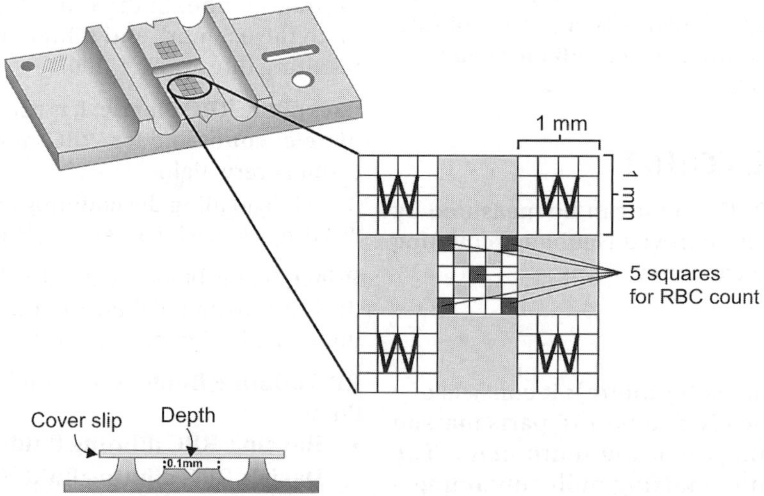

Fig. 31.2: Close-up view of improved Neubauer counting chamber (Diagrammatic). WBC counting areas are marked W and RBC counting areas in dark small 5 squares in the middle square. The entire central square is used for platelet count

Manual Method

WBC pipette: It has a **white glass bead** in the bulb which facilitates mixing of the blood and the diluent. It has 3 markings of 0.5, 1 and 11. In the white cell pipette, blood is drawn up to the 0.5 mark and diluent up to the 11.0 mark. The dilution in this case is 1:20.

Uses of the WBC pipette: Manual **WBC count, absolute eosinophil count** (AEC), **sperm count** and **cell count in any fluid** (e.g. synovial fluid). It can also used when total platelet count is low.

Principle: Whole blood is diluted with WBC diluting fluid and the glacial acetic acid in the fluid lyses the red cells. The nuclei of white blood cells are stained by gentian violet, which are counted in the WBC areas in the improved Neubauer counting chamber.

WBC diluting fluid (Turk's fluid) (Table 31.3).

Technique

- Gently mix the blood in the EDTA vial and draw the **blood in the WBC pipette up to 0.5** mark. Wipe off the excess blood from sides of the tip of the pipette.
- Dip the tip of the pipette in the **Turk's fluid** and draw the fluid **up to mark 11**.
- Holding the pipette horizontally in its long axis, rotate it slowly to ensure thorough mixing of blood and diluent. This is facilitated by the white bead in the bulb.
- Place the cover slip on the ruled area of the chamber.
- Discard the first 2–3 drops (since the fluid has not mixed with blood) of WBC fluid from the pipette. **Charge the improved Neubauer counting chamber** by placing the tip of the pipette just under the cover slip and allow the fluid to flow by capillary action till the counting chamber is just filled.
- Wait for 2–3 minutes for the cells to settle in the chamber. Examine the WBC areas under the microscope using a high power objective.
- Count the total number of WBCs in the areas marked in the Figure 31.2 (in big squares, each area is divided into 16 medium-sized squares).
- WBC count = counted cells × 50 cells/cu mm (mm^3) of blood.

Sources of error: Improper blood collection, improper mixing of blood sample and improper charging of Neubauer chamber may result in inaccurate values.

Corrections of Total WBC Count for nRBC

Nucleated red cells are not lyzed by the diluting fluid and counted with WBCs. If nucleated red blood cells (nRBCs) are 5 or more per 100 WBCs (when observed on peripheral smear) in the differential leukocyte count, a correction for nRBCs should be made.

Corrected TLC/cu mm

$$= \frac{\text{Uncorrected TLC (per cu mm)} \times 100}{\text{No. of nRBCs per 100 WBCs} + 100}$$

Automated Analyzer

- **Advantages:** (i) Easy rapid and time-saving method, (2) large number of blood samples is counted rapidly, and (3) high level of precision.
- **Disadvantages:** (1) equipment is expensive (2) calibration error, and (3) giant platelets are counted as RBCs.

Normal range of WBC count is shown in Table 31.4.

Uses of WBC count: It is used to support diagnosis of various infections and inflammatory lesions, leukemias (a class of hematological malignancies of bone marrow cells in which immature blood cells continuously multiply at the expense of normal blood cells) and various other hematological disorders.

Leukocytosis (increased WBC count): Total leukocyte count of more than 11,000/cu mm (11×10^9/L) is termed as leukocytosis. The common causes of leukocytosis are shown in Box 13.9.

Leukopenia (decreased WBC count): Total leukocyte count of less than 4,000/cu mm (4×10^9/L) is termed as leukopenia. The common causes of leukopenia are shown in Box 13.10.

Neutrophilia: It is defined as an **absolute neutrophil count of more than 8,000/cu mm (8×10^9/L).** Causes of neutrophilia are shown in Box 13.11.

Neutropenia (agranulocytosis): It is defined as **reduction in the absolute neutrophil count (total WBC × %**

Table 31.3: Composition of WBC diluting fluid (Turk's fluid)

Constituents	Quantity	Action
Glacial acetic acid	2 mL	Lyses the RBCs
1% gentian violet	5 drops	Stains nuclei of WBC
Add water	100 mL	Diluent

Table 31.4: Normal range for WBC count

	Range
Adults	4000–11000 cells/cu mm
At birth	8000–22000 cells/cu mm
Childhood	6000–15000 cells/cu mm

segmented neutrophils and band forms) below 1.5 × 10^9/L (1,500/cu mm). Causes of neutropenia are shown in Box 13.12.

PLATELET COUNT

Manual Method

Equipment: Improved Neubauer counting chamber. RBC pipette. If platelet count is low a WBC pipette can be used instead of RBC pipette.

Principle: Anticoagulated blood is diluted with a diluent that lyses the red cells (e.g. 1% ammonium oxalate) leaving visible platelets. Dacie's fluid and Rees-Ecker fluid can also be used for RBC count.

Platelet diluting fluids

There are 3 types of platelet diluting fluids (Table 31.5).

Technique

- Gently mix the blood in the EDTA vial and draw the **blood in the RBC pipette up to 0.5 mark.** Wipe off the excess blood from sides of the tip of the pipette.
- Dip the tip of the pipette in 1% ammonium oxalate (Brecher-Cronkite fluid) and draw the **fluid up to mark 101**.
- Holding the pipette horizontally in its long axis, rotate it slowly to ensure thorough mixing of blood and diluent. This is facilitated by the white bead in the bulb.
- Place the cover slip on the ruled area of the chamber.
- Discard the first 2–3 drops (since the fluid has not mixed with blood) of fluid from the pipette. **Charge the improved Neubauer counting chamber** by placing the tip of the pipette just under the cover slip and allow the fluid to flow by capillary action till the counting chamber is just filled.
- Keep the charged improved Neubauer counting chamber in a petri dish with wet filter paper at the bottom for 5 minutes for the platelets to settle down.
- Platelets are counted in the entire central 1 × 1 mm square.

Platelet count = Total counted cells in the central square × 2000 per cu mm of blood (If WBC pipette is used, platelet count = Total counted cells in the central square × 200/cu mm of blood).

Box 31.1: Various causes of thrombocytosis

Idiopathic/primary (autonomous production)
- Essential thrombocytosis
- Polycythemia vera
- Chronic myeloid leukemia

Secondary (reactive thrombocytosis)
- Malignancy
- Following splenectomy

Normal Range

It ranges from 1,50,000 to 4,50,000 platelets per cu mm (150 – 450 × 10^9/L) (150 – 450 × 10^3/μL).

Thrombocytopenia (Decreased Platelet Count)

Definition: Thrombocytopenia is the term used when the platelet count is less than 1,50,000/cu mm (150 × 10^9/L).

Causes of thrombocytopenia are shown in Box 13.21.

Thrombocytosis (Increased Platelet Count)

Definition: Platelet count of more than 4,50,000/cu mm (450 × 10^9/L) is known as thrombocytosis.

Causes of thrombocytosis are shown in Box 31.1.

ABSOLUTE EOSINOPHIL COUNT

Manual Method

Equipment

- Improved Neubauer counting chamber.
- WBC pipette.

Diluting Fluid

Dunger's fluid composition is shows in Table 31.6. It should be preserved in the refrigerator.

Technique

- Gently mix the blood in the EDTA vial, so that the cells mix well with plasma.

Table 31.5: Composition of platelet diluting fluids

Dacie's fluid	Rees-Ecker fluid	Brecher-Cronkite fluid
Sodium citrate dihydrate (5 g)	Sodium citrate (3.8 g)	1% ammonium oxalate solution
0.2% brilliant cresyl blue (0/1mL)	Brilliant cresyl blue (50 mg)	
Formalin (1 mL)	Formalin (0.2 mL)	
Distilled water (100 mL)	Distilled water (100 mL)	

Table 31.6: Composition of Dunger's fluid

Constituents	Quantity	Action
Eosin	200 mg	Stains the eosinophil granules orange red
Acetone	10 mL	Fixation of eosinophils
Water	80 mL	Lysis of red cells and white cells (except eosinophils which are resistant)

- Draw the **blood in the WBC pipette up to mark 1.** Wipe off the excess blood from sides of the tip of the pipette.
- Dip the tip of the pipette in the **Dunger's fluid** and draw the fluid **up to mark 11.** The dilution is 1 in 10.
- Holding the pipette horizontally in its long axis, rotate it slowly to ensure thorough mixing of blood and diluent. This is facilitated by the white bead in the bulb.
- Place the cover slip on the cleaned ruled area of the counting chamber.
- Discard the first 2 to 3 drops (since the fluid has not mixed with blood) of WBC fluid from the pipette.
- **Charge the chamber** by placing the tip of the pipette just under the cover slip and fluid flows under it by capillary action. Allow till the counting chamber is just filled.
- Wait for 5 minutes for the eosinophils to settle in the chamber.
- **Count the number of eosinophils in the 4 corner squares** under the microscope using a low power objective. Eosinophils are identified because of their bright red granules and count should be done within 30 minutes.

Absolute eosinophil count (AEC) = Total number of eosinophils in 4 squares × 25.

AEC using Fuch's Rosenthal chamber: It is preferable to do AEC using Fuch's Rosenthal chamber, where the depth of chamber is 0.2 mm compared to 0.1 mm in improved Neubauer chamber. This increase in depth means more cells will be counted thereby increasing the accuracy of AEC.

Normal Range of Eosinophil Count

Eosinophils constitute 1–6% of circulating WBCs. The range of absolute eosinophil count is 40–450 cells/cu mm ($0.04–0.45 \times 10^9$/L).

Use

Absolute eosinophil count (AEC) in blood is useful in diagnosis, treatment and follow-up of cases of eosinophilia.

High AEC (Eosinophilia)

Definition: Eosinophilia is defined as an absolute eosinophil count of more than 450/cu mm (mm^3).

Causes: Refer Box 13.13.

Automated Analyzer/Cell Counters

RBC count, WBC count and platelet count can also be obtained by electronic particle counters. These have presently replaced the manual methods.

SELF-ASSESSMENT EXERCISE

I. Short Notes

1. WBC count.
2. RBC count.
3. Platelet count.

CHAPTER 32

Hematocrit, ESR Estimation and Peripheral Blood Smear Examination

CHAPTER OUTLINE

HEMATOCRIT

Hematocrit (packed cell volume) is the **ratio of the volume of red cells** to that of the **whole blood**. It indicates relative volume of red cells and plasma (e.g. in anemia red cells are reduced with corresponding reduction in the hematocrit).

Methods of Estimation of PCV

- Macromethod using Wintrobe tube
- Micromethod using capillary tube
- Automated analyzer

(Macromethod and micromethod: Both are direct estimations)

Wintrobe Method

Wintrobe tube (Fig. 32.1)**:** It is a special thick walled glass tube calibrated at 1 mm intervals upto 105–110 mm with bold markings from top as 0, 10, 20, 30,...100 for ESR and 100, 90, 80,...10, 0 for PCV. The markings are in descending order from the top for PCV estimation and marking in ascending order from the top for ESR determination.

Anticoagulants used: EDTA, heparin or double oxalate.

Principle

Anticoagulated whole blood is centrifuged at a standard speed (3500 RPM). RBCs which are heavier than white cells, platelets and plasma, sediment at the bottom and the volume of red cell mass denotes the hematocrit.

Method

Collect the blood in an EDTA vial and mix the blood sample properly.

With the help of a Pasteur's pipette (dropper with long, thin capillary tube like nozzle) draw the blood from the vial and fill the Wintrobe tube till the top mark of 100.

Centrifuge the tube at 3,500 RPM for half an hour.

Take the reading of packed red cells from bottom. It is expressed as a percentage.

Different Layers (Fig. 32.1)

Other use of Wintrobe tube is for ESR estimation. However, the Westergren method is preferred as it is more accurate.

Microhematocrit Method

A heparinized capillary tube is used and the blood is filled by capillary action. One end is sealed and it is centrifuged in a special centrifuge. As the tubes are not graduated, the PCV is measured using a special chart.

Advantages

Easy, small quantity of blood is needed (useful in pediatric patients), capillary blood is sufficient, less time and amount of plasma trapped in the red cell column is less, thereby minimizing the error.

Disadvantage

It requires a special (expensive) centrifuge.

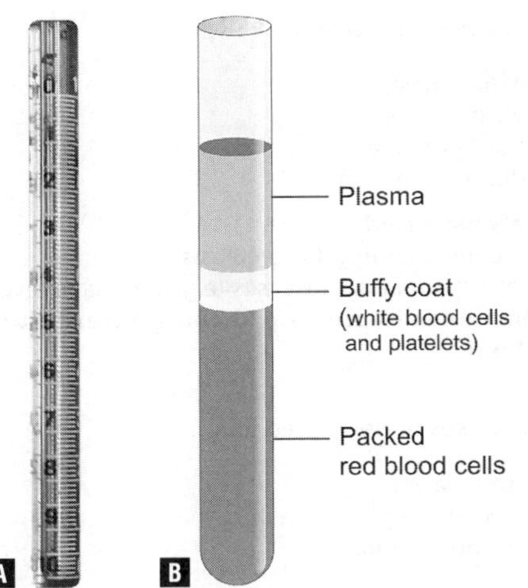

Figs 32.1A and B: (A) Wintrobe tube and (B) diagrammatic appearance of different columns after the blood is centrifuged

Table 32.1: Normal range of packed cell volume (PCV)

	Range
Males	40–50%
Females	36–46%
Infants	45–70% (cord blood)

Box 32.1: Causes of increased PCV

Absolute
- Primary: Polycythemia vera
- Secondary: Lung disease, cyanotic heart disease, living in high attitude

Relative: Reduced plasma volume, e.g. dehydration due to diarrhea, vomiting

Automated Analyzer

Nowadays, automated analyzers are available for estimation of hematocrit.

Normal range for PCV (Table 32.1): Hematocrit is expressed as a percentage (e.g. 45%) or as a decimal fraction (e.g. 0.45). It is useful for evaluating absolute values like MCV and MCHC.

Causes of increased PCV are presented in Box 32.1.

Decreased PCV is seen in anemia.

ERYTHROCYTE SEDIMENTATION RATE

Erythrocyte sedimentation rate (ESR) estimation is a commonly used nonspecific test in routine clinical practice.

Principle: When anticoagulated blood is placed in a vertical tube and is allowed to stand, RBCs settle toward the bottom of the tube. The speed of sedimentation of red cells in plasma over a period of 1 hour is measured by the length of the sedimented RBC column and is expressed in millimeters. RBCs have net negative charge on their surface and tend to repel each other. The repulsive forces are partially or totally counteracted if there is an increase in the positively charged plasma proteins.

Stages of ESR

Sedimentation occurs in three stages:
- **Stage of aggregation/rouleaux formation:** In the initial 10 minutes, there is little sedimentation as rouleaux form and the size of the rouleaux formed influence the speed of sedimentation.
- **Stage of settling:** For about 40 minutes, settling occurs at a constant rate.
- **Stage of packing:** Packing of RBCs occurs in the final 10 minutes.

Methods

The two commonly employed methods are: Westergren and Wintrobe methods.

Westergren Method

Equipment (Fig. 32.2): Westergren tube is a straight glass pipette (open at both ends) 30 cm in length, bore of 2.55 mm and calibrated in millimeters from 0-200. The capacity of tube is about 1 mL. The tube is vertically placed on the Westergren rack.

Anticoagulant used: The anticoagulant used is 3.8% trisodium citrate. Ratio of blood and anticoagulant: 2 mL

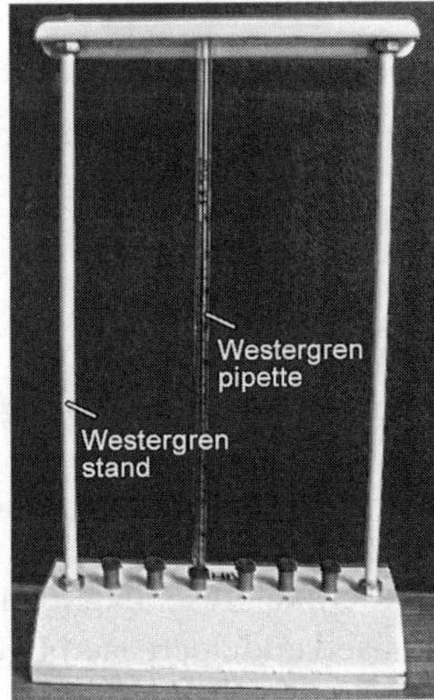

Fig. 32.2: Westergren pipette placed vertically in the rack

Table 32.2: Normal range for ESR

	Range
Adult males	0–10 mm 1st hour
Adult females	0–12 mm 1st hour
Children	0–10 mm 1st hour

of whole blood in 0.5 mL of 3.8% trisodium citrate. Blood to anticoagulant ratio should be 4:1.

Procedure: A Westergren pipette is filled up to the 0 mark and placed vertically in the Westergren rack at room temperature. After 60 minutes, the distance between the top of the red cell column and 0 mark is noted in millimeters as ESR reading.

Result: ESR is expressed as mm at the end of 1 hour.

Normal range: (Table 32.2).

Advantages: This is a more sensitive and accurate method when compared to the Wintrobe method. This is because the column is longer, i.e. 200 mm.

Disposable Methods

Disposable ESR kits are more convenient, where the ESR pipette sucks the blood to fill precisely to the zero mark. This eliminates risky mouth pipetting of blood.

Wintrobe Method

Wintrobe tube can be used first for estimation of ESR and then it is centrifuged for estimation of hematocrit.

Alternative Methods

Capillary method (micro ESR method) is useful in pediatric patients.

Zeta Sedimentation Rate

Automated ESR (e.g. Ves-Matic bench top analyzer): Results are obtained within 30 minutes and are comparable with Westergren 1 hour reading.

Significance of ESR

ESR is a **prognostic test** rather than a diagnostic test. It is useful in monitoring disease activity.

Note: ESR may be rarely normal in patients with neoplasms, connective tissue diseases and infections. A normal ESR cannot be used to exclude these diagnostic possibilities.

Causes of increased and decreased ESR are shown in Box 32.2 and 32.3 respectively.

Box 32.2: Causes of increased ESR

Markedly increased
- Multiple myeloma
- Macroglobulinemia
- Hyperfibrinogenemia

Moderately increased
- Infective diseases (e.g. tuberculosis)
- Chronic inflammatory diseases (e.g. rheumatic fever)
- **Autoimmune diseases (e.g. rheumatoid arthritis, SLE)**
- **Neoplasia**

Box 32.3: Causes of decreased ESR

- Polycythemia vera
- Sickle cell disease
- Hypofibrinogenemia

PERIPHERAL BLOOD SMEAR EXAMINATION

Peripheral smear (peripheral blood film) is the most important, valuable and frequently asked investigation in hematology laboratory. It provides the following information:

- **Red cell morphology**, which is important for diagnosis of anemias.
- **WBC disorders and differential leukocyte count** (DLC).
- **Platelet number and morphology** useful in the diagnosis of bleeding disorders.
- **Cross check the CBC parameters** derived from automated cell counters.
- **Detection of blood parasites** (hemoparasites).

STAINS FOR BLOOD SMEAR

- The blood cells contain cellular structures which vary in their reaction (pH), some are acidic and others being basic.
- The aniline dyes used in staining blood smears are of two general classes: basic dyes such as methylene blue and acidic dyes such as eosin.
- All stains which are made of combinations of acidic and basic dyes are called **Romanowsky stains.** The differences between the various Romanowsky stains are mainly in the proportion of the reagents and in their preparation.

Romanowsky Stains

A mixture of methylene blue (basic stain) and eosin (acidic stain) was first prepared by Romanowsky in 1891 and employed on his work on malarial parasite. The action of these stains depends on compounds formed by the interaction of methylene blue and eosin. Methylene blue on oxidation produces colored compounds called azures that have the ability to combine with eosin. Oxidation is achieved during maturation/chemical treatment of the stain. The azures are responsible for different shades of staining in the smears (i.e. RBCs pink, granules of eosinophils red-orange, granules of basophils bluish black, granules of neutrophils-lilac).

- Nuclei and structures in the blood which are stained by the basic dyes are called basophilic.
- Structures that take up only acidic dyes are called acidophilic or eosinophilic.

Romanowsky group includes the following stains:

- ***Leishman stain*** which contains Leishman powder and acetone free methyl alcohol (methanol).
  - **Preparation of stain:** Dissolve 1 g of Leishman powder in 500 mL of acetone free methyl alcohol in a conical flask. Warm it at 50°C for 15 minutes. Keep it for ripening by exposing to sunlight for 2 days. **Acetone free methyl alcohol** acts as a **fixative**. Since acetone destroys the cells, methyl alcohol should be free from acetone.
- ***Giemsa stain*** contains Giemsa stain powder, glycerol and acetone free methyl alcohol.
  - **Preparation of stain:** Dissolve 1 g of Giemsa stain powder in 66 mL of glycerol at 60°C for 2 hours. After cooling add 66 mL of acetone free methyl alcohol and mix it. Keep it at 37°C for one week for ripening.
- ***Wright stain***
- ***Jenner stain***
- ***Jenner-Giemsa stain***
- ***Field stain***

PREPARATION OF THE PERIPHERAL BLOOD SMEAR (FIG. 32.3)

- A drop of blood is placed on a clean grease free glass slide 1 cm away from one end.
- Take a spreader (either another slide or a narrower piece of slide with smooth edge) and place its smooth edge over the drop of blood so as to spread the blood along its edge.
- Place the slide at about 30–40° angle and make the smear with a smooth (not jerky) forward movement. The resulting ideal smear should be about 2.5–3.5 cm in length.
- Allow it to dry at room temperature and label.

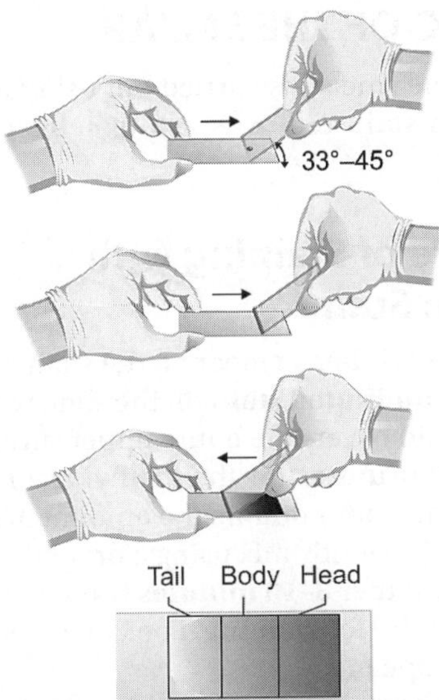

Fig. 32.3: Different steps in the preparation of peripheral blood smear and appearance of a well-made smear

Features of a Well-made Peripheral Smear

- Length: Smear should be 2/3 to 3/4 of the length of the slide.
- Shape: The smear should be either tongue or finger-shaped (smooth without any irregularities or holes).
- Well made smear has three parts namely, head, body and tail (Fig. 32.3).

Sources of Error

- Presence of grease on the slide causes blank oval areas in the smear.
- If spreader edge is not smooth, the tail of the smear shows ragged edges and most of the neutrophils accumulate in the tail end. The rest of the smear shows paucity of neutrophils, a process termed as tailing of the smear. This results in erroneous differential counts.

FIXATION OF THE SMEAR

- The blood smears should be fixed within 4 hours for good staining.
- Blood films are 'fixed' by **acetone-free methyl alcohol** which is present in most of the commonly used stains, namely Leishman or Wright or Giemsa stain.
- It can also be fixed by dipping the slide 8–10 times in a coplin jar with methyl alcohol.

STAINING OF THE SMEAR

Staining of the smears is carried out using Romanowsky stains which stain red cells, white cells, platelets and parasites.

Procedure of Staining with Leishman Stain

- Keep the peripheral smear on the staining rack.
- **Pour the undiluted stain** on the slide with a dropper so that stain covers the entire upper surface of slide.
- Wait for **2 minutes** for the methyl alcohol to **fix the smear**. Then pour double the amount of buffer water on the slide. Gently mix using a dropper.
- Wait for another **8–10 minutes** (time depends on the batch of stain) for **staining**. Look for greenish metallic scum to appear.
- Displace the stain by pouring running water from one side of the slide so that the stain scum is drained off the slide and no more stain is left on the slide.
  - Precaution: Do not discard the stain from slide by just tilting it, since it will result in stain precipitates over the smear.
- Remove the slide from staining rack and keep it in slanting position to dry it up.
- Examine the slide under microscope.

Sources of Error

- Buffered pH of 6.8 is important for good quality of staining.
  - Acidic pH red cells appear pink and WBCs takes up very light stain.
  - Basic pH red cells appear blue and WBCs appear bluish-black.
- Staining errors:
  - If smear is overstained (due to more alkaline pH/ too long period of staining), wash the smears with undiluted Leishman stain or methanol for few seconds.
  - If smear is understained (due to more acidic pH/ too short period of staining), restain by adding both Leishman stain and buffer for required period depending on the extent of understaining.

Procedure of Staining with Giemsa Stain

- Peripheral smear prepared is fixed by dipping 8–10 times in a coplin jar containing methanol.
- Allow the slide to dry.
- Pour the diluted stain (1 in 10) and wait for 20–30 minutes.

Note: The amount of dilution and time for staining varies with each batch of stain.

- Wash the slide (as in staining by Leishman) and dry it.

Thick film for malarial parasite: Thick film method is preferred for mass surveys, quick diagnosis and when malarial parasites are likely to be few. It is advisable to make both thin and thick films on the same slide. Thick blood films can be stained by **Field's rapid method** or **Jaswant-Singh-Bhattacherji (JSB) stain.**

Examination of a Peripheral Blood Smear

- **Red blood cells:** Red cells are examined for (1) size, (2) shape, (3) color, (4) inclusions and (5) other abnormalities.
- **White blood cells:** Number and distribution. At least 100 white cells should be counted. Normal range of differential leukocyte count is shown in Table 13.4.
- **Platelets:** Number and distribution.
- **Hemoparasites** (such as malaria, microfilaria).
- **Any abnormal cells.**

SELF-ASSESSMENT EXERCISE

I. Short Notes

1. Packed cell volume.
2. Erythrocyte sedimentation rate.
3. Peripheral smear examination.

CHAPTER 33

Reticulocyte Count

CHAPTER OUTLINE

- Methods of Reticulocyte Count

Reticulocytes are immature, non-nucleated RBCs released from bone marrow. They are slightly larger than the mature RBCs. They continue to synthesize hemoglobin after loss of the nucleus.

METHODS OF RETICULOCYTE COUNT

- Visual method
- Automated method.

Visual Method

Principle: Staining in living state is known as **supravital staining**. Reticulocytes contain ribosomes and RNA, which can be stained by supravital stains like brilliant cresyl blue and new methylene blue in the live and unfixed state. When blood is briefly incubated in new methylene blue or brilliant cresyl blue solution, the RNA is precipitated as a dye-ribonucleoprotein complex. On microscopy, the complex appears as a dark blue network (reticulum or filamentous strand or granular material). Reticulocytes stain ***polychromatic*** with Romanowsky stains and hence the term "***polychromatophil***" is used to indicate their presence in peripheral smear (Table 33.1).

Brilliant Cresyl Blue/New Methylene Blue Stain (Figs 33.1A and B)

Procedure

- Take two to three drops each of supravital stain and blood in a test tube and mix.
- Incubate for 15 minutes at room temperature and remix.
- Take a drop of mixture on the slide and prepare a thin smear. Air-dry the smear.

Table 33.1: Composition of supravital stain for reticulocyte count

Contents	Quantity	Action
Brilliant cresyl blue/new methylene blue	1 g	Stains reticulocyte RNA and ribosomes
3% sodium citrate solution	20 mL	Anticoagulant
0.9% sodium chloride solution	80 mL	Isotonic saline

- View under the microscope with an oil immersion lens. At least 1,000 red cells are counted and percentage of reticulocytes is calculated. A Miller disc ocular inserted into the eyepiece of microscope allows rapid estimation and reduces counting errors. **Reticulocytes should be distinguished from Heinz bodies, Pappenheimer bodies, HbH inclusions, Howell-Jolly bodies.**

Normal reticulocyte count: Reticulocyte count is expressed as percentage of total red cells.

- Normal 0.5–2.5%
- Newborn (cord blood) 1–7.0%

Absolute reticulocyte count = Reticulocyte percentage × red cell count.

Normal is 50,000–85,000/cu mm.

Reticulocyte Count Correction for Anemia

- In patients with anemia, the reticulocyte count does not reflect the true marrow response. So, the reticulocyte count obtained must be corrected for the severity of the anemia. The corrected reticulocyte count is calculated by multiplying the reticulocyte percentage by a factor adjusting for the degree of anemia (i.e. actual PCV divided by normal PCV for the age). Corrected reticulocyte count >2% suggests that the reticulocyte release is appropriate to the degree of anemia and <2% is inappropriate.

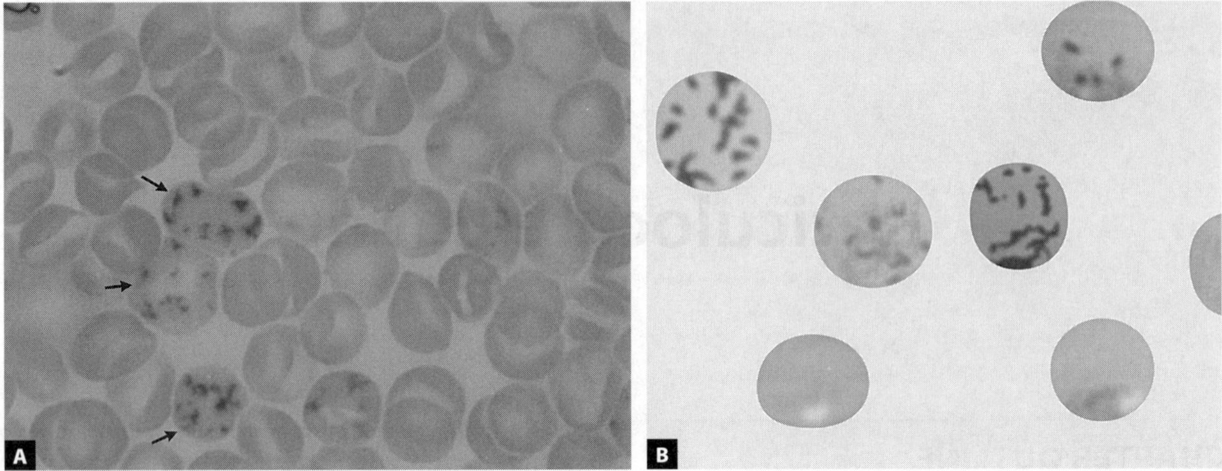

Figs 33.1A and B: Smear shows reticulocyte with blue filamentous/granular material (new methylene blue stain)

Table 33.2: Causes of increased and reduced reticulocyte count

Causes of increased reticulocyte count	Causes of reduced reticulocyte count
Hemolytic anemias • Hemolytic crisis • Hemorrhage • Following treatment in iron/folic acid/vitamin B12 deficiency anemias. Highest counts are found on 6th/7th day of treatment and indicate marrow response to hematinics	Due to decreased erythropoietic activity • Aplastic anemia • Aplastic crisis due to parvovirus (hereditary spherocytosis and sickle cell disease) • Pure red cell aplasia • Fanconi anemia • Myelofibrosis

Corrected reticulocyte count (Reticulocyte index)

$$= \textbf{Reticulocyte count} \times \frac{\textbf{PCV (hematocrit) of patient}}{\textbf{Normal PCV (hematocrit) for the age}}$$

- **Reticulocyte production index (RPI):** Early-released reticulocytes enter the circulation a day earlier than normal reticulocytes and the corrected reticulocyte count is further multiplied by 0.5 to obtain the reticulocyte production index (RPI).

  Reticulocyte production index (RPI)

  $$= \textbf{Reticulocyte count} \times \frac{\textbf{Hemoglobin}}{\textbf{Normal hemoglobin for the age}} \times \textbf{0.5}$$

  - If RPI is greater than 2%; it indicates adequate erythropoietic response of the bone marrow and suggests that anemia is either due to acute blood loss or hemolysis.
  - If RPI is less than 2%; it indicates that the anemia is due to defective bone marrow production.

Automated Method of Reticulocyte Count

Reticulocyte count can also be performed in automated cell counters or by a flow cytometer. It is superior and accurate to manual count. However, Howell-Jolly bodies, Heinz bodies, Pappenheimer bodies and giant platelets, when present may also be counted as reticulocytes.

Causes of increased and reduced reticulocyte count is listed in Table 33.2.

SELF-ASSESSMENT EXERCISE

I. Short Notes

1. Reticulocyte count its method of demonstration/stains used with procedure.
2. Various causes of increased and decreased reticulocyte count. Write its significance.

CHAPTER 34

Bone Marrow Examination

CHAPTER OUTLINE

INTRODUCTION

Bone marrow examination is essentially done to confirm or rule out a hematologic disorder. It also helps in evaluation of non-hematological disorders (e.g. metastasis). Bone marrow may be obtained by:

- **Aspiration:** Bone marrow aspiration is a simple, easy and safe procedure.
- **Trephine biopsy:** It is indicated in conditions where the aspiration either fails to yield marrow or to confirm some of the diseases (where biopsy findings are diagnostic).

BONE MARROW ASPIRATION

Bone Marrow Needles

Needles commonly employed for the aspiration of the marrow are Salah needle (Fig. 34.1) and Klima needle.

Parts of the Bone Marrow Needle

- **Stilette:** It prevents entry of soft tissue and bone fragments into the aspiration needle when it pierces through them.
- **Aspiration needle:** For aspirating the marrow, a syringe is attached after removing the stilette.
- **Guard:** It adjusts the depth of penetration of the aspiration needle.

Sites for Bone Marrow Aspirate

Usual sites for bone marrow aspiration are:

- Sternum
- Posterior superior iliac spine
- Iliac crest
- Anterior superior iliac spine
- Spinous process of lumbar vertebra.

In infants, upper end of the tibia is the ideal site for marrow aspirate.

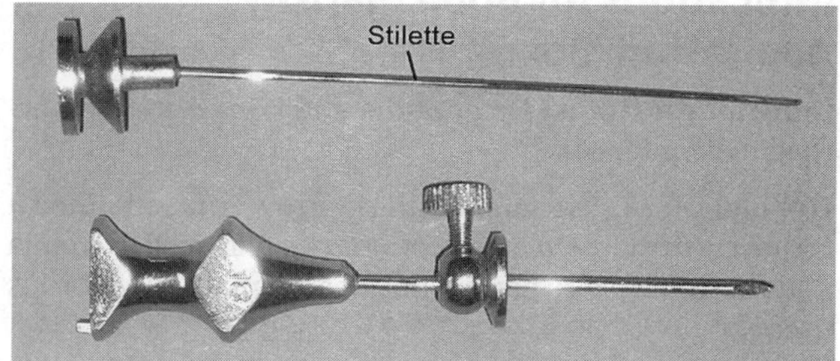

Fig. 34.1: Salah bone marrow aspiration needle with stilette (above)

Evaluation of Bone Marrow Aspirate

- **Cellularity:** The cellularity of the marrow is reported as normocellular/hypercellular/hypocellular. Cellularity of marrow should be correlated with the age of the patient.
- **Myeloid and erythroid (M:E) ratio:** This is done by counting at least 500 cells and expressing the cells as ratio of myeloid and erythroid cells. Normal M:E ratio varies from 2:1 to 4:1.
- **Erythropoiesis:** Erythroid precursors are examined for:
  - Marrow response: Normal/increased/decreased.
  - Maturation: Normoblastic/megaloblastic/micronormoblastic.
- **Myelopoiesis:** It is examined for:
  - Normal response: Normal/increased/decreased.
  - Maturation arrest.
  - Morphological abnormalities: Hypergranular/absent granules.
  - Abnormal cells/blasts.

- **Megakaryopoiesis:** They are examined for:
  - Number
  - Morphology.
- **Lymphocytes:** Normal/increased/abnormal.
- **Plasma cells:** Normal/increased.
- **Others:** Metastatic tumor cells, parasites (malaria, *Leishmania donovani*) and fungus or any other abnormal cells.
- **Iron stores:** Iron stores are evaluated by Prussian blue reaction (Perl's stain). Iron stores are commented as normal/increased/decreased or nil.
- **Cytochemistry/special stains**.

Indications for Bone Marrow Aspiration (Box 34.1)

Contraindications: Hemophilia and congenital hemorrhagic disorders.

Dry tap: During aspiration, if the marrow is not obtained it is called a dry tap. Dry tap is common in hairy cell leukemia and myelofibrosis (marrow has been replaced by fibrous tissue).

Box 34.1: Indications for bone marrow aspiration

Diagnostic
- Primary hematolymphoid disorders
  - Red cell disorders: Nutritional anemia (e.g. megaloblastic anemia)
  - White cell disorders: Diagnosis and classification of acute leukemias
  - Megakaryocytic disorders: Idiopathic thrombocytopenic purpura (ITP) and other thrombocytopenias
  - Myeloproliferative neoplasms: Polycythemia vera, chronic myeloid leukemia
  - Myelodysplastic syndromes
  - Plasma cell neoplasms: Multiple myeloma
- Systemic diseases
  - Storage disorders: Gaucher, Niemann-Pick disease
- Staging of lymphoid malignancies and solid tumors
  - Lymphoma
  - Metastatic deposits (e.g. carcinoma prostate, breast, lung, kidney)
- Detection of infection and/or source of pyrexia of unknown origin (PUO)
- Parasitic disorders: Kala-azar
- Fungal disorders: Histoplasma
- Mycobacterial infection

Post-treatment follow-up: To know the response to therapy and follow-up in cases of leukemia, aplastic anemia and agranulocytosis

Therapeutic: Bone marrow transplant

BONE MARROW TREPHINE BIOPSY

Marrow trephine biopsy is performed by one of the trephine biopsy needles like, Jamshidi needle or Westerman-Jensen needle or Islam needle. The biopsy obtained consists of a core of bone with marrow. Trephine biopsy tissue is decalcified and processed like other histopathological tissue containing bone. Sections are stained with hematoxylin and eosin stain, reticulin stain, Masson's trichrome stain (for fibrous tissue). Immunocytochemical staining can be performed especially for acute leukemias.

Sites of Trephine Biopsy

- Posterior superior iliac spine (most commonly used site).
- Anterior superior iliac spine.
- Spinous process of vertebra.

Box 34.2: Indications for trephine biopsy

- Aplastic anemia
- Myeloproliferative neoplasms—to study reticulin fibrosis in myelofibrosis
- Myelodysplastic syndromes
- Pre and post bone marrow transplantation
- Pyrexia of unknown origin (granuloma of tuberculosis).
- Bone morphology in chronic renal failure, osteoporosis and osteomalacia
- Staging: Lymphoma and to detect metastasis in cancer patients
- Human immunodeficiency syndrome (AIDS)

Indications for Trephine Biopsy (Box 34.2)

SELF-ASSESSMENT EXERCISE

I. Short Notes

1. Examination of bone marrow.

CHAPTER 35

Cerebrospinal Fluid Examination

CHAPTER OUTLINE

INTRODUCTION

Importance of CSF examination: Analysis of the cerebrospinal fluid (CSF) is of diagnostic importance in conditions like meningitis or primary/metastatic tumor of CNS with CSF involvement.

Collection of CSF: CSF is usually obtained by lumbar puncture (LP) using an LP needle under strict aseptic conditions (Fig. 35.1).

Sites

Lumbar puncture: In **adults**, CSF is normally collected in the midline of the lower back in the 3rd lumbar space and in children in the 4th lumbar space.

METHOD OF COLLECTION

Procedure

- An lumbar puncture can be performed with the patient in the lateral recumbent or prone positions or sitting upright. The patient is instructed to remain in the fetal position with the neck, back, and limbs held in flexion.
- The overlying skin should be cleaned with alcohol and a disinfectant; the antiseptic should be allowed to dry before the procedure is begun.
- A sterile drape (a covering, usually of cloth, plastic, or sterile paper, used to cover body parts during surgical procedure) with an opening over the lumbar spine is placed on the patient.

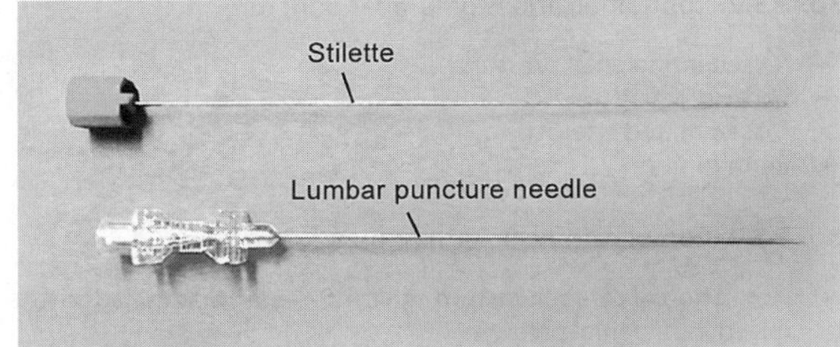

Fig. 35.1: Lumbar puncture needle with stilette

- Local anesthesia is infiltrated into the previously identified lumbar intervertebral space and a 20 or 22 gauge lumbar puncture needle (Fig. 35.1) containing a stylet/stilette (a small, sharp-pointed instrument for probing) is inserted into the lumbar intervertebral space. The lumbar puncture needle may be advanced slowly until the subarachnoid space is entered. Once CSF appears and begins to flow through the needle, the patient should be instructed to slowly straighten or extend the legs to allow free flow of CSF within the subarachnoid space.

Normally, CSF is submitted to the laboratory in three or occasionally four sterile test tubes. The amount of CSF collected should not exceed 6 to 8 mL.

- **Tube 1:** For estimation of protein and glucose and serology.
- **Tube 2:** Used for preparation of smears to stain with the Gram stain or other stains and for culture and sensitivity.
- **Tube 3:** For cell counts and differential counts.
- **Tube 4** (if indicated): For special tests such as the cryptococcal antigen, serologic test for syphilis, molecular tests or other serologic studies, and cytology.

Indications, contraindications and complications of lumbar puncture are presented in Boxes 35.1, 35.2 and 35.3 respectively.

Box 35.1: Indications for lumbar puncture

Diagnostic indications
- Infection
- Meningeal infection: Bacterial (pyogenic, tuberculosis) syphilitic, viral, fungal
- Encephalitis
- Subarachnoid hemorrhage
- Primary or metastatic malignancy (e.g. acute leukemia, lymphoma)
- Demyelinating diseases: Multiple sclerosis, Guillain-Barré syndrome

Therapeutic indications
- Spinal anesthesia
- Intrathecal injection of chemotherapeutic drugs for CNS prophylaxis/relapse of ALL, lymphomas

Box 35.2: Contraindications of lumbar puncture

- Raised intracranial pressure
- Local infective lesion
- Disseminated sclerosis
- Brain tumor

Box 35.3: Complications of lumbar puncture

- Herniation of cerebellum through the foramen magnum due to raised intracranial pressure
- Hematoma, either extradural or subdural
- Introduction of infection by the LP needle through the infected skin or subcutaneous tissue

EXAMINATION OF CEREBROSPINAL FLUID

Physical Examination

Cerebrospinal fluid (CSF) pressure: The normal CSF pressure in adults is 90–180 mm of water in the lateral position, while in infants and children it ranges from 40-100 mm of water reaching the adult level by 6–8 years.

- **Causes of raised CSF pressure:** Meningitis, cerebral edema, mass lesions in brain.
- **Causes of decreased CSF pressure:** Dehydration, circulatory collapse.

Color and appearance: Normal CSF is clear and watery.

- Turbidity of CSF is due to pus or RBCs.
  - **Xanthochromia** (yellow CSF) results from old hemorrhage, obstructive jaundice or excess of protein.
  - Differentiation of subarachnoid hemorrhage from a traumatic puncture: After centrifugation, the supernatant fluid is clear with a traumatic tap, whereas it appears xanthochromic (a faint pink, orange or yellow color) in subarachnoid hemorrhage.

Clot formation: Normal CSF does not clot. When blood-brain barrier is disturbed, fibrinogen appears in CSF. Fibrinogen gets converted to fibrin and forms clot. Causes of fibrin clot are as follows:

- Meningitis
  - In **tuberculous meningitis,** the clot is fine, delicate and typically described as **cobweb** appearance.
  - In purulent meningitis, large clot is formed.
- Tumors of CNS.

Microscopic Examination

Total cell count: Normal CSF usually does not contain cells, although cell count of 0–5 lymphocytes/μL is considered as normal. An increased cell count is known as **pleocytosis**.

Significance:

- **Neutrophils** are increased in **acute pyogenic meningitis**.
- **Lymphocytes** are increased in **viral**, syphilitic, **tuberculous** and fungal meningitis.

India-ink preparation is used for diagnosis of cryptococcal meningitis.

In tuberculous meningitis, acid fast stain can detect tuberculous bacilli.

Biochemical Evaluation

- Proteins are elevated in meningitis and glucose level is reduced due to utilization by the microbes.
- Chloride reduction in tuberculous meningitis.
- Glucose estimation: CSF glucose is decreased in pyogenic meningitis, tumors of meninges, subarachnoid hemorrhage.

CSF findings in various types of meningitis (refer Table 28.2).

Microbiological Examination

It helps to identify the causative agent in cases of meningitis. The microbiological examination includes Gram-stain, AFB stain, serological examination, culture and sensitivity and PCR, etc.

Serological examination: Venereal disease research laboratory (VDRL) test can be performed for diagnosis of neurosyphilis.

SELF-ASSESSMENT EXERCISE

I. Short Notes

1. CSF examination.

CHAPTER

36

Body Fluids, Gastric Analysis and Sputum Examination

CHAPTER OUTLINE

- Introduction
- Examination of Body Fluids
- Examination of Synovial Fluid
- Gastric Analysis
- Sputum Examination

INTRODUCTION

Body fluids are lubricating fluids present within the body cavities. Body cavities include—pleural, peritoneal, pericardial and synovial. Normally, a small amount of fluid is present within the body cavities which keeps the surfaces moist and lubricated so that the movement of the adjacent or the opposing membrane surfaces occurs with minimal friction. **Increase in the volume of the fluid** in these **cavities** is known as **effusion**.

The commonly examined body fluids in the laboratory include pleural, pericardial, peritoneal fluid and synovial fluid.

Specimen Collection

The body fluid is collected in a clean, dry container under aseptic precautions and atraumatically to avoid mixing with fresh blood. The fluid is collected in the following three sterile test tubes:

- **Chemical examination:** Fluoride tube
- **Microscopic examination:** EDTA tube
- **Bacteriological examination:** Plain tube (without anticoagulant).

They should be examined as early as possible to prevent chemical changes, growth of bacteria and disintegration of cells.

EXAMINATION OF BODY FLUIDS

Physical Examination

Note volume, color and appearance.

Color: Pleural, pericardial and ascitic (peritoneal) fluids are usually clear and straw colored.

- Uniform **blood** stained **fluid suggests malignancy** involving the organs/tissues surrounding the respective body cavity.
- **Turbid** fluid may be **due to high cell count or high protein content**.
- **Chylous** with milky appearance usually indicates high lipid content **due to lymphatic obstruction**.

Transudate vs exudate: The effusion may be broadly divided into transudate and exudate. It is important to differentiate whether the fluid is a transudate or exudate (refer Table 3.2).

- **Transudate** is usually seen in all body cavities with diseases like heart failure and hypoalbuminemic conditions (e.g. nephrotic syndrome). Cirrhosis results in prominent ascites, but may also cause pleural effusion.
- **Exudate** usually suggests infection or malignancy.

Chemical Examination

- **Protein estimation:** This helps to differentiate transudate from exudate (refer Table 3.2).
- **Glucose estimation:** Low glucose in the body fluids usually suggests bacterial infection (including tuberculosis), malignancy or nonspecific inflammation.
- **Measurement of amylase in ascitic fluid:** It is useful in patients with pancreatic lesions.

Microscopic Examination

Cell count is done similar to total WBC count using improved Neubauer chamber. Normally, few mesothelial cells (lining cells of body cavities) and lymphocytes are seen.

Differential WBC Count

Procedure: Centrifuge the body fluid and from the sediment prepare the smears (at least 2).

Stains:

- **Leishman's stain:** Stain one smear with Leishman's stain and count 100 cells and express the differential count.
- **Gram's stain/acid fast stain:** These stains are useful in suspected cases of infective/tubercular infections.

Cytological Examination for Malignant Cells

Procedure: The body fluid is centrifuged; smears are made from the sediment and fixed immediately in absolute alcohol. The smears are stained by Papanicolaou stain. Hematoxylin and eosin stain or Giemsa may also be used.

Microbiological Examination

Culture is done to identify the organism in cases of effusion due to infections.

EXAMINATION OF SYNOVIAL FLUID

Uses: Examination of synovial fluid is useful in the diagnosis of joint disorders.

- Infective arthritis (septic arthritis, rheumatic).
- Gouty arthritis (metabolic disorder).
- Rheumatoid arthritis (autoimmune disorder).
- Degenerative arthritis.

Laboratory examination: It consists of (1) physical examination, (2) microscopic examination, (3) chemical examination and (4) microbiological examination.

Physical Examination

Color and Appearance (Table 36.1)

Table 36.1: Color and appearance of synovial fluid

Appearance	Condition
Normal	Clear, straw colored and viscous. It does not clot
Turbid	Infection and inflammation of the joint space, presence of crystals
Purulent	Septic arthritis
Red or brown supernatant	Hemarthrosis or in a traumatic tap

Viscosity Test

Synovial fluid is viscous due to the presence of hyaluronic acid. The viscosity of the synovial fluid decreases in inflammatory joint disorders due to the breakdown of hyaluronic acid by the enzyme hyaluronidase.

Mucin Clot Test

Hyaluronic acid forms a compact clot when mixed with acetic acid. Low concentration of hyaluronic acid does not allow the formation of a firm clot. Add few drops of synovial fluid to 20 mL of 5% acetic acid in a small beaker. A good clot is formed if the synovial fluid is normal.

- In inflammatory diseases of the joint, there is poor clot formation due to degrading enzymes from the inflammatory cells (e.g. tuberculous arthritis).
- Noninflammatory joint disorders show good clot formation, whereas hemorrhagic synovial fluid prevents clot formation due to dilution of fluid.
- Fair to poorly formed clot is seen in rheumatoid arthritis, gout and pseudogout.

Microscopic Examination

The total leukocyte count is estimated similar to total WBC count using improved Neubauer chamber.

Differential Leukocyte Count

If polymorphs are more than 70%, it indicates bacterial arthritis. Noninflammatory arthropathies (osteoarthritis) are associated with lymphocytes and macrophages.

Wet Smear Examination

Centrifuge the synovial fluid and take the sediment on a glass slide and cover it with a coverslip. Observe the slide first under low power objective, then under high power objective with reduced light and carefully note for the presence of following crystals:

- Urate crystals are seen in gouty arthritis.
- Rhomboid calcium pyrophosphate crystals are seen in pseudo-gout.
- Cholesterol crystals are seen in rheumatoid arthritis.

Crystals can be confirmed using polarized microscopy.

Chemical Examination

- **Glucose and protein estimation:** Significance is similar to glucose and protein in the other body fluids.

Microbiological Examination

Synovial fluid culture is recommended in suspected cases of pyogenic/tubercular arthritis.

GASTRIC ANALYSIS

Gastric analysis is performed in few diseases of the stomach. Gastric analysis include the laboratory tests to measure gastric secretions and serum gastrin.

Indications for Gastric Analysis

In gastric analysis, amount of acid secreted by the stomach is estimated on collected gastric juice. The indications are as follows:

- To determine the cause of recurrent peptic ulcer disease (PUD).
  - To detect Zollinger-Ellison syndrome
  - To decide the completeness of vagotomy nowadays not performed for PUD.
- To determine the cause of raised fasting serum gastrin level.
- To support the diagnosis of pernicious anemia.
- To differentiate benign gastric ulcer versus malignant ulcer.
- In patient suspected of PUD with normal radiological appearance.
- To determine the type of surgery in patient with PUD.

Contraindications for Gastric Analysis

- Conditions in which gastric intubation is contraindicated, e.g. esophageal stricture or varices, recent history of severe gastric hemorrhage, hypertension, cardiac failure.
- Pyloric stenosis.

Gastric Analysis

Tests for Gastric Secretions

Tests for gastric acid secretions

In these tets, the acid output from the stomach is measured in the fasting state and after injection of drugs that stimulates secretion of gastric acid.

Collection of sample:

- All drugs that affect the gastric acid secretion should be stopped 24 hours prior to the test. Proton pump inhibitors should be discontinued 5 days before the test.
- Quantitative analysis is performed after an overnight fast.
- Gastric juice can be aspirated through an oral or nasogastric (commonly used) tube or during endoscopy.
- **Basal acid output (BAO):** The gastric secretion collected in 4 consecutive 15-minute intervals. This unstimulated, one hour collection after titration for the acid concentration is called BAO. BAO is the amount of hydrochloric acid (HCL) secreted in the absence of any external stimuli.
- **Maximal acid output (MAO):** Subsequently, the stomach is stimulated to secrete maximal acid. The gastric secretion is similarly collected for 1 hour and the acid content called as MAO. It is the amount of hydrochloric acid (HCL) secreted by the stomach following stimulants (e.g. pentagastrin).
- **Peak acid output (PAO):** Two highest 15-minute acid outputs are added and then multiplied by 2. It represents the greatest possible acid secretion and is termed the peak acid output (PAO).

The tests for gastric acid secretion are named after the stimulants used for MAO. Some of the commonly used stimulants are:

- Histamine not used nowadays.
- **Histalog (Betazole)**.
- **Pentagastrin (Peptavlon)**.
- **Insulin meal (Hollander test)**.
- **Tubeless analysis:** In this a resin-bound dye is given orally. The release of dye by the action of gastric acid and its appearance in the urine indicates the presence of gastric acid.

Interpretation

- Conditions in which **higher values** are observed:
  - Duodenal ulcer
  - Zollinger-Ellison syndrome (gastrinoma)
  - Anastomotic ulcer.
- Conditions in which **low value** or achlorhydria are observed in:
  - Pernicious anemia (atrophic gastritis).
  - Achlorhydria in the patient with gastric ulcer is highly suggestive of malignant ulcer of stomach.

Test for intrinsic factor

- Intrinsic factor (IF) is required for the absorption of vitamin B_{12} from the small intestine.

- **Schilling test** (refer page 139) is used for evaluation of patients with suspected pernicious anemia.

Tests for Gastrin

Gastrin can be measured by the following methods:

1. Serum gastrin levels: Radioimmunoassay (RIA) is the commonly used method.

Causes of raised serum gastrin:
- Atrophic gastritis (with low gastric acid secretion)
- Zollinger-Ellison syndrome or gastrinoma (with high gastric acid secretion)
- Following surgery on the stomach.

2. Gastrin provocation tests: These tests are used to differentiate between hyper gastrinemia and gastric acid hypersecretion. These tests include:
- **Secretin test**.
- **Calcium infusion test**.

Cytological Examination for Malignant Cells

Brushing, lavage, aspirate or a biopsy material for examination may be obtained under direct visual control by endoscopic instrument from any area in the gastrointestinal tract. "Salvage cytology" is a technique consisting of washing the channel of the endoscopic instrument with saline and collecting the fluid for cytologic analysis into a suction trap. Smears are immediately made and fixed immediately in absolute alcohol. The smears are stained by Papanicolaou stain.

Hematoxylin and eosin stain or Giemsa may also be used.

SPUTUM EXAMINATION

Sputum is a highly specialized watery, colorless and odorless product of the respiratory tract. Expectorated sputum is always abnormal and it consists of mucus and a variety of cellular and noncellular materials. It is the most frequently received specimen from the respiratory tract. Both its collection and examination are advantageous as samples are easily obtained, cost effective and its cellular content is representative of the entire respiratory tract.

Sputum Collection

- The patient is instructed to cough up to get the sputum proper and the same is collected in a wide mouthed sterile, glass/plastic container with screw cap.
- In those patients who cannot produce sputum spontaneously by deep coughing, a specimen of sputum may be induced. This is done by inhalation of appropriate solvents which are aerosolized to stimulate sputum production.
- Early morning sputum sample is preferred for routine examination and 24 hours sample for the demonstration of tubercle bacilli by concentration method.

Sputum examination consists of (1) physical examination, (2) microscopic examination and (3) culture study.

Table 36.2: Different colors of sputum and its causes

Appearance/color	Causes
White, viscid, mucoid	Asthma
Serous, clear, watery	Pulmonary edema
Clear or mucoid, gray, glassy, tenacious	Chronic bronchitis
Yellow due to pus/neutrophils	Acute lower respiratory tract (pulmonary) infections
Green	Long-standing infection (bronchiectasis, lung abscess)
Rusty due to lysis of red cells	Pneumonia (e.g. pneumococcal) and pulmonary infarction
Bright red due to fresh blood	Pulmonary tuberculosis, lung tumors, pulmonary infarction
Black due to coal dust	Coal workers pneumoconiosis or in heavy smokers
Anchovy sauce (chocolate brown)	Rupture of amebic liver abscess into lung
Blood tinged sputum	Mitral stenosis, pulmonary tuberculosis, carcinoma lung, pulmonary infarction

Physical Examination

Quantity

- In bronchiectasis, large amount of purulent sputum is coughed out.
- Large amount of watery sputum with pink tinge suggests pulmonary edema.

Appearance/Color

Different colors of sputum and its causes are shown in Table 36.2.

Odor or Smell

Foul smelling sputum is observed in bronchiectasis and lung abscess and is due to anaerobic bacterial infections.

Microscopic Examination

Staining of sputum: Two to three smears are made on a clean dry glass slides and are stained with:
- Leishman stain or Wright stain for differential count.

Table 36.3: Type of cells in sputum and their significance

Type of cell	Significance
Pus cells (neutrophils)	Pyogenic infection of the respiratory tract
Eosinophils	Asthma and parasitic infections of the lungs
Lymphocytes	Early pulmonary tuberculosis
Red blood cells	Hemorrhage (bleeding) into the lungs or the bronchi
Heart failure cells (hemosiderin-laden macrophages)	Chronic venous congestion of the lungs, pulmonary infarction and hemorrhage
Anthracotic (carbon) pigment-laden cells	Coal workers' pneumoconiosis and those who live in smoky polluted atmosphere

- Other stains (depends on the clinical/pathological features):
  - Gram's stain for microorganisms.
  - Ziehl-Neelsen stain for acid fast tubercle bacilli.
  - Special stains for fungi.
  - Papanicolaou stain for study of malignant cells.

Cells

Normal sputum consists of a few neutrophils, few lymphocytes, carbon laden macrophages, occasional eosinophils and red cells. Various types of cells seen in sputum and their significance are shown in Table 36.3.

Other Structures

Curschmann's spiral

Found in the sputum of patients with bronchial asthma.

Charcot-Leyden crystals

Found in bronchial asthma.

Parasites:

- **Larvae of strongyloides stercoralis** and roundworms may be seen.
- ***Entamoeba histolytica*:** Cysts or the trophozoites may be found when an amoebic liver abscess ruptures into the lungs.
- ***Echinococcus granulosus*:** Scolices and hooklets of the larval form may be seen with the rupture of the hydatid cyst of the lungs into the bronchus.

Culture Study

Sputum culture may demonstrate the causative infectious agent.

SELF-ASSESSMENT EXERCISE

I. Short Notes

1. Examination of body fluids.
2. Synovial fluid examination.
3. Gastric fluid analysis.
4. Sputum examination.

CHAPTER

37

Semen Analysis

CHAPTER OUTLINE

- ➢ Introduction
- ➢ Semen Analysis

INTRODUCTION

Semen (seminal fluid) consists of spermatozoa (sperms) and the fluid part. About 40% cases of infertility are due to abnormalities in semen and therefore semen analysis is the first test to be performed while investigating for infertility. **Defect of sperms** may be **quantitative** (absence of sperms, lack of enough sperms) or **qualitative**.

Indications for Semen Analysis

- **Assessment of fertility/infertility**.
- Determine the **effectiveness of vasectomy**.
- Determine the **suitability** of semen for **artificial insemination**.
- **Medicolegal purpose:** In alleged rape cases, vaginal pool smears are examined to detect sperms.

Collection of the Sample

Patient is asked to collect the semen by masturbation after a minimum of 2 days and a maximum of 7 days of sexual abstinence. Specimen should be collected in a clean, dry and wide mouthed plastic/glass container. Collection of condom sample is not advisable because they often contain spermicidal agents which impair the sperm motility. Examination should be done within 1 hour of collection.

SEMEN ANALYSIS

Physical Examination

- **Liquefaction: Immediately after ejaculation**, the semen is normally a **semisolid coagulated mass**. At room temperature, the semen usually begins to liquefy (become thinner) within a few minutes and **completely liquefies within 15 minutes**. Within 30 minutes it becomes more homogeneous and watery.
- **Semen viscosity:** Fresh semen is fairly viscid and the viscosity can be estimated by gently aspirating semen into a wide-bore plastic disposable pipette, allowing the semen to drop by gravity. **Normal semen falls drop by drop** and if viscosity is abnormal, the drop will form a thread more than 2 cm long.
- **Appearance:** Freshly ejaculated semen is an **opaque, white-gray and viscid** fluid. After liquefaction it has homogeneous gray-opalescent appearance. Semen may have red-brown color when red blood cells are present (hemospermia) or yellow in patients with jaundice or ingestion of certain vitamins or drugs.
- **Semen volume:** Normal volume is **≥2 mL per ejaculate**. Low semen volume may be due to obstruction of the ejaculatory duct, congenital bilateral absence of the vas deferens or can also be due to difficulty in collection. High semen volume may be due to active exudation in cases of inflammatory lesions of the accessory organs.
- **Semen pH:** Alkaline and ranges from **7.2–8.0** (>7.2). The pH should be measured after liquefaction, preferably after 30 minutes.

Microscopic Examination

- **Assessment of sperm motility: Motility** of the sperms **helps in penetration of cervical mucus** and **migration of the sperms into the fallopian tube**. In normal semen, **>50%** of sperms should be motile (progressively motile and non-progressively motile). This is assessed by placing a drop of liquefied semen on a clean glass slide with a coverslip placed over it and examining under microscope.
- **Total sperm count:** Sperm count is carried out in an improved Neubauer chamber using a Thoma pipette in a dilution of 1 in 20 (as for total leukocyte count).

Table 37.1: Composition of semen diluting fluid

Constituents	Quantity
Sodium bicarbonate	5 g
Formalin	1 mL
Distilled water	100 mL

The composition of semen diluting fluid is shown in Table 37.1.

Normal sperm count: >40 millions/ejaculate.

- **Sperm morphology** (Fig. 37.1)**:** Smear prepared from semen is fixed and stained with Papanicolaou stain to identify the morphological features.

  Normal: Spermatozoa have a head, neck, middle piece (midpiece), principal piece and endpiece. Normally more than 30% of sperms have normal morphology.

  Head: It is oval in shape with smooth outline.

  Neck and midpiece: It is slender, regular and has the same length as the sperm head.

  Tail (principal) piece: It has a uniform caliber and is thinner than the midpiece. It is about 10 times the head length and may be looped back on itself.

Table 37.2: WHO (2010) reference values

Semen characteristics	Reference range
Volume	≥ 2 mL
pH	7.2–8.0
Color	Translucent, gray-white or opalescent
Liquefaction	<30 minutes
Sperm concentration	>20 millions/mL
Total sperm count	>40 millions/ejaculate
Morphology	>30% normal
Vitality	>75% live forms
WBC	<1.0 x 10^6/mL
Motility within one hour of ejaculation	>50%
Total acid phosphatase	≥200 U/ejaculate
Total fructose	≥13 μmol/ejaculate

Morphology of normal and abnormal forms of sperm is shown in Figure 37.1.

- Sperm aggregation or agglutination:
  - **Aggregation of spermatozoa:** Should be noted

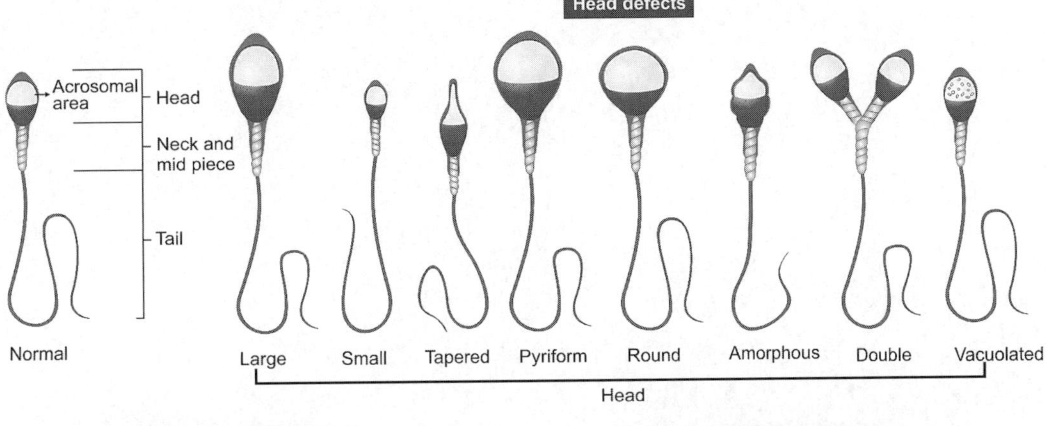

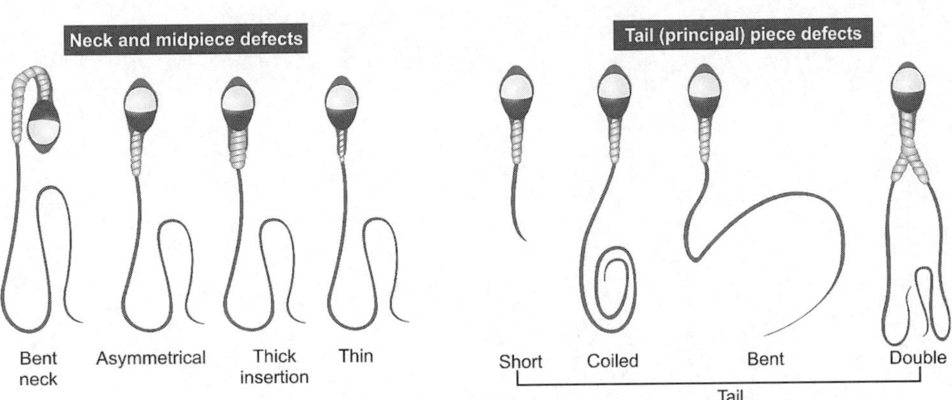

Fig. 37.1: Sperm morphology of both normal and abnormal forms

- **Agglutination of spermatozoa:** Refers to motile spermatozoa sticking to each other.

- **Cellular elements other than spermatozoa:** includes epithelial cells from the genitourinary tract and "round cells" (leukocytes and immature germ cells).
- **Sperm vitality:** It is important to know whether immotile spermatozoa are alive or dead. Normally, >75% live forms are observed and detected using eosin stain.

WHO (2010) reference values for semen analysis are mentioned in Table 37.2.

SELF-ASSESSMENT EXERCISE

I. Short Notes

1. Semen analysis.

CHAPTER

38

Urine Analysis

CHAPTER OUTLINE

- Introduction
- Physical Examination
- Chemical Examination
- Microscopic Examination
- Urine Culture and Sensitivity

INTRODUCTION

Urine analysis (urinalysis) reflects the state of function of the kidneys and urinary tract. It also provides information about metabolic or systemic (nonrenal) disorders.

Collection of Urine Specimen

Urine should be collected in a clean, dry and preferably sterilized container.

Containers Used

- Clean, dry wide-mouthed glass bottles
- Disposable plastic containers
- Polythene bags for collecting urine from infants.

Methods of Collection

- Freshly voided urine should be collected in a clean container either directly or into a clean dry bed pan from which it can be transferred to a clean container. Specimens from infant and children can be collected in disposable collection apparatus.
- **For bacteriological examination** (culture and sensitivity) clean-voided midstream specimen is required. To avoid contamination of the specimen with organisms from distal urethra, the initial stream of urine is discarded and the subsequent sample which constitutes midstream is collected. In males, the sample is collected after retracting the foreskin of penis and cleaning the glans with soap water. In females, the labia is spread and cleaned with soap and water.

Types of Urine Sample

- **First morning specimen:** The first-morning (8 hours concentrated)/any fresh random urine specimen are suitable for routine examination.
- **Random specimen:** It is most convenient and suitable for chemical analysis and microscopic examination.
- **Twenty four hours sample:** It is used for quantitative estimation of protein, sugar, electrolytes, hormones and acid fast bacilli.
- **Postprandial specimen:** Collection of urine specimen 2 hours after lunch or meal is used for detecting glycosuria.

Preservation of Urine

Urine sample should be **examined within 2 hours** of collection. If delay is likely to occur, it should be preserved either by refrigeration (without any preservative) or by use of preservatives like toluene, concentrated HCl, thymol and formaldehyde.

Examination of Urine

Urine examination consists of: (1) physical examination, (2) chemical examination and (3) microscopic examination.

PHYSICAL EXAMINATION

Volume: A healthy adult excretes about 600–2000 mL of urine in 24 hours. In infants, the volume is 300–600 mL/day. Volume is measured by collecting 24-hour urine samples in a measuring cylinder.

- **Polyuria:** Increased urine output (more than 2 liters in 24 hours). The causes of polyuria are mentioned in Box 38.1.

Box 38.1: Causes of polyuria

- Diabetes mellitus
- Chronic renal diseases
- Diuretic therapy

Box 38.2: Causes of oliguria

- Excessive loss of fluid: For example, in hemorrhage, burns, dehydration and shock
- Acute glomerulonephritis
- Acute tubular necrosis

Table 38.1: Conditions associated with color changes in urine

Color	Condition
Dark brown	Oliguria
Smoky (red or red-brown)	Red blood cells (hematuria)
Yellow-brown	Bilirubin

Table 38.2: Causes of different odor

Odor	Cause
Fruity (sweet)	Presence of acetone (ketonuria)
Ammoniacal	Bacterial decomposition
Putrid or foul	Severe urinary tract infection

- **Oliguria:** Decreased urinary output (less than 500 mL in 24 hours). The causes of oliguria are mentioned in Box 38.2.
- **Anuria:** Markedly diminished urine output, usually less than 125 mL in 24 hours. It may be caused by mismatched blood transfusion, renal ischemia, tumors, etc.

Color (Table 38.1)**:** Normal urine is straw to amber colored due to the presence of urochrome pigment, excretion of which is generally proportional to the metabolic rate.

Transparency and turbidity: Normal urine is usually clear when passed fresh. It may become cloudy, hazy or turbid with the presence of mucus, phosphates, pus, crystals, blood, casts or bacterial growth.

Odor (Table 38.2)**:** Normal urine has a faintly aromatic odor because of volatile acids.

Reaction (pH): Normal urine is usually acidic with pH varying from 4.6–8. The reaction of urine is determined with blue and red litmus paper. The urine when examined must be fresh as it turns alkaline on standing due to bacterial decomposition.

- Acidic urine turns blue litmus paper red.
- Alkaline urine turns red litmus paper blue.

Specific gravity: Specific gravity is used as a measure of concentrating power of the kidney. Normal specific gravity of a 24-hour urine sample is 1.003–1.035, average being 1.016. Specific gravity (SG) is measured by: (1) urinometer, (2) refractometer and (3) dipstick method.

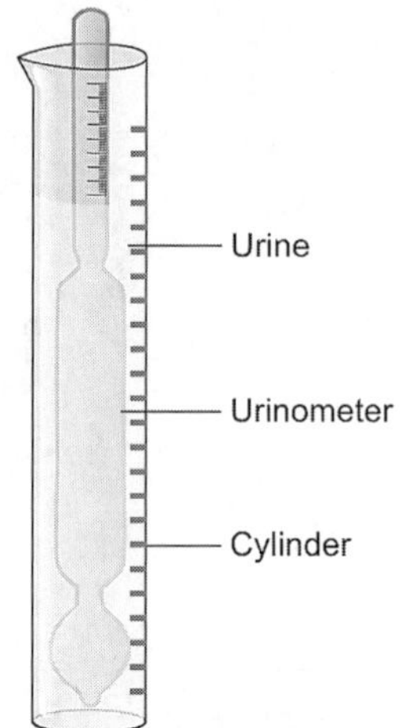

Fig. 38.1: Urinometer for specific gravity measurement

Box 38.3: Causes of increased, decreased and fixed specific gravity

Increased specific gravity
- Glycosuria
- Dehydration: Restricted fluid intake, diarrhea, vomiting, fever and excessive sweating

Decreased specific gravity
- Excessive fluid intake
- Diabetes insipidus
- End stage kidney: Chronic glomerulonephritis, chronic pyelonephritis, bilateral polycystic kidneys, hypertension

Low and fixed specific gravity
- Chronic renal failure

Urinometer (Fig. 38.1) is a specialized hydrometer. It consists of a glass cylinder which floats in urine and has a calibrated stem to measure specific gravity at a given temperature.

When specific gravity is fixed at 1.010, this is known as isosthenuria. It is indicative of severe renal damage (chronic renal failure) with disturbance of both the concentrating and diluting abilities of the kidney.

Interpretation: Specific gravity provides information about the renal status and hydration.

The various causes of specific gravity variation are shown in Box 38.3.

CHEMICAL EXAMINATION

Proteinuria

The presence of detectable protein in the urine is known as proteinuria.

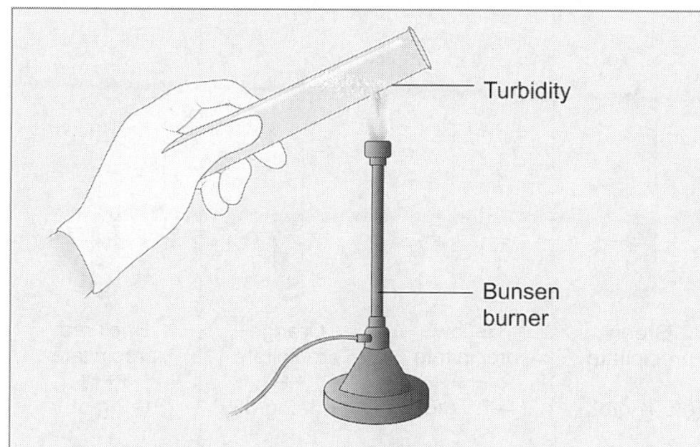

Fig. 38.2: Method of performing heat and acetic acid test

Table 38.3: Interpretation of heat and acetic acid test

Description	Result
No cloudiness/precipitate	Negative
White cloudiness	+
Granular white precipitate	++
Floccular precipitate	+++
Thick opaque precipitate	++++

Tests for protein: These include—heat and acetic acid test, sulfosalicylic acid test, Heller's test and dipstick method.

Heat and Acetic Acid Test

Principle: Heat induced **coagulation of proteins** and precipitation. Coagulation can be further enhanced when drops of acetic acid are added.

Procedure (Fig. 38.2):
- Fill three-fourth of a test tube with clear urine.
- **Heat the upper part (1/3) of the urine** (the lower part of the urine acts as a control for checking turbidity in the heated upper part). The development of turbidity may be due to coagulation of proteins or due to phosphates.
- **Add a few (3–5) drops of 10% glacial acetic acid** and if turbidity persists, it is due to proteins (phosphates will dissolve).

Interpretation: Depending on the amount of precipitate, results are interpreted as shown in Table 38.3.

Sulfosalicylic Acid Test

This test detects all types of proteins (albumin, globulin, glycoproteins and Bence Jones proteins).

Principle: Cold precipitation of proteins by a strong acid.

Procedure: Take 2.5 mL of urine in a small test tube. Slowly pour 2.5 mL of sulfosalicylic acid. Wait for 5 minutes.

Box 38.4: Causes of proteinuria

- Glomerular damage: Nephrotic syndrome, acute and chronic glomerulonephritis
- Tubular damage: Pyelonephritis, acute tubular necrosis
- Prerenal: Multiple myeloma (Bence Jones protein)

Interpretation: Presence of a cloudy precipitate indicates the presence of proteins in urine.

Other tests for detecting proteins in urine include Heller's test and dipstick method.

Quantitative Estimation of Proteins in Urine

Protein excretion in a 24-hour urine sample is required in suspected cases of nephrotic syndrome (>3.5 g/24 hours). This may be carried out by Esbach's albuminometer method.

Causes of Proteinuria (Albuminuria)

They are presented in Box 38.4.

Reducing Substances in Urine

Reducing substances in urine may be sugars or nonsugars.
- **Sugars:** Glucose, fructose, pentose, galactose, lactose, maltose and sucrose. The presence of detectable amounts of glucose in urine is termed glycosuria and is one of the reducing substances.
- **Nonsugars:** Ascorbic acid, uric acid, urates, salicylates, streptomycin, phenol, etc.

Tests for reducing substance: These include: Benedict's qualitative test and dipstick method.

Benedict's Qualitative Test (Semiquantitative)

This test detects the presence of reducing substances in urine and is not specific for glucose.

Principle: The cupric sulfate present in the Benedict's reagent reacts with the reducing substances in the urine which convert cupric sulfate to cuprous oxide in hot alkaline media. Thus, this test is based on the **reduction of cupric ions in Benedict's solution to cuprous ions.** In the absence of reducing substances in urine, the color of the reagent remains blue.

Procedure (Fig. 38.3):
- Take 5 mL of Benedict's (qualitative) reagent in a test tube.
- Boil to exclude presence of reducing substances in reagent.
- Add 8 drops (0.5 mL) of protein-free urine. Boil the mixture for 5 minutes and allow to cool. The ratio of 5 mL **Benedict's reagent and 8 drops (0.5 mL) of urine ratio is important because it is a semiquantitative test.**

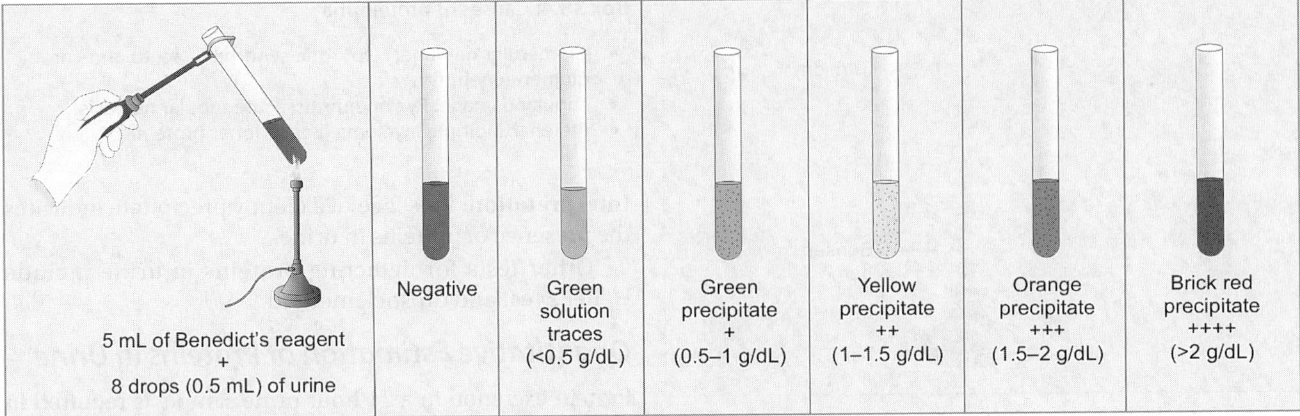

Fig. 38.3: Method and interpretation of Benedict's test

Table 38.4: Causes of glycosuria and causes of false positivity by nonsugar reducing substances

Causes of glycosuria	Causes of false positivity by nonsugar reducing substances
Diabetes mellitus	Ascorbic acid
Renal glycosuria	Salicylates
Alimentary glycosuria	Phenylketonuria

- Note the color of the precipitate which is cuprous oxide formed due to reduction of cupric sulfate of Benedict's reagent to cuprous oxide.

Interpretation: The change of color from blue to green, yellow and orange/red depends on the amount of sugar present (Fig. 38.3).

Causes of Glycosuria (*Table 38.4*)

Ketone Bodies

The presence of ketone bodies in the urine is a measure of the metabolic rather than renal function. Whenever there is a defect in carbohydrate metabolism, there is increased production of ketone bodies which begin to accumulate in the blood and are subsequently excreted in the urine.

Ketone bodies are three metabolically related compounds namely: **Acetoacetic (diacetic) acid, β-hydroxybutyric acid and acetone**.

Tests for ketone bodies: These include: Rothera's test, Gerhardt's test and dipstick method:

Rothera's Test

Principle: Acetoacetic acid (diacetic acid) and acetone react with sodium nitroprusside in presence of an alkali to form a **purple color compound.**

Box 38.5: Causes of ketonuria

- Diabetic ketoacidosis
- Starvation
- Prolonged vomiting or diarrhea
- Prolonged febrile illness
- von Gierke's disease
- Eclampsia

Procedure

- Take 4 mL of urine in a test tube.
- Add a few crystals of sodium nitroprusside and saturate the urine with ammonium sulfate by mixing vigorously.
- Overlay with few drops of liquor ammonia along the wall of the tube.

Interpretation: Development of a purple ring indicates the presence of acetoacetic acid/acetone or both. A brown or red color is of no significance.

Causes of Ketonuria (*Box 38.5*)

Bilirubin (Bile Pigment)

Tests for bilirubin in urine provide information concerning metabolic or systemic disorders, especially liver function. Bilirubin is a breakdown product of hemoglobin and is normally not present in urine.

Tests for bilirubin: These include: Fouchet's test and dipstick method.

Fouchet's Test

Principle: Fouchet's reagent contains trichloroacetic acid and ferric chloride. **In an acidic medium, ferric chloride**

oxidizes bilirubin to produce a **dark green colored biliverdin**.

Procedure
- Take 10 mL of urine in a test tube and add 3 mL of 10% barium chloride solution.
- Mix the two and filter the mixture through a filter paper. Bilirubin along with barium salt remains on filter paper.
- Add a few drops of Fouchet's reagent onto the filter paper.

Interpretation: Green or blue color indicates bilirubinuria.
Note: **Foam test** is a simple test to detect bile pigments at the bed side. Take urine in a test tube and shake the urine. If bile pigments are present in the urine, the foam on top will be yellow in color.

Causes of Bilirubinuria

- **Obstructive jaundice:** Urine shows bilirubin without urobilinogen.
- **Hepatocellular jaundice:** Bilirubin is absent in urine of patients with hemolytic jaundice.

Urobilinogen

It is normally present in urine in trace amount (1–2 mg/dL) and is insufficient to cause a significant positive reaction. Whenever the liver is unable to efficiently remove the reabsorbed urobilinogen from the portal circulation (e.g. liver diseases, hemolytic anemia) more urobilinogen than normal is routed through the kidney and hence excreted in the urine.

Tests for Urobilinogen

These include: Ehrlich's test and dipstick method.

Causes of Decreased/Absent Urobilinogen in Urine

In obstructive jaundice, bilirubin does not reach the intestine and hence is not converted into urobilinogen.

Causes of increased urobilinogen in urine are shown in Table 38.5.

Table 38.5: Causes of increased urobilinogen in urine

Hemolytic anemias (without bilirubin in urine)	Liver diseases
Thalassemia	Preicteric phase of infective hepatitis
Sickle cell anemia	Drugs or toxic hepatitis
Hereditary spherocytosis	Cirrhosis

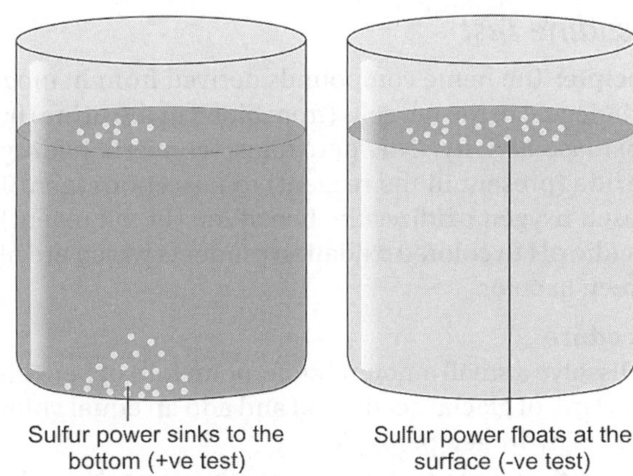

Fig. 38.4: Positive (left) and negative (right) Hay's test

Bile Salts

Bile salts are composed of mixture of bile acids and glycine or taurine. Normally, bile salts are not present in urine.

Hay's Sulfur Test

Principle: Bile salts have unusual property of **lowering the surface tension of urine** markedly even when present in small concentrations. This property is made use of in the Hay's test.

Procedure: Take 10 mL urine in a wide bore test tube (2 cm in diameter or more) or a small beaker. Sprinkle sulfur powder over its surface, watch for 5 minutes.

Interpretation: Sulfur powder sinks to the bottom of test tube (Fig. 38.4) in the presence of bile salts in urine.

Precaution: Since, soap can give false positive result, the test tube should be clean.

Causes of Bile Salts in Urine

Hepatocellular and obstructive jaundice.

Tests for Blood in Urine

These tests include: Benzidine test, orthotoluidine test and dipstick method. They detect hematuria, hemoglobinuria or myoglobinuria.

Hematuria: It is the presence of **blood in the urine**. Urine is red colored in severe hematuria and smoky in mild hematuria. RBCs are demonstrable in urinary sediment. Causes of hematuria are presented in Box 38.6.

Tests for blood: These are: benzidine test, orthotoluidine test and dipstick method.

Benzidine Test

Principle: The heme compounds derived from hemoglobin molecule in the red cells (from blood in the urine) have peroxidase activity. This peroxidase converts hydrogen peroxide (present in the reagent) to nascent oxygen. The released oxygen oxidizes the benzidine (in the regent) in an acidic pH to colored oxidation products which are blue or green in color.

Procedure

- Dissolve a small amount (knife-point full) of benzidine in 2 mL of glacial acetic acid and add an equal volume of 3% hydrogen peroxide.
- From the above, take 2 mL in another test tube and add 2 mL of previously boiled and cooled urine and mix.

Interpretation: The appearance of blue color indicates the presence of blood.

Multistix Reagent Strips for Urine Testing

These have single/multiple discrete cellulose squares which are impregnated with reagents for testing glucose, protein, pH, specific gravity, hemoglobin, ketone bodies, bilirubin and urobilinogen. There are single test strips, e.g. diastix for glucose and multistix for multiple tests.

Automated Urinalysis

Fully automated urine analyzer provided with automatic functions are presently available, e.g. Uriplus.

MICROSCOPIC EXAMINATION

Microscopic examination of urinary deposit or sediment is an essential part of urine examination. The deposits are mainly organized deposits which consists of: (1) cells [blood cells (red cells and white cells) epithelial cells (renal, transitional, and squamous)], (2) casts (with or without inclusions), (3) crystals and (4) other abnormal cells or formed elements.

Cells

They are expressed as number of cells per low power or high power field.

- **Red blood cells (RBCs):** Presence of RBCs (more than 2/hpf) in the urine indicates bleeding at any point in the urinary system from the glomerulus to the urethra and is known as hematuria. Causes of hematuria are listed in Box 38.6.
- **White blood cells (WBCs):** Increased number of WBCs (mainly neutrophils more than 5/hpf) in urine is known as pyuria. It is indicative of urinary tract infection. The causative organism of infection may be identified by bacteriological examination. Causes of pus cells in urine are shown in Box 38.7.
- **Epithelial cells:** These are derived from the urinary tract (transitional and renal) or genital tract (squamous). A few (0–2/hpf) transitional cells from the bladder may be present in the normal urine and squamous cells from the vulva and vagina usually contaminate a routine specimen from women.

Box 38.6: Causes of hematuria

Renal diseases
- Renal stones (nephrolithiasis)
- Renal cell carcinoma
- Acute glomerulonephritis
- Renal tuberculosis
- Trauma (including renal biopsy)
- Bacterial endocarditis with kidney involvement
- Malignant hypertension
- Hydronephrosis
- Renal infarct

Lower urinary tract/prostatic diseases
- Bladder stones (lithiasis)
- Cystitis
- Urethritis
- Carcinoma bladder and prostate

Blood disorders
- Bleeding disorders: Coagulation disorders, severe thrombocytopenia
- Acute leukemia
- Sickle cell disease

Miscellaneous
- Instrumentation of urinary tract

Box 38.7: Causes of pus cells (Pyuria) and glitter cells in urine

- Pyelonephritis
- Urethritis
- Cystitis
- Urinary tract infection (UTI)

Casts

They are one of the organized elements which are formed only in the kidney and are indicative of a renal disease. They are formed by solidification of Tamm Horsfall protein, a glycoprotein secreted in the distal convoluted tubules and

Cast	Appearance	Cast	Appearance
Hyaline casts	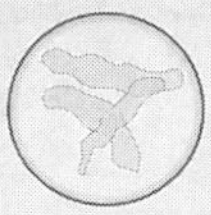	Leukocyte (WBC) casts	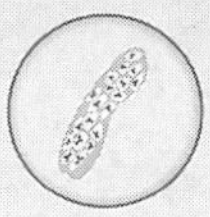
Waxy casts	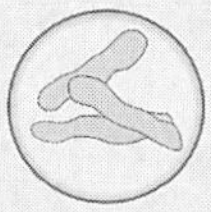	Epithelial casts	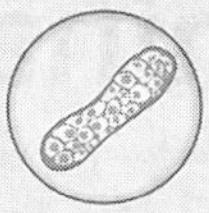
Granular casts	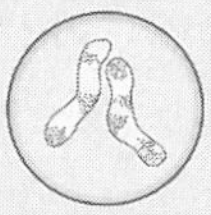	Fatty casts	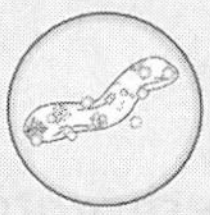
Red blood cell (RBC) casts	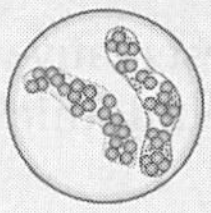	Broad casts	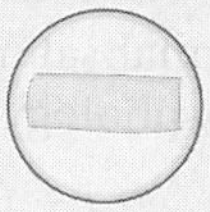

Fig. 38.5: Casts in urine

Crystal	Diagram	Crystal	Diagram
Amorphous urates	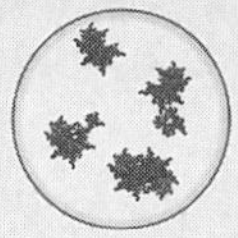	Amorphous phosphates	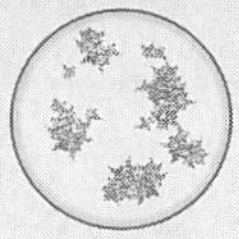
Crystalline urates	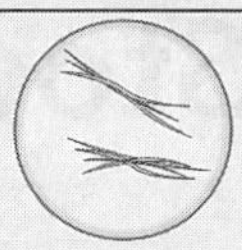	Crystalline phosphates-triple phosphates	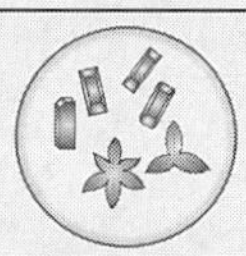
Crystalline uric acid	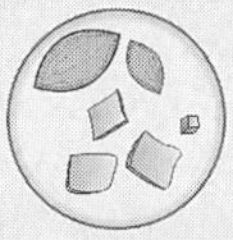	Calcium carbonate	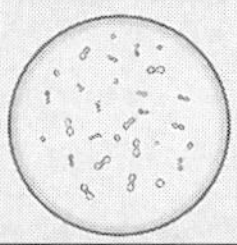
Calcium oxalate	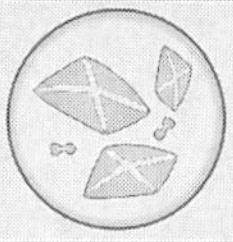	Ammonium biurate crystals	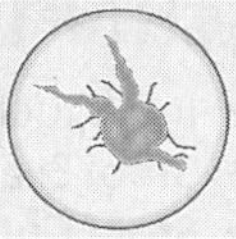

Fig. 38.6: Crystals in urine

collecting tubules. These proteins can trap any elements including cells, cell fragments or granular material (Fig. 38.5). Casts are cylindrical structures with parallel sides and rounded ends. The casts may have only proteins (hyaline and waxy casts) or have trapped granular debris (granular casts), epithelial cells (epithelial casts), leukocytes (leukocyte casts), red blood cells (RBC casts) or fat droplets (fatty casts).

Crystals (Fig. 38.6)

These are not usually present in urine. Crystals of oxalates, urates and cystine are present in patients with history of renal stone, while urates alone are present in gout. Oxalates, urates and cystine are present in acidic urine while phosphates, calcium carbonates and ammonium urates are present in alkaline urine.

Others

Includes abnormal cells (malignant cells, fungi, parasites) and other formed elements.

URINE CULTURE AND SENSITIVITY

Collection: Midstream urine sample/catheter specimen/suprapubic specimen.

Culture media used: 5% sheep blood agar and MacConkey's agar.

Procedure:

- Urine is cultured on plates by using standard loop.
- Fixed amount of urine is cultured on to the media and incubated at 37°C for 18–20 hours.
- Number of colonies is counted at the end of the incubation period.
- The causative organisms are identified by using biochemical tests.
- Antibiotic sensitivity testing is done for the identified pathogenic organism.

Interpretation: Diagnosis of urinary tract infection depends on quantitative urine culture yielding greater than 100,000 colony forming units per mL of urine and is termed as "significant bacteriuria".

SELF-ASSESSMENT EXERCISE

I. Short Notes

1. Routine examination of urine.
2. Physical characteristics of urine.
3. Chemical analysis of urine.
4. Culture and sensitivity of urine.

CHAPTER 39

Stool Examination

CHAPTER OUTLINE

- Introduction
- Stool Examination
- Stool Culture and Sensitivity

INTRODUCTION

Examination of sample of stool is easily done and is very useful in the evaluation of diarrheal diseases, parasitic infestations, colorectal carcinoma and malabsorption.

Collection

- **Container:** Stool sample is collected either in a wide mouthed glass or plastic jars with a screw cap. Container should be clean and dry.
- **Method of collection:** The sample is transferred from a clean bed pan or toilet into the container.
- **Amount of sample:** Stool required is small and about 2–5 g of the stool sample is adequate.

Precautions in Collection

- Morning sample is preferred.
- Sample should be labeled and the time of collection to be mentioned.
- The container after sample collection should be closed to avoid drying.
- Contamination with either urine or other substances in the bed pan or toilet should be avoided.
- Stool must be fresh. Examine within 1 hour of collection.
- If blood/mucus/any other abnormal gross features are present in the stool, it should be included in the sample collected.

Preservation

Formal-saline can be used as preservative which preserves morphology of protozoa and helminthic eggs.

STOOL EXAMINATION

Physical Examination

1. **Quantity:** The quantity of stool varies from 100–250 g/day depending on the type of diet consumed.
2. **Consistency and form:**
   - Normal feces is well-formed.
   - Extensively hard stool is observed during constipation.
   - Large bulky, frothy, pale, foul smelling stool which floats on water is characteristic of steatorrhea (poor fat digestion).
   - Rice water stool is typical of cholera.
   - Watery/semisolid stool in diarrhea, dysentery and following use of a laxative/enema.
3. **Color:**
   - **Normal:** Golden brown due to stercobilin, a pigment derived from bilirubin metabolism.
   - **Black tarry stool:** It is usually due to altered blood in stool and known as **melena**. The source of blood is bleeding from the upper gastrointestinal tract (GIT). But black tarry stool may also be observed following iron administration.
   - **Bright red color:** It is due to bleeding from the lower GIT like bleeding piles.
   - **Clay colored stools:** They are observed in obstructive jaundice.
4. **Odor:** Normal odor of stool is due to indole and skatole formed by intestinal fermentation and putrefaction. The odor varies according to the pH of the stool.

5 **Blood and mucus in stool:** This is observed in either amebic dysentery or bacillary dysentery.
6. **Parasites:** Stool sample may show adult worms/segments of worms (e.g. roundworm, pinworm, whipworm, hoodworm or tapeworm).

Chemical Examination

The chemical examination of stool includes:

Reaction and pH

- **Normal stool pH:** It ranges from 5.8 to 7.5.
- **Strongly acidic stool:** Observed with excess carbohydrate diet or fermentation due to lactose intolerance.
- **Strongly alkaline stool:** Observed with excess proteins in diet.

Occult Blood

Small amount of blood in stool cannot be seen on gross examination. Chemical test is necessary to detect occult blood in stool. Presence of blood/hemoglobin in the stool which is detected by a 'chemical test' and not by the naked eye is known as 'occult (hidden) blood'.

Test for occult blood

Benzidine test: It is a sensitive test for detecting occult blood.

Principle: The heme compounds derived from hemoglobin molecule in the red cells (from blood in the stool) have peroxidase activity. This peroxidase converts hydrogen peroxide (present in the reagent) to nascent oxygen. The released oxygen oxidizes the benzidine (in the regent) in an acidic pH to colored oxidation products which are blue or green in color.

Procedure:

- The benzidine reagent consists of 4 g benzidine base in 10 mL glacial acetic acid. It is stable for 2–4 months.
- Emulsify a bit of stool in 5 mL water.
- Mix 1 mL of emulsion with 1 mL of benzidine reagent in a test tube.
- Add several drops of 3% hydrogen peroxide.

Interpretation: The appearance of blue color indicates the presence of blood.

Precaution: Benzidine is carcinogenic.

Apart from benzidine, other test to detect occult blood is **Guaiacum test** using gum guaiacum.

Various commercial tests are available for testing occult blood.

Causes of false-positive reactions:

- Presence of substances like myoglobin and hemoglobin (present in red meat) in diet.
- Presence of vegetable peroxidases (e.g. horse radish, bananas, black grapes, pears, plums, melons).
- Leukocytes and bacteria.
- Drugs like boric acid, bromides, iodine and oxidizing agents.

Causes of false-negative reactions: Use of vitamin C and other oxidants.

Significance

- Determining the cause of **microcytic hypochromic anemia** due to chronic blood loss. Causes of chronic blood loss may be:
  - Gastrointestinal tract (GIT) neoplasms (e.g. colon, stomach cancer)
  - Ulcerative diseases of the GIT
  - Hookworm infection
- Drugs like aspirin, steroids and indomethacin can be associated with increased gastrointestinal bleeding.

Other Chemical Tests

- **Quantitative fecal fat estimation:** Increase in fecal fat (more than 6 g per day) is found in malabsorption syndromes or diseases of pancreas.
- Presence of reducing substances like lactose in stool may be found in infants with diarrhea.

Microscopic Examination

A fresh sample of stool without any contamination with disinfectants is used for microscopic examination. On microscopy, examine the stool for:

- Leukocytes (pus cells), red blood cells, muscle fibers, fat globules, crystals, cysts and yeast cells and are expressed as number seen per high power field.
- Protozoa, eggs, larvae and cysts of parasites, flagellates and ciliates. They are reported as scanty, few, moderate or many.

Methods for the Preparation of Stool for Microscopy

Saline preparation

A small amount of stool sample is picked up with the help of tooth prick and taken on a glass slide. Mix with normal saline to make a thin emulsion so that the fine print can be seen through it. Cover with a cover slip. This is useful for the demonstration of motility especially of *Entamoeba histolytica*.

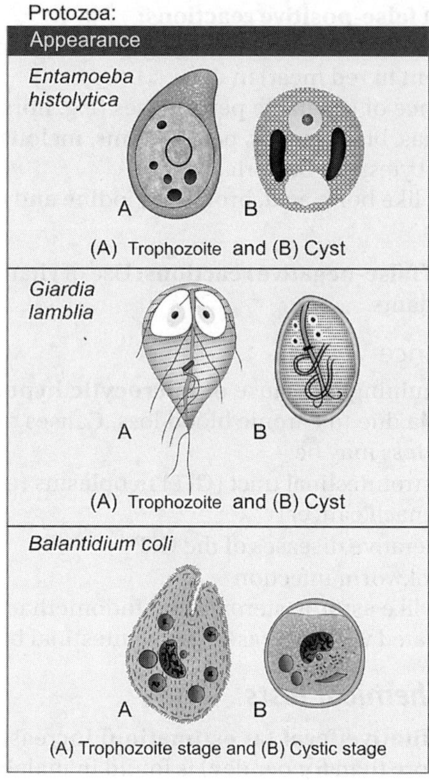

Fig. 39.1: Diagrammatic appearance of various protozoa in stool

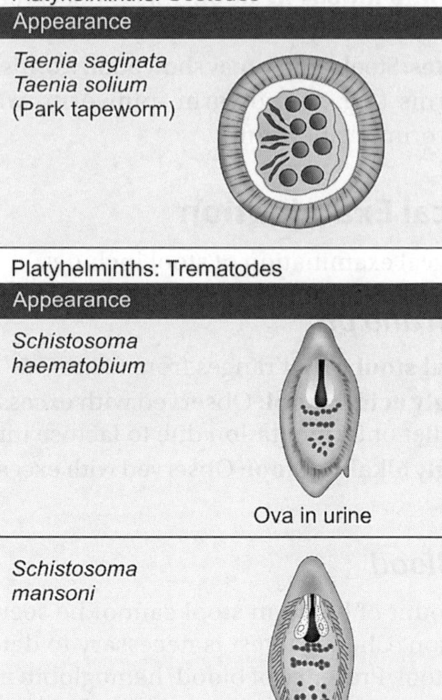

Fig. 39.2: Diagrammatic appearance of cestodes and trematodes in stool

Iodine preparation

In this, Gram's iodine is used instead of saline. Iodine imparts brown color to chromatin granules (nuclei) of amoebic cysts and also glycogen vacuole. But iodine kills living parasites thereby preventing identification of motility.

Stool concentration methods

When ova and cysts are few in number and are not detected by routine methods, concentration method will be of help. These methods are as follows:

- **Floatation method:** The stool sample is mixed with either zinc sulfate or magnesium sulfate which has a high specific gravity and causes the parasite to float in the solution. It is used for concentration of cysts, larvae and most of the helminthic eggs.
- **Sedimentation methods:** In this method, the parasites sediment and get deposited at the bottom by centrifugation. It can be done by either simple sedimentation method or by formal-saline ether sedimentation method.
  - **Simple sedimentation method:** A small amount of stool sample is mixed with saline in a tube or bottle and sieved through a strainer. The sieved contents are centrifuged and the supernatant fluid discarded. The deposit is resuspended in more saline, mixed and centrifuged. This is repeated till the supernatant fluid appears clear. The deposit is examined directly on a glass slide.
  - **Formal-saline ether sedimentation method:** This yields a good concentration of parasites and is recommended for routine work. But this method cannot be used to concentrate living parasites because the formalin used kills the parasites.

The appearances of various trophozoite/egg/ova/larva are shown in Figures 39.1 to 39.3.

STOOL CULTURE AND SENSITIVITY

Collection

Stool sample for culture should be collected in a sterile wide mouthed container.

Culture Media Used

MacConkey's agar, nutrient agar or selective media depending on the suspected organism.

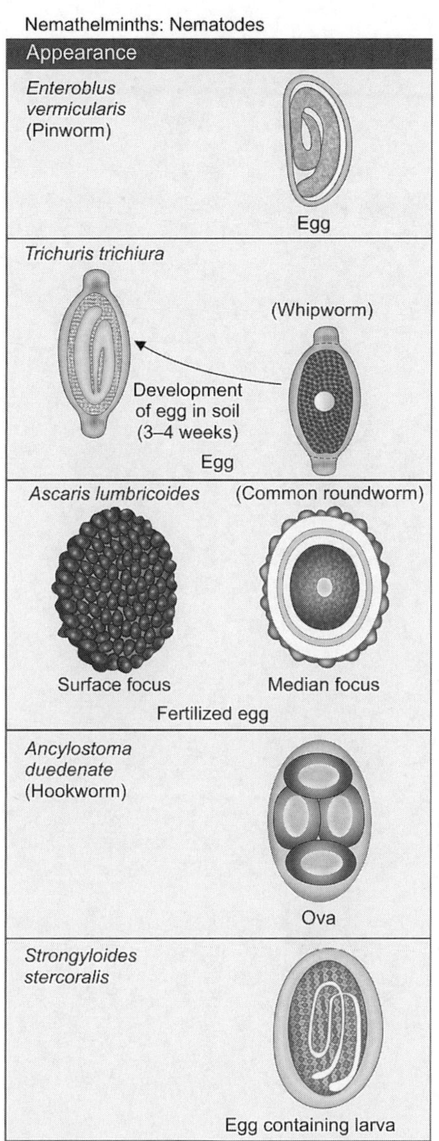

Fig. 39.3: Diagrammatic appearance of various nematodes in stool

Procedure:

- Take stool in culture media and incubate at 37°C for 18–20 hours.
- Suspected colonies are tested by using oxidase test.
- The causative organisms are identified by using biochemical tests.
- The organism may be confirmed by agglutination using specific antisera.

Antibiotic sensitivity testing is done for the identified pathogenic organism.

SELF-ASSESSMENT EXERCISE

I. Short Notes

1. Stool examination.
2. Occult blood.
3. Ova, parasite and cyst in stool.

Index

Page numbers followed by *b* refer to box, *f* refer to figure, and *t* refer to table.

C

F

I

J

K

Q

R

W

X

Z